GLAMOUR'S how to do anything better book

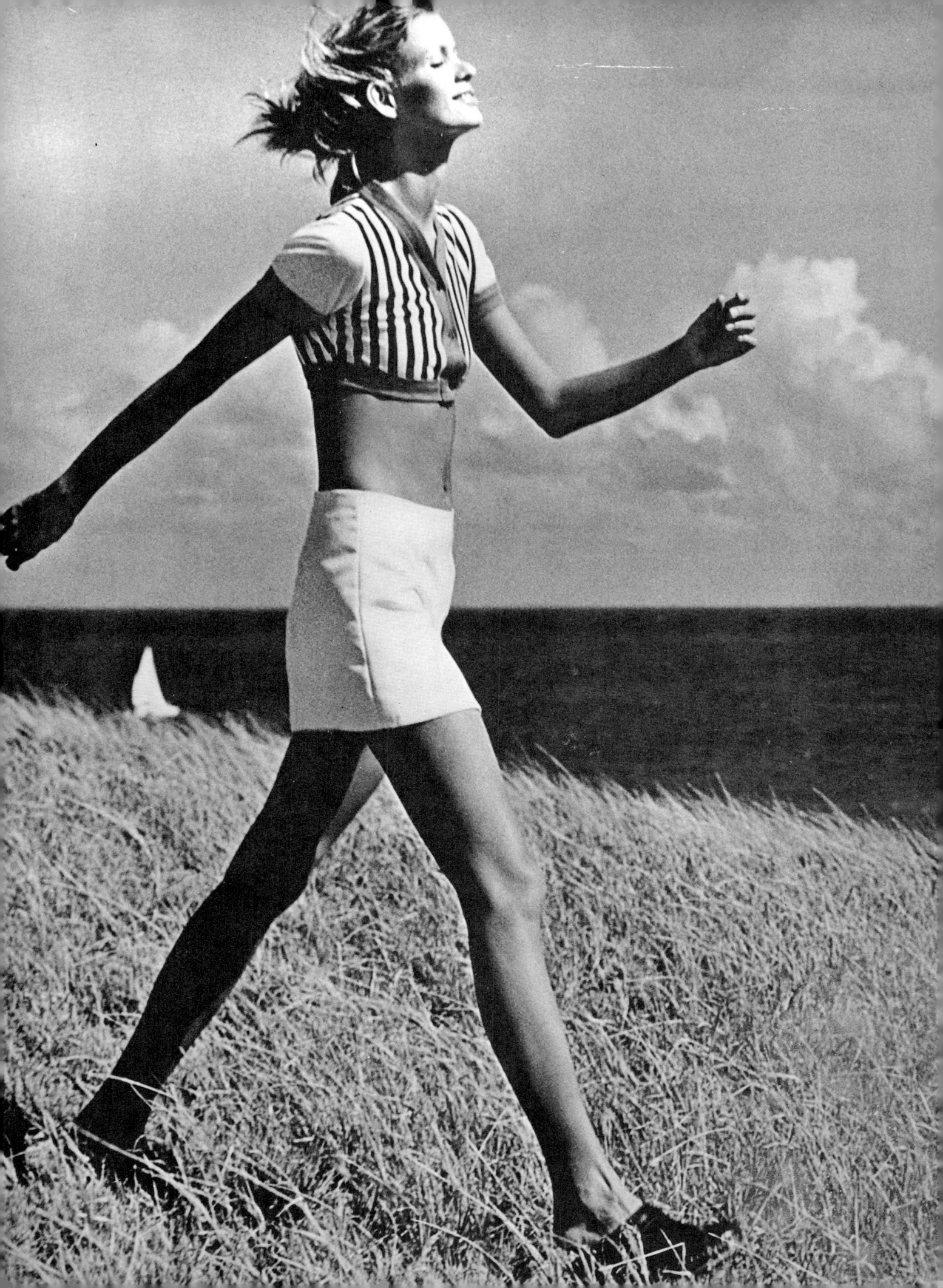

GLAMOUR'S
how to do anything better book

by the editors of *GLAMOUR* magazine

Edited by Nancy Young
Designed by Michelle Braverman
Illustrations by Durell Godfrey
A Rutledge Book   The Condé Nast Publications Inc. New York

Copyright © 1971, 1972, 1973, 1974, 1975, 1976, 1977 by The Condé Nast Publications Inc., 350 Madison Avenue, New York, N.Y. 10017. Produced by Rutledge Books, a division of Arcata Consumer Products Corporation, 25 West 43 Street, New York, N.Y. 10036. Published in 1977 by The Condé Nast Publications Inc. All rights reserved. Printed in the United States of America. Distributed by Charles Scribner's Sons, New York, N.Y.

Library of Congress Cataloging in Publication Data
Main entry under title:
Glamour's How to do anything better book.
   Includes index.
   1. Women. 2. Beauty, Personal.
3. Women—Health and hygiene.
4. Home economics. 5. Women—Psychology.
I. Young, Nancy. II. Glamour.
III. Title: How to do anything better book.
HQ1221.G65   1977   158'.1'024042   77-77621
ISBN 0-87469-013-7

Photograph page 177: United Press International

contents

apartments 6 art 9 auctions 10 autumn 10
beauty products 11 bicycles 13 body 14 books 16
camping 17 careers 18 cars 20
children 23 Christmas 27 clothes care 30
college 31 complaints 35 conversation 36
cooking 37 crafts 42 credit 47
decorating 49 diet 52 dining out 56 drinks 58
exercises 60
fashion 65 flowers 73 food 74 foreign languages 78
games 79 glasses 80
hair 81 Halloween 88 health 89 home furnishings 95
insomnia 97 insurance 97 italic writing 98
jeans 99 jewelry 100 kites 103 knives 103
landlord/tenant 104 legal matters 105
lighting 107 living problems 108
mail 113 makeup 114 men 116 metric system 120
months 121 movies 127 moving 128
names 129 nature 130 Oktoberfest 131 outdoors 131
parties 133 pets 134 plants 137 pregnancy 141
quilts 142 records 143 romance 144
self-improvement 145 sewing 149 shoes 155
shopping smart 158 skiing 167 skin 170 sleep 172
smoking 174 sports 175 spring 183 sticky situations 184
summer 188 swimming 192
teeth 193 tennis 195 Thanksgiving 196
tipping 197 travel 198 TV 204
umbrellas 206 vacations 207 voice 208
weather 209 weddings 210 wine 214
winter 216 women's rights 217
Xerox art 219 X-rays 219
yogurt 220 zuppa inglese 221
index 222

a apartments

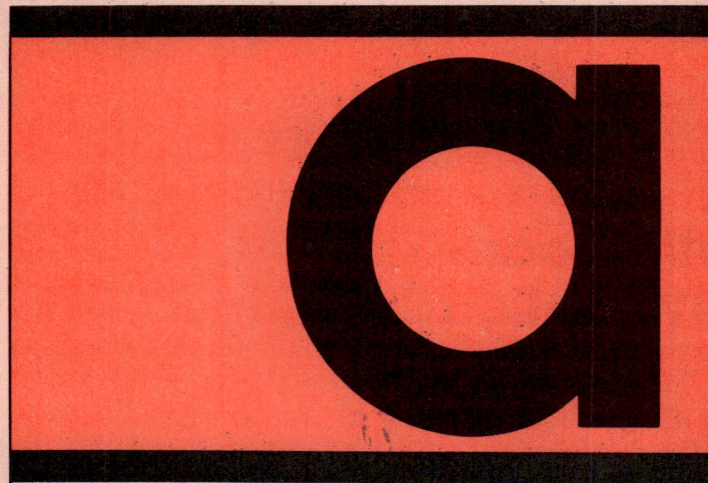

apartments
art
auctions
autumn

apartments

ads
a guide to rent ads

Apartment ads have a language all their own and vary from state to state. A "studio" in San Francisco is an "efficiency" in Philadelphia and a "buffet" in Denver. But some key abbreviations and phrases usually mean the same anywhere and are translated below.

A/C—air conditioning (an individual room unit, whose electricity costs you pay).

CEN a/c—central air conditioning (it's hooked into the whole building; you pay nothing extra).

Adults only; for mature-thinking persons only, come swing with us—ads containing information like this appear regularly in newspapers and may mean anything from not allowing children to expecting tenants to behave as if they had moved into a singles' bar.

Alc—alcove, a small area off a large room, also described as an *L-shape* or a *½ room*.

B—bathroom, but not necessarily with a bathtub. Some small bathrooms in older buildings have just a toilet, sink, and stall shower.

Bkr—broker. He charges a fee if you rent an apartment through him unless the ad says *fee paid*.

Bnstn—brownstone. Usually a three- or four-story older building without an elevator, often renovated with modern kitchen and bathroom fixtures.

Buf, stud, eff—buffet, studio, efficiency—all one-room apartments.

Cons—concession (something extra offered by the landlord to persuade you to take the apartment, like a month's free rent or free gas and electricity). This is common practice, for instance, in a few towns where available apartments outnumber people who want them, but it's almost unheard of in crowded cities.

Conver—conversion. A large house that has been divided into apartments.

Ctyd—courtyard.

Dup—duplex. An apartment with two floors.

Extras—special features from a dishwasher to a swimming pool.

Frplc—fireplace, which may be just for decoration unless the ad specifies *wbf* (wood-burning fireplace).

Gdn apt—garden apartment with entrance on the ground floor and the use of a garden.

1½, 2½—the half room can be an alcove, a foyer, or a bathroom.

Jr—very small (*Jr 3* means three small rooms).

Ldry—laundry facilities in building.

Lux—luxury, a debatable item. Usually it means at least an elevator, laundry room, and air conditioning.

Nudec—newly decorated. In a furnished apartment, this means new furniture; in an unfurnished apartment, it probably means a fresh paint job and possibly a modernized kitchen and bath.

Pr ent—private entrance. Apartment has its own front door.

Pull k—pullman kitchen. Basic kitchen appliances (sink, stove, refrigerator) are lined up on one wall but are not enclosed in a separate room (*sep k*).

RR—railroad flat. Several small rooms leading from one to another like railroad cars on a train.

Sec—security. Can be anything from a 24-hour doorman to an intercom. (Don't confuse with "security" deposit often requested by a landlord before he will rent an apartment.)

Slpg rm—sleeping room. A single room in a residential hotel or private home, often with only one bath to each floor.

Wk-up—walk-up; no elevator in building. *2 fl wk-up* means you walk up two flights of stairs.

W/W/C—wall-to-wall carpeting.

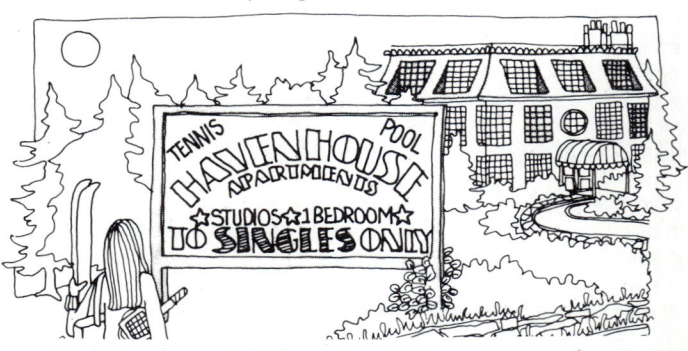

checklist
for apartment hunters

"Oh, it's cute. I'll take it!" But a week later, after you've hiked two miles carrying packages from the nearest grocery store, you know you have made a mistake about that apartment. Happiness or unhappiness with an apartment depends on many factors, some of which may not have occurred to you if you're not an experienced apartment-hunter.

● *Light, for instance. Some people can't be happy in dark apartments or those that get only north light. Check window exposures and make sure that no tall buildings block the sun if that is important to you.*

● *Air. Apartments that have only one exposure will give you no cross ventilation, and that can be a problem in warm weather. If you think you may need an air conditioner, make sure the building's wiring can handle one.*

● *Building maintenance and service. The best source of information for this is a tenant. Knock on a door and ask whether the building has roaches, whether the landlord responds to complaints, whether the heat and hot water are sufficient, whether the walls are so thin that your record player will bring complaints, and a party—the police.*

● *Rent. Is the rent that is being asked the legal rent for the apartment?*

apartments

Your local city rental agency will tell you.
- *Lease rights. Does your lease contain a sublet clause? Does it allow pets? Will the landlord paint; will he scrape the floors if necessary? How much will the rent be increased when the lease is up?*
- *Neighbors. It's nice to live in a place where your neighbors are friendly. Ask the superintendent what kind of people live in the building.*
- *The neighborhood. Will you feel comfortable on the streets late at night? How far away are services like public transportation, laundry, and markets?*

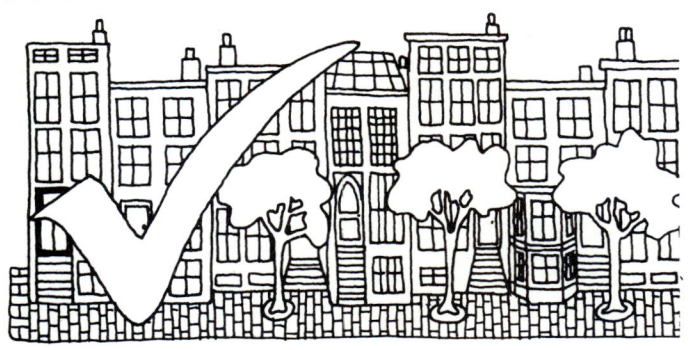

moving out
musts for moving out

- Most leases require that you leave an apartment in the same condition that you found it, allowing for normal "wear and tear." According to John Klotz, a tenant lawyer, a few smudged fingerprints on a door frame are an example of fair wear and tear. A hole in the wall made by a one-inch spike to hang a picture isn't—and you'll probably be required to plaster it or at least to pay for the work. You'd also be wise to give the place a once-over with a mop or sponge to play down as many signs of life as possible.
- Contributions you made to the apartment—built-in bookshelves, wall-to-wall carpeting, cabinets—can be taken with you only if they can be removed without causing structural damage. Some leases have clauses forbidding the removal of added "fixtures," so check before you start tearing yours down.
- If your lease required that you give your landlord a security deposit, be sure to arrange for it to be returned—after he's agreed that you don't owe it to him to cover damages in the apartment. In some states, you're entitled to bank interest on that deposit—ask your city or state housing administration. If your landlord has been consistently unreliable and you're afraid he won't reimburse the security, ask him to use it as the last month's rent. He may or may not do this, but it's worth an attempt. He's not legally required to accept your security as rent.
- If damages become an issue, work out what they are with the landlord and insist on seeing bills for the work required to repair them.

rental agencies
don't get ripped off by them

When you're apartment hunting, you need all the good leads you can get. But beware of agencies selling lists of fabulous-sounding, right-priced apartments. Their latest rental rip-off is offering rose-colored descriptions of closetlike apartments that make them sound like dream houses. These are listed along with a few really luxurious apartments that may have been for rent six months ago but are no longer available. This list can cost $25 or more.

When you get down to it, once you've been taken, there's not much you can do to get your money back—or the days you've wasted wild-goose chasing. So make sure before you buy that you're getting exactly what you're paying for. (Apartment hunting is exhausting and frustrating enough as it is without compounding it.)

Read the small print in the contract. Before you sign it, check out the agency with a local Better Business Bureau or ask consumer protection agencies in the area whether they've had any complaints about the companies that you're interested in. Your real-estate commission may also be involved in investigating such potential frauds. According to New York officials, if the agency is a licensed real-estate broker, it's most likely reputable—otherwise, it would fast lose its license—so check credentials.

If you do get taken, register a complaint with your state attorney general's office or other consumer protection official. You may also have some luck taking the agency to small-claims court, although rental agencies can often wriggle out of responsibility by way of small-print disclaimers on your contract.

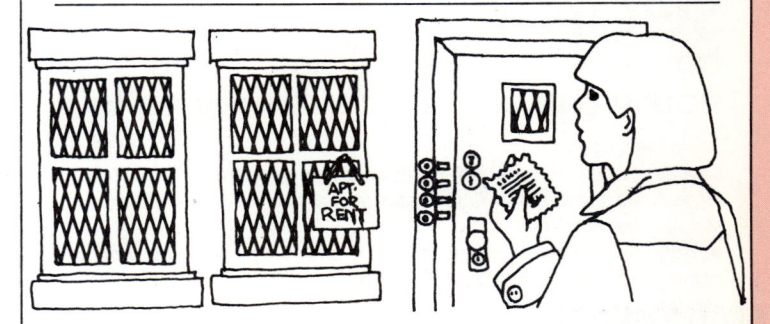

safety
how to tell which apartments are safe

The safety potential of an apartment you're about to rent can be deceptive. Any of the following clues should prompt you to double-check its reputation, by talking either to its former occupants or to others in the building.
- An apartment fortified like Fort Knox may be less secure than it appears. A string of *locks* on the door can mean that security in the building is slack and that a rash of burglaries has probably prompted tenants to be extra cautious. It may also mean that the apartment itself has been burglarized or that its location within the building could make it a likely target for break-ins. Either possibility is especially likely to be true when locks are teamed with other security precautions, such as a burglar alarm or attack-dog stickers on the windows. If you do move into one of these apartments, have at least one lock changed, regardless of the number of locks there are. How do you know who has keys to them?
- *Doors* that don't lie flush against their frames may have been pried open. If you decide to take an apartment that has a bent door, ask to have it fixed before you move in.
- A *window gate* is a must for maximum protection in any apartment having a window opening onto a fire escape. But more than one gate on any window probably means that one was not *enough* of a deterrent. Bent gates are usually an intruder's handiwork.
- Apartments facing the front of a building tend to be safer than less visible, back-of-the-building ones, and top- or ground-floor apartments tend to be more vulnerable than those in between, simply because they provide easy entrance and escape hatches for burglars via the roof or street.
- **what makes an apartment safe?**

If you can afford it, look for a building with a doorman or elevator attendant. In non-doorman buildings, look for an intercom connecting your apartment with the main lobby, a strong lock on the front door, peepholes on individual apartments, and buildings that are small enough that strangers are easily recognizable. Finally, a call to the local police station can tell you something about crime rates in the area—and perhaps even in your particular building.

a apartments

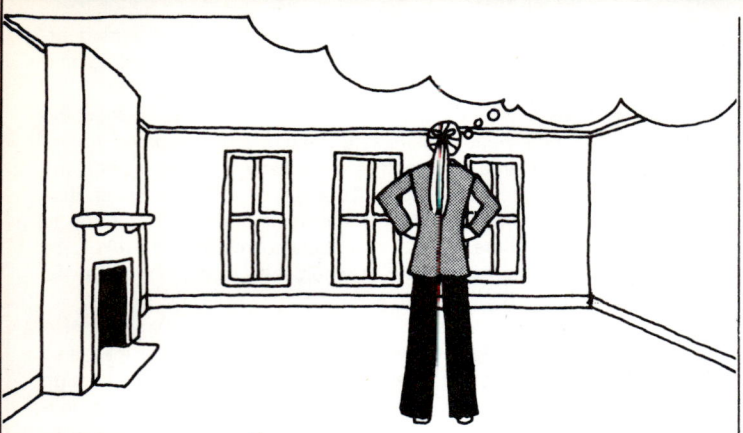

search
how to find an apartment in the city you live in or one you're moving to

The same ground rules apply to apartment hunting in any city. To be successful, you need equal parts persistence, legwork, and luck. In large cities, the search will probably take a little longer. And a systematic approach will help.

- Before you move to a new city, look into temporary living arrangements. If you can't camp on a friend's sofa for a few weeks, you can live inexpensively at a YWCA, women's residence hotel, or moderately priced transient hotel. Ask friends for their recommendations or write to the city's Visitor's Bureau for a list.
- You will need money for living expenses, plus the cost of renting an apartment. This usually includes the first month's rent, security (another month's rent), and possibly a rental agent's fee (another month's rent or up to 12 percent of the annual rental). These costs could amount to more than $600 in places like New York, Boston, and San Francisco. Whether you manage for less depends upon the kind of extras (doorman, elevator) that you expect and whether you're willing to share an apartment with a roommate.
- When you want to start looking, describe your situation to everyone you know or have been asked to look up in the city you're moving to. Include how much you want to pay, what size apartment you need, and the kind of neighbors you prefer—or simply say that you're desperate enough to investigate any lead.

One couple found a unique way to look for a big-city apartment. Three months before their wedding, they printed fliers that read: "If you, or anyone you know, are moving out from this or any other reasonably priced building, we would appreciate it if you would call us . . . we can't live on love alone." They distributed two hundred fliers, but you can be a little less enthusiastic.

- If you're moving to a city where you don't know a soul, a kindly employer or personnel officer might answer one or two basic questions, such as which newspapers carry the most comprehensive apartment listings. You might also ask for names of some reputable rental agencies.
- Comb real-estate advertisements in newspapers and act quickly on them. Don't wait until Wednesday to call about an apartment described in Tuesday's paper. Landlords and rental agencies expect almost instantaneous decisions. If you simply adore an apartment, let them know immediately that you want it. The usual procedure for holding an apartment so that it's not rented to someone else is to leave a deposit.
- Take a block-by-block approach to pounding the pavement in the areas that you like. Query doormen and building superintendents about vacant apartments. Some people leave $5 or $10 with a scattering of doormen, hoping they will call when an apartment becomes available (fairly risky—and expensive).
- Consult unconventional sources. The bulletin board in a local supermarket often displays rental notices among the circulars and baby-sitting offers. A gregarious druggist, cleaner, or liquor store owner will occasionally drop a good lead. Keep an eye on bulletin boards where you work—they're gold mines, too.
- Visit a nearby university. You'll find listings of inexpensive apartments on bulletin boards in the student union and advertised in the school paper. To rent most, you don't need student status.
- Look clean and presentable. A good approach is to dress as you would for a job interview, and if you travel with a partner, make sure he or she does, too. Scruffy jeans, tattered jackets, and unkempt beards may dissuade a superintendent from letting you in the door . . . let alone renting you an apartment.

survival
ideas for the first week alone in a new apartment or town

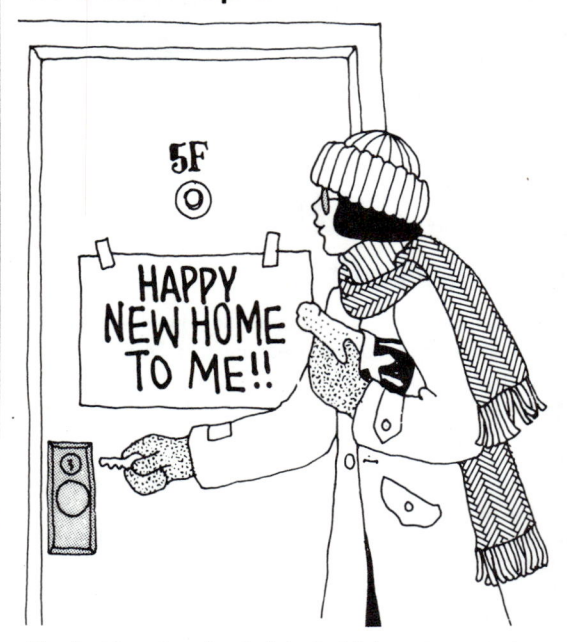

The first few days (and nights) of living alone can be quite unsettling, especially if the only company you've got is a whistling tea kettle. If you're about to move into your first apartment, here are some suggestions that will help you get that home-sweet-home feeling quickly.

- Have your phone installed on or prior to your moving day so that you'll have access to it on that first night alone. Arrangements should be made in advance because the telephone company might need anywhere from three working days to two weeks' notice for installation.
- Fill out in advance a change-of-address form with your old post office and indicate the effective new address date. What's more comforting than your favorite magazine or a friend's letter in the mailbox? Change-of-address notices for magazine subscriptions should be sent in at least three weeks in advance. If you're moving to a new town and haven't yet found a permanent residence, try to arrange for your mail to be sent to the local post office and pick it up there.
- If your new apartment is going to be vacant for a day or so before you move in, use this time to take a second look at the place, get rid of any items left by former tenants, and make a list of things you might not have realized you needed—extra lighting, extension cords, shades. Ask your landlord if you may put up your curtains then, too.
- Ask friends or family to give you a hand with moving and then have a pizza and champagne picnic on the floor when everything's settled. Even if you have to move by yourself, still treat yourself to a little split of champagne.
- Be sure to arrive at your new place with a marked survival kit containing all the essentials for the first night: light bulbs, radio, clock,

bedding, towels and washcloths, soap, toilet paper, eating utensils, food, and a book.
- Though the first days are bound to be chaotic, try to confine boxes and clutter to one room or area and make another area comfortable and livable. Set out photographs, knickknacks, and plants.
- Invest in a night light so you won't be disoriented if you have to get up suddenly.
- Be sure you're known to at least one person nearby in case of a crisis.

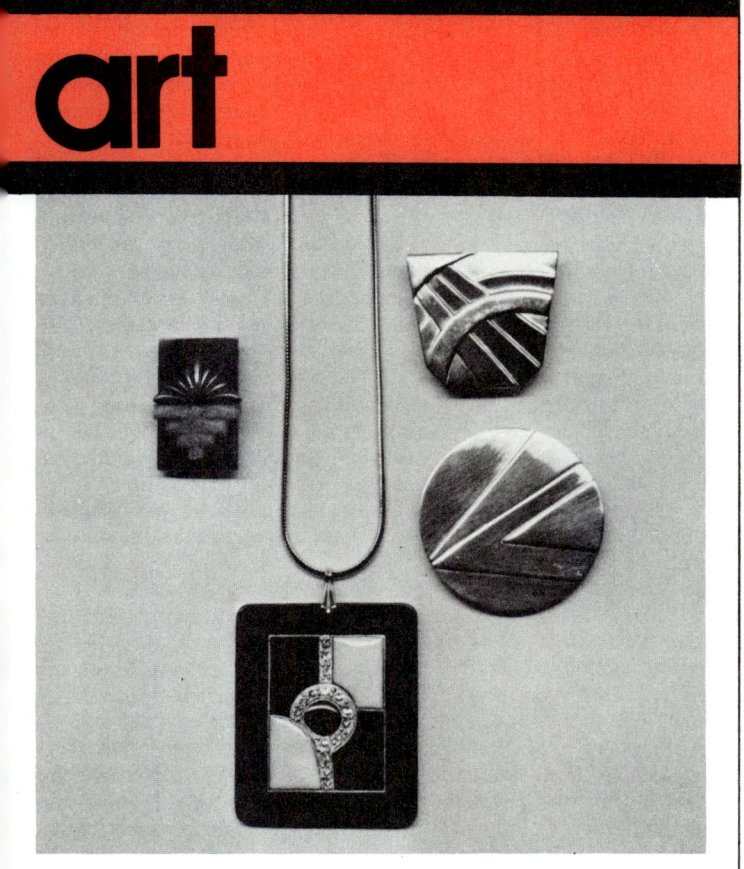

art

deco — how to know art deco when you see it

Art deco has had noticeable influence on fashion and decorating, but could you tell—if put to the test—what is art deco and what isn't?

Look at some of these designs. You'll notice that they are all in some geometric pattern based on a semicircle or a right-angled triangle. These two forms are the basis of most art deco design.

Art deco was popular in the 1920s and 1930s, so if you want to see some pure examples, catch an old Fred Astaire-Ginger Rogers movie or a romantic comedy of the Jean Harlow era. The furniture, jewelry, fabric, everything about these movies has an art deco look. More recently, "Lorelei," the musical revival of "Gentlemen Prefer Blondes," used art deco sets.

The height of the art deco movement was in 1925 at the Paris Exposition. This event gave rise to the American popular and commercial forms now referred to as art deco—a term, by the way, that didn't exist at the time.

Don't confuse art deco with art nouveau. Art nouveau, another style of art design and architecture, dates from the 1800s to 1905. It is a style marked by the use of flowing lines, interlaced patterns, and whiplash curves. Plant and flower motifs are common, too. Tiffany lampshades are art nouveau, for instance, as well as some poured concrete forms.

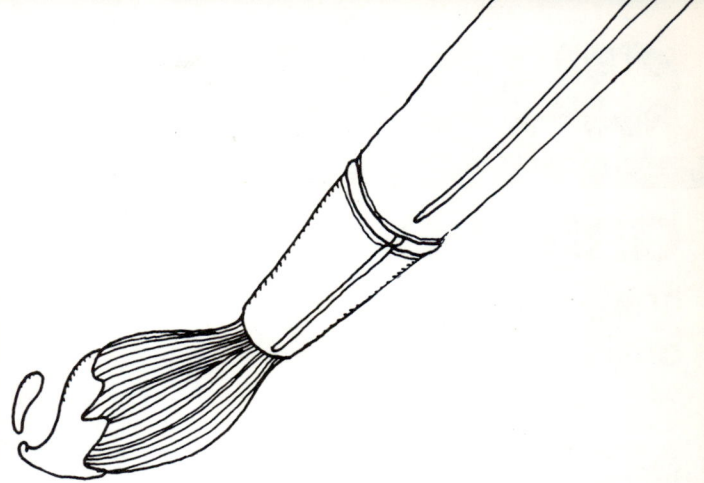

originals

think you can't afford art "originals"?

Owning paintings and sculpture runs high in dollars, but you can find woodcuts, etchings, lithographs, and other original works of art reasonably priced.

You should, however, know what artists and art dealers mean by original. For paintings and sculpture, it means one-of-a-kind. For etchings, woodcuts, etc., it doesn't necessarily apply. Many copies can be made from the same metal or wood plate, and they're all considered "original" if the artist designed the plate and supervised the quality. Print is also a tricky word for the beginning art buyer, since there are print reproductions and print originals. Your Mona Lisa poster, for example, is a printed reproduction of an original painting. But a Picasso woodcut made directly from the artist's plate is an original "print."

Before you buy, first visit museums and commercial art galleries to develop a feel for different media, quality, and price. Jeffrey Wortman of Sotheby Parke Bernet Galleries in New York suggests you focus on one period or one group of artists and first buy prints in your "specialty."

A reputable art dealer who specializes in original prints is your best source of purchase; ask a local art museum to recommend someone. Old books, newspapers, and magazines also turn out original prints— mass-produced on poor paper, perhaps, but designed by the artist who made the plates and supervised the printing (e.g., you might find an engraved Daumier cartoon on newsprint for under $10). Also consider art lending-buying services offered by some museums. Monthly or bimonthly rents vary from several dollars to about $100 for prints that are worth from under $40 to many thousands. You can live with the print before buying it, and the rental fee is deducted from the buying price.

- **glossary of basic terms**

Lithographs: A drawing is made on limestone with greasy crayon. Sponged wet, the limestone absorbs water, while the greasy design repels it. Greasy ink is applied; it sticks to the design but rolls off wet stone. Paper pressed on stone transfers the print.

Relief prints—woodcuts, wood engravings: A plate with a raised design is inked and then pressed with paper to make print.

Intaglio prints—engravings, drypoints, etchings: Design is cut into a metal plate with tools or acid. Ink is applied to fill the grooves or pits, and the rest of the plate is cleaned. Paper is pressed on it to make a print.

Limited editions: Old masters didn't limit impressions (the number of prints made from a plate), but modern artists may. A print that is numbered 6/21 means 6th print of an edition of 21.

Signed prints: Old masters didn't sign their works of art; modern artists usually do.

a auctions

auctions

antique
how to buy at your first antique auction

An antique auction is a delight—tables heaped with enough gleaming china and silver to serve an army, graceful sofas with slightly faded covers, and the tangy scent of wax and varnish. However, auctions can be intimidating to the uninitiated, so here are some tips to help you prepare for and enjoy an auction.

Inspect the merchandise to be sold before attending any auction. A day is usually set aside for this just before the actual sale. Look carefully for chips, cracks, breaks, and so forth in any pieces you're interested in and remember that at auction time, you'll be given only a one-word description of the item—such as "fair" or "good" condition.

Ask in advance about the pedigree of anything you're interested in and whether it's owned by the auction gallery or by an individual. You should be aware that anything owned by the gallery is, in general, less likely to be a runaway bargain or a "steal," since the gallery knows what it paid for an item and will protect the selling price, especially for a valuable item, by putting a "reserve" on it. This means simply that the item won't be sold for less than a specified, or "reserve," price. An individual owner can also put a reserve on an object, but sometimes he or she isn't aware of this option or may choose to sell for whatever price the bidding happens to bring.

If you're interested in a particular item and want to know approximately what it will go for, ask the auction gallery beforehand. They'll usually give you an estimate and may even tell you if there's a reserve on it.

When you go to the actual sale, be prepared to pay in cash—checks are usually not accepted—and be ready to take your buys home immediately. If you leave a deposit and pick up the goods later, you'll have to pay storage.

Bidding practices are set by the gallery, but in general, the increments by which a bid increases depend on the starting price of the item. For example, if the bidding starts at $500, the next bid won't be $505; it will more likely be $550. But if an item starts at $10, the next bid could be $15 or even $12.50. Listen carefully to the auctioneer for cues. He'll say, "I have $35, do I hear $50?" Chances are he means he really wants $50 and if you raise your hand now, he'll assume you're bidding the $50. An auctioneer must recognize your bidding, however. So you really needn't worry about being like the victim in all those auction movie scenes in which someone unintentionally bids a fortune for something simply by scratching his head.

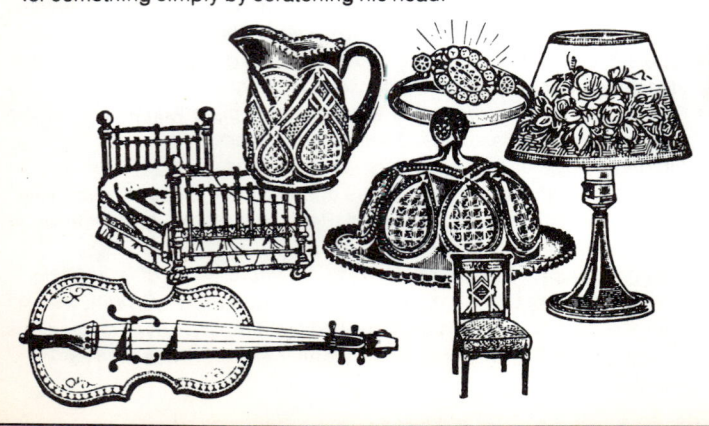

country
bidding at your first country auction

A country auction is a circus, a bingo game, and a treasure hunt all rolled into one. Lawnmowers to antiques may be sold for a song. But even in the backwoods, valuable items usually bring high bids.

So go just for fun. Bid on items you like and leave the "investments" to dealers. Set price limits, and don't buy anything uninspected.

- **where and when**
- Most country auctions are held Saturdays, spring through fall, nationwide (especially in New England, Pennsylvania, Connecticut, and New York). Announcements appear in trade publications like the *Newtown Bee* or *Antiques Monthly* (libraries and newsstands have copies). Also check local newspapers or those of a nearby city for listings.
- **the presale examination**
- It's usually held hours before the sale. Bring a tape measure to be sure that a particular piece of furniture can fit through your doorway; a magnet to tell bronze from iron (bronze isn't magnetic, iron is); a magnifying glass to spot small imperfections or quality hallmarks on china, silver, and so forth. Check first for serious damage. Cracked glass or china—even well-repaired—may be worth 75 percent less. See whether furniture legs or tops will have to be replaced. If you still want a defective item, bid less for it.
- You'll probably be given just a list of sale items, not a newsy catalogue, so ask the auctioneer for extra clues to an item's condition or origin. Try to get an estimated sale price from him—so you don't wait hours for something out of your range.
- Use a notebook (bring it to the sale), listing what you want in order of preference. For each item, write down the lot number, description, estimated price, and your limit.
- **the sale**
- You usually register at a reception desk and get a numbered card to identify yourself if you win the bidding.
- If you want an item, bid immediately. The auctioneer will know you're in the the race and won't stop bids before you're out.
- Auctions can last all day, so wear comfortable clothes and shoes.
- Bring cash or a certified check. Personal checks very often aren't acceptable. If you buy, ask for a purchase receipt noting the sale date, payment, and the item's description. Items are auctioned "as is," but reputable auctioneers accept returns on things mistakenly represented (e.g., if your receipt says sterling but your teapot is plated).
- You must cart away purchases the same day or next, so bring newspaper and cartons to pack small items. For large things, the auctioneer may suggest a mover or a trailer-rental service. Check fees before the sale so a bargain $10 breakfront doesn't cost $150 to move.

autumn

flowers tips on gathering and keeping fall flowers

Dried arrangements of fall flowers usually cost a mint at most shops, but you can make your own dazzling displays for pennies.

Florists say that the biggest mistake beginners make is trying to combine too many "ingredients." Your display will look more professional if you stay with one or two items in each container. For example:

beauty products

- Big armfuls of dried wheat, bullrushes, or dune grass in a container shaped like a country milk can. (If you're gathering wheat, for example, in the country in summer, a good rule is to bring back twice as much as you think you'll need. Most people underestimate.)
- Masses of cedar, rhododendron, magnolia, or eucalyptus leaves, tied with a velvet ribbon, in a porcelain vase.
- Clusters of roadside flowers, first dried, then grouped in a jug or a brightly painted coffee can.

To dry flowers, rubber band them together, then hang them upside down for a few days in a spot with no direct sunlight or temperature extremes.

To keep any autumn leaves pliable after you pick them, pound the bottoms of the stems and let them stand for about one week in a mixture of one-half water and one-half glycerin, available in drugstores.

treasure hunt
great game at the beach in autumn

After the crowds have gone and you're not seeking a tan or a new man at the beach, it's time to hunt for buried treasure. All you need is a sandy beach, a sunny afternoon, and a metal detector. Many people spend pleasant fall afternoons on the beach with their metal detectors, listening for the hum (or other signal) that says they're near the discovery of anything from coins that slipped out of a sunbather's pocket to a watch or an old bottle cap. You probably won't find anything that will make you rich, but it's fun and good outdoor exercise. You can buy a metal detector at electronics shops for about $35.

Actually you can use your metal detector to hunt for loot in any unpaved area, but a beach is ideal because sand is easy to dig in, and considering all the people who crowd the beach during the summer, you are sure to find a few goodies here and there.

For a free booklet on treasure-hunting tips and information and—on request—names of clubs in your state or area, write for "Treasure Hunting Pays Off" from Garrett Electronics, 2814 National Drive, Garland, TX 75041, enclosing $1 for postage and handling.

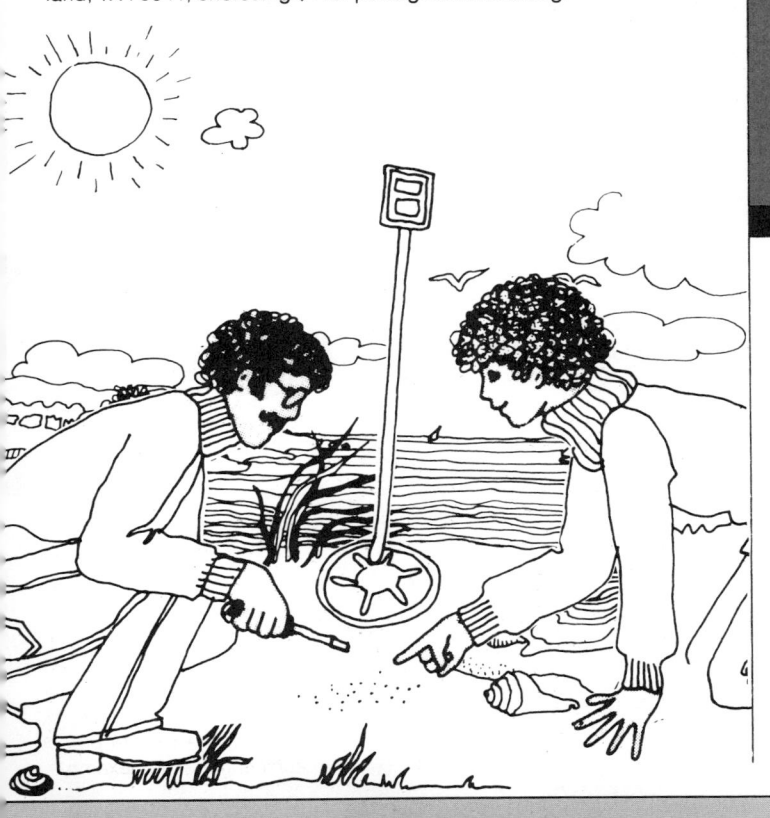

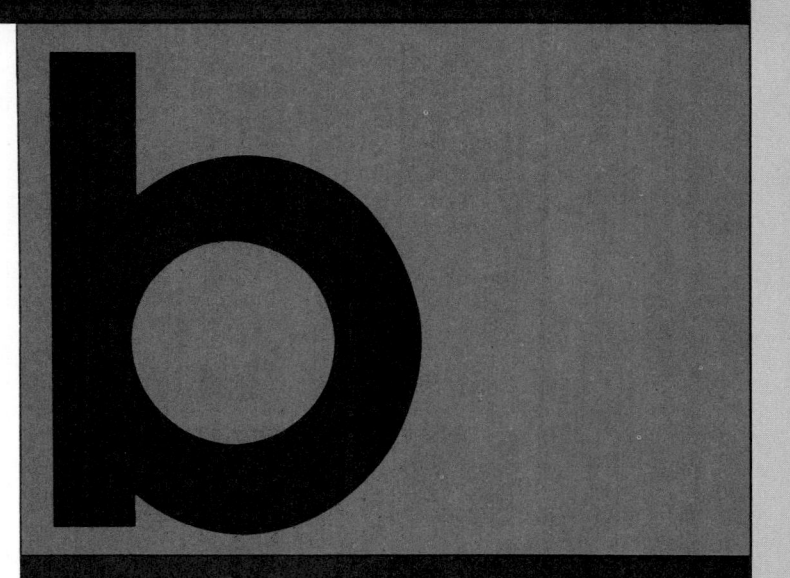

b

**beauty products
bicycles
body
books**

beauty products

cosmetics which ones do what

Most any woman can find her way through the lipsticks and eye shadow, but after that, the decisions can be tough. The confusion starts with what are usually called "treatment" products, those that help keep your skin in good shape—like toners, astringents, moisturizers, and so on. Which product does what and which ones do you really want? Here's a brief glossary of the most common treatment products to help you in your search:

- **cream or lotion cleansers**
  These products are usually a combination of ingredients that loosen dirt and makeup, so they can be tissued or wiped off. Some are water soluble, which means they should be rinsed off.
- **cleansing grains**
  A mildly abrasive grainy product that helps remove the uppermost layer of dead skin and dirt. Grains are not an alternative to cleansers but are used in addition to them, usually once or twice a week—and only on oily areas.

b beauty products

- **astringents**
  They are liquids usually made from a combination of alcohol, water, and glycerin. Astringents are used to cool or refresh the skin and to remove any soap residue after cleansing. Some astringents, usually those made for oily skins, have additional ingredients that give the skin a tightened feeling.
- **fresheners or toners**
  These are lotions that are made basically of the same ingredients as astringents, but usually with less alcohol. They do the same job as an astringent, but since they generally contain less alcohol, they are good choices for women with dry or sensitive skin.
- **moisturizers**
  These products deposit a light film on the skin that helps slow down the evaporation of natural moisture. They also provide a protective barrier between your skin and the environment and make a smooth base for makeup.
- **night creams**
  Basically the same ingredients as in moisturizers, but with a heavier consistency. Special eye and neck creams usually contain these same ingredients, along with a higher percentage of oil.
- **depilatories**
  Foam, cream, or liquid products that chemically remove hair—one formula for facial hair, another for body hair.
- **leg waxes**
  Specially formulated waxes that, when warmed, can be easily applied to legs. When the wax cools, it hardens and can be pulled off, taking hair with it.

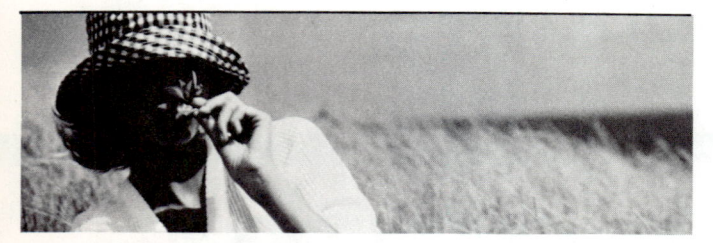

perfume
if you can't pronounce the name, how can you tell him you want it?

Maybe you can get along happily, even in Paris, without a knowledge of French, but Perfume French is another matter. Sooner or later you're going to fall in love with a scent that has a French name you can't pronounce and then where are you? The following list gives some of the favorites with French names, the connotation of the name, and the pronunciation.

- **perfume**   ● **pronunciation**

Calèche (elegant carriage)   Cal esh
L'Heure Bleu (twilight hour)   Lerr bluh
Emeraude (emerald)   Em er ode
L'Air du Temps (balmy air)   Lair du tohn
Ma Griffe (my signature)   Ma grief
Le Dix (the ten)   Le dees
Calandre (racy)   Kal on druh
Audace (daring)   Oh dass
Aviance (no meaning)   Ah vee aunce
Ciara (no meaning)   Sea are ah
Amour Amour (love, love)   Ah moor ah moor
Infini (without end)   An fee knee
Je Reviens (I return)   Zhuh ruh vee en
Ecusson (shield, or crest)   Ek que sohn
Courant (contemporary)   Coo ronn
Rive Gauche (Left Bank)   Reeve goche
Quelques Fleurs (tiny bouquet) Kel ka flerr

storage
where to put all those cosmetics

If all your cosmetics are so jumbled together that finding the right eye shadow is like looking for a contact lens in a crowded elevator, any of the ideas here are bound to help you. They're simple, inexpensive ways to organize your makeup and make that early-morning rummaging a thing of the past.

1. Stash your various cosmetics on a hanging plastic wall organizer, the kind with molded sections to hold kitchen utensils, desk things, whatever. Or make your own wall organizer from felt or pretty fabrics and fasten it to the back of a closet door. If you do this, you can make all the "pockets" just the size you need and even add a mirror.

2. Baskets make great cosmetic holders. Long, skinny ones, stacked on top of each other, fit right into the medicine cabinet. Filled with related cosmetics, they can be pulled out by category as needed. Small, cylindrical baskets can also go into the medicine cabinet and are ideal for tubes, brushes, and other "stand-up" cosmetics. Larger baskets, especially colorful ones with lids, are also terrific and look great when displayed on a dresser top or a shelf. Or line a small wall basket with bright vinyl or fabric and hang it near the bathroom sink.

3. An ordinary fishing tackle box, with storage sections, is a perfect catchall for all those makeup brushes, pots, compacts, and tubes. Keep it in a drawer or closet or paint it a bright, snappy color and set it out on your dresser or bathroom shelf.

4. Small plastic boxes, both clear and colored and in different sizes, are ideal for organizing makeup because you can see exactly what's in each one. Nest the boxes together on a clear plastic tray in the bathroom or put them all in a clear plastic box and keep in the closet, ready to pull out as needed.

5. If you like the idea of storing all your makeup in a drawer, buy some different-sized "snap-together" drawer sections in a dime store. They will keep things neat and easy to find. Or use the plastic divider tray from a fitted overnight case. The overnight case itself can be used as a portable vanity when storage space is limited.

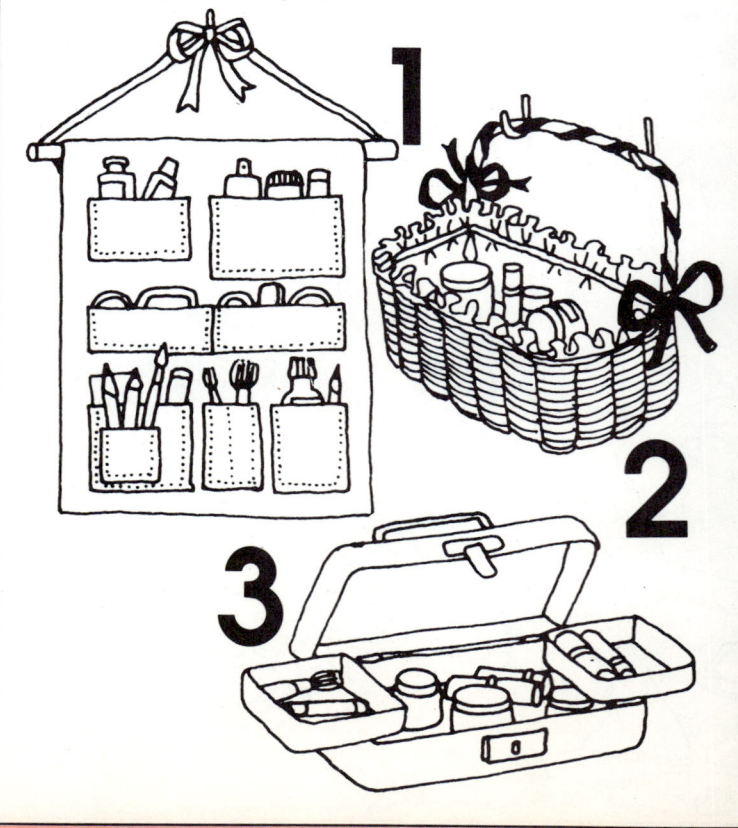

bicycles

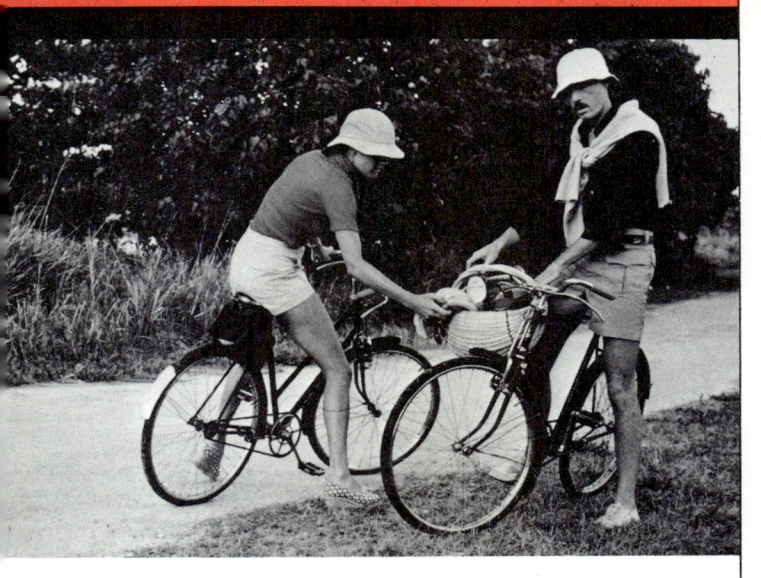

buying
tips on buying a bike

If you're in the market for a bike, investigate your area for a good bike shop. Most bikes have anywhere from a 3-month to a 4-year guarantee, but the best guarantee is dealing with a bike store equipped to make the adjustments necessary for safety.

● Your three main bike choices are: 1-speed bikes (30 to 60 lbs., $50 to $70); 3-speed tourist models, or "English racers," (35 to 40 lbs., $60 to $90); and 10- or 15-speed racers (under 30 lbs., $80 and up). For average use, your best bet is a 3-speed or 10-speed bike that combines lightness with the extra gears you'll need to cope with various road conditions. Pay at least $100 to $120 for a passable 10-speed bike or stick to a good 3-speed.

● The frame is the most important part of any bike and the best ones are light but strong. A sales clerk can help you choose the right frame size for your build. To check the fit yourself, have a friend hold the bike while you sit on it and push the pedal with the ball of your foot until your leg is at the six o'clock position. If your knee bends slightly, the bike fits; if you stretch any more, it's unsafe; any less, you'll work hard at peddling. (Scouts for second-hand bikes should be wary of damaged frames, which are hard to fix, and should have the bike checked by a reliable shop first.)

● You can choose a bike with coaster (foot) brakes or caliper (hand) brakes. Calipers require more frequent care but grip faster in dry weather. Down-turned handlebars allow you to ride bent over—awkward for city riding but more comfortable and efficient on long trips.

● "Take-apart" bikes with quick-release wheels and handlebars can be tricky to reassemble. Folding mini-bikes—with small 16" or 20" wheels—tend to be less stable and require more peddling to cover a given distance. Before you buy any extra-portable, be sure you can dismantle it easily.

● The most reliable American and imported bikes carry a label from the Consumer Product Safety Commission, which certifies their quality. Among the well-known American bikes are AMF, Huffy, Columbia, and Murray Ohio. Some top foreign makes are Gitane, Peugeot, Fuji, and Raleigh.

safety
dos and don'ts for bike safety

Whether you're simply a Sunday cyclist or depend on a bike for getting to work or around campus, the safety dos and don'ts below can help you steer clear of trouble. They're from Harold Heldreth, Coordinator of Bicycle Activities for the National Safety Council.

● DO check special bike regulations with your Department of Motor Vehicles. Some areas require bike registration and licensing and ban sidewalk driving. Also remember that most traffic rules for cars apply to bikes as well—from obeying road signs to driving on the right.

● DON'T ride an oversized bike—it's as tricky as walking in shoes three sizes too big.

● DO buy a safe bicycle. New models have to meet safety standards set by the Consumer Product Safety Commission regarding brakes, wheels, steering system, and frame.

● DO map out the safest bike route even if it ups travel time. Ride on scenic back roads, not freeways—many ban bikes anyway—and choose city streets with light traffic.

● DO watch for potholes, loose gravel, and other road hazards. If it's wet, go slowly and brake with small stops and starts to avoid skidding.

● DO drive straight, single file, and defensively. Watch for opening car doors and for cars (or pedestrians) bolting into the street from between parked cars. Don't just stare at the car in front of you; anticipate traffic movement further ahead, too. Be alert to sudden stops by the cars ahead of you.

● DON'T double up. Only "tandem" bikes are built for two. If you ride with a child, hitch his or her seat behind yours so that you can still see and move easily, and be sure the seat has a guard to keep the child's feet out of the moving spokes. Check also that the child's size and age match the requirements of the seat you use.

● DO safety-check your bike wardrobe. Avoid long coats, skirts, or scarves that can catch in wheels. Secure pants legs with ankle clips. Wear low-heeled shoes with slip-resistant soles to keep feet from sliding off pedals. At night, use clip-on leg lights and wear light-reflective clothing or sew-on reflective tape.

● DO invest in a horn or bell; front and rear lights (visible for about 500 feet); front, rear, and side reflectors; reflectorized tires; and a basket.

tuning up
how to get your bike in top shape

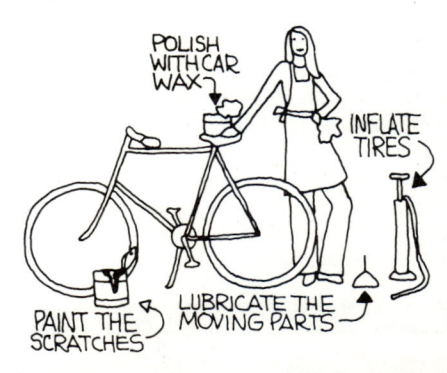

Whenever you're bringing your bike out of hibernation, remember that it takes lots of steady cycling to build up the stamina required for an expert's 50-mile day trip. So if you're out of shape, pedal an hour or so, then picnic. And before starting, follow these tips:

● Take your bicycle to a bike shop for an annual checkup and tune-up. They'll inspect gears, brakes, wheel alignment, hubs, pedals, and

b bicycles

tires plus tighten nuts and bolts. Cost is about $10 to $15 for a simple tune-up.
● Between tune-ups, do simple maintenance routines yourself. Lubricate moving parts with light oil or kerosene. Inflate tires to air pressure as stamped on sidewalls (3 to 5 lbs. less on very hot days to prevent blowouts caused by hot air expanding). Use car wax to polish, and use auto touch-up paint to cover scratches but don't paint over company tags or decals or you might lose your guarantee.
● Ask any dealer about bike insurance (about $12 a year to cover damage or theft of a $100 bike).

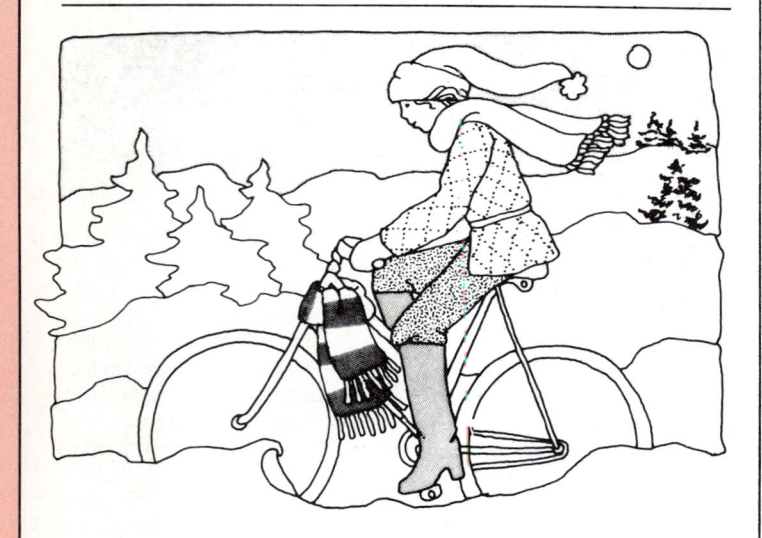

winter care
for bikes

Whether or not you plan to ride your bicycle this winter, now is a good time to give it a little extra attention, especially if you will have to cope with snow, slush, and salt.

● **using your bike during the winter**
The Bicycle Institute of America recommends using a light household-type oil on moving parts like gears and pedals, with an extra coat on the chain.
Check to see that the tires' air pressure conforms to the manufacturer's suggested pressure that is stamped on the tire. No adjustment is necessary in cold weather.
If you have to ride through puddles, be sure to dry your bicycle afterward to prevent rust.
You may find that in wet or foggy weather, the brakes squeak. It's nothing to worry about; the squeak is an indication that the wheel rim is wet. To make them work normally, apply the brakes gently before squeezing them hard. This removes the water from the rim.

● **storing your bike until spring**
Before you tuck away your bike, give it a routine cleaning. Then polish the paint with a paste wax preparation. Mechanical geniuses sometimes disassemble their bicycles, cleaning and greasing each part. They may even wrap each fixture separately in twill tape. If you're not up to this, just be sure to store your bike in a dry place.

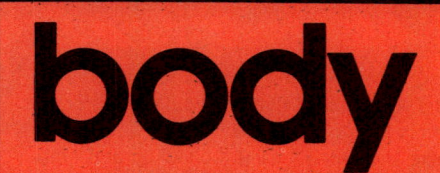

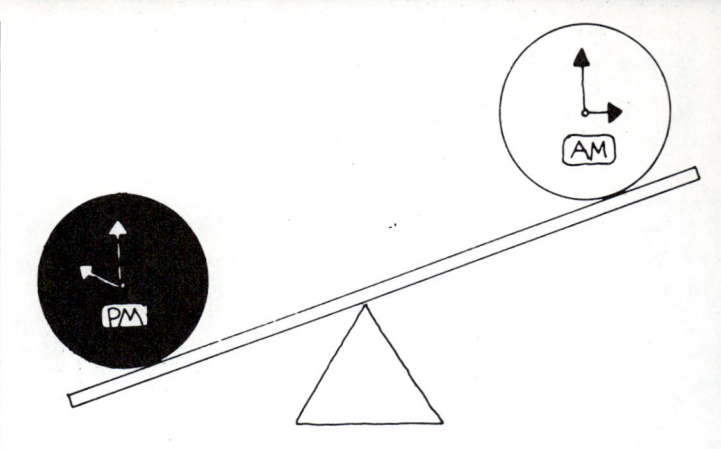

body

body rhythms
how to swing with your own

We all like to think we're consistent—the same person twenty-four hours a day—but actually, most of the body's internal systems are in a constant state of flux. Pulse, blood pressure, body temperature, and so on, all wax and wane in day-long cycles, cresting at one hour and bottoming out at another. As Gay Gaer Luce points out in Body Time, you're not the same person at midnight as you were at noon. Here are some suggestions to help you tune into your inner rhythms:

● Have you ever yawned through the last stages of a party only to find yourself wide awake immediately afterward? You were caught in the upsurge of an alertness cycle. Mounting evidence indicates that our waking hours are spent in roughly ninety-minute swings from feeling alert to feeling relaxed. If you can psych out your own body's rhythm, you will make better use of your alert hours and know the best time for drifting most easily into sleep.

● When you jet across time zones, traveling east to west, make allowances for fatigue. It's not just loss of sleep; it takes time for your body rhythms to adjust. Try going to bed progressively earlier each night for a few days before you leave and delay resetting your watch after you arrive, as a reminder that when it's the small hours of the morning back East, you can expect to feel low.

● Decide whether you're a lark or an owl—a morning person or a night one—then swing with it. You cope best when your body systems are functioning best, and everyone has a peak time of day. Chart your body temperature for a few days. From its nighttime low, if you're an owl, it will rise to normal an hour after waking; for a lark, an hour or so before waking.

● Couples who quarrel regularly should look for a pattern. Chances are the fighting hour occurs whenever dinner is late or after midnight. Those are the times when the blood sugar level is low and irritability, high. Another reason for dinner-hour irritability: sensory keenness increases for many people between about five and seven in the evening. So food tastes better then, but also children's voices and other noises seem to sound much louder.

● If you've been sleeping on a seesaw schedule, you're probably feeling frazzled. Keeping regular hours for a while will help put your body back in sync. The time you pick for going to bed "sets" your cycles and your inner time clock.

● If you're operating on little sleep, try eating more protein. The sleep-starved seem to need more.

● Dieting and plagued by hunger pangs? Relax. They come in four to six-hour cycles—they'll wane again.

● Keep a calendar record of your moods. Many people go through regular, cyclical mood shifts, as some women do when they experience premenstrual tension. Indications show that men, too, may experience a monthly hormonal and mood rhythm.

body b

massage
how to massage away tension

The next time he comes home uptight, maybe even with the headache that often accompanies tension, give him a massage. You can do it by using a relaxation technique from Sidney Zerinsky, director of the Swedish Institute School for Massage in New York.

This massage is for the neck and back, the areas that tension usually attacks. Mr. Zerinsky suggests that you massage groups of muscles together—the neck first, then the shoulders, and finally the lower back along the spine.

There are two massaging motions involved. The first is effleurage, a stroking motion. It is done with the palms of the hands, one or both together, and involves a gentle gliding motion. The hands should always work toward the heart to aid the vascular circulation, and gentle pressure should be applied as you stroke. See sketch for hand position.

The next movement is that of friction or kneading. This is a circular rolling motion over a muscle. It is easiest to do by placing one palm on the muscle, the other palm on top of your hand, and moving both in a circular motion, applying a gentle pressure.

Here is the sequence of motions that Mr. Zerinsky recommends. Starting with the neck (see sketches), use the stroking motion for a few minutes, then proceed to the kneading (use fingertips when kneading on the neck). Finish with the stroking again. Then do the same thing to the shoulders and the back. When you've finished, use the stroking motion over the entire neck and back for a few minutes. The whole massage should take fifteen or twenty minutes. If you'd like to use a moisture lotion, pick one that's not too runny and warm it a bit in your hand before applying.

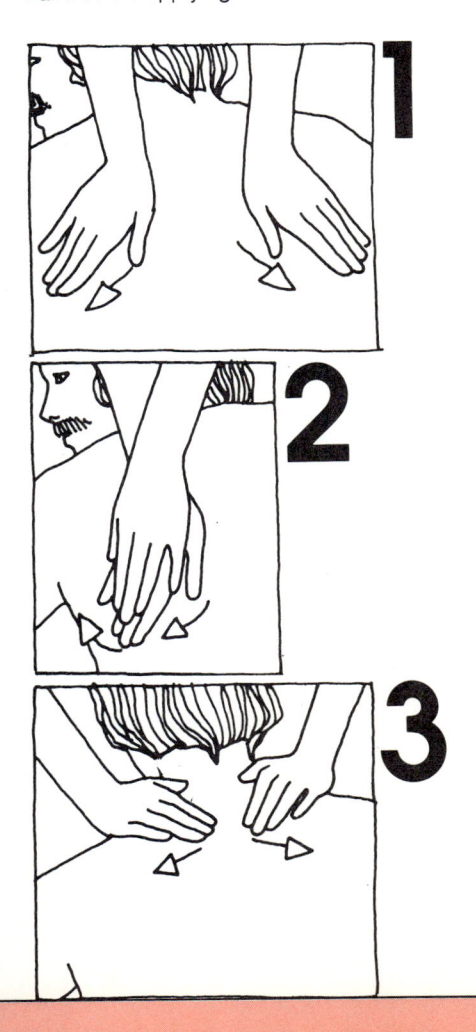

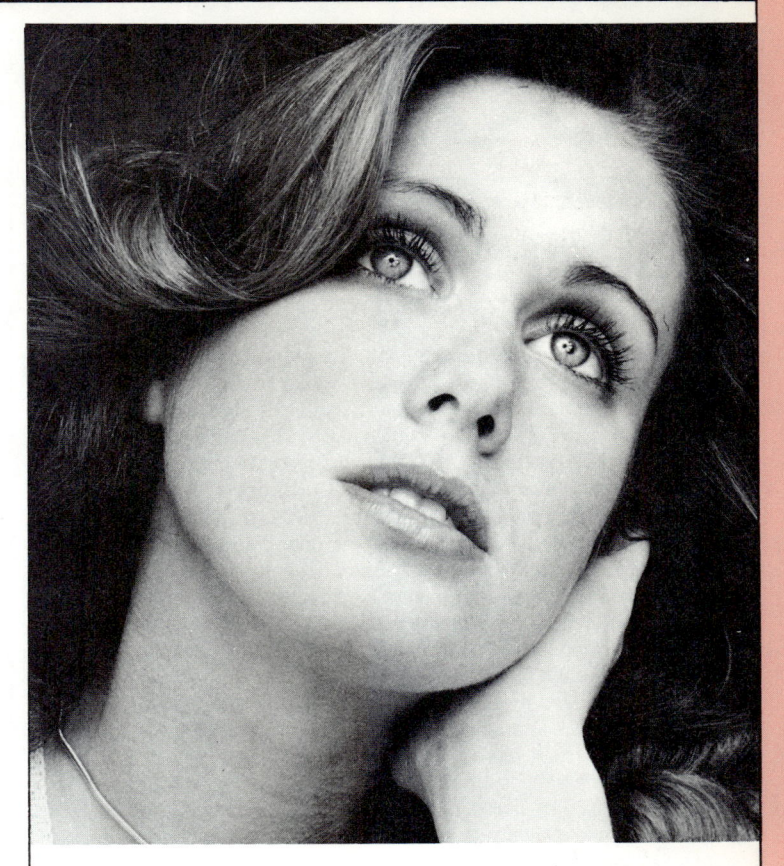

quirks
sounds, shivers, itches, and other body quirks—what do they mean?

Your body will often send you messages, but they don't necessarily mean anything exciting. To find the reasons for certain physical occurrences, we spoke with Dr. Michael Schmerin, an internist with The New York Hospital.

Ringing ears: No, you're not the hot topic of conversation somewhere. You've merely experienced a brief irritation of the eardrum.

"Sparks": After you get into bed at night, you may sometimes be entertained by a whole light show inside your head. These "sparks" are a consequence of closing your eyes tightly and thus putting pressure on blood vessels in the retina.

An itch: If your hand itches, don't count on a bundle of cash coming your way. The occasional, sudden urge to scratch is usually the result of a mild irritation of the nerves in the skin—or it can be a nervous reaction to a certain situation. (Chronic itching can be the manifestation of an underlying allergy.)

Lightheadedness when you get up quickly: In your blood vessels there are valve and pressure receptors that make adjustments to changes in your blood system. If you jump out of bed too fast and some of the blood suddenly leaves your head, those receptors won't be as quick as you are—and you will feel dizzy.

Foot asleep: That numbness or tingly feeling you may get occasionally in your leg or foot is the result of pressure on a nerve or on a blood vessel supplying a nerve—which happens when you cross one leg tightly over the other.

Shivering: Whenever you begin to get cold, the temperature regulator in your brain sends out warning signals to your body. Your shivering is the subsequent reflex of the small muscles in your skin that are designed to help generate heat.

If any of these occurrences persist, consult a physician.

b books

books

children's
books for 3- to 90-year-old children

Some children's books are enchanting enough to entertain anyone, any age. Here is a brief list of old and new favorites:
- *The Velveteen Rabbit* by Margery Williams. A story about a stuffed toy rabbit who, through the power of love and time, becomes real.
- *Star Mother's Youngest Child* by Louise Moeri. A curious young boy drops in from heaven to find out what Christmas is like.
- *The Little Prince* by Antoine de Saint-Exupéry. A prince from another planet meets an airplane pilot, who is marooned on a desert, and tells him about seeds that grow into dangerous giant trees, about taming a single rose, and his attitudes toward all these.
- *George & Martha* by James Marshell. Five very, very short stories about two hippopotamuses who are best friends and prove it with their truthfulness to each other.
- *The Giving Tree* by Shel Silverstein. As a little boy grows up, he takes all that his best friend, the tree, has to give. At the end of his life, he learns there is still more.
- *Zlateh the Goat* by Isaac Bashevis Singer. Servants who pretend to be angels, plus a bed full of sisters who can't unmix their feet are part of seven Jewish folk tales that show how the most difficult problems in life are solved with the simplest understanding.

clubs tips about them and some you might want to join

Joining a book club is a great way to expand your home library inexpensively. After sifting through an avalanche of new releases, a club offers quality selections and provides information about many more current books than you could possibly check out. If you're thinking of joining a club, read these tips first and then have a look at the list that follows.

Study carefully the book club ads and contracts that appear in newspapers or magazines. Most clubs bind you to a certain minimum purchase, and many operate on "negative option," which means you must return a card within ten days if you *don't* want their monthly selection . . . tricky if you're absentminded.

Remember that it takes usually four to eight weeks to receive a monthly selection, two weeks for an alternate.

Take into account that postage/handling is usually an additional expense and can add about 50 to 75 cents to book price.

In order to give substantial discounts, some clubs print their own editions using less expensive paper and bindings than in original publishers' editions.

The list below includes some large, general book clubs plus some interesting specialty ones. Key to abbreviations follows listing.
BOOK OF THE MONTH CLUB (280 Park Ave., N.Y., NY 10017). Current general fict./non-fict. IO 4 bks $1, must buy 4 in a year; D 40%; Book Dividend Plan.
QUALITY PAPERBACK BOOK CLUB (Book of the Month Club address). All categories, classic/current paperbacks; IO 3 bks $1 each; D 20%; SS to 40%; B.
- THE LITERARY GUILD (501 Franklin Ave., Garden City, NY 11530). General current fict./non-fict. IO 4 bks $1, must buy 4 more anytime; D to 40%; SS 50%–75%; B.
- THE DOUBLEDAY BOOK CLUB (Literary Guild address). Mostly current fict., some non-fict. (Many selections same as LG but offered a bit later at higher discount.) IO 6 bks 99¢, must buy 6 in a year; D mostly 50%; SS 70%–90%.
- COOKBOOK GUILD (Literary Guild address). IO 3 bks $1, must buy 4 more in 2 yrs.; D to 40%.
- AMERICAN GARDEN GUILD (Literary Guild address). IO 3 bks $1, must buy 4 more in 2 yrs.; D to 30%.
- MYSTERY GUILD (Literary Guild address). IO 6 bks $1, must buy 4 more in a year; D fixed price; $1.98/book.
- SCIENCE FICTION BOOK CLUB (Literary Guild address). IO 4 bks 10¢, must buy 4 in a year; D to 60%, but most books $1.98.
\# TIME-LIFE BOOKS (Time and Life Bldg., Chicago, IL 60611). Not strictly a club but 16-book series on special subjects—food, photography, gardening, art, etc. Enroll in a series and receive a book every other month for 10-day trial. No minimum purchase required. Can cancel enrollment anytime.
THE MOVIE BOOK CLUB (51 West 52 St., N.Y., NY 10019). IO 3 bks $1, must buy 4 more in 2 yrs.; D 25%–40%; SS; B.
WOMAN'S HOW-TO BOOK CLUB (44 Hillside Ave., Manhasset, NY 11030). Crafts, home repairs, cooking, gardening; IO—various joining offers; e.g., 1 bk 25¢, must buy 2 more in a year; D 30%–60%.
POPULAR SCIENCE BOOK CLUB (Same basics and address as for Woman's How-To Book Club). House building and remodeling, furniture making, plumbing, auto repair, etc.
OUTDOOR LIFE BOOK CLUB (Same basics and address as for Woman's How-To Book Club). Fishing, hunting, personal outdoor life accounts.
PSYCHOLOGY TODAY BOOK CLUB (1 Park Ave., N.Y., NY 10016). Mostly non-fict. Broadly concerned with the human condition; IO 3 bks for $3.95, must buy 4 more in 2 yrs.; D 15%–40%.

Key to abbreviations
IO—Introductory offer
D—Standard discount
SS—Special higher discount sales
B—Bonus plan (usually you earn bonus credits from items bought after your initial commitment and these set books at super discounts—70% or more)
(•) Clubs not offering original publishers' editions
(#) Clubs not operating on negative option (all others do)

mystery
4 grown-up replacements for Nancy Drew

Norah Mulcaheney is the sleuth in Lillian O'Donnell's adventures: *Don't Wear Your Wedding Ring*, *Dial 577-R-A-P-E*, *Baby Merchants*, and *Leisure Dying*. Norah is a concerned sleuth; she doesn't ask anyone to bleed, just to care. Kate Fansler detects in Amanda Cross's (pseudonym) adventures: *In the Last Analysis*, *The James Joyce Murder*, *Poetic Justice*, *The Theban Mysteries*, and *A Question of Max*. Kate takes the intellectual approach to murder—not surprising since she's also an English professor. Christie Opara is Dorothy Uhnak's detective in *The Bait*, *The Witness*, *The Ledger*, and *Law and Order*. Christie is a policewoman on the New York City D.A.'s Special Investigations Squad. Cordelia Gray was created by P. D. James (pseudonym) in *An Unsuitable Job for a Woman*, the first of a promised series of mystery books featuring Cordelia, a 22-year-old British private eye. We found our female sleuths in New York City's intriguing bookstore, Murder Ink, which is devoted entirely to you-know-what.

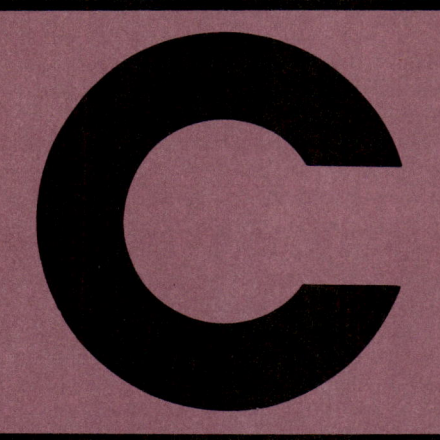

camping

camping
careers
cars
children
Christmas
clothes care
college
complaints
conversation
cooking
crafts
credit

what any new camper should know about sleeping bags and tents

Doug Kreeger, of Kreeger & Sons camping and backpacking equipment store, recommends that for your first camping expedition you borrow a sleeping bag and tent from an experienced camper to get an idea of your own likes and needs. When you're ready to buy your own gear, follow these guidelines that he suggests:

● **sleeping bags**

Shape: Sleeping bags are available in two basic sizes—average and large; and two basic shapes—semirectangular and modified mummy. Mummy bags usually have a hood and are tapered toward the bottom, making them extra warm and a bit lighter than rectangular bags.

Insulation: Most sleeping bags are made of lightweight, easy-to-care-for nylon and are insulated with goose down, duck down, or synthetic fiberfill. The thickness and resilience of the insulation is called the "loft," and the greater the loft, the warmer the bag will be. A high-quality, well-made goose-down bag has high loft and is extremely lightweight. These bags are priced from $70. Less-expensive, synthetically insulated bags can be as warm as down (like those filled with Polarguard®) but are bulkier. If you're planning on only warm-weather camping (as cool as 45 degrees), a synthetically filled bag (about $40) is adequate.

Construction: The stitching of a bag greatly determines its durability, so check for straight, even stitches. Look for about ten to twelve stitches per inch of fabric.

● **tents**

Shape: The two basic tent shapes are the "I" and the "A" frames. If you want an inexpensive tent or one that you can carry on a backpack, you'll do better with an I-frame, which has few poles and is light to carry and easy to erect. (Two-person I-frames start at about $25; A-frames start at about $55.)

Fabric: Most lightweight tents today are made of nylon rather than canvas. The strength of a tent is gauged not by weight but by thread count—the number of threads per square inch of material. The higher the thread count, the tighter the fabric will be and therefore more resistant to the elements. Consider also whether you want a single- or double-layer tent. A double (starting at about $70) has an inner layer of ventilated nylon as well as a water-resistant outer layer, or "fly." A single-layer tent is less expensive (starting at about $35), but on a hot, muggy night the condensation that forms on the inside can make you miserable.

Construction: As in bags, there should be ten to twelve stitches per inch of fabric. Be sure there are no gaps around door or window areas, where bugs and mosquitoes can enter.

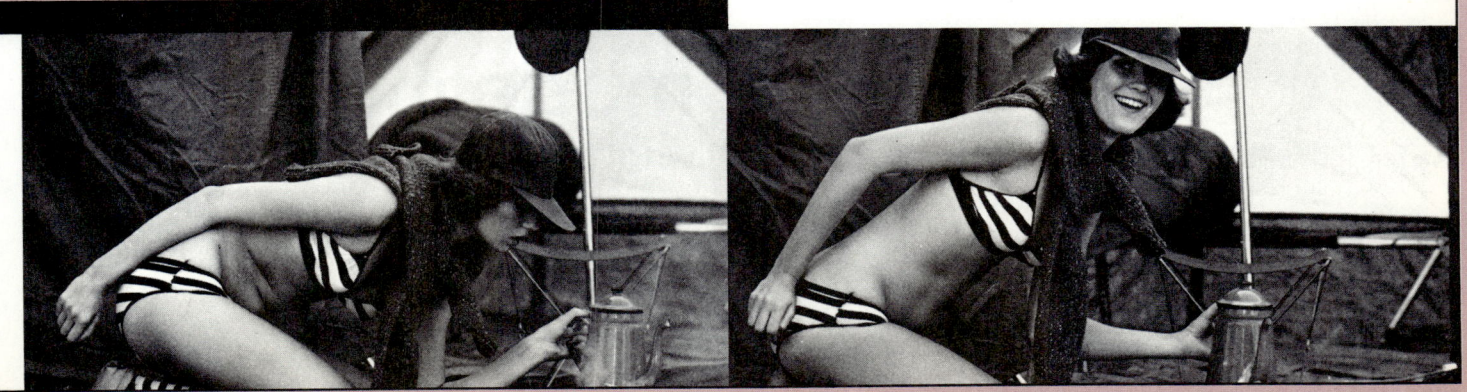

careers

careers

agencies
what you need to know about them

1. Register with only those agencies that have been in business for a while, preferably ones that have been recommended by friends or, better still, by personnel workers in your field.
2. Check the newspaper ads. You'll not only find out which agencies have a greater concentration of jobs in your area, but will also gain some insight into the agencies themselves. Do they give solid facts or simply rave reviews like "Exciting Job! Fascinating people! Great future! Lots of fun!"? Generally, the quality of an agency declines as the number of superlatives increases.
3. Judge the salaries that are offered. Are they in line with current rates or are they obvious come-ons? Check the salary range for comparable jobs at several agencies.
4. At the agency interview, be observant and critical. Are the interviewers people with whom you'd like to work? How do they speak? How do they dress? Remember that agencies often mirror their clients.
5. Be skeptical of agencies that are consistently evasive about why they won't send you on an interview for a job for which you're qualified. (You may have answered a phony ad placed just to bring in a flood of marketable applicants.) Be equally wary of those that send you out to see anyone and everyone. A bad match between job and applicant can happen occasionally, but after three or four time-wasters, drop the agency (they're playing the percentages at your expense).

interviews
how to psych out a job interview

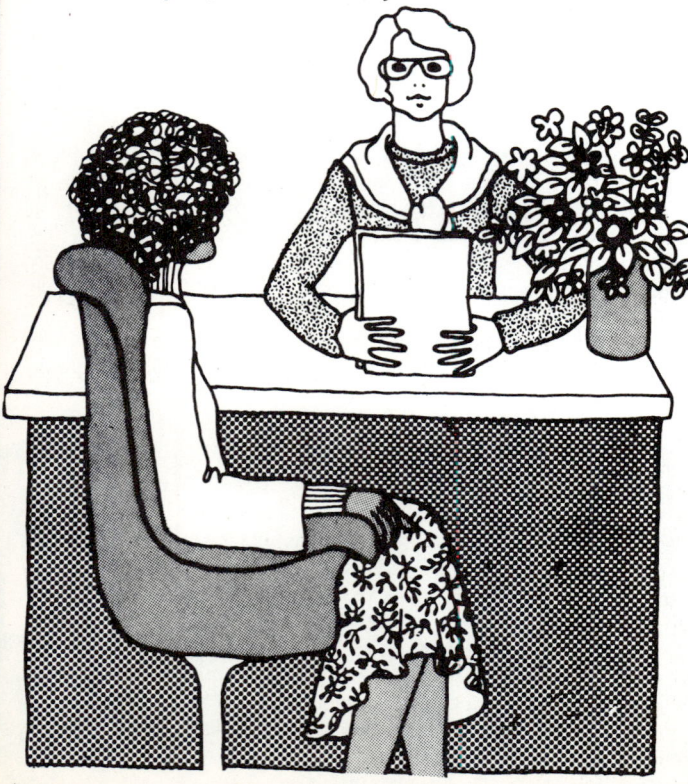

After a few job interviews, your palms may be less sweaty, but you still may not feel confident about your approach. Here's how to come up with honest answers to an interviewer's questions—answers that will prompt your own questions about the job.

- Remember that a job interview involves two people talking together, and a good interview results mostly from their liking each other. So relax, be yourself, and show an interest in what that other person is saying to you. Look him or her straight in the eyes and keep your posture open. Crossed legs and arms indicate—if the interviewer knows anything about body language—that you're either bluffing or likely to hide out in an office cubicle.
- It is illegal for an employer to ask questions, no matter how subtly phrased, about your status as a woman, mother, or wife—the same applies for your religion and nationality. However, some employers or interviewers either do not know all the laws regarding discrimination or they ignore them, and if you want the job, it isn't advisable to enlighten them. It is logical to anticipate their concern over such problems as the health of your children and the running of your household. You might state from the beginning that you are, say, married, with two children, have an excellent housekeeper or babysitter, a well-run house, and free to travel. You thereby eliminate an employer's fears about frequent absences because of sick children, family problems, and so on.
- Your interview is your chance to scrutinize the job but be selective about the questions you ask and to whom you ask them. Questions about the company, if they are objective, show interest; for example, asking about company philosophy regarding promotions and opportunity. You might ask the interviewer to give you a rough sketch of the department or organization and explain where you would fit in, making sure you see room to move up.
- If you are talking to a peer, perhaps the person you are to replace, you might ask what he or she likes about the company, how many people have held the job before, and for how long. But these same questions, if posed to a department head who would be your superior, could be considered inappropriate. You are expected to ask about your salary and salary policy in general, but don't plunge in with "When would I get a raise?" It is essential that you request to meet your potential boss to see whether you are mutually compatible.
- Even when you are not looking for a secretarial job, some counselors advise that you do not refuse to take a typing test. They believe that a refusal is a negative move that inevitably weakens your chances. You can, however, often avoid the issue if your résumé states clearly what skills you have, or if you settle this at once by saying, of course, you have adequate typing skill. Remember, having the skill doesn't mean you're looking for a job as a typist.
- Research the organization and field ahead of time to get an idea of the related needs and problems. Talk to a school placement counselor or faculty member who knows the field. Possibly they could refer you to someone who is active in that type of work who might be familiar with the specific company you're interested in. Finally, read a few recent issues of its trade magazine, if it has one. Or check the public library for a copy of the company's annual report or *Dun and Bradstreet's*. An informed approach usually prompts fresh insights and interest, and that spells a job.
- For more tips, read *Go Hire Yourself An Employer* by Richard K. Irish.

modeling
do you have what it takes to be a model?

"A fashion model is a girl who, through a piece of good luck, was born with the special physical requirements needed to become a model." That's what Eileen Ford, who runs one of New York's top model agencies, says in her book, *Secrets of the Model's World*. But how does an ordinary girl know what it takes to "make it" as a photographic model, and most of all, whether *she* can make it?

careers

Ms. Ford is very specific about the physical requirements her models must meet, mainly because a model must fit a manufacturer's sample clothes. (If too much pinning and altering are needed, it's not worth it.) Most clothes fall into three categories—junior, misses, and high fashion—and a model can be successful in any one or a combination of these areas. Here are Ms. Ford's requirements for each:

- **junior**
  Height: 5'7" to 5'8", stocking feet
  Bust: 32–34"
  Waist: 20–23"
  Hips: 32–34"
  Average weight: 105–116 lbs.
- **misses**
  Height: 5'7" to 5'8", stocking feet
  Bust: 33–33½"
  Waist: 20–23"
  Hips: 33–34"
  Average weight: 106–116 lbs.
- **high fashion**
  Height: 5'8" to 5'9", stocking feet
  Bust: 33–34"
  Waist: 22–24"
  Hips: 33–35"
  Average weight: 115–120 lbs.

There may be some slight deviation from these figures, but Ms. Ford says that if a girl doesn't fit these requirements, her chances of success are fairly slim.

Even girls who measure up to these basics still aren't assured of success. And as you might guess, being pretty isn't enough. In fact, Ms. Ford says, "The ideal face for photography needn't be a pretty one. If the brow is broad, the cheekbones high, the contours definite, and the chin not too prominent or receding, facial beauty doesn't matter." Good legs, good hands, a long neck, and healthy hair are important—and Ms. Ford also looks for a girl with large, wide-set eyes. Eyes can be enlarged with makeup, but if they're too close together, they tend to appear cross-eyed in the camera. A nose shouldn't be too broad or long, and the camera exaggerates any little bump or flaw. Lips are another problem area. Thin lips can be made to appear fuller, but not much can be done for an overly full mouth.

The competition in the modeling field is fierce. But the one thing that girls with real model potential have on their side is the fact that agencies *want* them. These girls will be moneymakers for anyone they work for. If an agency spots that potential in a particular girl, it will usually go out of its way to help her advance. She, too, must cooperate and this can mean long working hours and months and months of frustration. But . . . she just might make it big, and that's what it's all about.

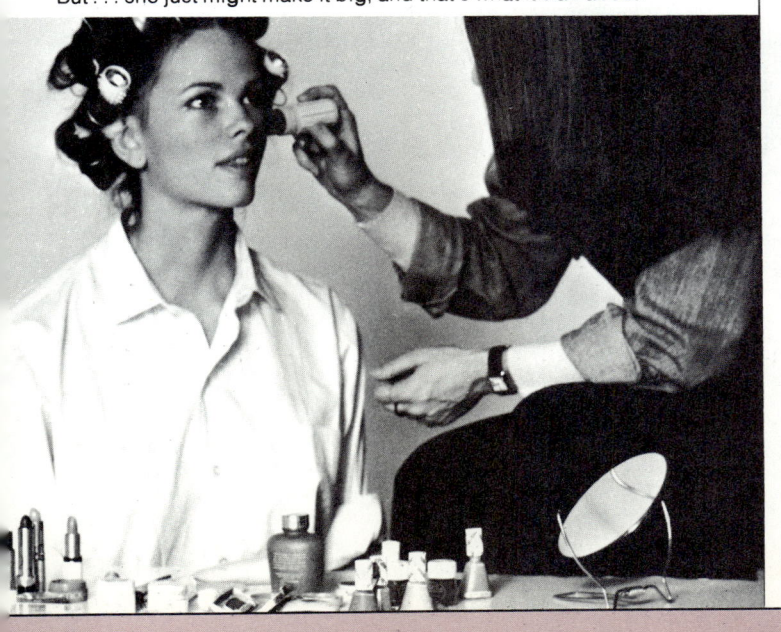

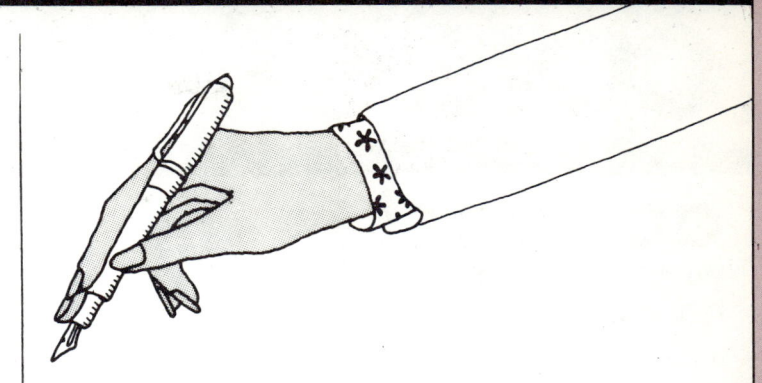

résumé tips for women
with or without work experience

A résumé can earn you a chance at a job, or it can dead-end you into the nearest wastebasket. Although an interview may clinch the job, your first crucial impression is made on paper. Here's how to write an eye-catching, door-opening résumé in the functional form. It works well for the "unemployee" with little or no professional experience.

- Be neat and succinct, using one or at most two pages. Put your name, address, and telephone at the top. Follow with your job objective.
- Now, instead of listing paid work experience chronologically by jobs, categorize all work experience, including unsalaried jobs, by skill. Under functional subheads, such as "Sales" or "Writing," describe your related work experience in short-paragraph style. Avoid information about salaries, dates, even job titles. For instance, a housewife should not show a potential employer at first glance that her only paid job was part-time during college on a newspaper copy desk. The functional résumé concentrates on capabilities, says Kathi Wakefield of MORE for Women, a career counseling service (at Gramercy Park Hotel, 2 Lexington Ave., New York, NY 10010). For example, this "housewife" can draw on the campaign material she wrote for a local political candidate, and the display window she designed for a friend's new culinary shop.

The functional résumé also works for the June graduate with four summers of lifeguarding and is surefire for the woman who is changing fields or turning a job into a career. Talking in terms of skills and accomplishments—not position titles—makes it easier for a potential employer to envision you in a new job situation.

- Warning: There are certain fields, such as law and education, that require the chronological résumé form, according to Today's Woman, a nationwide executive and professional placement service (at 21 Charles St., Westport, CT 06880). In any case, to avoid negative reaction from an employer who wants "statistics" immediately, end your résumé with a straight biography (firms' names, employment dates, schools, degrees).
- A final plus for the functional résumé: organizing your experience as it relates to a job goal prepares you with a strong self-image for the interview.
- **general tips**

These tips apply to both functional and straight, chronological-type résumés.

- Limit personal information to just what is needed to contact you. Do not include marital status. Except in the field of theater, never attach a picture. Also, don't mention salary expectations, and don't narrow down a job objective to a single position; just indicate a field.
- A tip for the recent college grad: Employers like someone who has financed his or her education. So include that information if you earned 70 percent of your college bills even if you did it waitressing.
- A dull, form cover letter weakens a résumé. Write a separate one pertinent to each potential employer. Show a genuine interest in each organization.

C cars

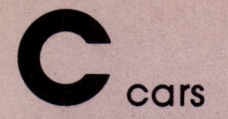

cars

accident
when you can't avoid one, how to minimize the damage

Accidents are by definition unexpected and sometimes by circumstances unavoidable. Even when faced with the unexpected and unavoidable, you can alter the severity of an accident. Despite newspaper accounts, drivers do not "lose" control of their car nearly as often as they "give up" control. You can choose the results of some accidents.

The choice an emergency presents is often a matter of degree. For instance, you might choose to plow into a stand of lilac bushes rather than hit a car that's jumped the divider and is headed straight at you. Or you might choose to bounce along a darkened ditch rather than into a wall of stalled cars.

Purposely going off the road or intentionally hitting anything might awe you, but we are dealing with crisis matters here. If you are driving, refuse to accept the inevitable, choose to mow down a length of fencing, to plunge into a snowbank, to use the roadside bushes as an impact-absorbing cushion.

It's unlikely you and your car will emerge unscathed from your chosen accident, but it is quite likely that you will not emerge at all from the one forced on you. Use your adrenaline and your determination. Keep selecting the lesser of the evils as they arise in the rapid sequence of an accident. Here are some guidelines:

- Drive off the road on purpose rather than skid off.
- Hit something soft rather than something hard.
- Hit something going your way or stationary rather than something coming toward you.
- Hit anything stationary with a glancing blow.
- Do anything to avoid a head-on.

driving tips for staying awake at the wheel

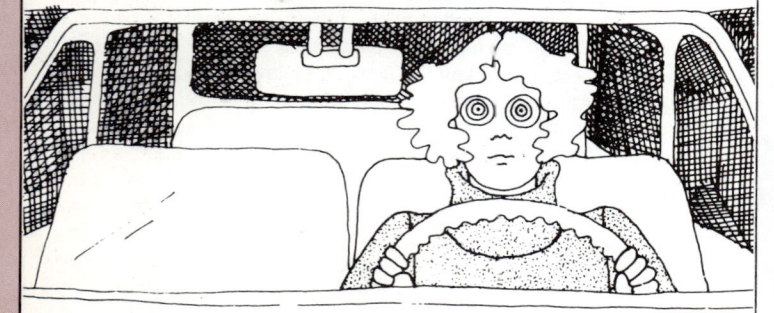

When you have to drive long distances, don't let fatigue or boredom cause an accident. Get enough sleep before you start a long trip, and limit your trips to a maximum of six to eight hours of driving a day. Here are some tips to help you prevent and/or counteract the fatigue that comes from the boredom of highway driving.

- Make rest stops every ninety minutes or so when possible. Never drive for more than two and a half hours or about 150 miles without a break. Better to arrive where you're heading a couple of hours later than to run into trouble.
- During rest stops, get blood circulating by jogging, walking quickly, stretching, exercising hands, and splashing cold water on face and wrists.
- Heavy meals can make you drowsy, so opt for many smaller snacks.

Fruit is refreshing; take chewing gum and hard candy, too, for behind-the-wheel snacking.
- Bring a friend along for company and conversation. It will be less fatiguing to both of you if you alternate driving shifts. If you must travel alone, keep occupied by singing, whistling, or talking to yourself.
- Listen to lively music on the radio or tape deck and sing along.
- Don't drive near large trucks for any length of time. And don't maintain the same speed in the same lane for long periods of time. Drive with variety.
- Keep the air in the car cool and circulating. Warm, stale air can make you drowsy, and cigarette smoke reduces the oxygen level inside the car. In cold weather, dress warmly and leave a window slightly open.
- Don't become too comfortable or inactive. Change your position, open and close windows, and inhale deeply at intervals.
- Finally, at the first sign of drowsiness, take a break and don't start up again until you feel alert. Knowing when to stop may be the most important driving skill you'll ever acquire.

extras
which extras do you really need on your new car?

The "bottom line" is nowhere more important than on the window sticker of a new car. That's where you read the price after all the extras are toted up: the vinyl this, the chrome that, and the Whatever Package. But which extras are right for you depends on many factors. If you're unclear about any, you might rent or borrow a car that has the options you're considering, and give your extras a test run first.

Engine—If you do most of your driving on flat, straight roads with no heavy loads in your car, you'll probably prefer the economic virtues of the smallest engine (usually a six-cylinder, not an eight) available. However, if you pile the car with people and objects, live where roads pitch and curve, have air conditioning, and drive with a little *brio*, you will be unhappily frustrated with the least powerful engine. It's unlikely that you'll ever need the "hottest" (highest horsepower) engine offered and, in these energy-crunch days, you'd hardly ever want it.

Heavy-duty suspension—If you tend to carry heavy loads or drive in a sportive fashion, by all means choose the heavy-duty option. It's not expensive and will take the mush out of cars too softly sprung. However, if you tend to be a moseying driver who rarely taxes the car's load capacity, you can probably manage with the standard suspension.

Trailer-towing package—Don't try to tow a camper or a boat without it.

Power windows—Look at the price. For that you can't crank? It's handy at toll booths and when adjusting the ventilation, but such power-assists all cost in terms of gas mileage.

Power disk brakes—Generally standard, but valuable if you have a choice.

Power steering—Not only does it ease the effort of steering a car, it can also improve your control. Power-assisted steering makes possible a steering ratio that makes the car more responsive. Parking is sometimes easier, too, with power steering.

Air conditioning—A car's resale value is certainly enhanced by it, but keep in mind that because of the extra weight it adds, you pay in gas to tote it around even when it's not in use.

Heavy-duty battery—If you make starts in cold weather, opt for the heartier version.

Rear window defogger—A great option.

Automatic speed control—This will keep your cruising speed constant on highways without a foot on the gas pedal. It should not even be considered unless you spend endless hours on superhighways.

Exterior trim strips—Their purpose is more than a cosmetic one. They protect the sides of your car from the constant assault by doors of other cars.

Remote control outside mirror—You can adjust your side mirror without

cars

having to roll down the window. Decide for yourself if the extra cost is worth the convenience to you.

Undercoating—Not to be confused with "rustproofing." Although undercoating can retard rust while it is still new and free of cracks, it's primarily for sound-deadening. Remember that engine and road noises can be fatiguing.

Rustproofing—It's a thorough chemical treatment that is guaranteed to prevent rust for a certain number of years. True rustproofing can cost $100 or more and is worth it if you live in an area where salt and the like are used for ice control; if you intend to keep the car longer than three years; or if you are concerned about the resale value in a heavily salted area.

Whitewall tires—If your aesthetic standards cry out for them, fine, but know that for the same amount extra, you could be buying a safety margin and possibly greater wear in a heavy-duty tire.

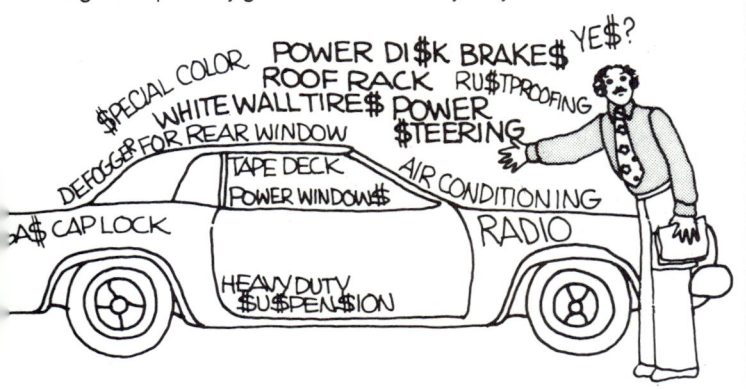

gas   squeeze more miles out of every gallon

Clearly, the best way to use less gas is to drive less; the next best way is to stop *less*. Think about it. Every time you step on your brake you are, in effect, wasting the gas you expended to get you moving at that speed in the first place. This isn't to suggest that you keep your foot clamped to the accelerator, horn blaring, and blunder ever on. But you might be surprised at how a little anticipation can decrease the times you have to come to a full stop.

For a start, when you have a choice, drive when the traffic is on the ebb. Fewer cars on the road mean fewer slows and stops. Maybe you could travel a route that has fewer stop signs. Also, if you sharpen your eye, you can read the traffic flow and benefit from it. For instance, if a traffic light ahead has been red for a spell, certainly it's due to change soon. If you slacken off on your speed a little now, you might be able to synchronize your arrival with green-up time and avoid a complete stop altogether. And when you park at a shopping center, choose a parking place midway between your errand spots or closest to the one with the greatest loading-logistics problem. Walk to the shops rather than drive to one and then another.

Letting the engine idle is wasteful, too—at least for any length of time. If you are waiting for someone and the engine is going to be idling for much more than a minute, it's better to turn it off. Here again anticipation will help—wait until everyone is in the car before stoking up the engine.

You can probably get the best mileage from a gallon of gasoline by driving a steady 45 miles per hour. Even up to 55, your gas consumption is fairly efficient. Faster than that, though, and economy takes a sharp plunge. The villain is air resistance. The faster a car goes, the more energy is required to shove the air out of the way. If you drive a sleek little sports car that is designed to slip through the air like wet soap, your higher-speed gas mileage will not be much different from that at lower speeds, but if you drive a big car with a broad beam, countering the air resistance can use a third as much gas going 70 instead of 50.

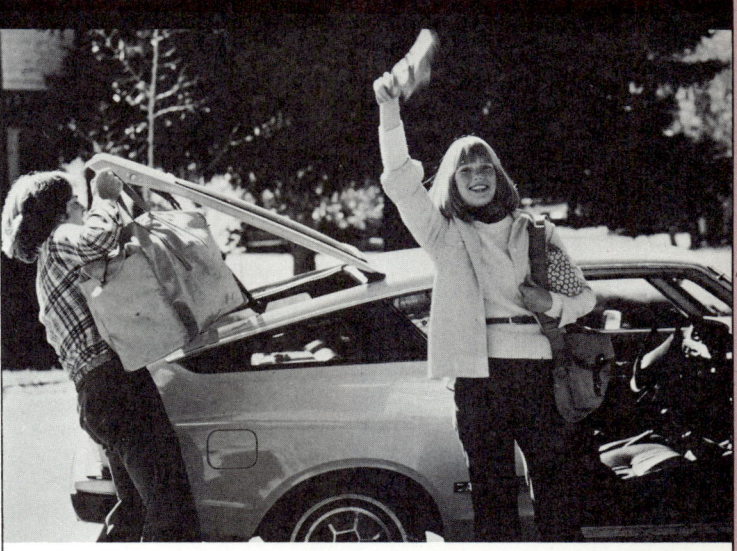

Remember, too, that a car with an automatic transmission gets about 6 percent fewer miles to the gallon than does the same car with a standard one. Using the air conditioner on a hot day in heavy traffic can take a further 20 percent chunk. (And emission controls, not exactly convenient but required, take another 6 to 7 percent.) But the real gas thief is weight. It takes gas to move poundage, and many cars are fat with options and opulence.

If you have always been a devotee of the small, lightweight car or perhaps more recently made the switch from a plush gas hog, consider yourself lucky or foresighted—but don't relax your vigilance. Gas is not only scarce, it is alarmingly expensive and the pocketbook you save is your own. So remember: Don't let your car idle to warm up, run on underinflated tires, speed, perform dragstrip starts from stop lights, or race your engine. Do consider car pools, drive with a light foot on the gas pedal, stop and start less, keep your engine in proper tune and the wheels aligned; consider riding a motorcycle, riding a bicycle, roller skating, or walking.

owner's manual
the foolproof guide to your car

If there were a foolproof guide to your car—the very same year, make, and model—written and illustrated so simply that anyone could understand it, would you buy it? You probably don't have to. It's most likely sitting untouched in your glove compartment right now. It's called the owner's manual and comes free with every new car.

"There seems to be no way we can induce people to read their owner's manual," lamented a Detroit public relations man. "One year

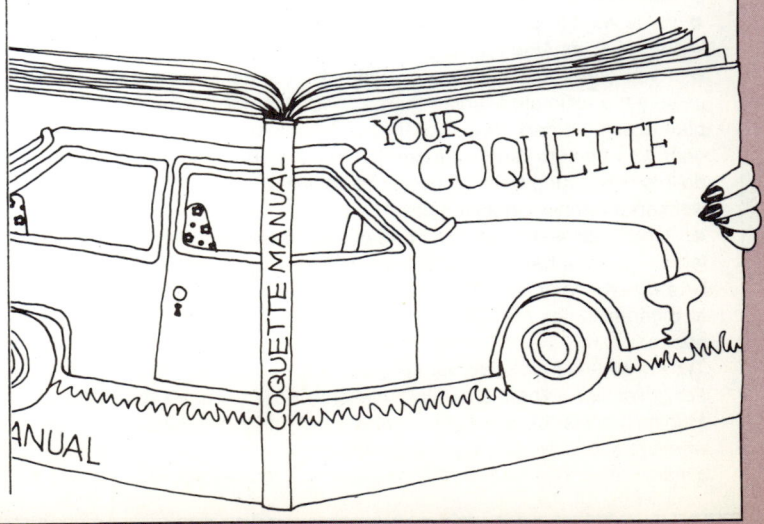

21

C cars

we wanted to put stickers on the dashboard—'Read Your Owner's Manual'—but the sales department said it would insult buyers. So we just keep answering questions on expensive long-distance calls, all of which are answered in the manual. For instance, how to start the engine in cold weather, how to care for the paint job, the numbers you need to know to put oil in the right place at the right time—and a lot more."

But what if your glove compartment is bare? It can happen, especially when you buy a used car. First check with the dealer who sold you the car to see if he has any extra manuals on hand. Or ask any dealer who sells your type of car for the address of the manufacturer's regional or zone office. Drop a note asking for the owner's manual for your year and model. If you have an imported car, a dealer can give you the address of the distributor in your area.

Some companies charge a small fee for the owner's manual. Here are some pertinent addresses for owners of American cars:

- **Chrysler**
Owner's manual, $1.50; Chrysler Corp., P.O. Box 40, Detroit, MI 48231.
- **American Motors**
Owner's manual, 60¢; Consumer Relations Dept., American Motors Sales Corp., 14250 Plymouth Rd., Detroit, MI 48232.
- **Ford**
New car owner's manual, $1.50; Ford Motor Co., Parts and Service Div., Owner Relations Dept., 1 Parklane Blvd. West, Dearborn, MI 48126.
Old car owner's manual, $2; Helm Inc., P.O. Box 07150, Detroit, MI 48207.
- **General Motors**
Owner's manual, approximately $1. Each division has its own appropriate address. Ask your dealer or write to General Motors Service Section, Detroit, MI 48202.

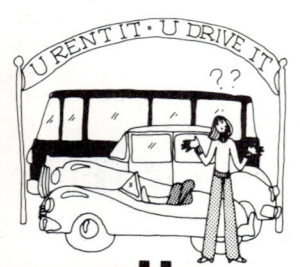

renting what you should know about renting a car

- To rent a car, you must be at least twenty-one—in some places twenty-five—years old.
- You must show a valid driver's license.
- If you want to pay by credit card, plan on using one that is widely known, such as American Express or Master Charge.
- If you prefer to pay by cash or check, you must leave a deposit—usually the estimated rental charge (based on the length of time you plan to use the car). When you pay by check, the rental agent usually calls your bank to verify your credit. However, the agent obviously can do this only during banking hours, so don't plan on paying by check on weekends or on nonbanking days.
- Rental plans—always read prices—are based on a combination of factors (see list below), and unless you are aware of them, there could be a difference of, say, $15 to $20 in charges for renting different cars at different times from the same company. Ask the agent questions about:

Type of car—A sedan is cheaper than a station wagon.
Length of time—There are daily, weekend, weekly, and monthly rates.
Mileage costs—A weekend rental may offer unlimited mileage, whereas a daily rental may charge anywhere from 15 cents to 20 cents a mile.

Gasoline charges—Some plans include gas while others require that you pay for your own.
Rent-it-here/Leave-it-there privileges—Some plans allow you to pick up a car in one spot and return it to another; other plans charge an additional fee when you leave the car in a different location.
- Do not rent from a firm that does not offer proper insurance. A standard policy offers $100,000 to $300,000 for bodily injury; $25,000 for property damage; full protection in case of fire or theft; and $100 deductible on collision damage (for about $2 extra a day, you can get full collision protection). *Note*: Make sure the insurance covers fine-print items like driving out of state; insuring a driver other than the renter; leaving a car unlocked; or returning it late.

signals make sure other drivers get your signals

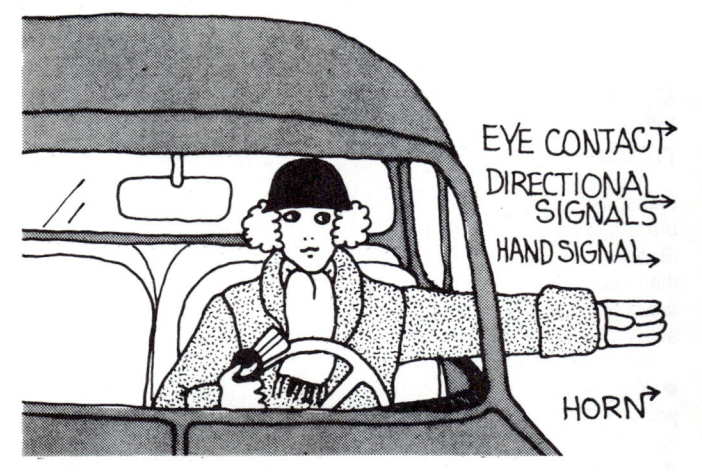

People have little trouble communicating when they are passengers in a moving vehicle. But when they become drivers, things seem to change. Perhaps the metal and glass that surround each driver fuzzes effective communication with others on the road.

But you can break down some of these barriers by using the means of inter-car communication available to you. Here are some of the most common and often overlooked ways.

Horn—Because of its misuse, the horn has fallen into disrepute; it is somehow considered rude to honk. However, whether or not your horn appeals to you aesthetically, do not neglect to use it at the appropriate time. When you are passing another car on a highway and you are not certain whether your presence is known, make it known with a toot, which is not to say a blast. Learn to get different tones from your horn, using a light tap, a quick twin touch, or a long lean when it's absolutely necessary.

Lights—In the daytime, flash your headlights as a warning, such as "Don't pull out of that driveway now; I'm closer than you think." Or use the flash to alert a pileup of oncoming cars; maybe there's a car stalled in their lane or a child on a wobbly bike. The drivers won't know exactly why you are flashing, but they will perk up and be that much more prepared for whatever awaits them.

The stop lights that flare red when you brake can be better used, too. If you are slowed sharply on a highway, put your brake on in short stabs to make those lights blink-blink a red warning to cars behind. Or, in extreme emergencies, put on your hazard lights.

When you intend to turn, use your directional signals well ahead of the time you brake to make the turn. When you signal a turn, the driver behind knows you will be slowing down for it and therefore anticipates your braking. That's much more effective communication than flashing your brake lights and leaving others to wonder why until they see your directional signal appear. If you are following a car that signals a turn, drop back instantly—unless, of course, you are being closely followed

children

by another car. In that case, move to the far side so that the car following you can see the signal clearly, too.

The four-way flasher, which is a light-signal system with quite specific meanings, should be used in emergency or unusual situations, such as when the vehicle is stopped or moving at a speed considerably slower than the general flow of traffic. Using your flashers for purposes other than these will only confuse others.

Hand signals—Don't overlook this simple old technique. For instance, using only your directional signal for a turn might be interpreted by the driver behind you as an indication of your turning at the next intersection, when in fact you want to turn into a driveway before that. If the other driver is following too closely, roll down the window and emphasize your intention with a hand turn signal.

Eye contact—This is a subtle technique, but an effective one. Look other drivers in the eye. It isn't easy but keep trying. For example, if you are waiting to pull into a long slow-moving stream of traffic, look at each of the oncoming drivers. If you catch an eye, the impact will often stop the driver cold, and you'll be waved into the stream. Don't forget to show your appreciation with a nod and a smile.

small car
how to drive a small car

Statistics indicate that the occupants of small cars are more susceptible to grievous injuries in the event of an accident, but don't be misled. Statistics also show that small cars are less often involved in accidents than their numbers might indicate. Reduced to the simplistic: Big cars are better-equipped to survive accidents, small cars are more likely to avoid them.

Here are some safety hints for drivers of small cars:

● *Keep in mind that you can be easily overlooked, so strive to make yourself more visible. You might try to drive with your low-beam headlights on even during the day.*

● *Don't drive along in someone's blind spot—at an angle off another car's rear quarter. Stay well back in rearview-mirror range or pull up from behind and pass quickly.*

● *Don't be shy about flashing your lights or giving a toot on your horn if you think another driver is unaware of your proximity.*

● *Avoid passing on the right on multiple-lane highways, even in places where the law allows it. That's the blindest of blind spots for other drivers.*

● *Show yourself. When you are on a heavily traveled two-lane highway, for instance, move about in your spot—near the center line for a while, then near the edge of the road. It's often difficult for drivers of large cars, especially station wagons, to see low, small cars that are following directly behind.*

● *Find your car's strong points and make use of them. Small cars are lighter, usually more maneuverable, and are quicker to stop than big cars. Use your size to turn onto a highway's shoulders for a possible escape route—something big cars cannot do as well. Use your maneuverability to dodge trouble. Use your shorter stopping distance to avoid a rear-end collision but always be aware that the car behind you may take longer to stop.*

● *Realize that because of the car's weight, your brakes might lock easily, so apply them by pumping rather than by one steady push. If your small car is not a sports car, its acceleration rate is probably more tortoise than hare; keep this in mind when you are merging with traffic.*

● *Be aware that big cars are likely to tailgate small cars more closely than they do cars their own size, because the driver can see over and around small cars more easily. So it is up to you to carry a cushion of space for them when you are driving in a long line of traffic. Leave more room than usual between yourself and the car in front of you. Then if an emergency develops, you have extra stopping space in front of you that you can "lend" to the car in back. Don't forget that the tailgating car needs more stopping room than you do! Allow for that. Pull far to one side as you slow down to allow him more room.*

clothes size
how to be sure of buying the right size for babies and little kids

For babies, your best bet is to jot down their height—it's the best guide to the right size. Weight and age by months, if you know them, are a further help. The size guide below was prepared by Sears for their catalog customers.

● **babies**

Size	Newborn	S	M	L	XL
Lbs.	to 14	15–20	21–26	27–32	33–36
Ht. (in inches)	to 24	24½ to 28	28½ to 32	32½ to 36	36½ to 38

● **toddlers – little children**

Size	1	2	3	4	5	6	6X
Ht. (in inches)	29½ thru 32	32½ thru 35	35½ thru 38	38½ thru 41	41½ thru 44	44½ thru 47	47½ thru 49

"Toddler" sizes are cut much fuller than are "regular" sizes to account for baby fat or diapers on boys and girls from about ages one and a half to four years. But whether you want toddler or regular sizes, height is still the most important factor in getting the right size. In the Sears guide above, sizes 1 through 4 come in "toddler," sizes 2 through 6X are regular. Remember, too, that sizes may vary among the different brands, so when you have to guess, buy one size larger than you think the baby needs. Babies won't shrink into anything, but eventually they will grow into the clothes. Probably the best idea is to ask the mother what size *she* buys—most will help you happily.

dressing
how to teach children to dress themselves

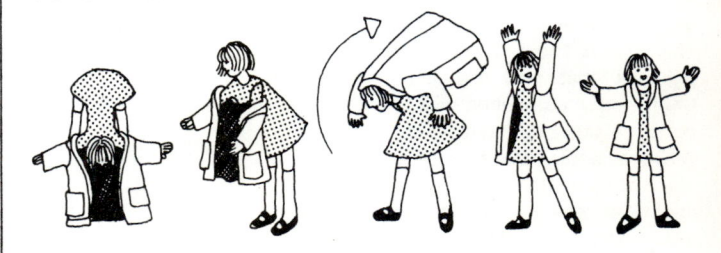

When a child first goes off to nursery school, you're doing everyone involved a favor if your child is dressed as self-sufficiently as possible. A child feels proud to be able to manage his or her own clothes, and the teachers are relieved to have six less buttons to fasten, two less mittens to retrieve, and so on. Use these tips to teach a child how to dress.

To put on a coat, cardigan, or anything that opens all the way down the front, teach your child to spread the garment on the floor with the neck nearest her, the hem farthest away. Your child can then insert both arms in the sleeves and swing the garment up and back, over-

C children

head; as this is done, the garment is pulled down into place (see sketches (p. 23). A zippered coat is much easier for small fingers to handle than one with buttons or snaps.

Boots slide over shoes quite easily if you put small plastic bags over the shoes first. It's a bit sweaty, but most three-year-olds can manage it. Make sure to warn the child to keep the bags away from the face.

Leggings with an elasticized waist are much simpler to put on than those that have to be fastened or have shoulder straps. Pull-on pants help small boys who have difficulty with fly-front trousers.

To keep mittens from disappearing, first crochet a long string, using a simple chain stitch in heavy wool. Attach it to the left mitten near the wrist and stretch it along all the way up the left sleeve, across the child's back, down the right sleeve, and onto the right mitten at the other end. It will invariably stretch, so keep it on the short side. When in place, a mitten dangles securely at the end of each sleeve.

early development
9 quick guidelines to start a child out right

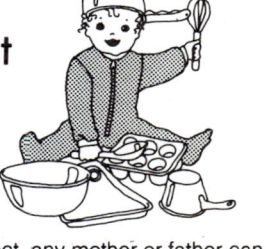

According to the Harvard Pre-School Project, any mother or father can help a young child grow up to become a more competent, confident, and independent human being. What it takes is neither a lot of time nor money, but a certain physical environment and attitude toward the child. The Harvard people (a group of behavioral scientists studying mothering techniques at Harvard University) came up with these guidelines to help mothers of preschoolers, especially those between the ages of five and seventeen months.

- Provide physical access to as much of the home as possible. Let the child satisfy his or her curiosity and explore the physical world. Of course, you might need to baby-proof some areas of your home.
- Provide a variety of things for exploration besides toys. Plastic jars, ice cube trays, pots, and pans all provide new shapes and textures to examine.
- Be available to your child for at least half of his or her waking hours. This does not mean that you should devote all your attention to mothering, just be available for encouragement, answering questions, and enthusiasm. The Harvard project calls it "on the fly" teaching and points out that many very effective mothers rarely spend five-, ten-, or twenty-minute stretches with the child, but stop for a minute or so dozens of times during the day.
- Occasionally use words that the child will find difficult to understand, then help the child grasp the meaning. For reinforcement, you might also repeat the explanation under different circumstances.
- Don't confine a child for long periods of time. Try to give as much free rein as possible.
- Don't allow your child to concentrate his or her energies on you all the time; encourage independent behavior and "pretend" activities.
- Don't worry that your child won't love you if you have to say no from time to time.
- Don't be overprotective; give your child as much freedom as possible.
- Don't worry about the speed at which a child learns to read, count, say the alphabet, etc. Don't worry about the child's slowness in learning to talk, so long as he or she continues to understand more and more words in time.

haircuts
tips for cutting your child's hair

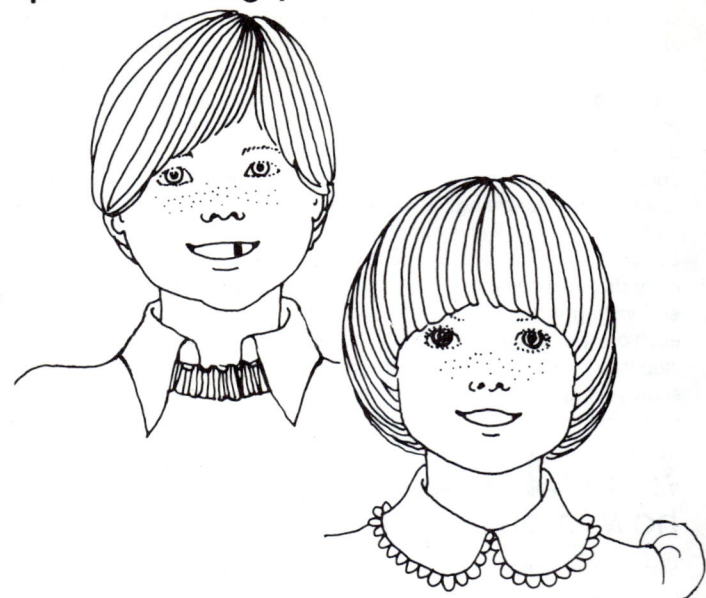

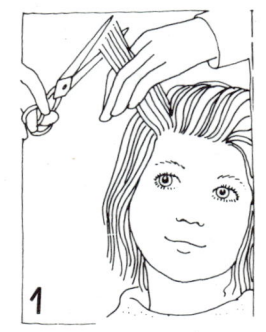

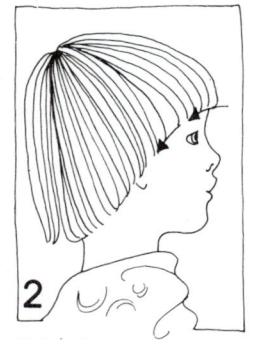

Getting a haircut isn't likely to be your child's favorite activity, but he or she will be more inclined to endure it if the cutter is someone familiar—like you. Here's an easy, step-by-step way to cut a young child's hair in a simple style.

Start by sitting the child comfortably on a chair that is facing a mirror. Use a couple of pillows on the chair if necessary so that you won't have to bend over too far. Try to interest the child in what you're doing so that he or she will look straight ahead into the mirror.

Now comb the clean, wet hair straight back, away from the face. Starting at the center back of the head, lift a section of hair (about two inches wide and an inch deep) straight up. With a good pair of small scissors, cut whatever length of hair you've decided on. Make a straight cut across the section. For the finished shape shown here, the hair should be at least three inches long. Continue cutting in this way, moving up the head. If you like, you can pin the hair you've already cut to keep it out of the way. Finish the top of the head, cutting exactly the same way. Now move to one side, but this time pick up vertical sections of hair instead of horizontal ones, and cut at a slight angle so that the hair at the bottom of the section is slightly shorter than that at the top (see Sketch 1). Then do the other side.

Now you're ready to cut the lower back section. Remove any clips, and comb through the hair to smooth. Moving from one side across the head to the other, lift up horizontal sections and cut the same amount as for the rest of the head. Use the hair you've already cut as a guide for length. Now comb all the hair straight down, away from the crown of the head, and trim off the edges by moving the scissors all around the head (see Sketch 2). You can make this cutting even or ragged. Making it slightly ragged will give a nice pixie effect.

If you'd like to find other styles to try on your own or a child's hair, you might look at *How to Cut Your Own or Anybody Else's Hair* by Bob Bent and Jack Bozzi.

children C

nightmares
how to handle your child's nightmares

Sometimes it's a tossup as to who's more upset by a child's nightmare—the child or the parent. So if your youngster has a midnight battle with tigers, walruses, and other assorted "monsters," here are some ways to handle his or her feelings . . . and your own.

● **how "normal" is a nightmare?**
Experiments have shown that even infants dream. These first dreams are probably pleasant. But once a child faces frustrations and problems—by eighteen months or so—occasional nightmares occur.

"A nightmare is a 'normally abnormal' state. It's a safety valve, an attempt by the psyche to have some healthy resolution to a problem. Unless your child is having a particularly rough time with one, it's probably not a good idea to stop the process and wake him or her up," says Dr. Martin Weinapple, assistant professor of child psychiatry and chief of adolescent services at Rutgers Medical School.

● **what to do when your child wakes up from a nightmare**
"Young children—up to about age three or four—have a hard time distinguishing between reality and fantasy, even when they're awake. In a dream context it's more difficult and scary. So a parent shouldn't even try to reason a dream out with a child," says Dr. Richard Granger, associate professor of clinical pediatrics at the Yale Child Study Center. "The parent can accept it as a reality for the child without accepting it as a reality for herself."

Treat any nightmare seriously—not as silly or babyish—but try to deal with it in a way that your child can understand. For example, if it's a dream about a tiger under the bed, you might look under the bed to reassure the child that the tiger isn't there. Only a youngster who is five years of age or older can begin to understand that he or she was "only dreaming."

After a nightmare it's crucial to let the child express his or her fears on the spot, unrushed. And for immediate comfort, young children are most responsive to touch and holding. Warm milk may be soothing as well.

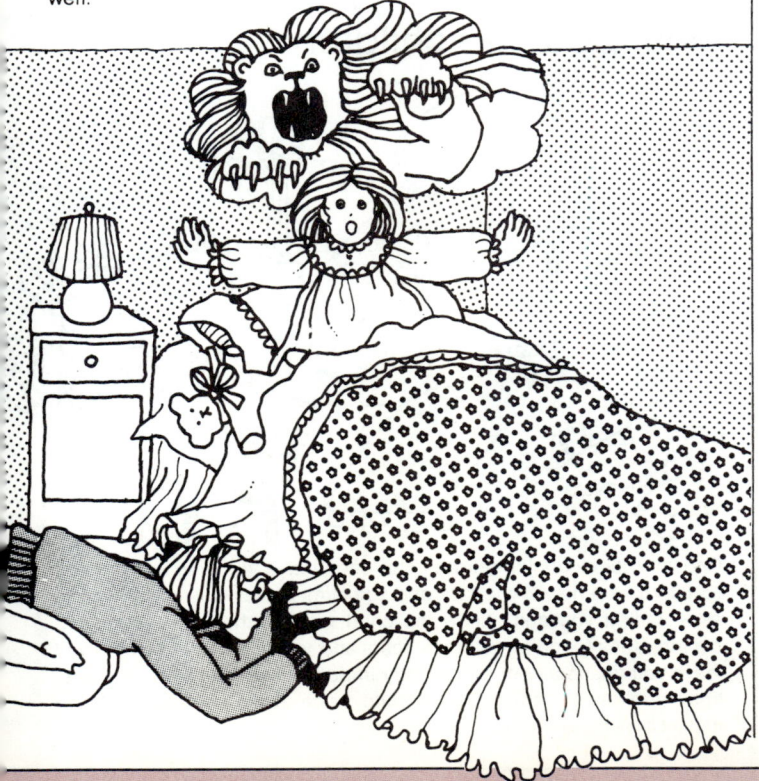

photographs
dos and don'ts for photographing children

● *DO ask a child to make funny faces to get him or her to loosen up. Just remember that the relaxed expression that immediately follows a "face" often provides a more natural shot than the "face" itself.*
● *To coax a natural smile out of a child, DON'T ask him or her to say "cheese." (What's funny about cheese?) Ask him to say "Cookie Monster," or the name of a favorite cartoon character.*
● *DON'T try to adhere too rigidly to the old rule about always having the sun shining into the face of your subject. The reason for this was that older cameras were not as "fast" (light sensitive) as those in use now. Some people still prefer front lighting, but today many cameras give good results using light on the sides of your subject.*
● *DO give a small child a new toy to distract him or her from the camera.*
● *DON'T expect a natural expression if you dress a child in stiff or unfamiliar clothes. As a general rule, the fewer the clothes, the happier the baby.*
● *DO whisper a happy "secret" to a child just before you snap his or her picture, and record the response to it; or, for a charming picture of two small children, ask one to whisper a secret to the other.*
● *DO record your child's growth photographically, by taking an annual photo of her in the same spot—say, standing next to the same dresser—to show how his or her size increases in relation to that of the object's.*
● *DO move in as close to the child as your camera will permit once he or she has relaxed a little. Too much background, not enough baby is a common problem in many albums.*

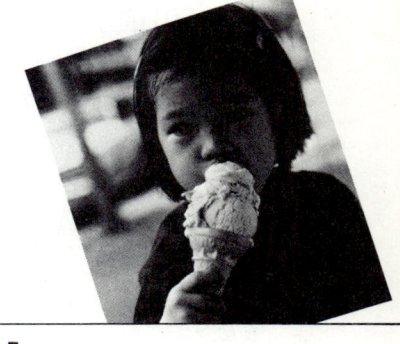

puppet make a dragon
puppet from a mateless mitten

When your child comes home with just one mitten *again*, don't throw it away. In just a few minutes, you can turn that mitten into a dragon puppet, inspired by Steven Hansen, "The Puppet Man," a talented young puppeteer who has performed in many places, including New York's Central Park.

To make the puppet, you'll need one knitted mitten, red felt, red yarn, a tapestry needle, two Ping-Pong balls, white glue, and a felt-tipped marker.

For the mouth, cut a piece of red felt that will fit the underside of the mitten from the tip to just where the thumb begins. Cut another piece in the shape of a forked tongue, big enough to cover the thumb. Glue both in place.

To make "scales" for the dragon, thread a tapestry needle with a 6" strand of red yarn. The ends of the yarn should be the same length, but left unknotted. Insert the needle on the top side of the mitten; pull the yarn half-way through. Then cut off the yarn just at the needle and

25

children

secure the double strand with a knot. Repeat this process until the dragon has enough scales.

Now glue the two Ping-Pong balls to the mitten so that they rest on top of the child's knuckles when the mitten is on. You must apply glue to *both* the Ping-Pong balls and the mitten to ensure a strong hold. Allow the glue to dry for several hours; then draw "eyes" on the balls with a felt-tipped marker.

If you have a mateless glove, make a spider puppet with bulging eyes. Glue on Ping-Pong balls at the knuckles.

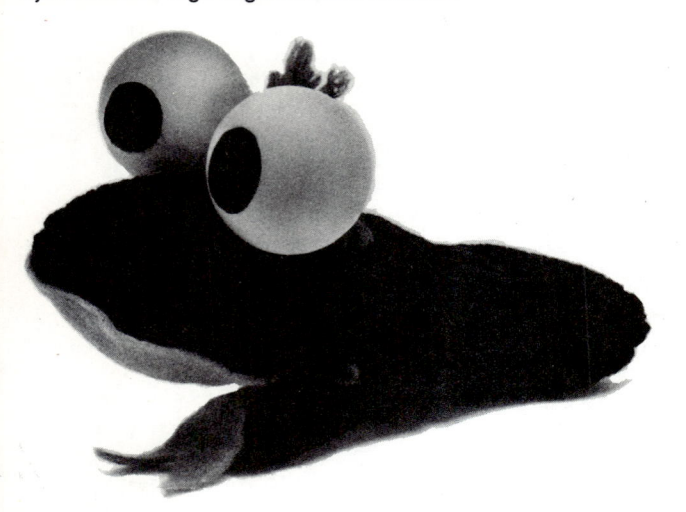

sneakers
7 ways to jazz them up

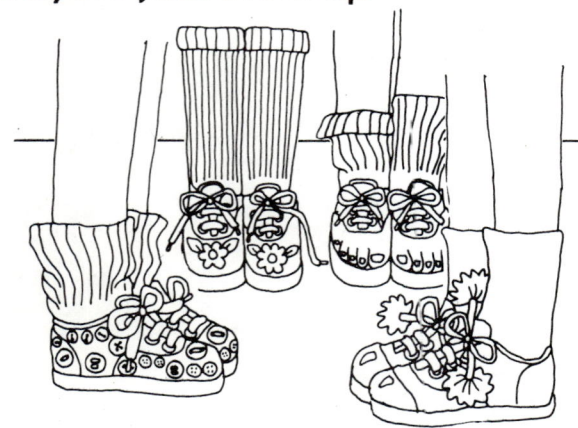

Plain white sneakers are fine, but we'll bet any kid will flip for jazzed-up, colorful, decorated sneakers. Either make them yourself or let the kids do their own. Here are some ideas to start:

1. Using waterproof felt-tipped markers is about the easiest, quickest way to zap up a sneaker. Draw on flowers, initials, stripes, whatever. Or, make the sneaker look like a shoe by doing a saddle-shoe or wing-tip design. You could also draw on "toes."
2. Sparkle a pair of sneakers with glitter. Do an allover random pattern or simple designs like arrows, geometrics, or initials. (Do remember, however, that the glitter will probably come off when washed, so wash by hand.)
3. Sew on buttons of different shapes and colors in any pattern you like. Use a fairly thick needle and heavy-duty thread.
4. With an embroidery needle, thimble, and bulky yarn, stitch initials on the front of each sneaker.
5. Stitch Witchery®, available in fabric and notions departments, is a super and inexpensive way to create an appliquéd effect. Just pick a fabric, cut out a shape, and iron on according to directions.
6. Decorate the sole where the canvas meets the rubber with different-colored narrow stripes, cut from adhesive tape that is available in art supply stores.
7. Do something with the laces. Substitute twine or hemp for a summery look, add a tassel to the laces, or lace up each sneaker with two laces, each going in a different direction, and tie at each end in a big bow.

time away
ideas for making time pass for small children when you have to be away from them

Tell your three-year-old that you're going away for a week, and you might as well call it a year. Preschoolers don't understand time well. When you have to leave for more than a day or two, try these ideas:

● *Tape small strips of paper, one for each day you'll be away, to the wall next to the child's bed. He or she can remove one each morning and see that the number gets smaller each day, knowing that you will return from your trip the day the last strip is removed.*

● *If you have to be away for several weeks, draw a calendar for a young child. Each day he or she colors in one square and knows you'll be back when the last square is colored. Another variation: In each calendar square, include a small drawing of something special that will happen that day (dinner with an aunt, a visit to a friend's house).*

● *Before you leave, fill a "surprise bag" with small wrapped presents, one to be opened each day. Include goodies like a tiny magnet, new crayons, plastic scissors, a cloth book, an animal-shaped sponge.*

● *Is your child one who just can't get to sleep without a story read by Mommy or Daddy? Some parents tape-record a favorite story or two that a baby sitter can play.*

toys a nonparent's guide to buying toys for other people's children

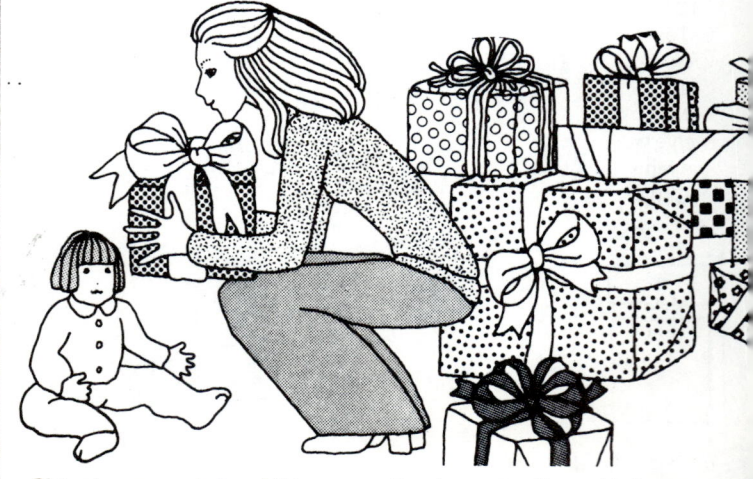

Choosing presents for children can often leave you limp with frustration if you are new to the task and sometimes even if you aren't—and especially if you don't know the child well. So here are some gift-buying ideas for children of ten years and younger. None of them will leave you financially or emotionally impoverished. But first a suggestion—don't try to "educate" the child since everybody else is doing that. FUN is the byword.

Christmas

- For a child less than a year old, anything that is squashy, bright, and squeaky is appealing. Consider socks with tethers, such as bunnies attached to the toes. Bright trapezes with hanging loops and balls designed to extend across cribs are intriguing to young exercisers and pullers. Obviously, avoid sharp-edged toys or anything that can be detached and swallowed.
- One- to three-year-olds are more discriminating as well as more sound-oriented. They usually respond to anything that can be pulled or pushed, provided it makes a noise. This age group also likes surprises like jack-in-the-boxes and toys with hidden parts.
- Three- and four-year-olds like toys that can be taken apart and put back together again, as well as building blocks. Indian headdresses, wigs, or any kind of disguise are also fun. Paste-on decals for the fingernails or body are attractive to the younger of this group. A real treasure is a bag containing his or her very own transparent and colored tapes, note pad, and blunt-tipped scissors.
- If you're gift buying for any child over four, you're dealing with a connoisseur who has not only definite tastes but usually a staggering collection of playthings. Since that age generally wants to be the whole show anyway, give something that will ensure star billing, like a magic-tricks kit or a box of disguises.
- By the time a child is six, he or she has acquired very special treasures. A strong box or any container with a lock and key is worth considering. Plastic or punch-out cardboard villages, forts, farms, etc. appeal to this age group.
- Older children, over eight, are fascinated by superlatives—the tallest man, the deepest river, and so on. An ideal gift would be the *Guinness Book of World Records*, full of super facts for the inquisitive mind.

toys
that are nonsexist, nonracist, and nonviolent

Today a parent can find many toys that are designed to help nip social stereotypes in the bud. A consumer watchdog group called the Public Action Coalition on Toys (PACT) gave awards to the manufacturers of ten such toys, all "safe, nonviolent, nonsexist, and nonracist." The list below will give you an idea of the kind of toys to look for.
- **the ten manufacturers and their toys that received awards from PACT:**
- Teaching Concepts, Inc. for their games, *Space Hop, Super Sandwich,* and *Read Around,* which teach astronomy, nutrition, and language arts.
- Milton Bradley Company for its stand-up figures, *Our Helpers,* twelve male and female workers of various races. Figures include male and female doctors, mail carriers, and even a female "hardhat."
- Childcraft for its *Toys by Antonio Vitali,* superbly crafted wooden puzzles and shapes.
- Bell Records for "Free To Be, You and Me," a recording that celebrates the uniqueness of each child.
- McGraw-Hill Book Company for the book version of "Free To Be, You and Me."
- Instructo for its *Non-Sexist Community Careers Flannel Board Set,* an "equal opportunity" toy showing both sexes in a wide range of occupations.
- Questor Education Products Company for its *Giant Tinkertoy,* a durable toy with a package illustration, that is notably nonsexist and nonracist—with different races and sexes shown.
- Child Guidance for *The Anything Muppet,* an attractive hand puppet.
- Fischer-Price Toys for its *Play Family Sesame Street,* based on the popular TV characters.
- Parker Brothers for its *Con Struct-o-Straws,* a "simple design concept translated into an open-ended play experience."

bow   tie the perfect bow

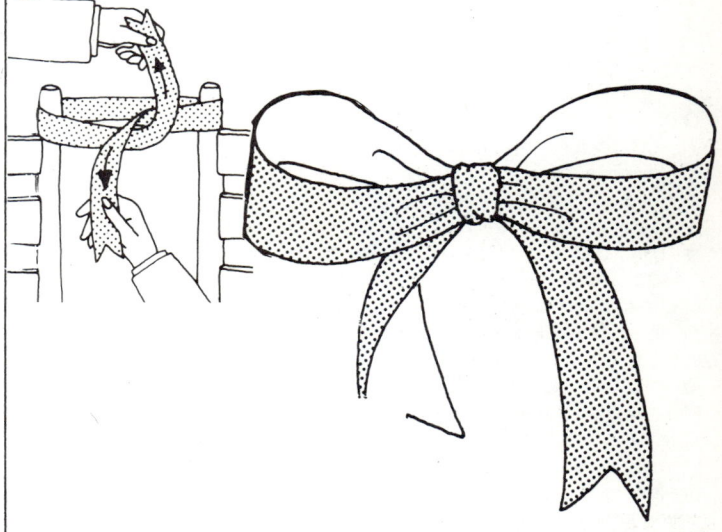

If you're all thumbs when it comes to tying Christmas bows, try this: Have a friend stand facing you with index fingers pointing up, hands as far apart as the size you want the bows to be. Loop the ribbon around his or her fingers, crossing in front, then bring around to the back and knot (see sketch). You can also do this with two ladder-back chairs, placed side by side, or anything else around the house that provides you two polelike objects to wrap around. Fabric bows, made this way, can be used as ornaments for the tree. Make a batch in all colors and patterns and maybe stick a bit of holly in the middle for a really pretty look.

calorie wipeouts
calorie counts of holiday foods

You probably won't be able to resist these tempting and traditional Christmas foods, high calorie count and all. But try giving your figure a break by not overindulging.

	calories
Brandied eggnog (1 cup)	455
Candied yams (6 oz.)	295
Candy cane (1¼ oz.)	138
Cranberry sauce (1 cup)	368
Fruitcake (1 oz.)	115
Gingerbread (2 oz.)	157
Mince pie (1 slice)	365
Mulled wine (1 cup)	345
Peanuts, roasted (1 cup)	840
Plum pudding (4 oz.)	340
Popcorn balls (½ cup)	130
Pumpkin pie (1 slice)	275
Roast goose meat (4 oz.)	265
Roast turkey meat (4 oz.)	215
Stuffing, bread (4 oz.)	236
Walnuts (1 cup)	790

Christmas

dinner 6 steps to help you organize Christmas dinner

Follow these easy, foolproof steps and you'll be a cool, calm, and festive hostess come Christmas day—even if this is your first holiday dinner.

- **suggested menu**

  Turkey with Stuffing
  Cold, Crunchy Green Vegetable
  Sweet Potatoes
  Cranberry Sauce
  Creamed Onions (optional)
  Pie: Apple, Mince, or Pumpkin

- **a week before Christmas**

Order your turkey.

Tips: Order a freshly killed or frozen turkey. Rather than buying a self-basting one, try our recipe for roasting instead; it produces a much juicier bird. If the bird is frozen, defrost it in your refrigerator two to three days before cooking.

- **the week before Christmas**

Make whole cranberry sauce from the recipe on cranberry package or one that you prefer from any basic cookbook. This can be done as much as a week ahead, as the flavor of the sauce improves from standing a few days.

- **the day before Christmas**

Make stuffing, bake pie, and cook green vegetable.

Tips: One easy and very tasty way to dress up stuffing is to use the crumbly type of commercially prepared herb stuffing and add to it a peeled, cored, and chopped baking apple and ¼ cup toasted slivered almonds or ¼ cup raisins. Double or triple these quantities if you use two or three bags of stuffing. Follow package directions for preparing the stuffing and refrigerate until you're ready to use it. *Never* stuff bird until just before cooking; stuffing will become soggy, unappealing, and thus spoil the turkey.

If you plan to bake a pie for dessert, do it now. Pick your recipe from a basic cookbook. You might also consider buying a frozen pie and heating it while guests eat dinner. Other options are buying a frozen crust or a pie-crust mix, then making your own filling.

We suggest serving a cold green vegetable as a crunchy and cool contrast to all the warm food. Broccoli, green beans, asparagus, or snow pea pods are good choices. Steam the vegetables a day ahead, drain, and refrigerate. Frozen vegetables can also be used.

- **early Christmas day**

Clean and prepare turkey for roasting.

Tips: Wash turkey under cold water, using a handful of salt for scouring. Dry bird. Rub with a split garlic clove. Sprinkle with salt and pepper. Massage half a stick of softened butter or 3 T. olive oil well into turkey skin. Stuff cavities loosely. Place breast-up on a rack in a shallow pan. Cover with a tent of heavy aluminum foil. Roast in 350° oven, removing tent for the last half hour. Allow 4 hours for a 4- to 8-lb. bird, 4½ for 8 to 12 lbs. Add a half hour more if stuffing was cold when used. Let turkey "rest" out of oven for a half hour before carving and serving.

- **while the turkey roasts**

Start gravy.

Tips: Boil giblets in salted water to cover until tender. Chop and save giblets and save water. When turkey is done, finish gravy by adding giblets and giblet water to pan drippings. Heat pan with drippings on stove top. To thicken gravy, use cornstarch, not flour, dissolved in a little water. Season to taste.

- **a half hour before you eat—while turkey "rests"**

Prepare sweet potatoes as below and "dress" green vegetable with oil and vinegar. Cook frozen creamed onions.

Tips: To make an easy, sensational sweet potato dish, mash canned sweet potatoes with can juices, ½ stick melted butter, and ¼ cup brown sugar per 17-oz. can of potatoes. Add salt and pepper to taste. Pour mixture into a buttered ovenproof dish and bake uncovered at 425° for a half hour. Serves 4–6.

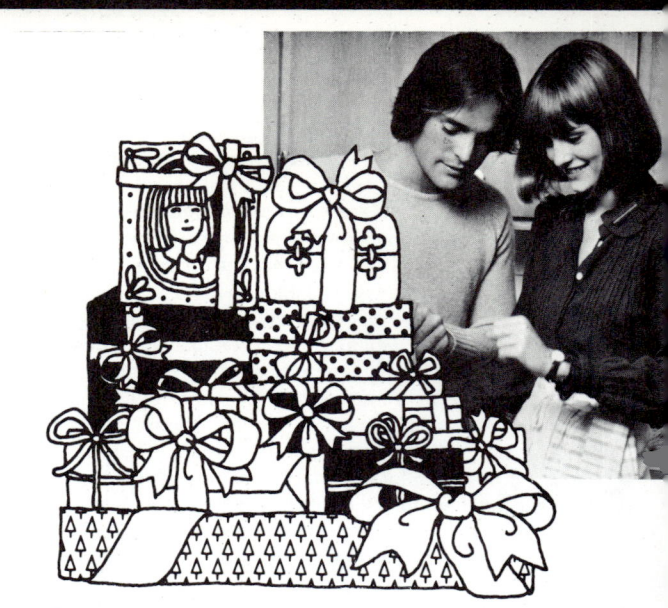

men great gift ideas and where to find them

Is it true, as many people believe, that it is harder to choose gifts for men than it is for women? The answer is yes if your thinking tends to get stuck in the ties-and-belts section of the nearest department store. But not if you can widen your shopping horizons to include a variety of stores or even different departments of the same store. For example:

Drugstores are often underrated as a source of gifts. Don't knock them; where else could you find a "Moustache Grooming Kit" for moustache, beard, or sideburns (with comb and natural-bristle brush)?

Army/Navy stores can outfit an outdoors or indoors man with anything from a canvas backpack to an epauletted Air Force shirt.

Gourmet food stores can yield a windfall of gifts, especially for the man whose cuisine might best be described as "haute can opener." (As long as he's wedded to his can opener, give him something great to open up.) A recent visit to one gourmet food shop turned up hefty cans of authentic French *cassoulet* and *tripes à la mode de caen*, Australian green turtle soup, and Norwegian reindeer meatballs. For less adventurous palates, there are also tins of cream of coconut (for making *piña coladas*); jars of *tartare, béchamel,* and *béarnaise* sauce (for his hamburger or steak); and the ultimate in seductive desserts, crêpes suzette in Grand Marnier.

Toy stores carry gifts for funny bones of all ages. How about a plastic model of Superman, Tarzan, Aquaman, Captain America, or the Amazing Spider-Man for the person on your list who most nearly resembles one of them? Or, for easing exam-week frustrations, offer a spongy, feather-light Nerf Ball.

Hardware stores are more than tool suppliers for the handyman or woman. True, there are jigsaws and dual-action finishing sanders, but there also may be a 99-cent paper chef's hat for his next barbecue.

Thrift shops or flea markets offer an unpredictable array of old and almost-new gifts. Hunt in particular for old campaign buttons (I LIKE IKE, HHH) or hundred-year-old pages from, say, *Harper's Weekly*, ready for framing.

Factory outlet stores may require an out-of-the-way trip, but it's worth it when you can buy things like 14k-gold men's jewelry, Tiffany-type lighting fixtures, and leather vests or ponchos at a 40 to 50 percent discount.

Museum gift shops sell more than calendars and postcards. They're an especially good source of old maps or prints of the city they're located in and decorative art—say, Indian boxwood owls or Ecuadorian carved wood skulls.

Rare or secondhand book, magazine, and print shops have quaint-looking finds for less money than you might expect. If you're hunting for

Christmas

a gift for a doctor or lawyer, check out old medical or legal texts or political cartoons and humorous prints of old English barristers or statesmen. For a man with a special hobby, there are also inexpensive early woodcuts or engravings.

Finally, if you're still stumped, ask him what store he's always wanted a present from—and go buy one.

shopping
at the dime store— more fun than money

You've got a Christmas list a mile long and a shoestring budget to work with. The solution just may be the local dime store. Here are some of the things you'll turn up.

Plants—Dime stores are a great source of inexpensive small plants. An attractive grouping in a decorative container makes a terrific gift. Or for someone who already has many plants, give a Lucite® hanging pot or a couple of macramé hangers, a mister, or a pretty watering can.

Jewelry—Best buys are golden and silvery chains, some of the best-looking with tiny charms hanging from them. There are also leather bracelets, bangles, and more.

Toys—Games, trains, puzzles, dolls, model cars—they're all here. You can even buy a small pool table at some large dime stores.

Fashion accessories—Every woman can use another scarf. You'll find square challis scarves, silky squares and oblongs, crunchy knit mufflers, smooth brushed wool scarves, and fabulous crocheted shawls. Berets, knit caps, and felt brimmed hats are even more terrific ideas, as are brightly colored knee socks. Army-type knapsacks and satchels are other steals.

Gadgets—For the chef's stocking, pick a jar opener, apple corer, egg slicer, vegetable chopper, ketchup squirter, corks, scoops, or a kitchen scale. For the bar, there's an ice crusher, jigger measures, stirrers, and tongs. Or go to the hardware department, where you'll find all the tools and gadgets you need around the house—a screwdriver, a small hammer, files, sandpaper, washers, wrenches, nails, and picture hangers. You might try assembling a small tool chest.

traps holiday tinsel
traps not to fall into

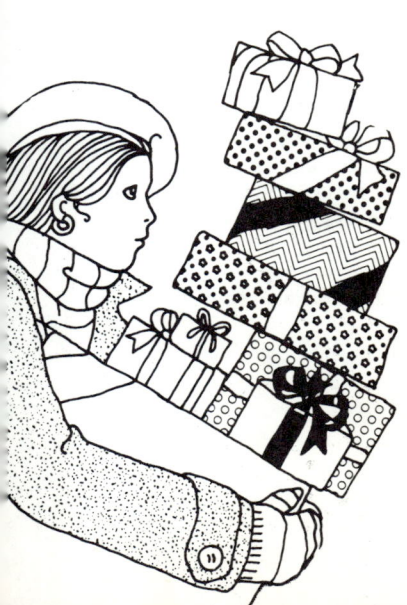

If there's one time to remember that all that glitters is not gold, it's at Christmas—when heaps of tinsel strung over holiday specials and displays can keep you from seeing that what's inside isn't all it's claimed to be.

- Take a careful look at those intriguing displays. Or once you get your purchase home, you might discover that it was really the display, not the gift, that was so eye-catching.
- Check gift "kits" carefully—things like baskets stuffed with boxes of tea or a bunch of wooden kitchen utensils wrapped in ribbon. You might find that if you bought the items separately and assembled them yourself, it would cost less than the kit.
- Read the figures on packages of wrapping paper, ribbon, and decorations. Check footage of rolls of ribbon, tape, and paper. Some rolls of wrapping paper can turn out to be no longer than they are wide. And don't feel you have to trim your tree with one of everything from the decorations display. Think simple—and economical. A string of 15 regular Christmas tree lights uses 105 watts of electricity, but a string of 15 "midget" lights uses only 18 watts.
- Be careful how you handle holiday store money—some department stores offer charge-account customers special holiday coupons with dollar values printed on them. You use them, instead of cash or charge card, for purchases—the benefit being that billing is delayed for several months. Remember that after validation, the coupons are a credit advance and should not be treated like play money. You'll be charged for any coupons that are lost, stolen, or not returned to the store by a certain date. Check other limitations.
- Be wary of unfamiliar charities that come to your door or mailbox, hoping to draw on your seasonal good will. Before making any donations, check via your state's secretary-of-state office to determine whether the organization is registered as a legitimate charity.
- Don't worry about how to deal with unsolicited boxes of Christmas cards or decorations that may arrive at your home—followed shortly thereafter by the bill. You are not required to pay for or return any item that you have not ordered.

tree
tips on buying a tree and keeping it fresh

If you've ever wondered whether a brittle, scraggly Christmas tree was even worth the time you spent decorating it, you may profit from the following reminders from the National Forest Products Association:

- A tree is too dry, and you should look for another one if: its needles break off easily when gently bent; the butt end is dry instead of wet and sticky; or a shower of needles falls off when the butt end is tamped sharply against the ground.
- Once your tree is home, make a diagonal cut in the butt end and put this end in a stand with water covering the top of the cut; then check water level daily. Keep the tree away from heat.
- Try putting 1 tsp. of turpentine in the water the tree stands in. This dissolves resin that can seal off the tree's water-absorbing vascular system. Or buy a commercial product to help keep the tree moist.

tree ornaments
you can make in 2 minutes flat

Make a candy airplane using a peppermint stick about 4" long, a stick of foil-covered chewing gum, 2 Life Savers®, and a 2" rubber band. Thread band through holes of Life Savers®, looping both ends over gum. Slip peppermint stick between Life Savers® and gum, perpendicular to it (see sketch). Put an S-shaped hook through rubber band to hang it on tree.

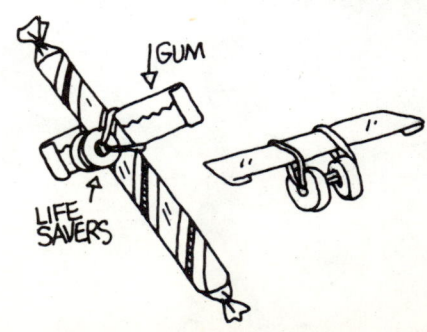

C Christmas

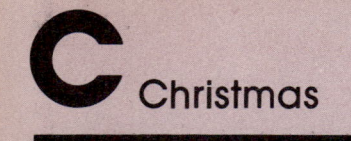

wrap-ups
7 fresh Christmas wrap-ups to make your gifts stand out

1. Try wrapping a gift box in the Sunday comics or a foreign language newspaper—maybe French, Hebrew, or Chinese—preferably one using cheerful headlines. Then spray with an acrylic fixative to keep the newsprint from smudging. Stencil on a bright Christmas greeting, using felt-tipped markers, and add some shiny geometric stickers for accents. Finish with a clear plastic spray if you'd like a glossy look. (If you're using simply an English language newspaper, you might liven it up a little by circling appropriate words or phrases—your name or the recipient's, for example—so that the box contains a message as well as a gift.)
2. Use pink butcher's paper for wrapping; then, instead of real stamps, ribbons, or bows, draw on your own with a felt-tipped marker. Or if you wish, decorate plain paper with small sketches of the person the gift is for and yourself, instead of using a conventional to-from tag.
3. Spruce up a plain brown wrapping paper by crossing it with thick bands of brown satin ribbon covered with other bands of gold-metallic, hole-punched ribbon. Or use ribbon in a vibrant color, such as orange, rich pink, or red.
4. Wrap your package with a remnant of a bright fabric instead of with paper, or maybe use a bandanna scarf. For ties, use shoelaces, yarn, or heavy, braided wool and add a small note tag on a string. If you're a seamstress, you might stitch together a group of bright patterns and checks for a crazy-quilt effect and tie with yarn. Of course, the wrapping would be too good to throw away and can be used again.
5. For the simplest whip-together package, use a shiny, colored box to which you've applied fruit or flower decals. Tie with cotton ribbon you've made from strips of gingham, calico, or another gay pattern and cut with pinking shears.
6. To lend a pop-art or "Early Warhol" effect to a homemade gift box, recycle cardboard or tin containers from common household products like Quaker Oats, Wheaties, coffee, or family-sized Tide. Spray with clear plastic for a high-gloss finish. And if you like, cover less-interesting backs or sides of containers with shiny, colored paper. Trim with solid-colored grosgrain ribbon. Again, these wrap-ups can be used on other occasions or serve as household organizers.
7. Pack posters, calendars, etc. in shiny, pencil-yellow mailing tubes (sold in art supply stores); trim with a barber pole spiral of colored tape. Or cover the tube with paper or cloth to be gathered at both ends with ties, pillow-bolster style.

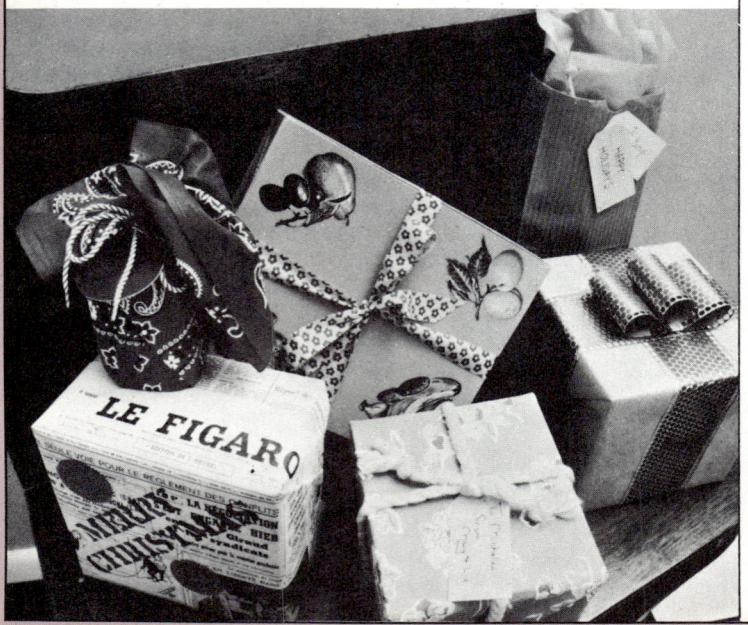

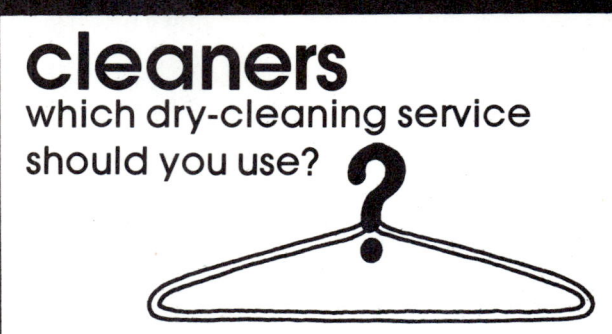

clothes care

cleaners
which dry-cleaning service should you use?

Right in your own neighborhood you've probably noticed more than one type of dry-cleaning shop—what makes one place different from another?

● **the work-done-on-the-premises shop**
The one sure thing this shop can promise is control over how your garments will be treated. When you do business here, the proprietor will be able to explain exactly what he can and cannot do, and he generally supervises most of the work. In the back of the store are the machines that saturate garments with chemical solvents in order to remove dirt; then they purge out the solvents with heat (dry cleaning is not actually a dry process but rather a water-free one). After cleaning comes the "finishing" when your clothes are pressed and steamed.

This type of dry cleaner can usually give your clothes special attention. You can ask to have particular stains treated, buttons replaced, lapels pressed flat, and there's probably same-day service if you want it. Remember that the price will most likely reflect these conveniences.

● **the work-done-off-the-premises shop**
Some dry-cleaning shops are actually just drop-off points, from where your clothes are sent to a central location shared by several stores. The cleaning is basically the same process as previously described, but because the main plant may handle a huge volume of garments every day, there isn't the same control over how your clothes are cleaned and "finished." But if you've found a shop of this kind that does consistently good work, there's no need to change. And you may be getting the job done for less than it would cost at an on-the-premises shop.

● **by-the-pound service**
Many laundromats now offer a dry-cleaning-by-the-pound service. Work is done right in the laundromat, sometimes by self-service. And you can't beat the price—it's usually about $2.50 for 4 lbs.; $4.25 for 8 lbs.—for the same dry-cleaning process used elsewhere. However, these services usually don't offer "finishing" or pressing, and sometimes the machines are overloaded, preventing clothes from coming out as clean as possible. It's ideal for blankets and hard-wear items, though.

Here's how three dry-cleaning shops in the New York City area varied in price:

	on-the-premises	off-the-premises	by-the-pound (rough estimate)
pants	$1.25	$1.10	$ .53
skirt	$1.25	$1.10	$ .53
sweater	$1.25	$1.10	$ .42
dress	$2.50	$2.20	$ .85
coat	$3.50	$3.50	$2.12
blanket	$3.00	$3.50	$2.12

down taking care of your down-filled vest or jacket

That soft, cozy, feather-filled vest or coat that's been keeping you warm all winter will continue to keep you warm for many more winters if you follow a few simple rules provided by the Feather & Down Association.

- Down, or feather-filled, garments shed a few feathers from time to time. When you see feathers protruding through the outer covering, don't pull them out. Instead, push them back into the garment. Pulling them out only enlarges the hole they've pushed through and can cause more feathers to leak out.
- Leave a bit of space on either side of your coat or vest in the closet. If it's bunched too tightly, the down gets packed together and reduces the warmth you get when wearing it.
- If the down does get flattened, you can fluff it by putting your garment—only if it's marked washable—in your dryer on low speed for a few minutes.
- Down can be either washed or dry cleaned, depending on what kind of fabric the down is encased in. Follow the care instructions on the label. If your garment is washable, you can dry it in your dryer. Many manufacturers suggest putting an old sneaker in the dryer along with the down garment. The sneaker "beats" the down and fluffs it. If your coat or vest must be dry cleaned, have it done professionally. The kind and quality of fluid used in some coin-operated machines could injure your garment.

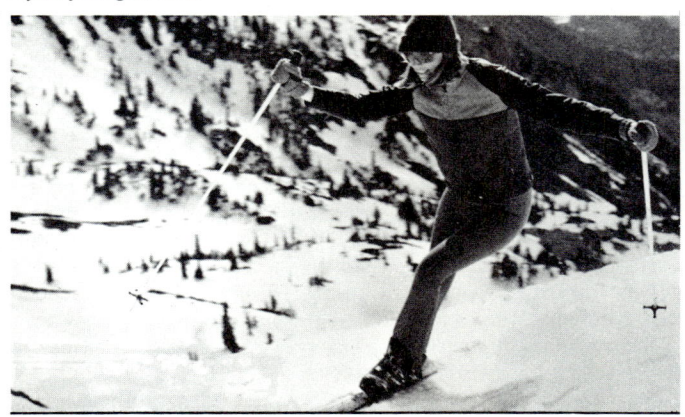

fabrics
can you wash it, iron it, pack it? what to expect from fabrics

Every garment you buy bears a label or hang tag that tells you what it's made of, but that doesn't necessarily inform you how the fiber or combination of fibers will perform when it comes to washing, wrinkling, and so forth. Following is a brief guide to acquaint you with the treatment and behavior of common fibers and fiber combinations.

Cotton knits: Wash in cool water, air dry. Expect some shrinkage, needs some ironing. They pack well.
Woven cottons: Machine wash and dry. Expect a small amount of shrinkage. Needs ironing unless fabric is specially treated.
Polyester* blends (with cotton, nylon, etc.): Machine wash and dry. The higher the percentage of polyester, the less wrinkling. Good travelers, drip-dry candidates.
All polyester*: Machine wash and dry. Little ironing. Drip-dry.
Acrylic* & acrylic blends: Machine wash and dry. Acrylic knits need little if any ironing. Expect to iron acrylic wovens.
Nylon*: Machine wash; dry or drip dry. Little or no ironing. Travels well.
Acetate*: Dry clean only, unless hang tag says hand washable.
Arnel triacetate: Machine wash and dry. If you iron at all, use low temperature. Travels well.
Metallics (Lurex, Mylar, etc.): If hang tag doesn't say washable, dry cleaning is best. Good travelers.
Rayon*: Dry clean only, unless tag says hand washable. Good travelers.
Wool: Follow instructions on the hang tag—lightweight wools and sweaters can be hand washed and laid flat to dry. Other garments might not be completely washable and should be dry cleaned. Good travelers.

*Note: We've listed commonly trademarked names for synthetic fibers so that you can recognize them and know what kind of performance to expect.
Polyester: Dacron, Fortrel, Kodel, Avlin, Spectran, Encron, Trevira.
Acrylic: Acrilan, Orlon, Creslan.
Nylon: Arnel, Antron, Enkalure, Crepeset, Blue C., Formelle, Qiana.
Acetate: Avisco, Estron.
Rayon: Avril, Avron, Fibranne.

college

abroad if you want to study in London, Rome, Tokyo, you probably can, even if you speak only English

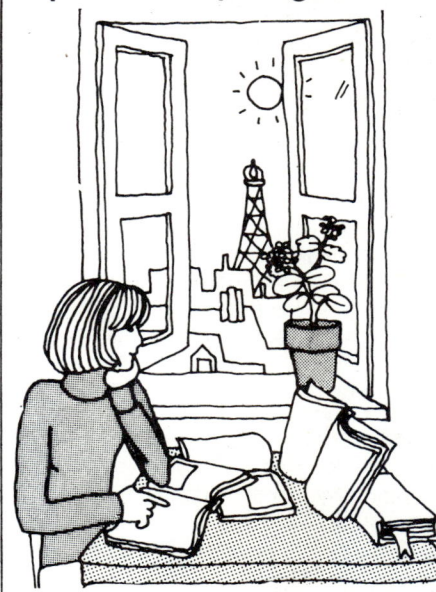

If you're a college student who dreams of studying abroad, it's not too early to start planning for next year's studies on a foreign campus.

The Institute of International Education (IIE) has probably the most helpful study-abroad library and also administers study-abroad grants. It publishes a four-volume, clear and comprehensive "Handbook on International Study for U.S. Nationals" ($6.95 each) and "U.S. College-Sponsored Programs Abroad: Academic Year" ($4.50). So first contact the IIE at 809 U.N. Plaza, New York, NY 10017 for information, or consult a study-abroad program officer on your campus.

With IIE's help, we've come up with some tricks for avoiding red tape. If you're an undergraduate, don't apply directly to a foreign university unless it has an established program for foreigners. First check U.S. college-sponsored programs—and look outside your own school if you're not satisfied with its offerings. Under these programs, credit is virtually assured, you travel and study with other Americans (or internationals), and occasionally you'll study with foreign students on a comparable academic level.

If you speak only English, you don't have to limit yourself to Great Britain. The Experiment in International Living, Brattleboro, VT 05301, offers many independent study programs abroad in English. The University of Stockholm also has an Institute for English-Speaking Stu-

college

dents with undergraduate and graduate social science courses. The American Academy in Rome offers to graduates the classics and fine arts. In Tokyo, the International Christian University has a sprinkling of the liberal arts plus graduate schools in education and public administration. Whatever you're considering, find out in advance whether credits you earn at the school will be accepted by your university.

Don't plan on working your way through school. Many countries restrict rights of foreigners to work for pay, and wage rates are often low. But if you're determined, check with the consulate before leaving.

If you plan to sightsee between exams, you are eligible for numerous discounts if you have an International Student Identity Card ($2.50). For the free "Student Travel Catalog," which has an application for the Identity Card, write to: Council on International Educational Exchange (CIEE), 777 U.N. Plaza, New York, NY 10017.

clothes
what to pack for college

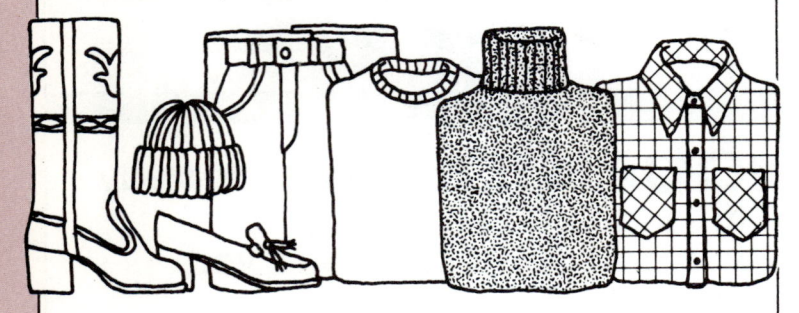

We polled hundreds of college women all across the country to find out what kind of clothes they wore the most and what they needed but forgot to bring along. Here's what we found:

Denims: Anything denim—jeans, skirts, overalls, jumpers, jumpsuits, vests—is the number 1 item everywhere. Jean skirts are very popular, and as for jeans themselves, no matter how many pairs you plan on packing, add another.

Tops: T-shirts and sweaters (all styles) seem to be the most frequently worn tops, with a big bulky sweater high on the list for outdoors. Shirts (flannel, cotton, solids, and plaids) complete this category.

Dresses and skirts: Most college women found they needed only a couple of dresses and relied on skirts (corduroy, wool, denim, cotton) when they wanted a change from wearing pants. If you are headed for an urban campus, however, you may want to include more dresses.

Pants: Besides jeans, a couple of pairs of corduroy or wool pants (or cotton blends in warmer climates) will add a bit of variety.

Coats: Of course, much depends on the particular climate, but down-filled jackets and/or vests seem to be popular everywhere for cold weather. If you have a warm winter coat, however, do bring that. And whatever you do, don't forget a raincoat. Many, many women said that they didn't have one and regretted it. Their recommendation: Pack a classic trench coat that you can use anytime.

Shoes: Boots are a necessity on most campuses. Negative-heel shoes and short boots run a close second. Also bring along sneakers, slippers, a pair of moccasins, and espadrilles or sandals.

Evening wear: A good-sized sampling of women found they needed some type of evening wear, so it might be wise to pack a long skirt or a long dress if you have one.

Accessories: The more scarves you have, the better. Get them in different lengths so you can wear them on your head, at your throat, or around your waist. Jewelry is a matter of personal choice—if you're a jewelry lover, by all means bring it with you. The same applies for hats. Handbag styles depend on individual taste, but canvas knapsack types are practical.

Sleepwear: Bring your favorite nighties (don't worry about the condition they're in—no one will care).

cramming
procrastinator's guide to exam cramming

When exams creep up on you, procrastinating your studies will only add panic to the situation. Chocolate chip pounds start slipping on and you become a victim of the caffeine jitters. Relax. Cramming (once in a while) is a fact of college life. Here are some tips to help you beat the two-tests-and-three-papers-this-week crunch:

● **cramming**
● Don't waste time with excessive underlining of text material. Circle names, dates, etc., in neon-colored inks; put "blaring" yellow boxes around passages the prof mentioned. Bracket key material and indicate extra significance in the margins, using a one-to-five asterisk rating system.
● A common poor reading habit is to skip chapter titles and subtitles. Reading them the night before an exam, however, will tie loose ends and illuminate the "big picture."
● For those books you didn't quite finish (or start), skim for the author's "idea" and skip his "proof" or interpretive detail. You can really bungle an exam if you blur several authors' interpretations into a fog of facts. But if your test shows you know the experts' opinions, it's understood that you have grasped the details (even if you haven't).
● Another trick is to memorize verbatim a couple of quotations from each book and work them into the exam.

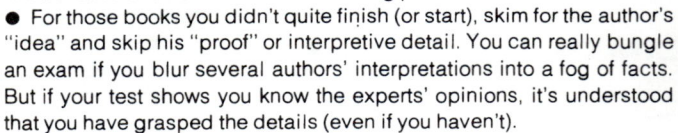

● **physical survival**
You've also got to survive the cramming ordeal physically (so you're not too wiped out to take the exam). Experienced "all nighters" know . . .
● Munching cookies and sipping colas between the lines will not energize you; relaxing during a regular mealtime will.
● It's a good idea to vary your study spots. It's going to be a long stretch, and boredom with the same four walls will make you feel even more tired.
● You should make sure your study area is cool, well-lighted, large enough to allow organization, and far enough away from your latest love interest to avoid distraction. Team studying works only if you handpick your company and don't waste time trying to impress anyone with your flirtatious lack of facts.
● Your most valuable lesson now may be knowing how to get a few hours of really deep sleep. Take your temperature every four hours for a few days to find out when it's at its 24-hour-low—that's the time to grab your deepest, most restorative "nap" during a study marathon. For most people who are night sleepers, this period usually falls in the wee hours of the morning. Also try setting your alarm for a three-hour nap. Sleep cycles repeat every 90 minutes, according to *How to Avoid Insomnia* by Gay Gaer Luce and Dr. Julius Segal, so three hours usually ensures a natural wake-up—you'll feel better if you don't have to stop the alarm in the middle of a dream.
● If you can bear some motherly advice, don't push yourself too hard. Going two or three days without sleep puts you into a "drunken" state (without the party).

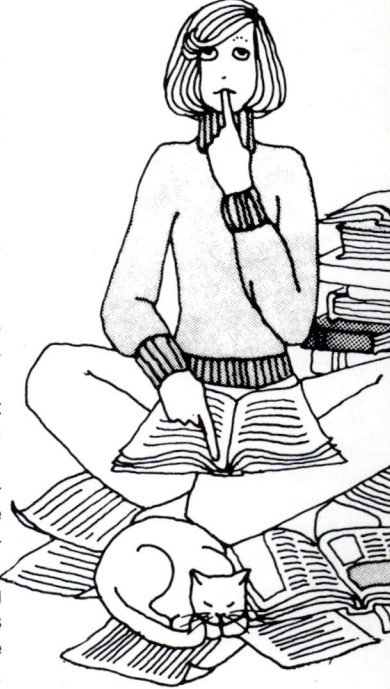

college

- A cool astringent face cleanser and ten-minute facial mask are quick refreshers during these brain-racking, eye-bagging days and nights.
- To relieve headaches and eyestrain, gently massage your forehead, temples, and the area around your eyes, using a light circular motion. Or apply pressure for one minute to two points between your eyebrows just above your nose; your head will feel marvelously cleared and light. Don't work under one small bright light while your roommate sleeps in an otherwise dark room; an evenly lighted room will reduce eyestrain. Unshaded light sources in the field of vision are also taboo.

diet
how to eat right and stay fit on cafeteria food

- Maintaining a well-balanced diet and avoiding fattening snacks is the best way to ensure good health and keep your weight down, says Miriam Katz, Assistant Director of Nutrition at New York University Medical Center.
- If you don't have the time or ambition to get up for breakfast, keep some nutritious food on hand—cans of fruit or vegetable juice, all-bran or granola cereals, yogurt, bran or corn muffins—so you don't go to class with an empty stomach.
- Get a copy of the cafeteria's weekly menu from your service office and preselect what you're going to eat so that you won't be tempted by junk food when you're going through the line.
- Work out a regular eating pattern that suits you and your schedule. Try not to skip meals. Snacking is fine as long as it doesn't become a substitute for regular meals.
- Avoid vending-machine snacks as much as possible; it's better to munch on fresh or dried fruit. You may want to rent a refrigerator (cost: about $5.50 per month) so that you can keep a wider variety of healthy snacks and breakfast foods on hand.
- Whenever possible, eat fresh fruit and vegetables instead of cooked ones, which lose many of their vitamins through overcooking or warming.

essentials
18 lifesavers to take to college

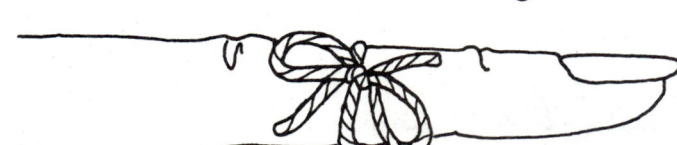

Check out our list of little things that make a big difference in campus survival.
- A calculator can help you pass that required statistics course or keep your first checkbook in order.
- An alarm clock.
- A pocket dictionary for in-class reference and a thesaurus to help you find just the right words to express yourself.
- A small jar or change purse well supplied with dimes, nickles, and quarters for phone calls and washing machines.
- A bottle of cold-water detergent for washing sweaters and underwear.
- An extension cord and a small lamp to dispel the "overhead depression" of many dorm rooms.
- One well-loved poster or picture to make the first days livable.
- A pack of cards or a board game.
- At least one plant so you know there's one other friendly living thing in your room.
- A small throw rug for "bedside feet."
- A small drying rack for hand washables.
- A small sewing kit full of emergency supplies.
- Electric curlers, curling iron, or blow dryer, and a small immersion heater for making tea or soup in your room.
- Two settings of inexpensive flatware, a can opener, and corkscrew.
- A camera to make a photo record of your experiences.
- Your favorite pillow from home.
- A child's pail from the dime store, to be used to transport toiletries from your room to the shower.
- A diary or notebook to serve as a friendly, dependable confidant through it all.

going back
if you left college and want to go back, here are areas to investigate

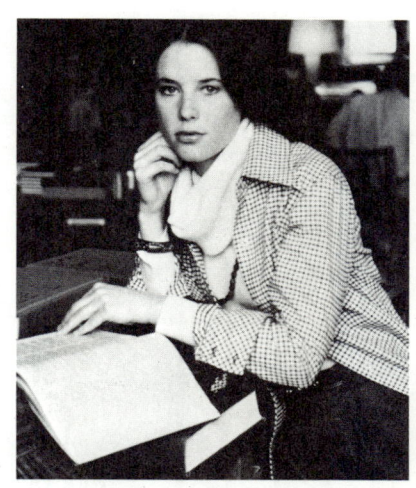

- Going back to college after you've been away for several years takes some planning. First you should seek advice from a counseling service at the college you want to attend or at another school in your area.
- Also investigate the possibility of entering a special program for adult women, if one exists at your college. It might be the better choice from both a financial and academic point of view.
- Some schools will let you take courses as a non-matriculated student before you are formally admitted. Consider taking one or two courses next semester to ease yourself back into the academic routine.
- If finances are a problem, investigate the feasibility of a bank or government loan, scholarship, fellowship, or work-study plan with the financial-aid office of the college you're thinking of attending.
- Find out if your prospective college will give credit for the College Level Examination Program (CLEP). This system affords you academic credit for your knowledge of college-level material, even though you may never have taken a formal course in the subject. For information, send a stamped, self-addressed, business-sized envelope to College Level Examination Program, Box 1824, Princeton, NJ 08540.
- You might be interested in sending for "General Information for the Returning Student," Catalyst Publications, Box G, 14 East 60 St., New York, NY 10022 (90¢, check or money order).

health
6 health mistakes not to make on campus

The bad habits regarding health that students develop are more likely to be those of omission rather than commission. It's the things you *don't* do that are more likely to make your body rebel.
1. Don't skip real meals and become a victim of "snack malnutrition." Many students fall into the trap of surviving on snacks—a soda and cheese and crackers from a vending machine or a sweet roll and coffee. If you can't avoid snacking, supply yourself with high-nutrition, low-calorie snack bars or instant-meal drinks. Buy a reputable book on

C college

nutrition and calories to help you restructure your eating habits.

2. Don't fail to recognize stress as a big college health problem. College has its own built-in stresses—exams, grades, and new social situations. This stress often manifests itself physically in headaches, stomach upsets, and fatigue. The recognition that stress is provoking the symptoms can make them less frightening.

3. Don't ignore a recurrent physical symptom. Although stress may be at the root of a great many physical complaints, if you frequently have headaches, frequently suffer from stomach upsets, or you always seem to be tired, see your doctor.

4. Don't let fear keep you from getting help if you think you've caught VD. Help is a toll-free phone call away—800-523-1885, seven days a week between 9 A.M. and 9 P.M. (Eastern time). Pennsylvania residents can call 800-462-4966. You'll reach Operation Venus, which gives free advice and clinic referrals for treatment in your area. Your call and any treatment will be kept confidential.

5. Young women account for the greatest increase in cigarette smoking in this country, and women are beginning to figure more prominently in heart attack statistics, so think before you start to smoke. Once you're hooked, it's very hard to stop. New evidence indicates that while filter-tipped cigarettes may decrease your cancer risks, they may increase your heart problems.

6. Should you contract mononucleosis, don't assume the whole semester or even the whole year is lost. The anxiety of students when they learn they have "mono" more often causes the need for prolonged bed rest than the disease itself. See a doctor if you have the classic symptoms of sore throat, severe headache, swollen glands, and fatigue, and above all, keep calm.

notes
the art of taking good notes

Efficient notetaking is a skill you can use throughout your life in any learning experience. Here are some ideas to help you take more concise, effective notes:
- Don't write too much. Professionals say you should spend about 80 percent of your time listening and only 20 percent writing.
- Record your notes in simplified outline form. Write key points in the margin, followed by a sentence or two of explanation. Indent minor points and ideas further in.
- Invent your own shorthand system for taking notes. For example, use W for "with"; TH for "the, these, those, them," etc.; a dot after a word to represent its ING form. Here are some useful symbols for common words from the School of Speedwriting textbook: is = $\wedge$; for = f ; are, our = π ; would = d ; have, very, of = v ; why = y ; was, as = z ; can = c ; to, it = i ; in, not = n ; will, well = l.
- Don't overlook the speaker's anecdotes and illustrations. Writing down a brief phrase about the story may jog your memory and bring back useful fact associations.
- Employ the 5 Rs of notetaking: *Record*. *Reduce* the main ideas or facts to a few key terms. *Recite* the meeting or lecture mentally while it's still fresh. Fill in any points you may have missed in class. *Reflect* over concepts and thoughts on your own while reviewing. *Review* periodically, especially notes from a class that meets only once or twice a month.

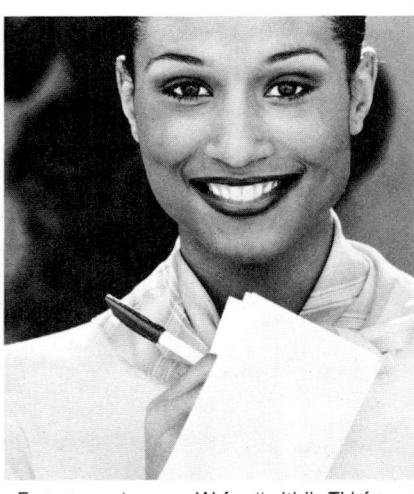

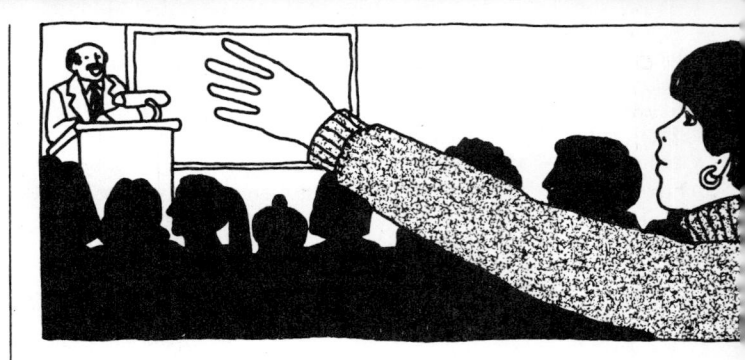

questions
how to ask good questions in class

Here are tips on how to ask questions from Professor Richard Brown, who teaches large lecture classes at The New School in New York City.
- *Edit your question mentally before you ask it and/or jot down a few key words to help you phrase the question as you go along. Make your questions simple and to the point.*
- *Don't ask a question that is only vaguely related to what's being taught or discussed unless you think that the answer will be interesting or worthwhile to the entire class.*
- *Eliminate verbal gingerbread in your questions, including big words and unnecessary lead-ins, such as, "Yes, I just wanted to ask you a question about...."*
- *Project your voice so that the professor doesn't have to repeat your question for the rest of the class.*
- *Never hesitate to ask a professor to explain a point; if you've done the reading and have been listening, you're probably not the only one who's missing what he or she is saying.*
- *Time your clarification questions so that they don't interrupt the rhythm of the class.*
- *Don't ask a question just to impress the professor or other students with your knowledge about the subject, but don't start a question by apologizing for asking it.*
- *Don't hesitate to take issue with your professor's opinion, but word your challenge in a tactful rather than hostile way or you'll end up alienating both the professor and the class.*

tests how to pass multiple-choice tests when you don't know the answers

How much do you have to know to pass multiple-choice tests? Less than you might expect, says Stuart Hoffman, a researcher in testing and education and a former math teacher. He says you can psych out any multiple-choice test by means of a few common sense rules and the knowledge that the test was devised, in most cases, by a human. Here are Mr. Hoffman's rules:

Remember that the teacher who constructs the test has a few principles he generally works from. One is that he tries to bury the correct answer among the alternate choice distractors. The first rule then is: The correct answer tends to be the third choice if there are five alternatives and second or third choice if there are four alternatives. One student claims he got through college by answering "C" to every question on "multiple guess tests."

An alternative that is much longer or shorter than the others tends to be the correct answer. Often the teacher will make an answer very long to include all possible exceptions, as, for example, "C" in: *America was discovered by: A) the Canadians, B) the Irish, C) either an Italian sailing for Spain or the Vikings, D) the Ukrainians, E) the Chinese.*

On the other hand, the teacher may leave out just one word from the lead-in sentence and make that word the correct alternative, as "C" in: *Biology is the study of: A) plants and chemicals and falling bodies, B) cells and protoplasm, C) life, D) numbers and their geometric applicabilities, E) the heavens and earth.*

When the stem and alternative do not make grammatical sense, that choice is wrong. Only "C" completes a grammatically correct sentence in: *The opposite of an optimist is a: A) optimetrist, B) reactionaries, C) pessimist, D) fatalists, E) altruist.*

Alternatives that use the words *All, Always, None,* or *Never* tend to be wrong, but alternatives that include the words *Most* or *Some* tend to be correct. The reason: Very few things in life happen *never* or *always.*

Look for clues in other questions. One question might read, *Who invented the cotton gin?* Three questions later there might be the phrase, "Whitney's cotton gin...."

If two alternatives are exactly the same except for one word, one of them is usually the correct answer. The answer is "C" in the question: *Supplementary angles are: A) 2 angles that are opposite each other, B) 2 angles that are formed by a transversal cutting parallel lines, C) 2 angles adding up to 180 degrees, D) 2 angles adding up to 90 degrees.*

"None of the above" is usually a wrong answer. The teacher may use that phrase as an alternative simply for lack of a better choice.

If you are sure that two given alternatives are correct and another is "All of the above," that is usually the correct answer.

Find out before a multiple-choice test if it is worthwhile to guess. If the teacher says there is no penalty for guessing, answer every question. If a penalty will be in effect, however, guess only when you can eliminate a few choices as being obviously wrong.

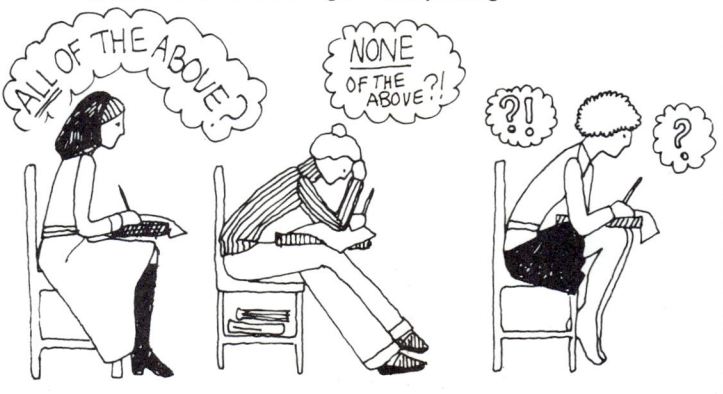

complaints

hotline toll-free consumer hotline on product safety

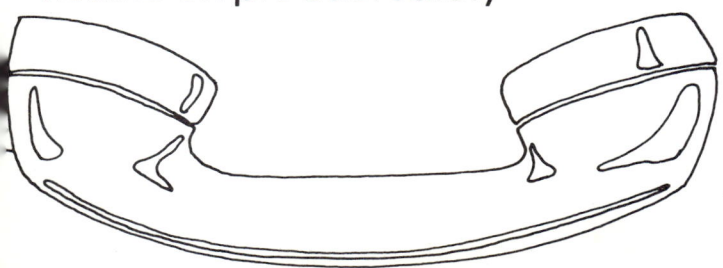

If you've recently bought a new consumer product that you think is unsafe, officials at the U.S. Consumer Product Safety Commission want to know about it—and have set up a toll-free hotline to assist you. Residents of all states except Alaska, Hawaii, and Maryland may call 800-638-2666 (Maryland residents may call 800-492-2937) any time, twenty-four hours a day, seven days a week, to complain about the safety of any product except food, drugs, medical devices, cosmetics, pesticides, cars, boats, planes, firearms, tobacco, or alcohol. The Commission will use complaints to evaluate safety standards for categories of products. It will also send, on request, free information about a wide variety of consumer products to anyone who calls the toll-free number. For example, the Commission offers free leaflets on the safety of cribs, toys, TV sets, kitchen ranges, bicycles, bathtubs and shower stalls, and a variety of other items.

where to complain when you don't get what you've paid for

How do you get action on your complaint when, for example, a department store fails to deliver merchandise you mail-ordered months ago? Obviously, you should complain first to the store or company that is responsible. Next, you should take your complaint to a reliable third party, such as your local Better Business Bureau, city or state consumer-action agency, or newspaper or TV "action line." But what if you still can't get action—or simply feel that the problem should be brought to a higher authority's attention? Then you may want to write to an industry agency capable of pressuring its own members into action. Check the list below for the products or services you want to protest (or praise!), then write to the appropriate group, sending a copy of your letter to the store or company involved.

● **airlines**
Send complaints about regularly scheduled domestic airlines to: Office of the Consumer Advocate, Civil Aeronautics Board, 1825 Connecticut Ave. N.W., Washington, DC 20428.

● **appliances**
The Major Appliance Consumer Action Panel listens to—and usually resolves—complaints about major home appliances (like dishwashers and refrigerators). Write to: MACAP, 20 North Wacker Dr., Chicago, IL 60606. Or call (toll free) 800-621-0477. Illinois residents can call (collect) 312-236-3223.

● **automobiles**
When your car turns out to be a lemon or when you have trouble with your dealer, ask your city or state Automobile Dealers Association about the AUTOCAP (Automotive Consumer Action Program) nearest you. If there isn't one in your area, contact the National Automobile Dealers Association, Consumer Relations Office, 8400 Westpark Drive, McLean, VA 22101.

● **book clubs, record clubs, subscriptions, and other mail-ordered items**
If you have a problem regarding a mail-ordered item, write to: Direct Mail Marketing Association, 6 East 43 St., New York, NY 10017.

● **cleaners**
There are about two dozen state and regional cleaners associations that often serve as middlemen in disputes between service shops and patrons. For example, the Neighborhood Cleaners Association conducts lab tests on ruined garments to determine what caused the damage. New York, New Jersey, Connecticut, Pennsylvania, and Delaware residents *only* can write to: Neighborhood Cleaners Association, 116 East 27 St., New York, NY 10016. Check your phonebook for other cleaning associations.

● **furniture**
If both the store and manufacturer ignore your complaints about, say, a new sofa with a warped frame, you can write to the Furniture Industry Consumer Advisory Panel, P.O. Box 951, High Point, NC 27261.

complaints

- **hotels and motels**

If a hotel or motel has thrown a damper on your holiday, find out if it is a member of the American Hotel and Motel Association, 888 Seventh Ave., New York, NY 10019. If it is, the association can refer you to a state branch that may be able to help resolve your complaint. Or you can always register your complaint with the local chamber of commerce or visitors bureau.

- **railroads**

Wish you'd flown home on your last trip? Complain to the individual railroad and to Amtrak, the national railroad passenger corporation. Write to: Adequacy of Service Bureau, Amtrak, 955 L'Enfant Plaza S.W., Washington, DC 20024.

- **restaurants**

Send your complaint to: National Restaurant Association, One IBM Plaza, Suite 2600, Chicago, IL 60611. Also advise your state or city restaurant association and the appropriate agency, such as the health department.

conversation

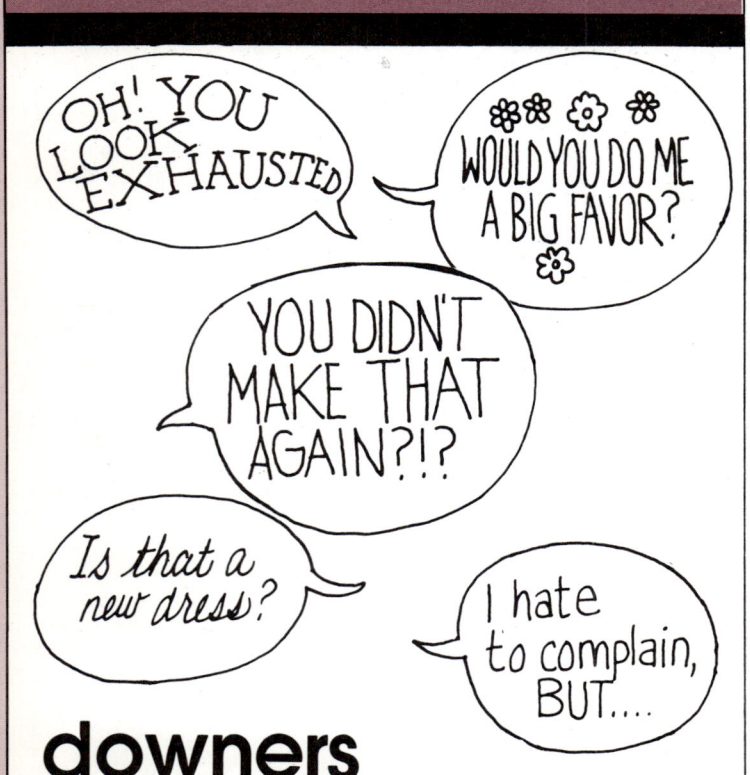

downers
how not to start a conversation

If you ever have the feeling no one wants to hear what you want to say, maybe it's not *what* you're saying, but *how* you're saying it that's the problem. The conversational openers that follow are turn-offs, because they're insincere or ambiguous, they lack directness, or they are downright annoying. Decide right now not to start another conversation this way and you'll attract a fascinated audience.

Shows of "concern"—"Oh, you look absolutely exhausted!" or "You look like you've been working too hard." (If either of these is the case, you're just adding insult to injury by pointing it out.)

Compliments?—"You've lost so much weight!" (This translates to, "Wow, were you fat!") "Oh, you got your hair cut!" (Well, do you like it or don't you, and why not say you like it or just not mention it?) "Is that a new dress?" (Saying "I like your new dress" or "I like your dress" is much more direct.)

Questions put in a negative way—All of these fall into the annoying category: "This isn't your little girl, is it?" "You're not the guest of honor here?" "You didn't make that dessert again?"

Telephone openers like . . . "I've been meaning to call you." "I really don't have time to talk, but . . ." (This kind of introduction puts your listener in a less than enthusiastic frame of mind.)

Pussyfooting—"Promise me you won't get mad when I tell you this . . ." (Say this and it's a sure thing she will get mad.) "This probably isn't a good time to ask, but . . ." (Then why ask?) "Are you in a good mood?" (She was until you asked!)

Questions that don't wait for an answer—"Hi, how are you? Now, what I need is . . ." (You don't want conversation here, you want to talk *at* someone.)

Cornering tactics—"Would you do me a big favor?" "You're the only person in the world who can do this." "Sweetheart, you want to do something for me?" (You've never called him "Sweetheart" before!)

Slow starts—"I hate to be a drag, but . . ." "I hate to complain, but . . ." "You're not going to like this, but . . ."

Self-deprecation—"I'm no expert, but . . ." "You may not be interested, but . . ." "This may not be what you're looking for, but . . ."

Real killers—"You're a nice guy, but . . ."

The ultimate bad start—"I hope I'm not interrupting anything."

starters
23 questions that will start a conversation when all others fail

Conversational dead ends can threaten almost any date or party, and even the most self-assured hostess may fumble in the clutch. There are, however, several ways to prevent such situations from arising, or to nip them in the bud when they do. One is simply to introduce the hottest item currently in the national, local, or campus news. You might ask your guests how they feel about the recent local or campus crime wave; does it make them feel any less at ease about going out at night? Another good way to fire a conversation is to first rethink the kinds of questions you ask. Instead of relying on the simple "yes" or "no" questions, you might try to ask more open-ended ones: "What kind of music do you like best?" rather than "Do you like the Stones?" and "What is the most enjoyable part of your job?" rather than "Do you like being a product manager?" You might also try to ask slightly more imaginative questions, such as any of those given below.

We can't tell you when to use which question—you'll have to decide that on the basis of the discussion at hand and your relationship with the person or group—but most likely none will earn a dull or one-word reply.

One caution, however: Relate to your friends, don't interview. If you ask questions, you should care about their answers—and be prepared to give your own.

- **on his or her job**

1. What are the most and least rewarding parts of your job?
2. What would you like to do if you could change professions?
3. If you could trade jobs with anyone in the world, who would it be and why?
4. What was your first job, and how did it influence your present career?
5. What would you like to be doing in five years? In twenty?

- **on movies and TV**

6. Do you think American movie and TV audiences get a "kick" from violence?
7. If not, why do you think violence in movies and on TV is so popular?
8. What are your all-time favorite movies and TV programs—or commercials?
9. Do newscasters give the public the whole story? How accurately do programs like "All in the Family" portray American families?

cooking

• on marriage and families
10. Who had more influence on you, your mother or your father?
11. Does marriage mean the same to you as it does to your parents?
12. Is fidelity obsolete?
13. Did you become who you are because of your parents or in spite of them?

• on life in general
14. Do you or did you ever have a "hero" or "heroine"? Who?
15. If not, why don't people seem to have heroes or heroines anymore?
16. What do you read and why?
17. What achievement in your life are you most proud of?
18. Did you have a favorite age or year?
19. If you could have lived in another era, what would it have been?

• ask at your own risk . . .
20. When was the last time you cried? Laughed till you cried? Got really angry?
21. When you can't sleep, what do you think about?
22. What was your favorite dream?
23. What would you like your epitaph to say?

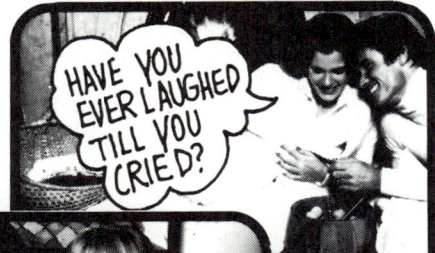

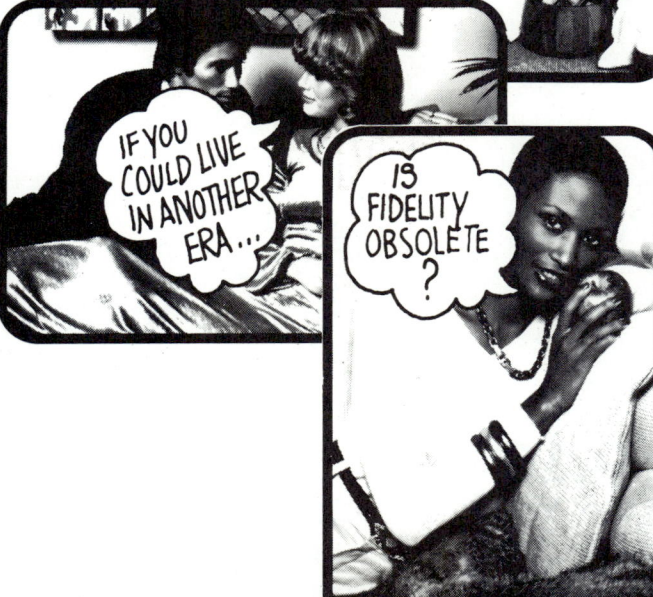

cooking

at his place
whip up a meal in his kitchen

After you and a friend spend the day bicycling in the country, whip up these delicious dishes for the two of you when you get home—in less than an hour. You can even make them at his place, where utensils may run to one bowl, two pans, and a can opener.

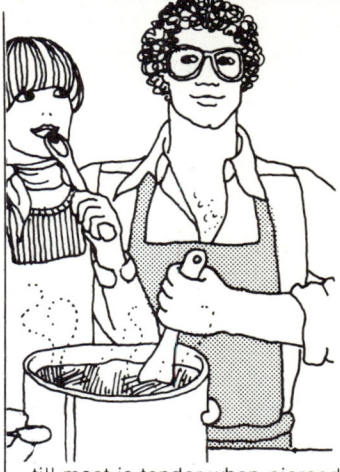

• chicken in beer
2 lbs. chicken legs, thighs, and breasts
Salt, pepper to taste
3 T. oil
7–8 small white onions, peeled
1 clove garlic, minced (optional)
1 3-oz. can sliced mushrooms, drained
½ c. tomato sauce
Pinch of sugar
¾ c. (½ can) beer
¼–½ c. heavy cream

Season chicken pieces with salt, pepper. Heat oil in a large skillet or wide saucepan and brown chicken on one side about 5 mins. Turn, add onions, and brown 5 mins. more. Stir in garlic, mushrooms, tomato sauce, sugar, beer. Cover and simmer 30 mins. (turn chicken after 15 mins.), or till meat is tender when pierced with a fork. Blend cream into sauce. Serve with rice tossed with grated Parmesan cheese and butter.

Or, if you're in the mood for hamburgers, try these with a special salad and dessert.

• Roquefort or bleu cheese burgers
2 T. (about 2 oz.) Roquefort or bleu cheese
2 tsp. butter
1 tsp. Worcestershire sauce (optional)
¾–1 lb. ground round or chuck beef
Salt, pepper to taste

Mix cheese, butter, and Worcestershire and, using a spoon, form into two balls. Chill. Season beef with salt and pepper and make four patties. Sandwich each cheese ball between two patties, pinch edges together to seal, then broil (or sauté in greased skillet) 3 to 5 mins. on each side.

• quick artichoke heart salad
1 small head of Boston or other lettuce, rinsed, dried, and chilled
1 6-oz. jar marinated artichoke hearts, chilled
1 tsp. lemon juice

Tear lettuce into bite-sized pieces. To serve, toss with artichoke marinade and lemon juice, and top with artichoke hearts.

• hot chocolate-nut sundae
3-oz. bar of milk chocolate with almonds
¾ c. heavy cream

Melt chocolate in a small pan set in a skillet of simmering water (or in top of a double boiler if you have one). Beat in cream until blended. Serve hot over coffee (or another flavor) ice cream.

beef sauce
a great one that can make any amateur cook look like a pro

If you were on the inside track of a reputable French restaurant, you'd discover that the "sauce chef" often has the most important job in the kitchen. So take your cue from this and work on a couple of impressive sauces—maybe the one below for beef and another for fish—and become an instant gourmet cook.

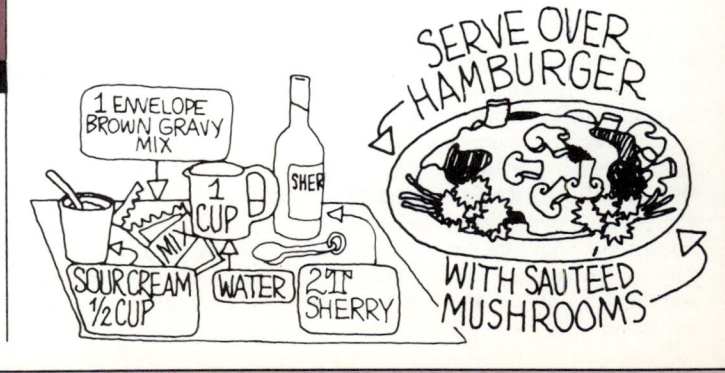

cooking

● easy brown sauce with sour cream and sherry

1 envelope prepared brown gravy mix
1 c. water
½ c. sour cream
2 T. sherry, or to taste

Mix the powdered gravy mix with water, and heat according to package directions. When sauce is bubbly and thickened, add sour cream and stir to mix. Add sherry and stir again. Makes about 1½ c. sauce.

Serve sauce over ordinary hamburger with sautéed mushrooms, over sliced flank steak, or London broil. You can make "instant stroganoff" by thin-slicing and sautéing any tender cut of beef, adding sliced, sautéed mushrooms and chopped sautéed onions, then pouring sauce over it all and simmering for a few minutes.

Try adding a teaspoon of dried, minced dill to the sauce and serving it with tiny cooked meatballs. Let sauce and meatballs simmer together for a few minutes to develop the flavor.

coffee how to brew the ultimate cup of coffee

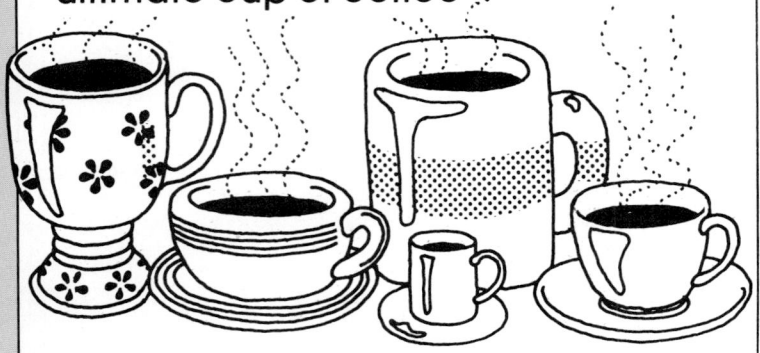

Coffee drinkers seem to fall into two basic groups. The first is the kind who'll drink any kind of coffee, instant or otherwise. The second is the kind who is always searching for a new way to brew *the* ultimate cup—and it's for this group (or the just curious) that we offer the following tips.

● making the perfect cup of coffee

A drip or filter pot is preferred by most experts. You use boiled water cooled a moment, then poured over coffee grounds in a paper or other type of filter. Water passes over grounds just once, so coffee isn't "over-extracted" and bitter. The filter removes grounds, oils, and waxes to yield a clear, smooth brew. Vacuum and plunger pots are also advisable.

Whatever the pot, your best formula for a serving of regular-strength coffee is 1 approved coffee measure (2 level T.) of ground coffee to 6 oz. (¾ c.) water. For extra mildness, add boiling water to the pot after brewing (cutting down on coffee before brewing makes the drink bitter, not mild). For stronger demitasse, use only 4 oz. (½ c.) water.

Choose top-quality fresh coffee. If you have a local gourmet coffee or food shop, try buying beans and grinding them yourself. No one coffee has the "best" of everything—aroma, body, "winey" or tangy taste, or strong, acidy flavor. So experiment with blends to concoct your favorite.

Use cold tap water, because hot water pipes release minerals that affect coffee taste. Try bottled water if tap water in your area has an unpleasant taste or odor. Avoid using artificially softened water that contains extra sodium (that too affects taste).

Don't reheat coffee or it will turn bitter. You can keep it warm by placing the pot over your stove's pilot light or in a pan of hot water.

● roasting and grinding coffee beans

Whatever brand of coffee beans you buy, taste will vary according to "roast"; the longer the beans were roasted, the darker and stronger they are. An American roast is mildest, then come Viennese, French, and finally, the strongest, Italian roast. Here, too, you might experiment with blends.

Different coffee makers are suited for either coarse, medium, or extra-fine grounds. Check pot instructions or follow this general rule: Grind 6 seconds for coarse grounds to be used in percolators and Chemex drips; 10 seconds for most other drips and filters; 15 seconds for vacuum pots; 30 seconds for a Melitta; and 60 seconds for powdery Turkish coffee. Your blender can be used on coarser grounds, but a special coffee grinder is advisable for anything finer.

● some coffee favorites and how to make them

● *Espresso*—Authentic espresso requires special equipment. If you don't have it, you can make a simple substitute by using Italian roast in demitasse proportions.
● *French*—Use French roast coffee alone. Or add 1 part chicory root to 7 parts coffee.
● *Café au lait*—Mix equal amounts of strong demitasse with scalded milk. For home-style cappuccino, sprinkle cinnamon on top.
● *Mocha*—For each serving, brew a mixture of 1 T. coffee and 1 T. instant chocolate.
● *Viennese*—Strong black coffee with dollops of whipped cream on top.

Another tasty combination is a strong demitasse laced with your favorite liqueur. Some possibilities are Vandermint, anisette, crème de menthe, or Kahlúa.

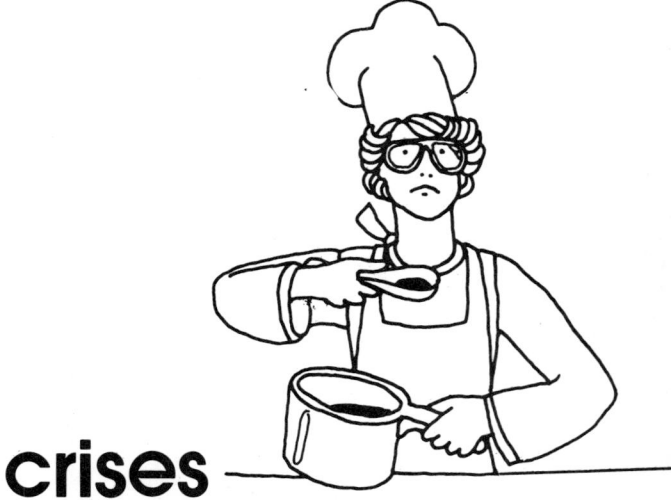

crises
what to do if the cake falls, the vegetables burn, the gravy gets lumpy — and other last-minute cooking crises

Following is a rundown of the most common kitchen crises and the quickest ways to deal with them. Most of the ideas have been adapted from *How To Be A Really Good Cook* by Dilys Wells.

● *Problem:* A cake that collapsed in the middle
● *Solution:* Fill the center with drained canned fruit and trim the edges with swirls of whipped cream.
● *Problem:* Scorched vegetables
● *Solution:* Disguise the burned taste by adding a tangy-flavored ingredient—barbecue sauce or curry powder. Or, transfer the vegetables from the scorched pan into a clean one and place a small metal cap (such as a ketchup bottle cap) filled with salt on top of the food. Cover and let sit a few minutes.

If the food isn't burned too badly, set the pan in a bigger pan of cold water till the steam escapes. The burned taste should escape with the steam.

● *Problem:* Underdone meat
● *Solution:* Slice the meat, place in a roasting pan, and cook in a hot oven (425° F.) for 10 mins. or under the broiler for 5 mins.
● *Problem:* Flavorless soup or gravy

cooking

- *Solution:* Add wine, tomato paste, mustard, or lemon juice to taste.
- *Problem:* Lumpy gravy or sauce
- *Solution:* Pour it through a fine strainer or liquidize it in a blender. Then reheat in a clean pan, preferably a double boiler, stirring constantly.
- *Problem:* Too much salt
- *Solution:* For an over-salted gravy, sauce, or soup, sprinkle in a small amount of instant mashed potatoes and stir thoroughly. Or, if you have cold mashed potatoes on hand, beat them right into the food.

  For over-salted vegetables, add a bit of lemon juice, cream, or sugar.
- *Problem:* Ruined icing for a cake
- *Solution:* Make a hot sauce from preserves. Put preserves through a sieve, thin down with a few teaspoons of orange or lemon juice, and heat gently. Pour over cake and serve immediately. Or smooth warmed honey over cake and top with chopped nuts, raisins, glacé fruits, or sprinkles.
- *Problem:* A disastrous dessert
- *Solution:* Serve ice cream with fruit preserves or a liqueur (e. g., vanilla ice cream with crème de menthe). Or substitute after-dinner liqueurs in place of dessert.

dessert a delicious one that won't shoot your diet

This cheese dessert is delicious, simple to make, and relatively easy on your diet. The main ingredients are cottage cheese and those ethereal Italian almond cookies called *amaretti*, which come wrapped two together in brightly colored tissue paper.

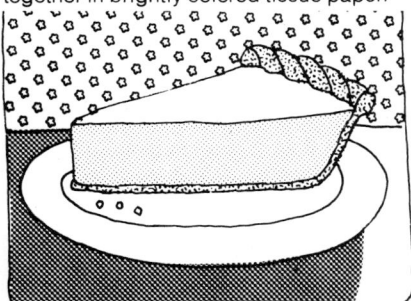

- ● **almond-crusted cheese pie**

1 ¾ c. creamed-style cottage cheese
4 tsp. cornstarch
5 T. sugar
1 tsp. vanilla
Grated rind of ½ lemon or lime
2 eggs, separated

- ● **pie crust**

24 individual amaretti*
¼ c. (scant measure) melted butter or margarine

Preheat oven to 400° F. With rolling pin, crush *amaretti* into fine crumbs. Pour butter over all but a tablespoon of crumbs. Stir to mix. Press crumbs into bottom and sides of lightly greased 9" pie pan and bake 4 mins. Remove pie shell, and turn oven to 350° F.

For filling, combine all ingredients except egg whites. Beat with electric beater until smooth. Beat egg whites till stiff. Fold into pie filling, then pour filling into pie shell. Sprinkle remaining crumbs on top. Bake 25 mins. Cool, but don't chill.

* You must use amaretti, *not* macaroons or other almond cookies. Conventional almond cookies are too sticky. Amaretti are available in tins or boxes at Italian grocery shops or at the gourmet department of large stores. We used Amaretti di Saronno.

gourmet forgeries
3 that nobody – except the experts – could detect

If you love hollandaise sauce but dread the last-minute risk of curdled or separated ingredients and fussing with the double boiler; if you're looking for a good-tasting, inexpensive pâté you can make in minutes or an impressive dessert you needn't slave over, you've come to the right place. Here we offer clever gourmet forgeries.

- ● **pâté**

4 strips bacon
2 4¾-oz. cans Sells Liver Pâté
1 large clove garlic
⅓ lb. mushrooms, uncooked and chopped fine
2 T. cognac

Fry bacon till only slightly crisp; drain. Mash together pâté from both cans with fork. Add pressed or very finely chopped garlic clove. Crumble the bacon strips into mixture. Add mushrooms and cognac and blend together with fork. Chill for several hours before serving with crackers or melba toast.

- ● **foolproof hollandaise sauce**

2 egg yolks
3 T. lemon juice
½ c. firm butter

Combine yolks and lemon juice in a small pan; stir with a wooden spoon until blended. Add half the butter. Stir over very low heat until the butter melts. Put in the remaining butter. Stir slowly until it melts and the sauce thickens. Take care that the butter melts slowly—this gives the yolks time to cook and thicken the sauce, which prevents curdling.

You can serve it hot immediately or later at room temperature. Pour over asparagus or other vegetable, eggs Benedict, or make a sauce Béarnaise for filet mignon or tournedos simply by adding 2 tsp. minced shallots, ½ tsp. dried tarragon, 1 tsp. minced fresh parsley, and ⅛ tsp. cayenne pepper. Makes 1 cup.

- ● **party pudding**

36 lady fingers
1 c. sherry or cognac
Raspberry jam
½ c. candied orange or ginger, chopped
½ pt. heavy cream

Dip 12 lady fingers in sherry or cognac and water. (Use ½ c. sherry mixed with 1 c. water; reserve ½ c. sherry.) Place the lady fingers in a crystal or china serving bowl. Spread the layer with a thin coating of raspberry jam; sprinkle with half the orange or ginger. Repeat layer of dipped lady fingers and spread again with jam and fruit. Cover with a top layer of lady fingers. Then pour the remaining ½ c. of sherry over all. Cover with a double layer of aluminum foil, then weight with a plate piled with canned goods or a heavy large jar. Put in refrigerator and leave overnight. Before guests arrive, whip the heavy cream and spread over top of pudding. Makes 6 servings.

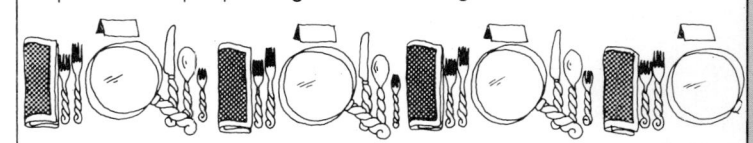

herb butters
to turn any vegetable or bread into a country treat

In about three minutes' time, you can make any kind of herb butter using your favorite herbs. Served on hot homemade bread or fresh, crunchy bakery bread or on almost any vegetable, herb butters evoke the delicious taste of real country cooking.

- ● **mint butter with baked potatoes**

¼ lb. butter
4 T. dried mint or ½ c. fresh, chopped
1 tsp. grated lemon rind
2 tsp. lemon juice

Allow butter to soften at room temperature, then mix well with other ingredients. Pour into a brown, glazed country crock if you have one, or any pretty, small serving bowl. Refrigerate until an hour before serving time, then remove from refrigerator to soften. Pass it around for guests to garnish their potatoes. Serves 4–6.

- ● **mint butter on toast with tea**

Spread mint butter generously on toasted slices of bread. Sprinkle 1

C cooking

tsp. of sugar over each buttered slice and heat them under the broiler for about a minute to melt and mix the butter and sugar. Serve with hot lemon tea.

● **tarragon butter on artichokes**

½ c. butter
2 T. dried tarragon
1 pinch garlic salt
2 T. lemon juice

Melt butter in small saucepan, then add remaining ingredients. Mix well and keep warm. When ready to serve, pour into 2 individual bowls and serve with boiled, drained artichokes for dipping. Serves 2.

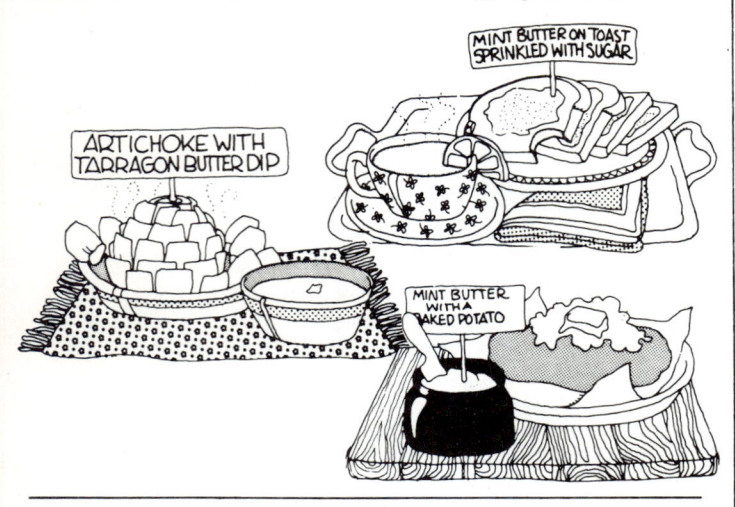

leftovers
what to do with the leftover sour cream, tomato paste, or 6 egg yolks your recipe didn't call for

The trouble with recipe extras—leftovers from dinner or any other cooking venture—is that usually only an expert can make them taste like anything but leftovers, plus it's extra work. Here are some ideas for the most common recipe leftovers that are worth the effort:

Egg yolks (from the cake that called for six egg whites): Try something different and whip up a delicious zabaglione. Beat the egg yolks until thick and pale in color. Gradually beat in ½ c. sugar. Then beat in ½ c. Marsala wine. Pour into the top part of a double boiler over pan of simmering water and continue beating till mixture foams and begins to thicken. Serve warm in sherbert glasses or over strawberries.

Egg whites: If you're left with egg whites, make some meringue shells to be filled with ice cream, topped with dessert sauce. Beat 6 egg whites, ¼ tsp. salt, and ¼ tsp. cream of tartar until foamy. Add 1½ c. sugar very slowly and continue beating till meringue forms stiff, glossy peaks. Beat in 1 tsp. vanilla or almond extract. Shape in cuplike forms and bake 55 to 60 mins. at 275° F. on a greased and floured cookie sheet. Cool.

Bread: Let rolls, croissants, or bread sit a few days till stale or dry in a slow oven (about 250° F.). Then, make bread crumbs by putting bread in a paper bag and crushing with a rolling pin. Add seasonings to taste. Or make croutons by breaking up the bread into bite-sized pieces, then sautéing in butter seasoned with herbs, garlic, and/or cheese.

Tomato paste: Make your own spaghetti sauce. First sauté onions, peppers, ground meat or sausage, mushrooms, salt, and pepper. In a saucepan, mix together tomato paste, tomato sauce, and canned or fresh tomatoes. Mix to the consistency you like. Add seasonings and a bit of sugar. Then add onion mixture and simmer for at least an hour. Freeze and use when needed.

Sour cream: For a delicious, cool side dish, mix the sour cream with sliced fresh cucumbers. Season with a touch of pepper, dry mustard, and salt. If you wish, add a little lemon juice, too.

Vegetables: If you are using fresh vegetables, cut up the extras and serve raw with a tangy dip—a great hors d'oeuvre or first course. Use leftover cooked vegetables in an omelet.

Last bit of ketchup: Add a bit of hot water, stir, and season gravy or meat with it.

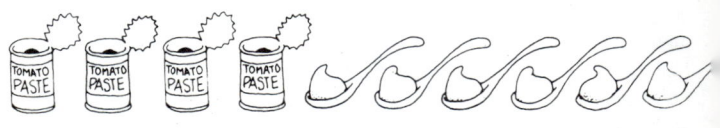

meat steamer
make your own meat steamer for tasty, low-calorie dishes

Steaming has always been a popular way to cook vegetables because it preserves their nutritional value and enhances their flavor by not diluting with cooking liquid. Meat is also delicious when steamed, but regular vegetable steamers cannot be used for meat because all the juice is lost through the holes in the steamer. The solution is the make-it-yourself steamer (see sketch). Remember, when you steam meat, you're not only getting more flavor but also fewer calories by not having to add a supply of cooking fat.

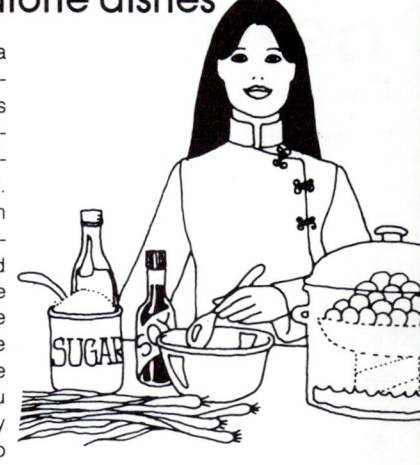

To make your steamer, simply remove both ends of a large, clean, empty can from peanuts or coffee. Place the can in a large pot that has an inch of water in the bottom. Put the meat you want to steam in a heat-proof dish or small saucepan, place this on top of the can, and cover with a lid. Follow any recipe for steamed meat. Chinese cookbooks usually have plenty of steamed dishes, or start with the following recipe for delectable steamed meatballs.

● **steamed meatballs**

½ lb. lean ground beef
1 T. fresh ginger, chopped or ½ tsp., powdered
¼ tsp. salt
¼ tsp. MSG (optional)
1 T. cornstarch
½ T. dry sherry
¼ c. cold water

In a mixing bowl, combine beef with ginger, salt, MSG, cornstarch, and sherry. Blend well. Gradually add water, stirring in a circular motion. Shape mixture into small balls. Bring water in steamer to a boil. Lightly oil a heat-proof dish and balance it on top of can in steamer. Arrange meatballs in dish. Cover steamer and steam 15 mins. Serve meatballs with following sauce:

2 tsp. soy sauce
2 tsp. sherry
½ tsp. sugar
2 scallions, finely chopped

Mix all ingredients and serve in a separate dish with meatballs. Each diner spears a meatball and dunks it in sauce. You can serve the meatballs for dinner with rice and a salad or as cocktail hors d'oeuvres.

cooking

mousse
a no-fuss gourmet dessert, plus lots of variations on the basic recipe

Even a meat-and-potatoes meal can turn into fancy fare when you top it off with a special dessert mousse. The recipe below can be flavored with anything from lemon, lime, or orange juice to coffee or your favorite liqueur. (Choice possibilities: Kahlúa, Vandermint, Amaretto, Calvados, or crème de menthe.)

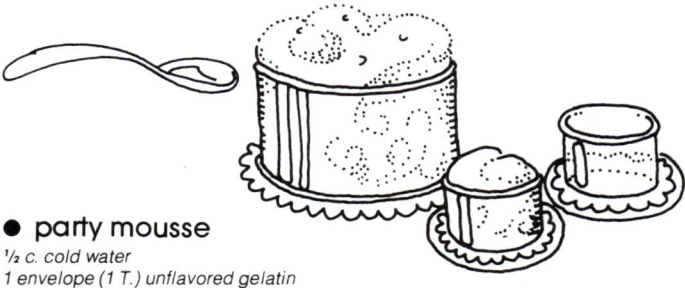

● party mousse
½ c. cold water
1 envelope (1 T.) unflavored gelatin
4 eggs, separated
½–¾ c. sugar (to sweeten lemon or lime juice or coffee)
½ c. citrus juice, strong coffee, or liqueur
1 c. heavy cream

Pour cold water in a heavy saucepan and sprinkle on gelatin to soften. Stir in egg yolks and sugar. Then turn on heat. Stirring constantly, cook over low flame until gelatin dissolves and mixture thickens enough to coat a spoon. (Don't boil or yolks will scramble.) Remove from heat. Stir in flavoring, taste for sweetness, and chill until mixture sets to the consistency of unbeaten egg whites. Remove from refrigerator. Beat egg whites until stiff and gently fold into mixture; whip heavy cream to soft peaks and fold in. Then turn into individual dessert dishes, wine glasses, or a large serving bowl. Chill several hours or overnight. Serves 6–8.

poundcake
how to turn a poundcake into a gourmet gift

This elaborate, gala Sicilian cake is based on nothing more than the simplest poundcake you can buy (even frozen), plus ricotta cheese and chocolate. It freezes well and keeps in the refrigerator up to a week. It serves many people, because the thinnest slivers are rich enough for the sweetest tooth. You'll need:

1 9" × 3" poundcake
1 lb. ricotta cheese
2 T. heavy cream
4 T. fine granulated sugar
3 T. orange liqueur (Grand Marnier, Triple Sec)
2 T. candied orange peel, coarsely chopped
1 T. candied lemon peel, coarsely chopped
2 sq. (2 oz.) semisweet chocolate, grated

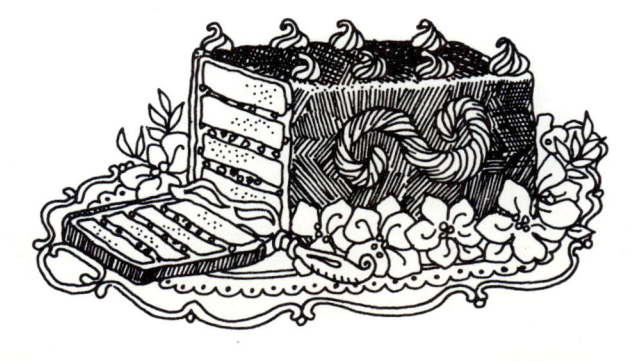

Place poundcake on its side for easy handling while you slice off end crusts, level the top, and slice in fourths lengthwise. Force cheese through a not-too-fine sieve into mixing bowl and beat till perfectly smooth. Continue beating and add cream, sugar, and liqueur. With rubber spatula, gently fold in candied fruit and chocolate. Spread a double layer of foil on a flat surface. Then put first slice of cake on foil and spread filling; layer another slice on top of that and again fill, repeating till last slice is added. Press together into boxy shape, smooth sides with spatula, and refrigerate overnight. Cheese mixture will be firm when cold. Make a rich European chocolate frosting to coat cake:

4 sq. (4 oz.) semisweet chocolate
2 T. whipping cream
1⅓ c. confectioners' sugar

Melt chocolate in top pan of double boiler over pan of hot water. Add whipping cream; beat well. Add confectioners' sugar till taste is sweet enough, beating till icing is smooth. Spread while still warm.

Put cake in a foil loaf pan and wrap with an outer layer of brightly colored or patterned foil. When you deliver it, make sure your cake is stored in the refrigerator right away.

restaurant
how to eat at a famous restaurant at home

The "21" Club, one of this nation's best-known restaurants, shared some of their recipes with us. Now you can surprise guests at home with a dinner from a famous restaurant. The meal here consists of cornish hens in a creamy sauce garnished with fresh grapes and served with rice. For dessert, there's delicate Sabayon sauce poured over the splurge of fresh strawberries. The final touch is Café Diable, a brandy-flavored coffee to remember dinner over.

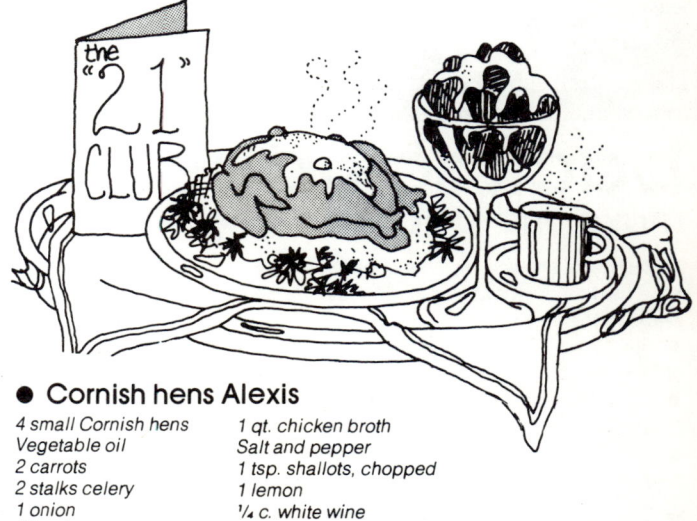

● Cornish hens Alexis
4 small Cornish hens
Vegetable oil
2 carrots
2 stalks celery
1 onion
2 bay leaves
Dash rosemary
¼ lb. butter, melted
1½ c. flour
1 qt. chicken broth
Salt and pepper
1 tsp. shallots, chopped
1 lemon
¼ c. white wine
4 T. sour cream
1½ c. white seedless grapes
Parsley, chopped

Preheat oven to 350° F. Roast Cornish hens in a covered casserole for 15 mins., basting occasionally with vegetable oil. While birds roast, dice all vegetables; after 15 mins. of roasting, add vegetables, bay leaves, and rosemary to birds. Roast an additional 20 mins. While birds roast, make a roux by melting the butter and sprinkling in the flour; stir continuously until the mixture is smooth. Gradually add hot chicken broth and stir until you have a smooth, fairly thick sauce. Season with salt and pepper. Simmer for 15 to 20 mins. While sauce cooks, sauté shallots in a little extra butter in a separate pan, add juice of lemon, wine, and sour cream. When mixture is hot, add to the sim-

41

cooking

mering sauce. Just before serving, add grapes to sauce. Pour over hens in the covered casserole and reheat in oven. Sprinkle with chopped parsley. Serves 4. Accompany the hens with herbed or plain rice, buttered and topped with parsley.

● **Sabayon sauce**

7 egg yolks
½ c. sugar
1 c. Marsala or sherry
1 pt. fresh strawberries*

In top pan of a double boiler, beat egg yolks and sugar lightly with whisk or beater. Add Marsala or sherry and beat. Place over simmering, not boiling, water. Cook, beating steadily until mixture thickens slightly and doubles in volume (about 20 to 25 mins.). Remove top of double boiler from hot water. Keep beating a few minutes longer. To serve, pile strawberries in dessert dishes; spoon sauce over them or pass sauce separately. Serves 4.

*If fresh strawberries are unavailable or they are too expensive, serve the sauce over drained canned pears—it's delicious.

● **café diable**

Coiled peel of whole lemon (removed in single strip)
Coiled peel of whole orange (removed in single strip)
24 cloves
2 sticks cinnamon
2 tsp. granulated sugar
4 oz. brandy
3 8-oz. cups espresso coffee
2 oz. kirschwasser

Stud lemon and orange peels with cloves and put them in a lined copper bowl (or a saucepan) along with cinnamon, sugar, and brandy. Set a match to the mixture so that the brandy flames for a moment or two, and then add the coffee, putting out the flame. Remove the peels and cinnamon; add kirschwasser. Serve immediately in demitasse cups. Serves 8.

crafts

back scrubber
make one in no time

If your daily shower involves a variety of contortions in order to wash your back, why not take a few minutes to make this handy terry cloth back washer?

● Buy ¼ yd. of bright-colored 45″ terry cloth fabric and two inexpensive plastic bangle bracelets—available at most dime stores.
● Cut off 5″ from the width of fabric so that it measures 40″ × 9″. Fold the edges in ½″ twice (to prevent raveling) and machine-stitch.
● Form handles at each end of the terry cloth strip by folding a small portion of cloth over a bracelet and then handstitching snugly in place.

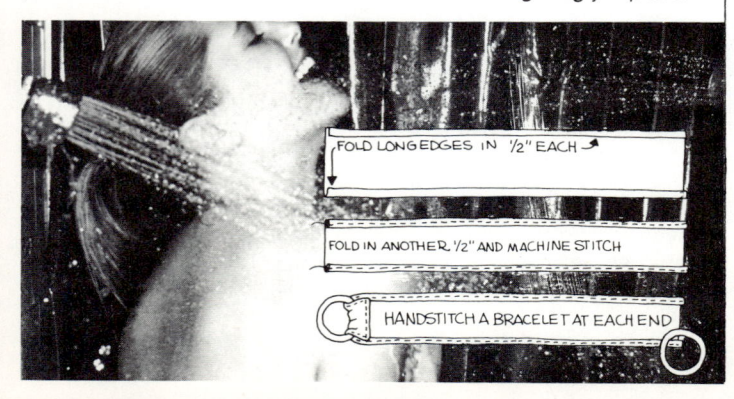

bath wrap
turn an ordinary towel into a pretty bath wrap

The pretty towel wrap below is just the thing to slip into after a shower or a bath. Even if you're a nonsewer, it's simple to make.

Use a standard-sized towel, 31″ of ¾″-wide elastic, and some VELCRO® fastener. Turn down one long edge of towel to form a 1″-wide casing for elastic (do this by hand if you don't have a sewing machine). Thread elastic through casing but do not push through the last 6″ of casing. Anchor the elastic firmly at each end by stitching through elastic and towel (see sketch). Now sew a 3″ strip of VELCRO® fastener on end of towel with no elastic in it. Try on towel to determine where to sew corresponding fastener—it should be at the spot where towel feels snug but still comfortable. Sew the corresponding fastener in place.

These measurements will suit an average-sized woman. If your bosom is especially small or large, adjust the elastic measurement by 1″ or so as needed. If you're over 5′10″ tall, modesty may compel you to sew a length of pretty ribbon on the bottom of the towel for extra length.

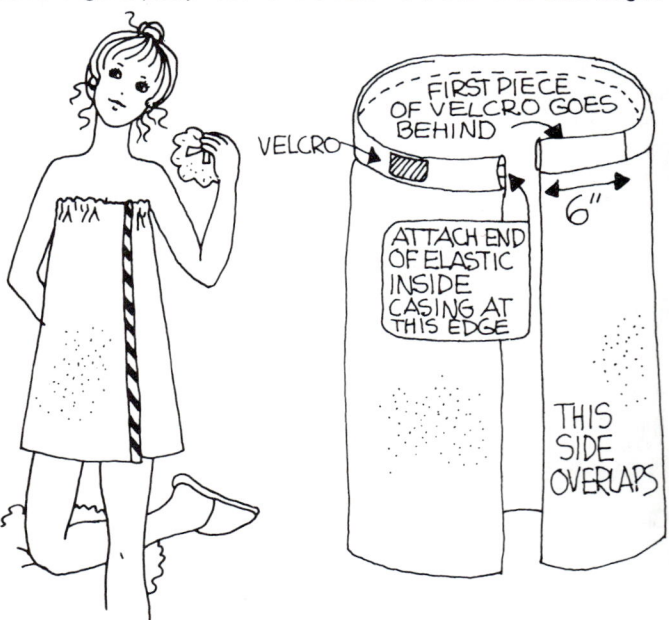

carryall
make your own beach or picnic carryall

The beach or picnic carryall, opposite, is about as practical and good-looking as any you'll find. The best fabric to use is a sturdy canvas or sailcloth in a weight that your sewing machine can handle easily. We used 1 yard of natural-colored 45″ canvas for the bag and ⅓ yard of awning-stripe canvas for the pockets. You'll also need approximately 2 yards of lightweight upholstery webbing for the handles, a package of gripper snaps, and an 18″ industrial or jacket-weight separating zipper.

Cut the canvas for the main part of the bag into a piece that measures 31″ long and 45″ wide. Now cut two pockets, one 18″ × 12″ and one 12″ × 19½″. Press under ½″ hem on all sides of the smaller pocket. Pin pocket in place on one 22½″ side of canvas (see sketch). Pocket should be centered widthwise and set 3½″ from bottom. Stitch pocket down on sides and bottom. Stitch down the middle of the

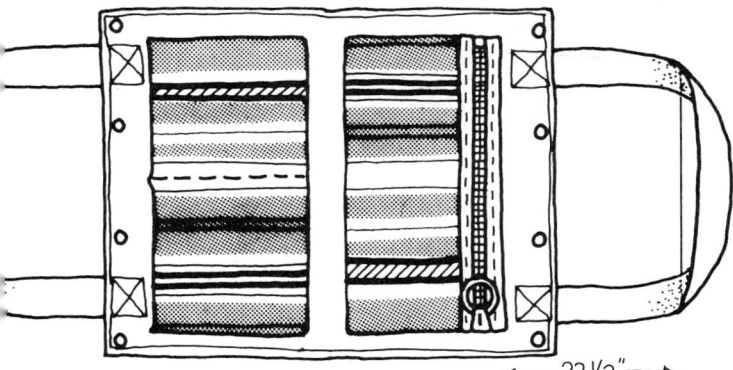

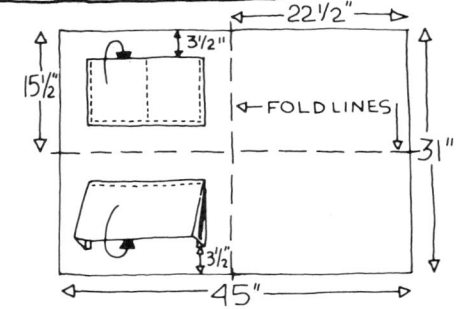

crafts

three sides, leaving 4" open to turn right side out. Iron a 1" pleat about 2" in from each side (see sketch). Then topstitch pocket to one of the two remaining sling pieces, centering it along the bottom seam. Cut eight 12" pieces of ribbon for the ties and pin down as shown. (The ends will be caught in the seams.) With right sides together, stitch the two remaining pieces together, leaving 4" free to turn right side out. Turn, press, and topstitch, catching the 4" opening. Slip over the back of your chair and tie.

Note: These dimensions fit most desk chairs but measure the back of yours for any necessary adjustments.

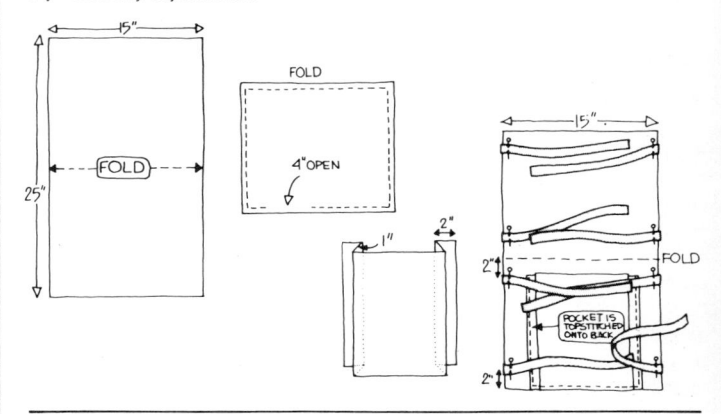

pocket if you want to make two compartments.

The second pocket has an accordion fold at the sides so that it will expand to hold more. First, press under ½" hem on all four edges. To make the fold, press a "W" on both short sides, with each leg of the "W" about ½" wide. Pin pocket in place, centering widthwise and 3½" from bottom. Mark spot where top of pocket reaches with a chalk or pencil line. Remove pocket and sew one edge of zipper over your line. Sew the other edge of zipper to top of your pocket. Now stitch pocket in place, catching only the bottom fold of the accordion pleat.

Now fold carryall in half lengthwise, right sides together (the pockets will be in the middle, out of sight). Stitch together on two sides: one long and one short. Turn bag right side out, turn under ½" on remaining unstitched edge, and top-stitch closed. Cut handles to desired length, either comfortable shoulder-strap length or shorter, and stitch down on bag. Attach four gripper snaps across top of bag.

You can slide your beach or picnic blanket in the center of your carryall and keep small items in the pockets. You might like to decorate your bag by stenciling on initials or embroidering it. One clever woman stenciled a backgammon board on hers.

chair-sling a great chair-sling in less than an hour

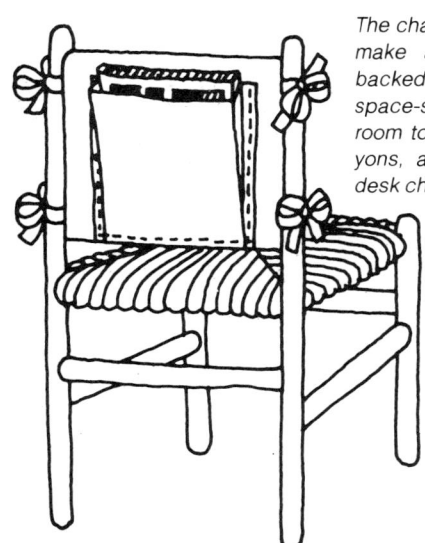

The chair sling, at left, is a snap to make and can turn any high-backed chair into an organizer and space-saver. Use it in a child's room to hold coloring books, crayons, and homework, or on your desk chair as a catchall.

You'll need ¾ yard of 45" fabric (you might want two colors, one for the sling itself and another for the pocket), plus 2⅔ yards of ribbon.

Cut three pieces of fabric, each 15" × 25" (two for the sling, one for the pocket). Fold your pocket piece in half, crosswise. With right sides together, stitch

desk folder
a handsome one for your — or his — desk

If your desk is a disaster area, cluttered with papers and more papers, what you need is a desk folder. Here is one that's easy to make and good-looking. You'll need: Two 9" × 12" pieces of cardboard; white glue; cloth tape, 1" wide, any color; and ½ yd. fabric or heavy paper (we used Skinner UltraSuede Fabric).

Place cardboard pieces side by side, ½" apart, and stretch the cloth tape over the ½" opening to form a binding (see sketch). Then cut one piece of fabric 4" longer and 4" wider than the total size of the folder. Cover the cardboard with glue. Center cardboard on the wrong side of fabric, overlapping 2" on all sides. Fold under fabric at corners and press firmly to adhere to folder. Cut another piece of fabric 1" shorter

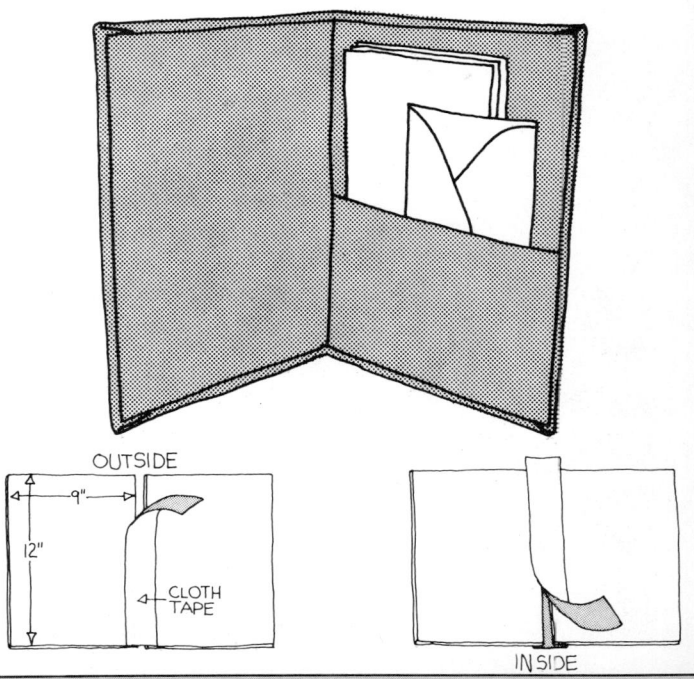

crafts

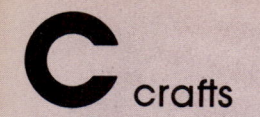

and 1" narrower than inside of folder. Glue in place as the inside cover. Cut the pocket the same width as the inside of the folder—to the desired depth—and glue on three sides. Press folder in open position under books overnight.

Note: The folder can be any size, but be sure to leave 4" of fabric to overlap. If you like, allow ¼" to turn under inside cover and pocket if fabric has unfinished edges.

frames
unique fabric-matted frames for your favorite photographs

- To make the frames photographed here, start with an inexpensive wood or plastic frame (maybe spray-painted a bright color) or use a chrome or Lucite® box frame.
- For the matting, you might use gingham, calico, or another small-print fabric that sets off your photo but doesn't overpower it. Cut a piece of fabric ⅛"–¼" larger on all sides than your frame's cardboard backing. Then place fabric on an ironing board and center photograph on top.
- Next, you'll need plain or embroidered ribbon plus iron-on bonding tape (like Stitch Witchery®) that measures about half the ribbon's width. Lay bonding tape along—but not touching—the top edge of the photograph and place ribbon on tape, top edges together. Iron ribbon very carefully by pressing and lifting, rather than sliding the iron back and forth, to keep the ribbon from moving while being bonded to the fabric.
- Complete the "tic-tac-toe" edging around the photograph by bonding three more ribbons along its bottom and sides (see sketch). Remember: Always fuse together outside edges of ribbon and tape so that the inside ribbon edges freely overlap and hold the photograph. Thus, you can slip the photo in and out—even switch pictures for a new display.
- Place fabric on the frame's cardboard backing, press against the glass, and hang your finished, personalized photograph.

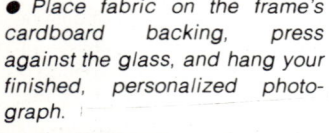

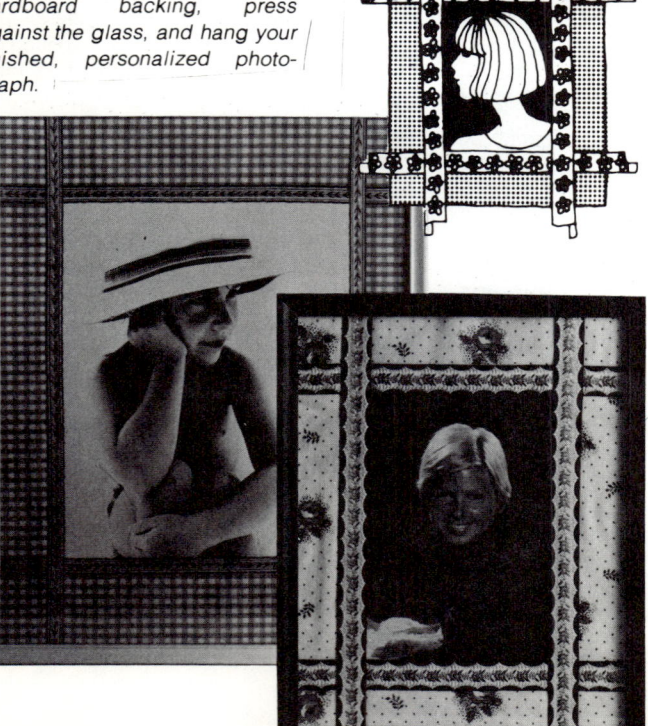

hammock
a good-looking one you can make

If you can sew a seam, you can make this hammock in about four hours with no trouble. Then all you need are two sturdy walls or shady trees to support your work.

- You'll need two wooden dowels, each 40" long, 1⅛" in diameter; two 3"-diameter metal rings (from a marine supply store); 67 yards of 2" webbing (from a hardware store); and shiny upholstery tacks.
- Since the hammock is woven with a natural white and a bright-colored webbing, dye 30 yards of webbing your choice of color (this allows for shrinkage).
- For the hammock's length, cut twelve colored webbing strips, each 83½" long, two white strips, each 81½" long, and two white strips, each 80" long. At both ends of each strip, fold a ¼" hem, then fold under 4" and sew down with zigzag stitching to form a loop (see sketch). Later you'll slip the dowels through these loops.
- For the hammock's width, cut thirty-one white webbing strips, each 35" long. At both ends of these strips, fold a ¼" hem and form a loop by folding under 2¼", sewing down with zigzag stitching.
- Arrange long strips on the floor so that colored strips are in the center, one 81½" strip on each side, and an 80" white strip on each end (see sketch). Using a dowel for each end of the hammock, slip dowels through loops of all long strips except the very end ones—labeled 1 and 16 in the sketch.
- Now cross-weave with the 35" strips. Start and end by slipping the loop of each 35" strip over the 80" strips, left off the dowel in the previous step.
- For the support, cut two 60" strips of webbing and slip the strips through one 3" metal ring. Center ring on webbing, and then stitch across the short ends of each pair of strips, forming two big closed loops. Cut two additional strips of fabric and repeat procedure for the second 3" metal ring. Then use each loop as a sling for the dowel, pinning two darts underneath so that the dowel lies snugly (see sketch). Remove dowel, turn dart inside, and stitch, leaving excess material. Finally, tap in shiny upholstery tacks along the dart to secure the sling to the dowel (see sketch).

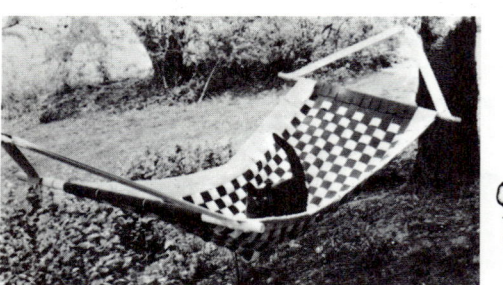

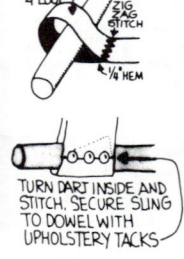

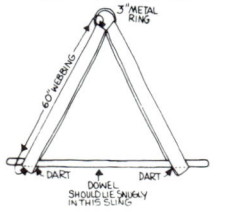

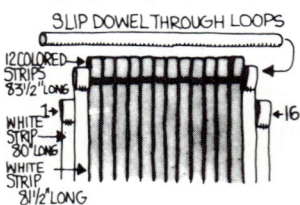

hassock
hassock that's a catchall, too

The patch-pocket hassock, opposite, is a convenient catchall for magazines, note pads, knitting projects, or your book of the week—and it takes little time to make.

You'll need a bottomless wood cube (ours was 16" × 16" × 12") and a foam seat about 3" thick, cut to fit the cube top. Glue foam to cube.

Then drape enough fabric over it to cover top and sides, allowing a couple of inches extra at the bottom.

With fabric draped over cube, decide where you'd like pockets and mark positions with pins. Cut patches from extra fabric and for each one, iron back a ¼" hem all around. Stitch one side with zig-zag stitching, then sew patch to fabric along its three remaining sides to form pocket. Make sections within the pockets as desired by zig-zag stitching through pocket to fabric.

Again, drape fabric over hassock and now wrap as you would a package. Smooth excess fabric under on one side (see sketch) and fasten bottom edge to inside of cube with a staple gun (or tacks). Do the same on the opposite side. Turn last two bottom edges under and staple.

Among the best fabrics to use are denim, canvas, or lightweight corduroy. You might vary the look by doing the background in one color or design, the pockets in another. Or try a different pocket arrangement for each side of the hassock—shallow or deep pockets, single or sectioned ones.

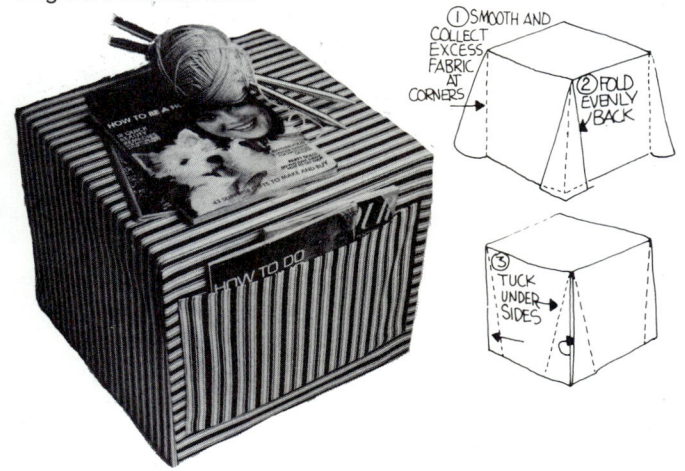

makeup case
sew your own makeup case

The little roll case sketched above right comes in handy at the office, the beach, or anywhere else. You can make it yourself for pennies in less than an hour.

The size of your case depends on the items you're going to carry—the biggest might be a small hairbrush. You can make the case from any bright fabric—polka-dotted, flowered, striped, whatever. A vinylized fabric is best for the beach. You'll need a half yard of fabric, any width, and about two yards of matching or contrasting grosgrain ribbon.

Cut two pieces of fabric to the size you want the case to be—either 7" x 8" or 6" x 7" is a good size. Now assemble the makeup you want to include in the case—probably mascara, lipstick or gloss, blusher, a small hairbrush and comb, and maybe a tiny mirror. Arrange the makeup in rows (see sketch) on right side of one of the fabric pieces. Now, lay ribbon over makeup. Mark places where the ribbon needs to be sewn down to form loops with straight pins. Remove makeup, stitch down loops, checking as you go that each loop is large enough to accommodate makeup. Cut off any excess ribbon.

Now cut a length of ribbon 30" long and place it lengthwise across the right side of remaining piece of fabric. Stitch down, starting at one end and stitching to within 3" of opposite end. The open 3" will form an overlap when you roll the case.

To finish case, stitch the two pieces of fabric together, *wrong* sides facing each other (turn in a ¼" hem all around as you go). If you wish, leave about 3" open at one corner on a long side to form a little pocket for money.

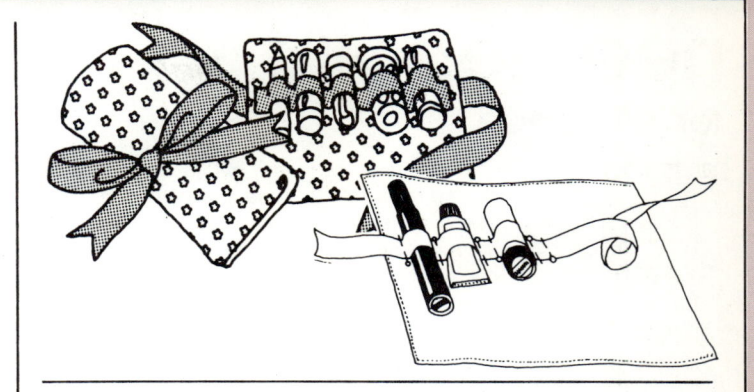

money
earn $$$ for your handmade jewelry, macramé, or anything you make

Your friends may ooh and ahh over your handmade pillows, macramé belts, and seashell jewelry—but could you actually *sell* those items to local stores? More often than you might expect, yes. Here are some tips to help you get started:

● Whether you're hoping to sell your crafts to a major department store or your corner gift shop, the most professional approach is to call the store first to find out who sees prospective "vendors" and when. (To a store buyer, anyone with goods to sell is known as a vendor.) In small stores, the owner may simply see anyone who drops in, but in department stores, each department (needlepoint, pottery, and so forth) usually has its own buyer, who sees new talent once a week, by appointment, on "vendor's day."

● Before you see the buyer, call your state Department of Labor to find out whether you need a license to sell your items. In some states, for example, you might need a license to sell quilts, pillows, or anything that is stuffed in order to ensure that your stuffing meets local health requirements. On the other hand, you might not need a license to sell candles or pottery. If necessary, you should be able to secure a license quickly and inexpensively.

● When you do visit a buyer, present your best cross section of the items for sale. You may be asked to try a slightly different approach before your work is accepted.

● Be prepared to give the buyer a definite idea of how much money you would expect to receive for each item the store accepts; this figure should include the cost of your materials, as well as how much you expect to be paid for the labor on each item. The store will then determine the item's price on the basis of its own mark-up policies and how much you will earn for each item. You should also give the buyer information regarding how quickly and in what quantities you'd be able to produce more.

● The buyer may ask whether any other store is selling your work. Some stores request "exclusives" on your line for a specified period of time, such as three months.

● Make sure you understand how you are to be paid for your work. In some cases a store will buy a group of items for a flat fee per item; others will accept your work only on consignment. This means that you leave your crafts in the store and are paid only for those that actually sell. There are obvious drawbacks to on-consignment selling—it ties up your merchandise, for one thing—but if you're a rank beginner, it may be the only way to start your trade.

● Get a written purchase order from the buyer for anything that you sell. This should include his or her signature, a complete description of the items ordered (including unit cost of each and the total cost), plus the terms of payment. For example, a department store may not pay you on receipt of your items, but within the first ten days of the month following receipt of them.

● If a buyer shows no interest in your crafts, try another store. . . one store's flop is another's hottest item.

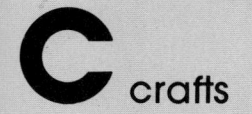

crafts

needlepoint
for left-handers

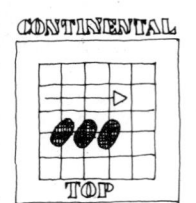

One easy trick can turn right-handed needlepoint directions into those any left-hander can use. Simply turn your canvas upside down and start your stitches on the lower left-hand corner, working across from left to right. When the canvas is turned right side up, the stitches will slant in the conventional direction. To follow usual needlepoint directions, turn the diagrams upside down too, and then do the stitches as diagrammed. Also make transpositions in the written directions: top becomes bottom, right becomes left, and so on. With a basket-weave stitch, up rows become down, and down ones up.

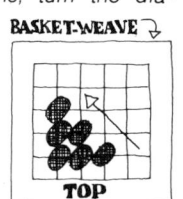

painting glass plates—fun art

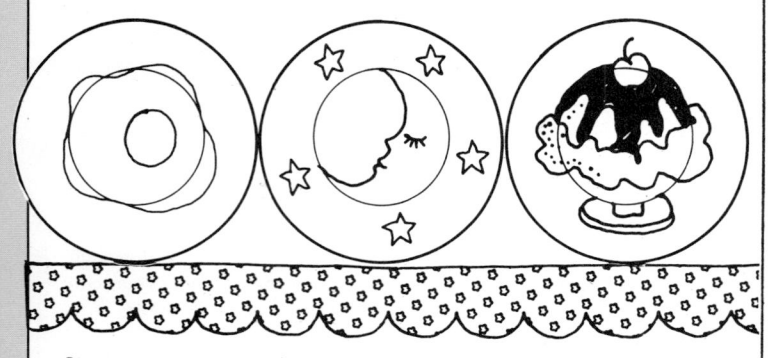

Clear glass plates make ideal natural backgrounds for a little color and imagination. Paint them on cold or rainy nights to cheer up your table.

Use glass stain or ceramic enamel and work on the back side of plate. Since your design will be reversed when you turn the plate over, you may want to draw the pattern on paper first, then cut and tape it to the front of the plate while you're working on the back. (Base your design on the center circle.) Here are some ideas:
- The "once-over-easy" breakfast plate is a yellow yolk painted in the center circle with the white spread egglike around its edges.
- The bedtime-snack plate is a dozing man-in-the-moon set inside the circle with stars shining around the border.
- The dieter's torture is a huge hot fudge sundae. When all your cottage cheese is gone, you face a luscious mound of chocolate and French vanilla. Again, use the center circle for the basic white scoop, drip brown down the sides, paint it in a sundae dish, and top it with a red cherry.
- For kids, make a "Clean Plate Champ" plate to get them through the "I hate everything but hamburgers" years.
- For light lunches, paint various fruits on a set of plates—a juicy giant strawberry, a bunch of pale green grapes, or a tart lemon.
- For the more adventurous, decorate with tropical fish or even a series on the household variety goldfish. Extend the nose and tails out from the circle, add a gill, scales, and a big beautiful pop eye. Show it breathing a few blue bubbles and use it to serve salmon plates, tuna sandwiches, creamed herring, or shrimp.
- French words, like *fromage* (cheese), *salade* (salad), and *omelette* (omelet), may be painted in the center circle or arched over the top of the plate. Simply use a stencil for painting the letters.

pillows you can design

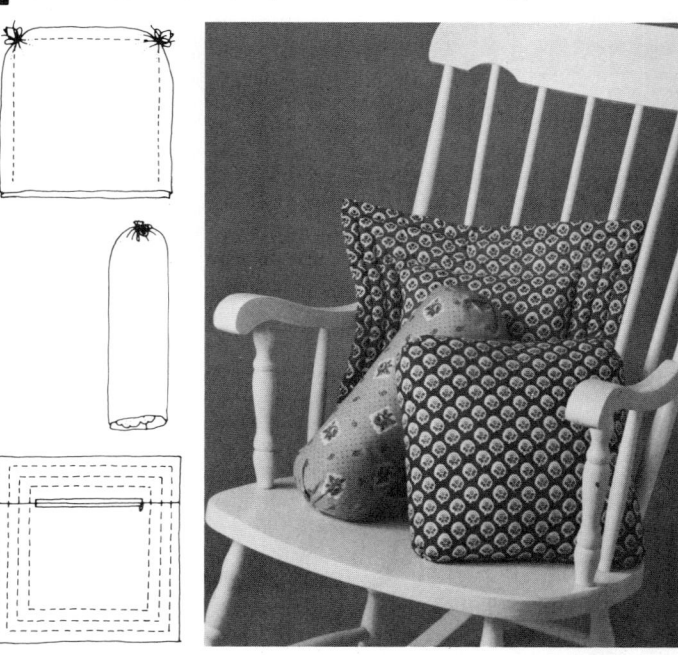

Pillows like the ones shown above can give a room a brand new look. Here's how to make them:

For the square pillow with gathered corners (front), buy or make a square-cornered pillow form. Then cut your outer cover of decorative fabric to the same size as your form plus allow for the depth of the pillow form, which should be added to both length and width. With right sides together, stitch the two cover pieces, leaving opening on one side to insert pillow form. Still on the wrong side, wrap and tie a drawstring around each of the four corners about 1" down from the seams (see sketch). Turn cover to right side, insert pillow form, and handstitch opening closed.

To make the bolster pillow (center), you'll need to make your own inner pillow form first, since most bolster forms in stores are too big for an occasional pillow. Start by sewing a length of muslin together to form a tube the diameter and length you want pillow to be, leaving an opening for the stuffing. Leave both ends open. Cut two circles the diameter of bolster. Stitch circles to ends of tubes, right sides together; turn tube to right side, stuff with fiberfill, and stitch opening closed. Now make the outer cover by sewing a length of fabric into a tube the same diameter as your finished inner bolster and the same length plus the diameter. For example, if your inner bolster is 12" long and 4" in diameter, your outer cover should be 16" long and 4" in diameter. Turn back a narrow hem on each end of the tube of fabric, leaving a tiny opening to insert a drawstring. Insert drawstring, pull tight and tie, pushing string ends into the hole in the center (see sketch). If you wish, finish each end with a decorative button.

To make the square pillow with quilted edging (back), start with a knife-edged square pillow form. Then cut one piece of fabric for cover 4" larger all around than form. Cut the other cover piece ¾" longer on two parallel sides. Now cut across this longer piece about a quarter of the way down from one short side. Stitch ends of the cut edges closed, leaving opening for a zipper that is slightly smaller than the size of your pillow form. Insert zipper (see sketch). Now take a piece of cotton batting and cut it to the size of the outer pillow cover. With right sides facing, stitch the outer cover together. Turn cover to right side through zipper opening. Insert cotton batting and smooth it flat inside cover. Now stitch all around the outer pillow edge to form quilting. Make at least two rows of stitching about 1" apart. The last row of stitching should enclose the opening for the pillow form. Insert pillow form and you're finished.

46

credit C

ribbon pillows and bags to make

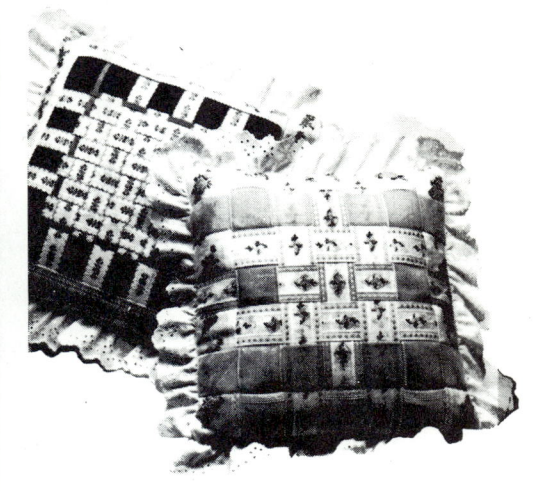

Ribbon is for tying in your hair, wrapping packages, lacing shoes—and for making the beautiful bags and pillows shown here.

You can easily master this ribbon-weaving technique by making the envelope clutch bag below. Start with a yard of lining fabric—any inexpensive cotton that coordinates with your ribbon color will do. You'll also need a yard of muslin and a yard of 18" fusible webbing, like Stitch Witchery®, plus 20 yards of one color ribbon, and one extra yard of color to make the stripe.

Cut the muslin and fusible webbing into a piece that matches the shape and dimensions of the sketch below. Place fusible webbing over muslin. Now begin covering the surface with ribbon strips in a vertical direction. Since the shape of the bag is irregular, it's easiest to cut the lengths of ribbon as you work. Lay each piece of ribbon vertically on the webbing and pin loose ends to hold securely. When you've covered the entire surface with ribbon, you can start weaving in the remaining ribbon horizontally in an under-over pattern. Again, cut your ribbon lengths as you go and pin to hold securely. You can add the colored stripe in the flap of the bag wherever you choose. Once you've woven all the ribbon, follow the manufacturer's directions for ironing fusible webbing into place. (The usual procedure is to lay a light pressing cloth over the ribbon, put the iron on steam, and press down the ribbon.) Pick up the iron and move it from spot to spot instead of sliding it, until you're sure the ribbon is fused to the muslin backing.

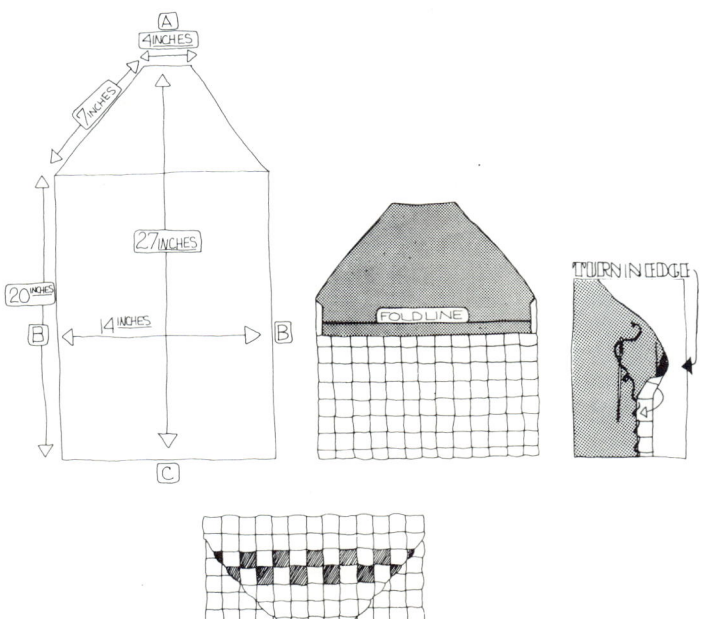

To finish your bag, pin lining to ribbon piece, right sides together. Stitch down by machine, leaving about ½" seam allowance and a 3" opening on side C. Turn bag to right side, handstitch opening closed. Now, with ribbon sides together, fold side C 8½" up toward A. Stitch both sides in place by machine. Turn bag to right side. Hand sew seam allowance just below flap so that flap is even with sides of bag (see sketch). Finish by sewing on snap or decorative closing.

Once you've learned this technique, you can also make beautiful pillows and place mats. Create a very handsome effect simply by using two colors of ribbon—one for the vertical stripes, another for the horizontal.

Pillows and bag were done with Century Ribbon, Stitch Witchery® by Stacy, and Franken ruffled eyelet.

credit

cards which credit cards are right for you?

These days the right credit card will pay for almost anything—your college tuition, a parking ticket, birth control pills, even a street-corner hot dog, or a dugout canoe ride up the Amazon headwaters. Check to see which of the three main types of credit cards suits your needs.

● **bank charge cards**

The best-known bank charge cards are Master Charge and Visa (formerly BankAmericard), and they offer perhaps the widest range of goods and services in the U.S. and overseas, including "cash advances," which allow you to obtain varying amounts of money simply by presenting your card at a participating bank. These cards are issued by banks to individuals who have proved creditworthy—often a matter of established credit with other cards or proof of steady employment. Standards of creditworthiness vary around the country and may include an age requirement. With a bank charge card, you receive a monthly statement covering all of the purchases you have made. If you pay your entire balance within a specified period, you usually have to pay no interest charges. But if you do not pay the entire balance, you must pay a certain minimum, and interest will be charged on the unpaid balance. Bank charge cards can be applied to all those items listed above, but most people use them primarily for clothing and major household purchases.

● **travel and entertainment cards**

These give you mainly what the name implies: meals, lodging, airplane tickets, car rentals, and the like, in the U.S. and around the world. The biggest "T&E" cards are American Express, Carte Blanche, and Diners Club, all of which are usually held by heads of families with incomes of $10,000 or more. However, this is not a hard-and-fast rule, and some, such as American Express, have special plans for women and for younger—and less affluent—cardholders. All three credit cards charge annual fees of $20. In most cases, you cannot stretch your payments over a long period and must pay the entire sum in one or two installments. (One exception is T&E transportation packages, in which extended payments are allowed, but there is a finance charge.) Perhaps the greatest advantage of T&E cards is that, because of their

C credit

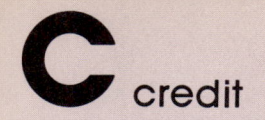

high standards and international recognition, many foreign countries accept them more readily than they do other cards. And in a monetary crisis, some foreign service establishments will accept credit-card charges more readily than cash.

● **private label or one-company cards**
Such cards are those issued by a department store or a gas company and are free, although you usually pay an interest charge on your unpaid balance each month. Requirements vary nationally. Some stores offer a "junior" card for teenagers upon the parents' consent. Others require that you be at least twenty-one and meet other requirements as well.

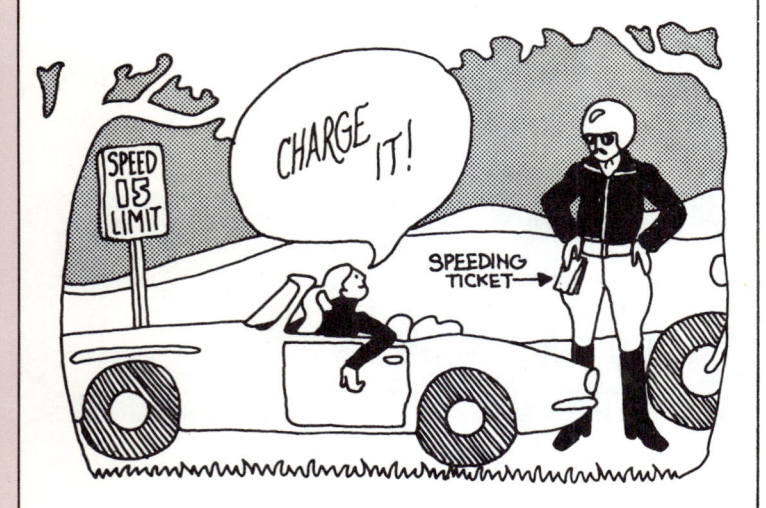

file
how to find out what's in your credit file and what to do if you're denied credit

If you've ever been denied credit and don't know why, or just wondered if there really is a secret file somewhere with your name on it, here are some facts you should be aware of:

Yes, there may be a file on you—if you've ever applied for credit. A consumer credit report is completed by a credit bureau and supplied to those firms where you have applied for credit. It contains basic identifying information about you as well as a record of your credit transactions, such as loans and charge accounts.

The 1970 Fair Credit Reporting Act gives you, the consumer, certain rights regarding information collected about you in such a report.

If you are denied credit, wholly or partly because of something contained in a credit report, the user of the report must inform you of this and supply you with the name and address of the reporting agency. (The information that affected the decision may be as simple as the length of time you've lived at your present address.)

You have the right to know the nature and substance of all the information in a credit report, as well as the names of those who have received reports for credit purposes within the past six months.

In most cases, adverse information regarding you that is more than seven years old may not be reported.

If you dispute an item in your file, the reporting agency must reinvestigate. Anything found to be inaccurate must be deleted and you can direct the agency to notify those who were sent the report. If the reinvestigation does not resolve the dispute, you may file a statement telling your side of the story.

If you haven't been denied credit but would still like to know what's on file about you, contact some of the larger credit-reporting agencies near you. You'll find them listed in the Yellow Pages. (A firm like TRW Credit Data has offices in many cities around the country.) By completing the proper request form, you can receive a transcript of your file, if one exists, for a small fee.

As a woman applying for credit, you should also be aware of the *1974 Equal Credit Opportunity Act. Under this law, a lender must reveal, if asked, the reasons for a denial of credit. The law also provides that a woman can apply for credit and credit cards using her maiden, married, or hyphenated name.*

problems
how to avoid rip-offs and other problems with credit cards

Newspapers have carried reports of people who had financed round-the-world trips or charged thousands of dollars with stolen credit cards. But because of the credit-card industry's use of increasingly sophisticated computer systems, such abuses are far less likely to occur. Here's how to steer clear of such problems:

● Treat your credit cards as you would cash; that is, don't leave them lying around on counters; don't carry more of them than you need; and don't pack them in your luggage when traveling.

● Don't throw away an expired card or one that you no longer want without first cutting it in half.

● Keep a list of your credit-card numbers—and the numbers to call in case they're lost or stolen—in a place apart from your credit cards. (See below for what to do when a card is stolen or lost.)

● Use any card at least once a year; don't keep it in your wallet merely for emergency or identification purposes.

● It may be a chore, but save the tissue receipts from each charge you make. Not only does this help you spot purchases you didn't make, it also can alert you to possible tampering with the receipts of purchases you did make. Unscrupulous merchants, for example, have been known to change $7 to $8, $9, or $17. And equally unscrupulous clerks have been known to run off two receipts when you charge an item. The first they return to you; on the second, they forge your signature and write up a "purchase" for themselves.

● Save monthly billing statements, too. They provide a record of all the interest (finance charges) you've paid for credit-card purchases, which is deductible on your income tax. In addition, keeping a record of what cards you use most and least often may indicate that you have a card you don't need or that you need a few more.

● Remember that a credit card can be invaluable if you run low on cash on vacation, because it will cover the cost of food and lodging and supply a cash advance as well. However, you need to apply for one at least six to eight weeks before any trip to make sure you get it on time.

● **if your credit card is lost or stolen . . .**

● *During business hours,* telephone the nearest office of the credit-card issuer or try the toll-free numbers you can call at any hour, seven days a week, set up by some card issuers (Master Charge, American Express). Then immediately send to the same office a registered, return-receipt-requested letter or the postcard provided by some companies upon issuance of your card to the same effect.

● *During the evening or weekend,* if the card issuer does not have a round-the-clock, toll-free number, send a telegram to the nearest office of the card company followed by a registered letter.

● *In a foreign country,* telephone the nearest office of your credit-card company or issuing bank and follow it with a registered letter to the same office. If you can't locate the office, ask for help at a hotel, store, or bank that displays the credit card decal.

When you notify the credit-card issuer at once, you are not responsible for any purchases you did not make. If you fail to do so, you could at worst be legally responsible for $50 worth of purchases. Generally, however, most credit-card issuers do not press to collect anything from owners of lost, stolen, or misused cards.

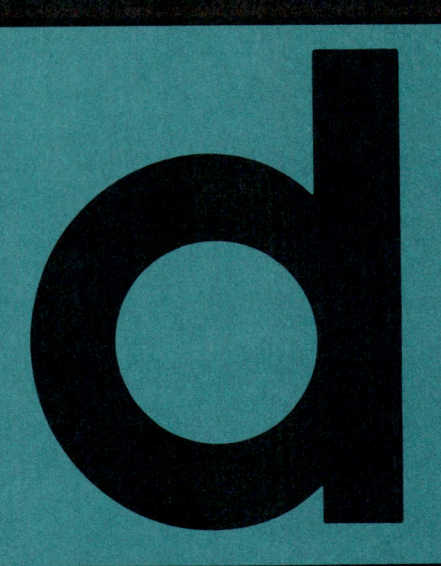

decorating

decorating
diet
dining out
drinks

decorating

candles
dos and don'ts for winter candlelight

How can you warm up a wintery room without hiking up your fuel bill? Try candles. Their cozy glow will warm the atmosphere even without raising the temperature. These dos and don'ts—most from Holly Scaringi at Bailiwick Candle Shop in New York—can make candles shine brighter and last longer.

- DO clean dusty candles by rubbing gently with a soft cloth moistened with lighter fluid or cleaning fluid.
- DO put candles in the refrigerator (*not* the freezer) a half hour before lighting to make them burn longer.
- DO prevent votive glasses from cracking by pouring in a teaspoon of water as a cooler. Remove the metal clip from an old votive before inserting a new one.
- DON'T sit candles in a draft or they'll drip, burn unevenly, and possibly collapse. For problem candles that start to smoke, try trimming the wick to 1/2".
- DO buy beeswax candles instead of paraffin. They cost double but burn two to three times longer, are smokeless, dripless, and glow translucently.
- DON'T fix candles to a holder with the usual melted wax—instead, try sticky candle adhesive. Wax hardens, so your candle may snap off with the first jolt, but adhesive stays pliable.
- DO try "bobêches," disks that you slip around the candle base to catch drippings.
- DO store candles flat in a drawer if you don't plan to use them for a while, or they may bend from the heat in an unventilated room.

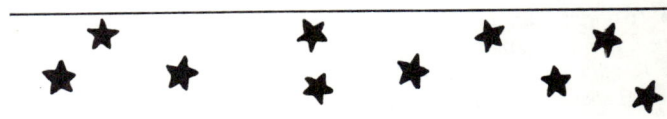

ceiling
for a great view of things— decorate your ceiling

If you're like most people, your ceiling is probably the last thing you consider when decorating. Too bad, because ceiling art can give a brand new look to a room. You don't have to be a Michelangelo to do it — just check out the projects below, all fairly inexpensive and easy to do.

How would you like waking up to a lovely "sky" ceiling, complete with wispy clouds? First paint the ceiling a soft sky-blue color (roller painting is the easiest and quickest way); let dry. Then dip a piece of terry toweling into white enamel (just enough to coat the cloth lightly) and dab clouds onto the background. This method creates a wonderful wispy effect that looks like real clouds.

For a starry, nighttime ceiling, paint with a deep navy blue. Then stick on stars that you've cut from silver- or gold-toned self-adhesive paper; or use precut stars (from a dime store) and apply with wallpaper paste. You can buy some that even glow in the dark. For the ambitious decorator, get a book on constellations and design your own "Ursa Major" and "Ursa Minor."

Colored adhesive tapes, available in most five-and-tens, paint, or stationery stores, are ideal for border stripes. Or use them in a child's room to make simple shapes like triangles, squares, or zig-zags.

Another idea that's fabulous for a child's room is using precut letters and numbers that you can buy at hardware or paint stores. Stick them on randomly or paper the ceiling with the alphabet. If you can't find colors you like, make them yourself from self-adhesive paper.

One of the easiest and prettiest decorating ideas is simply to cut and paste pictures along the edges or at the corners of a ceiling. Good motifs for a kitchen are fruit or vegetables; for a bedroom or bath, shells or flowers; for a nursery, animals or toys.

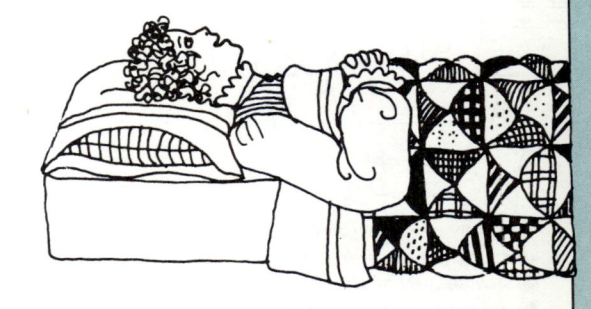

closet
give your closet a clean and new look

If cleaning your closet usually consists of rearranging the clothes you're still hoping will come back in style, take a new approach—do something special with the closet itself.

Think in terms of giving your closet a little class. If it's a hall closet that guests can peek into when you hang their coats, try coordinating the closet with the overall color scheme and tone of your entrance way

d decorating

or front room. For a bedroom closet, add some pizzazz so you'll look forward to opening it.
- Paint the inside a high-gloss white or a bright color, or apply self-adhesive paper—silver or blue Mylar would be dazzling. Consider covering the wall with fabric, using a staple gun. (If the closet rung can't be removed, slit the fabric up from the bottom to just above the rung, lift the fabric around it, and then staple the slit closed to the wall.) Lay an old piece of carpeting or stick-on tiles on the floor.
- To brighten up a dreary closet, have a light installed or investigate the "no wires, no plug" type at a hardware store.
- Get the most from available space by double-hanging clothes. Buy an expansion rod at a department store and stretch it halfway between the closet rung and the floor. Recycle extra hangers back to the dry cleaners.
- Utilize your closet door. Hang a mirror or narrow shelves with a raised, protective edge, or a shoe bag. (Even if you prefer keeping your shoes elsewhere, the shoe bag pockets are good for holding socks, pantyhose, and underwear.) A pegboard is great for storage—attach it to the door with special screws available from a hardware store; then use pegboard hooks to hang scarves, caps, and jewelry.
- Make a pretty pillowcase into a garment bag. Slit the top enough for hanger to fit through and you have a terrific cover for skirts, shirts, or jackets you want to store.

desk super ways to cheer up a dreary desk

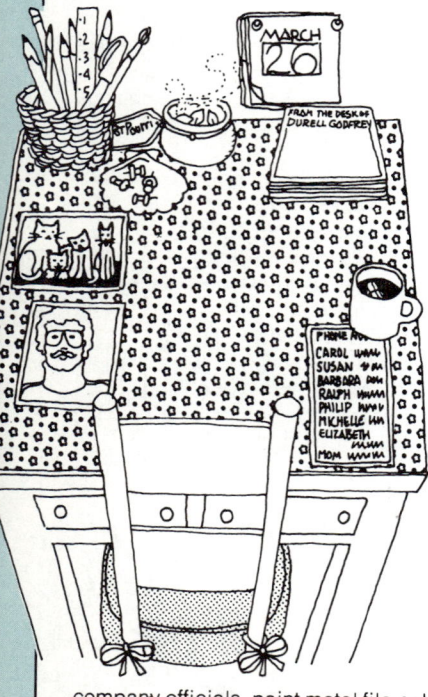

When your desk at the office or in your apartment becomes your second home, it's worth taking a little time to make it a cheerful one. Here are some ideas. (Of course, if your office has strict regulations, you'll have to check out your limitations.)
- Use wicker baskets instead of the usual pencil holders and catchalls. You might file a rainbow assortment of papers in a flat, plate-shaped basket, or a bunch of pencils in a narrow rectangular one.
- Cover a desk blotter with an attractive print fabric, taped to the back. Sew a matching cushion for your desk chair, attaching it to the back support with ties. You can also cover several file folders with the same fabric, using spray adhesive.
- If you have permission from company officials, paint metal file cabinets, in/out boxes, or wastebaskets a bright color. A soft yellow or blue can add a ray of sunlight to an otherwise gray affair.
- Put a collection of small framed pictures or treasures on your desk. A beautiful clam shell or carved wood box can hold paper clips or rubber bands; a piece of coral or a painted rock can be a paperweight. A small brandy snifter easily holds loose matchbooks, rubber bands, and other odds and ends.
- Keep an apothecary jar on your desk to store your personal treats—cookies, wrapped candies, or a mixture of raisins and nuts.
- To relieve desk-top overcrowding, think "up." You may be able to have your phone mounted on the wall, install a shelf over it, or find a wall-mounted in/out box. (You can also use two wall-mounted wicker baskets for in/out boxes.) An architect's lamp that clamps to the desk takes up less space than a lamp that sits on it.
- No place for plants on your desk? Try a terrarium-sized variety in a tiny straw basket or planter.
- If your typewriter takes up the lion's share of space on your desk, invest in a typing table or a small square Parsons table to use instead. Have casters put on so it can be rolled around easily.
- Let a slight but not overwhelming (some people are very sensitive to it) scent waft from your desk by keeping an aromatic potpourri in one corner.
- Cover the bulletin board near your desk with a bright fabric or a gift wrap. Attach with a staple gun or pushpins.
- Have a piece of glass cut to the size of your desk top. For color, place a sheet of fabric, gift wrap, or self-adhesive paper underneath the glass. Photographs or cutouts from magazines look good under glass, too, as do a child's artwork or your own collages.

fireplace romanticize your fire at home, ski lodge, or camp

The cheery, crackling glow of a fire is a treat in itself, but if you can make a good thing better, why not!
- Leftover orange or apple peels buried in the fire give a lovely homey scent. Stud the peels with a few cloves for an even spicier aroma.
- Increase the fragrance of your fire with the wood you burn. Although some varieties are more costly or scarce, their subtle fruity scent is worth the effort. You can also combine the more expensive woods with less expensive ones like pine. Try apple, cherry, cedar, hemlock, or maple for the fragrance.
- Pine cones, pine needles, or hickory chips are also inexpensive, sweet-smelling additions to any fire.
- Special fireplace incense is another idea to try. You'll find it wherever fireplace equipment is sold, or use regular incense.
- Add color works to your fire with color nuggets or chips—just toss them in and watch the colors shoot out from the flames.
- You can buy special logs that burn with brilliantly colored flames—a bit expensive, but worth the show.
- A less costly way to color your flames is to burn colored paper—magazine pages are perfect; the color section of the newspaper works too (the colored ink provides the color).
- You might make your own color logs by buying a gadget called the newspaper log roller, available in fireplace departments and hardware stores. Simply roll colored pages in with regular newspaper.

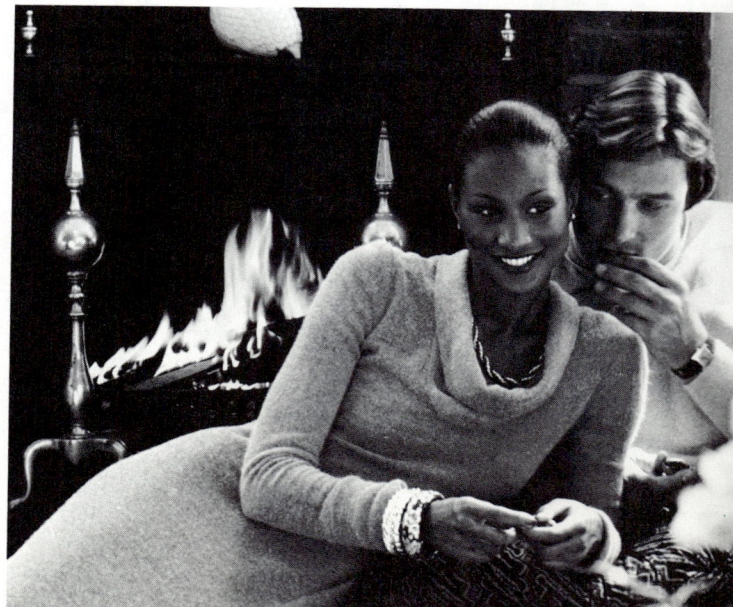

decorating

wall arrangements
how to arrange pictures and objects on a wall

Before you hang anything—pictures, pieces of sculpture, or china—first decide how much of the wall area you want to cover. Then cut newspaper or brown paper to the area size and plot the arrangement on the floor. For a room that is basically modern, an asymmetrical wall arrangement is often the most dynamic. Establish two sides of the grouping so as to form a right angle; this will give you two straight lines and will help in working out the asymmetry. With antique furniture, a simple arrangement works well—the largest object in the center, smaller elements on sides and bottom. For an eclectic taste, anything goes. To make sure that you hang your objects right where you want them:
1. Mark the exact center of the frame with a pencil.
2. Hold the frame where you want it on the wall and make a light pencil mark on the wall in line with the center of the frame.
3. With the back of the frame facing you, hang the wire on your finger and measure the distance between the top of the taut wire and the top of the frame.
4. Measure that same distance down from the mark you have made on the wall. This will give you the point at which to hammer in the nail or the bottom of the hook. (Put a small X of cellophane tape over the spot to help prevent the plaster from cracking.)

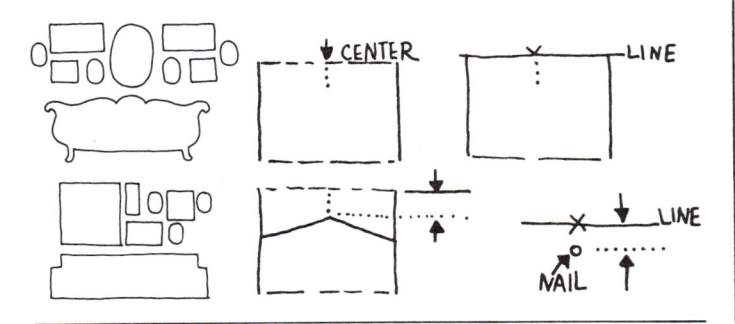

wall hangings
43 things to hang on a wall besides paintings and posters

If staring at the same four walls is driving you to boredom, why not brighten them with any of these inexpensive and ready-made hangings.
- *Campaign or other buttons, bead necklaces, pins, ropes of shells, bumper stickers, and almost anything not too heavy.* Either mount these on a piece of corrugated cardboard that is covered with felt or velvet, or work out your own unique display.
- *Baskets.* Suspend baskets with handles from cup hooks set into a shelf, molding, or wall. (You can bend cup hooks with pliers to slip baskets over them more easily.) Hang flat, loosely woven baskets from a nail that is slipped through a hole in the weave. Try different-shaped baskets grouped together, inside bottoms facing out.
- *Bicycles.* Yes, you can! Ask any hardware store for strong hooks that can be set into a ceiling—the kind used to hang swinging "basket" chairs. After a friend helps you install them, you can hang the bike from the hooks using chains, "stretch cords," or even pulleys.
- *Hanging rugs or quilts.* Both contribute to a warm and cozy atmosphere. Hang rugs by driving small nails through the corners or attaching picture wire and hanging as a painting. Sew small café-curtain rings to the top of a quilt and slip over a rod you can attach to the wall,

or hang the rings on picture nails.
- *Trays, trivets, place mats, door mats, or Japanese tatami (floor) mats.* Some are so unusual that no one will guess their true identity when hung in rooms other than the kitchen. You might mount or frame exceptionally beautiful mats.
- *Squares of exquisite fabric, gift wrap, wallpaper, or a scarf you'd rather hang than wear.* Glue fabric or paper to a white matting board from an art supply store, leaving a 2" to 3" margin all around; frame with a narrow wooden frame, painted a bright color if you wish.
- *Folding Oriental screens, mock road signs or billboards, and other heavy objects.* Rest any of these on L-shaped brackets (some can fill an entire wall by themselves).
- *Clothing such as floppy or slouch-brimmed hats, souvenir T-shirts, shawls, capes, ponchos, and Mexican serapes.* These can be hung in many ways—try displaying larger items on big "boutique" clothes hangers in different colors, clipping smaller ones with small plastic clothespins to a fishnet stretched across a wall.
- *Attractive shopping bags, menus, magazine covers, or maps.* Sand and shellac a piece of plywood a few inches larger than the item, then attach it to the wood with white glue. Add gloss by spraying with a clear plastic spray.
- *Kites, fans, clocks, plates, brass horns or anchors, sconces, plants (in macramé, leather, or ceramic planters), and hub caps or reflector lights from auto shops.* Any of these can enliven a wall that's too plain or break the monotony of a cluster of flat, framed prints. Take your item to any hardware store and ask for the appropriate mount or hook.

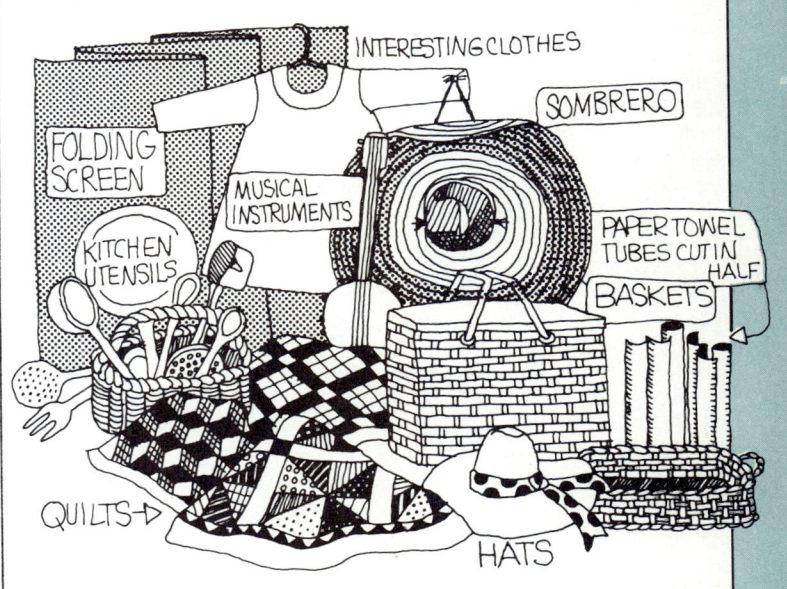

windows
11 choices for windows instead of curtains

If you want something more imaginative than curtains to make a window look special, here are some choices that will turn any window into a good-looking inside view.
- *Plants*—either hanging like curtains, in handsome pots held by chains or macramé, or sitting on shelves across the window. Both provide beautiful growing coverage, either foliage or flowering.
- *Baubles or beads*—make strings of beads (wooden, glass, plastic, or mixed) as long as your window, then tie to brass curtain rings, however many you need to span the window. Space at close intervals on a curtain rod. Or you could style a curtain by painting empty wooden spools of thread with bright colors and stringing them on ribbons or monofilament wire.

d decorating

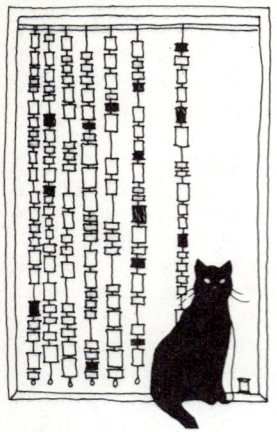

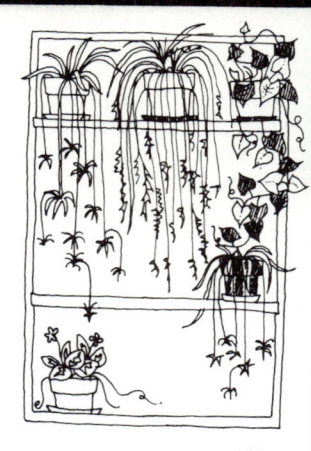

- **Pots and pans**—great idea for a kitchen window. Put curtain rods at several levels across the window and hang your pots and pans from them with S hooks. The better-looking and more colorful your pots, the prettier the window will be.
- **Prints or paintings plus storage**—don't overlook the possibility of covering a window (without much light or a view) to give yourself storage space with eye appeal. Build shelves across the window. Then hinge a big framed print or painting to one side of the window frame to cover the shelves. If the window frames are not deep enough and your shelves protrude, hang the painting from the top shelf so that it can be lifted up to give you access to the storage.
- **Stained-glass windows**—suspend one in front of any ordinary window for a stunning effect. You can use a brass hardware chain and eye hooks to do the job.
- **Stencils or murals**—you can either cover the whole pane or do several small designs that will allow more light in. Buy a stenciling kit or check art supply stores for individual stencils and paints for glass.
- **Shades**—pick up your wallpaper pattern or repeat pillow designs or coordinate with special colors in the room. You can glue any fabric or apply self-adhesive onto regular shades or buy do-it-yourself kits in stores.
- **Screens**—free-standing folding ones make dressy window fronts. Some of the most beautiful and inventive screens can be made from simple frames of wood hinged together, then filled in with leather, either in strips or solid decorated panels, with macramé, needlepoint, printed fabric, or shimmery heavyweight foil.
- **Books**—again if the view and the light are poor, don't hesitate to block a window. Shelves set up across a useless window make a good library extension, particularly a collection of cookbooks in a kitchen window.
- **Flags, pennants, or banners**—you can make your own or pick them up at auctions or in antique or thrift shops. For a festive air, hang them from wooden curtain rods just as you would curtains.
- **Wooden frames**—make a narrow plywood frame to go all around a window. Cover the frame with pretty fabric, self-adhesive paper, or even wallpaper for a handsome effect.

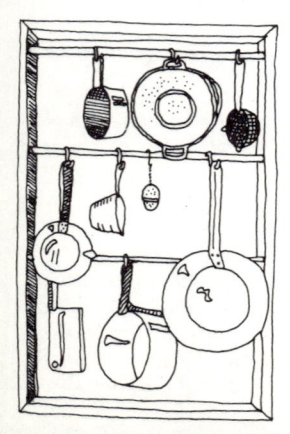

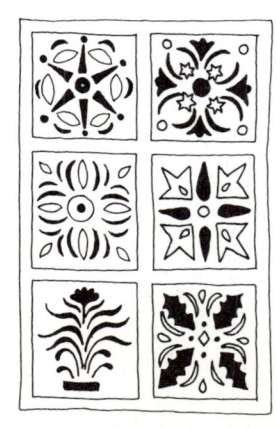

diet

ball games
eating during the game so you don't rack up more calories than points

While you're watching football or baseball games, you may be taking in more calories than action. To make sure you don't blow your diet from the bleachers, check the following list. If some calorie counts are too steep, why not bring your own low-calorie substitutes, such as fresh fruit or a container of clear soup?

snack	calories
1 hot dog on a roll with mustard and sauerkraut	290
3-oz. hamburger on a roll with ketchup	386
Ice-cream sandwich	173
Chocolate-coated vanilla ice-cream bar	162
½ c. shelled, roasted peanuts	400
4-oz. box of Cracker Jacks	434
10 potato chips	114
5 small pretzel sticks	20
1½-oz. bag of corn chips	249
1 c. plain popcorn	54
1 c. popcorn with 2 T. butter	254
8-oz. cola	96
8-oz. orange soda	117

boosters 3 easy boosters for dieters

Even the most successful dieter needs an occasional booster. Two doctors and their associates at the University of Pennsylvania's psychiatry department asked their overweight patients to try the following eating guidelines—which we think could work well for you, too:
- First, confine all eating, including snacking, to just one place. (This may help to break your straight-from-the-refrigerator snacking habit.)
- Second, to further discourage yourself from grabbing meals on-the-run, use a distinctive table setting, including a place mat and napkin of an unusual color.
- Third, make eating a pure activity that involves nothing else. Don't, for example, eat while poring over a newspaper. In addition, try counting every mouthful, and after every third mouthful, put the utensils back on the plate until the mouthful has been swallowed. These tips work like a dieter's string around the finger to remind you not only that you are on a diet, but also to slow down and think about what you are putting into your mouth.

diet

cheese — how to save calories on cheese

Nibbling on cheeses can mean taking in a heap of extra calories—or a little—depending on which ones you choose. For instance, cottage and farmer cheeses net you only about 30 calories per ounce, but Gouda has 120. Look over the ones listed below—you may be surprised at the 1-oz. calorie count:

● cheese	● calories
Camembert	85
Cheddar	113
Colby	111
Gorgonzola	112
Gruyère	110
Leyden	80
Mozzarella	79
Neufchâtel	70
Port du Salut	100
Sap Sago	76
Swiss	105

fast foods — can you have your diet and McDonald's, too?

The trouble with a scoop of Rocky Road ice cream is that it's a particularly rocky road to travel if you're on a diet. Still, the calorie count (204) might not be quite as high as you suspected—and it seems almost dietetic when compared with the count (557) for a McDonald's Big Mac. These and other fast-food calorie counts (approximate) may or may not confirm your worst suspicions.

Arby's: "Junior roast beef sandwich"—240; regular roast beef sandwich—429; turkey sandwich without Arby's dressing—337; with dressing—402; "ham 'n cheese"—458; Arby's "Super" roast beef sandwich—705.

Arthur Treacher's Fish & Chips: One piece of fish—172; one serving of chips—274; cole slaw—122.

Baskin-Robbins: One scoop (2½ oz.) with sugar cone: Chocolate Fudge—229; French Vanilla—217; Rocky Road—204; Butter Pecan—195; Jamoca Almond Fudge—190; Chocolate Mint—189; Jamoca—182; Strawberry—168; Peach—165.

Burger King: The "Whopper"—630; the "Whaler"—744; bag of French fries (2¾ oz.)—220; large shake—360; hamburger—250; cheeseburger—305; hot dog—291.

Carvel: A standard 3-oz. cup of Vanilla ice cream—148; Chocolate ice cream—147; Sherbet—105; Vanilla, Chocolate, or Coffee Thinny-Thin—55.5.

Chicken Delight: Average adult portion (one ½ chicken, 4 pieces)—625.

Colonel Sanders' Kentucky Fried Chicken: 15-piece bucket—3300; drumstick—220; "3-piece special"—660; "dinner" (with 3 pieces of chicken, cole slaw, mashed potatoes, gravy, roll)—980.

Dairy Queen: Average banana split—547; "Super Brazier"—875; "Brazier" French fries—200.

Dunkin' Donuts: Hole-in-the-middle "cake" donuts: plain cake—240; plain honey-dipped—260; plain with white icing—265; plain with chocolate icing—235; chocolate cake—240; chocolate honey-dipped—250. "Yeast-raised" donuts with jelly, custard, or cream fillings: sugared—205; honey-dipped—225 (add 40–50 calories for fillings).

Hardee's: "Huskee Deluxe"—525; "Huskee Junior"—475; fish sandwich—275; hot dog—265; apple turnover—290; average serving (2-oz.) French fries—155; milk shake (8-oz.)—320.

Howard Johnson's: Small cone: vanilla—186, chocolate—195; medium cone: vanilla—275, chocolate—291; large cone: vanilla—370, chocolate—390; any flavor sherbet—136. (Attention fans of fried clams and pecan pie: according to *The Brand-Name Calorie Counter*, 7-oz. pkg. Hojo's frozen fried clams—357; ⅛ of a 2-lb. pecan pie—474.)

Lum's: "The Ollie Burger" (5½ oz. ground beef "with secret herbs and spices")—calories are a secret, too, but 5½ oz. of broiled ground beef without a roll has 448. Average ounces in other Lum's portions, easily translated into calories with any pocket counter: fried onion rings—5½ oz.; hamburgers—4½ oz.

McDonald's: Egg McMuffin—312; Hamburger—249; Cheeseburger—309; Quarter Pounder—414; Quarter Pounder with Cheese—521; Big Mac—557; Filet-O-Fish—406; French fries—215; Apple Pie—265; Chocolate Shake—317; Vanilla Shake—332; Strawberry Shake—315.

Taco Bell: One taco—160; tostada—200; order of frijoles—230; enchirito—400; burrito—340; "Bellburger"—240.

White Castle: Hamburger—165; serving of French fries—219; cheeseburger—198; fish sandwich—200; milk shake—213; serving of onion rings—341.

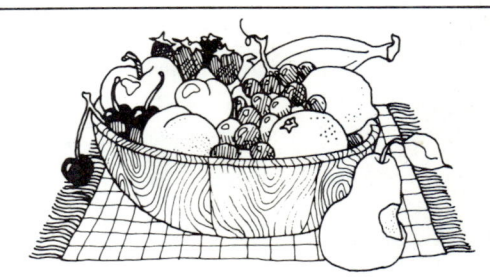

fruit — a calorie countdown on fruit

● fruit	● calories
Medium apple	80
3 small apricots	58
Medium banana	101
½ cantaloupe	40
½ c. whole sweet cherries	40
½ medium grapefruit	55
½ c. Concord grapes	33
½ c. white grapes	58
Medium nectarine	73
Navel orange	58
Medium peach	35
Medium pear	100
3-oz. slice pineapple	44
4 dried prunes	70
½ c. raisins	236
1 c. strawberries	53
4" × 8" slice watermelon	115

d diet

lo-cal substitutes
that taste good and satisfy

After lots of partying, a vacation, or holiday splurges, a diet can seem more difficult than usual to start or go back to. The chart below can help you ease into it naturally; fattening foods (both treats and staples) are listed, plus lower-calorie substitutes that look, taste, or satisfy almost as well.

for this	substitute this	calories saved
● **meat, fish, fowl**		
Roast duck (3 oz., 310)	Roast chicken (3 oz., 160)	150
Pork sausage (3 oz., 405)	Lean boiled ham (3 oz., 200)	205
Rib lamb chop (3 oz., 405)	Leg lamb roast (3 oz., 160)	245
Pork chop (3 oz., 340)	Veal chop (3 oz., 185)	155
Porterhouse steak (3 oz., 290)	Round steak (3 oz., 200)	90
Tuna, canned (3 oz., 165)	Salmon, canned (3 oz., 115)	50
● **fruits, vegetables**		
Potatoes, fried (1 c., 400)	Potatoes, mashed (1 c., 160)	240
Winter squash (1 c., 75)	Summer squash (1 c., 30)	45
Lima beans (1 c., 150)	Green beans (1 c., 30)	120
Creamed corn (1 c., 185)	Regular corn (1 c., 140)	45
Honeydew (½, 5″ dia., 65)	Cantaloupe (½, 5″ dia., 40)	25
Peach in syrup (2 halves, 80)	Peach, medium (50)	30
● **snacks, desserts**		
Potato chips (ten, 115)	Pretzels (10 small sticks, 35)	80
Apple Betty (1 c., 345)	Applesauce, no sugar (1 c., 100)	245
Cupcake/white icing (230)	Cupcake/no icing (115)	115
Cookies, assorted (3″ dia., 120)	Ladyfinger (35)	85
Lemon meringue pie (slice, 305)	Lemon gelatin (½ c., 70)	235
● **beverages**		
Whole milk (8 oz., 165)	Skim/buttermilk (8 oz., 80)	85
Orange juice (4 oz., 50)	Tomato juice (4 oz., 25)	25
Cocoa with milk (8 oz., 235)	Cocoa with water (8 oz., 140)	95
Coffee, 2 lumps sugar, 1 T. cream (1 c., 110)	Coffee, no-cal sweetener, nondairy creamer (1 c., 11)	99
Sweet wine, 20% alcohol (4 oz., 180)	Dry wine, 12% alcohol (4 oz., 100)	80
Old Fashioned (2 oz., 200)	Manhattan (2 oz., 140)	60
● **dairy, cereals, bread**		
Egg, scrambled (one, 110)	Egg, poached (one, 80)	30
Toast and butter (170)	Toast and apple butter (90)	80
Sour cream (1 c., 455)	Yogurt, plain (1 c., 135)	320
Ice cream, rich (4 oz., 250)	Ices (4 oz., 170)	80
Cheese—bleu, Cheddar, Swiss, cream (1 oz., 105)	Cottage cheese, uncreamed (1 oz., 80)	25
Bran flakes (1 c., 120)	Corn flakes (1 c., 95)	25

lunch
brown-bag lunches with more style and fewer calories

Brown-bagging it sounds at first like a great idea. It saves you both money and time on your lunch hour, but eventually you get bored with the fare. You can also find yourself consuming too many calories if you fall into the sandwich syndrome. There are many other good-tasting and thinning foods you can bring to the office and really enjoy eating.

● The one-serving size of frozen shrimp or crab cocktail is ideal for an office lunch. Take one from the freezer when you leave for work, and by the time you're ready to eat, it will be defrosted but still lovely and cool. With a piece of fresh fruit, it's satisfying and thinning.

● Marinate leftover vegetables—mushrooms, green beans, carrots, and asparagus—in low-calorie dressing. Let them sit in the dressing in the refrigerator overnight. Next morning, put them in a plastic container and bring for lunch. They'll be tasty and will keep through the morning without refrigeration.

● Make yourself a salade Niçoise. Drain a can of water-packed tuna and empty into a small plastic container. Add a quartered hard-boiled egg, a couple of tomato wedges, some black olives, and a generous squeeze of lemon juice. Add just a few drops of olive oil, close the plastic container, and shake gently to mix. Let it marinate all morning at your desk, and prepare for a delicious meal.

● Raw vegetable sticks and hard-boiled eggs are easy to pack and very low in calories. Although not the most inspired eating, they're fine when interspersed with more exotic fare, especially on mornings when you're in a hurry.

● If you're lucky enough to have some leftover broiled or roasted chicken, a bit of steak, or roast beef, these, too, can be brown-bag fare.

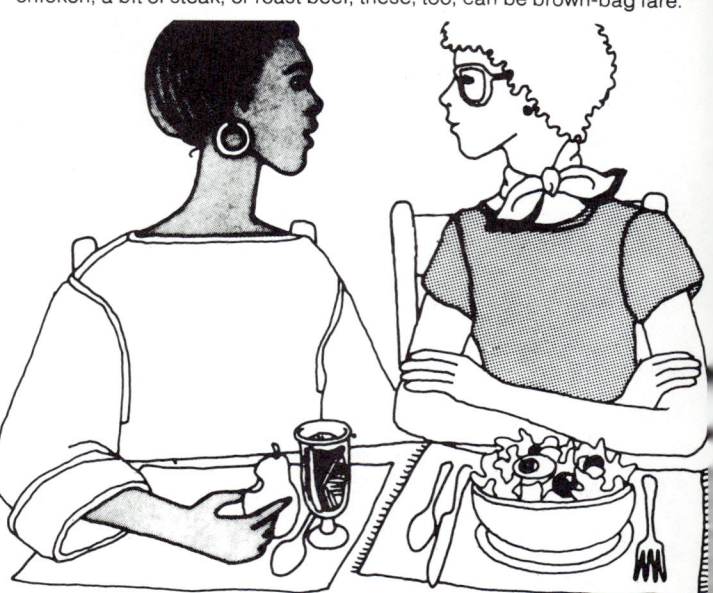

sandwiches
find the sandwich to fit your calorie budget

Few people, especially Americans, can resist a sandwich indefinitely, so be aware of these facts. Rather than eating a sandwich from a coffee shop, make it yourself on thin-sliced bread, knocking off 42 calories. The coffee shop alternative is to eat only one of the pieces of regular-sliced bread in your sandwich—you'll lop off about 60 calories. One tablespoon of mayonnaise adds 110 calories to any sandwich, but the same amount of mustard adds only about 10. Before you order your next sandwich, read this chart.

● sandwich (on regular white bread, no butter or mayonnaise)	● calories
Cucumber (6 med. slices)	126
Lettuce, tomato (1 lettuce leaf, 1 med. tomato)	153
Sliced chicken (1 slice 3″ x 3″ x ¼″)	199
Sliced egg (1 large hard-boiled egg)	200
Sliced turkey (1 slice 3″ x 3″ x ¼″)	200
Cottage cheese and tomato (4 T. cottage cheese, 1 med. tomato)	212
Ham (1 slice, baked)	220
Cheese (Swiss, 1 slice)	220
Roast beef (1 slice)	245
Bacon, lettuce, tomato (2 strips bacon, lettuce leaf, 1 med. tomato)	248
Hamburger (3-oz. patty with bun)	332
Chicken salad (4 T. with mayonnaise and celery)	367
Tuna salad (2 oz. tuna, 1 T. mayonnaise)	395

diet

Soups: (8-oz. can)
chicken noodle ... 125
split pea ... 265
tomato ... 160
vegetable ... 140
Beef stew (8 oz.) ... 155
Pork and beans (8 oz.) ... 280
Spaghetti with meatballs (8 oz.) ... 250
Ham sandwich ... 275
Hot dog with bun, mustard ... 270
Hamburger with bun, ketchup ... 440
Tossed green salad, French dressing ... 65

vitamin C
great low-calorie, high-vitamin-C foods

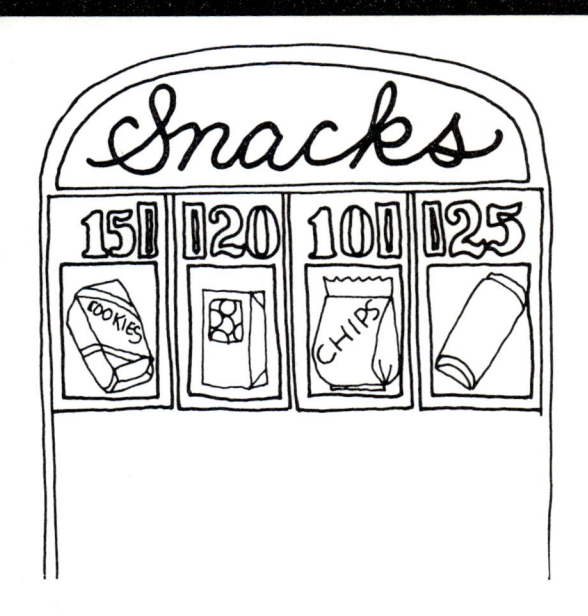

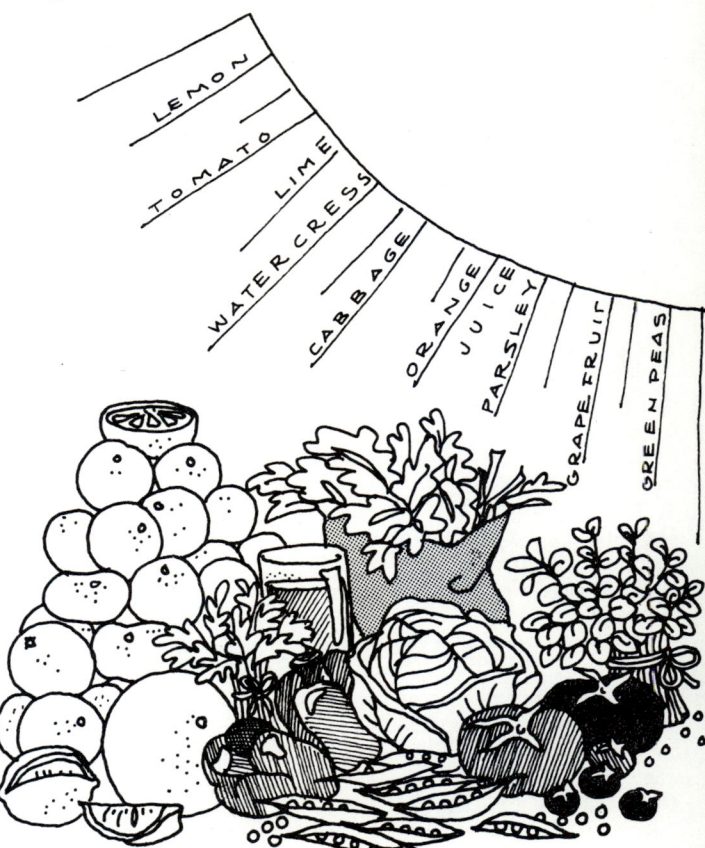

snacks calorie counts for what's in vending machines

If you can't pass a vending machine without whipping out spare change for anything from Life Savers to hot dogs, reading the chart below may help you break the habit. The chart lists approximate calorie counts for common vending-machine snacks. (Some may be actually *less* fattening than you expected and worth an occasional splurge.)

● cookies, chips, nuts   ● calories
Cheese Peanut Butter Sandwich Cookies (6, 1½ oz.) ... 210
Cheese and crackers (4, 1⅛ oz.) ... 125
Corn chips (1 oz.) ... 240
Fig Newton Cakes (2, 2 oz.) ... 208
Lorna Doones (6, 1½ oz.) ... 207
Oreo Creme Sandwich Cookies (6, 1⅝ oz.) ... 227
Peanuts (1¼ oz.) ... 225
Potato chips (1 oz.) ... 160

● candies, gum
Chocolate bar (plain, 1⅛ oz.) ... 160
Clark Bar (1⅛ oz.) ... 165
Fudgies (each one) ... 50
Gum (most brands, per stick) ... 10
Life Savers (per candy): cinnamon, peppermint, wintergreen, spearmint ... 7
   Other flavors ... 10
M & M's Plain Chocolate Candies (1.2 oz.) ... 168
M & M's Peanut Chocolate Candies (1.2 oz.) ... 169
Mars Almond Bar (1.5 oz.) ... 202
Milky Way Bar (1⅞₁₆ oz.) ... 203
Snickers Bar (1.4 oz.) ... 182
Vanilla Caramel Bars (each one) ... 50
Zag Nut Bar (1¼ oz.) ... 165
$100,000 Bar (1¼ oz.) ... 175

● ice cream
Orange cream bar (5½ oz.) ... 103
Vanilla ice-cream pop (5½ oz.) ... 150
Vanilla ice-cream sandwich (5½ oz.) ... 175

● lunch foods
Drinks:
   grapefruit juice (5.5-oz. can) ... 60
   orange juice (5.5-oz. can) ... 70
   pineapple juice, unsweetened (5.5-oz. can) ... 85
   tomato juice (5.5-oz. can) ... 30
   chocolate drink (½ pint) ... 150
   chocolate milk (½ pint) ... 205
   skimmed/buttermilk (¼ pint) ... 90
   whole milk (¼ pint) ... 160
Creamed cottage cheese (3 oz.) ... 90
Hard-boiled egg, 2 Saltines ... 115

If you believe in a hefty intake of vitamin C, you can eat a lot more of the fresh vitamin-C foods on this list happily, without piling up calories.

● food   ● calories
Watercress (1 cup trimmed) ... 6
Green pepper (1 medium) ... 15
Grapefruit (½) ... 55
Tangerine (1 medium) ... 40
Fresh orange juice (8 oz.) ... 110
Peas (1 cup cooked) ... 116
Tomato (1 small) ... 24
Spinach (1 cup chopped) ... 14
Parsley (1 T. chopped) ... 1
Cabbage (1 cup cooked) ... 32

55

d dining out

dining out

Chinese food
is more than chow mein and wonton soup

Be more daring in your choice of Chinese food and you'll be rewarded with some delicate and unusual tastes, plus a boost in the diet department. Chinese food, thanks to its emphasis on fresh, low-calorie vegetables and relatively uncaloric sauces, is much less fattening than most other restaurant food. It's fun to order a different dish for everyone at your table so you can sample a little of each. Try these:

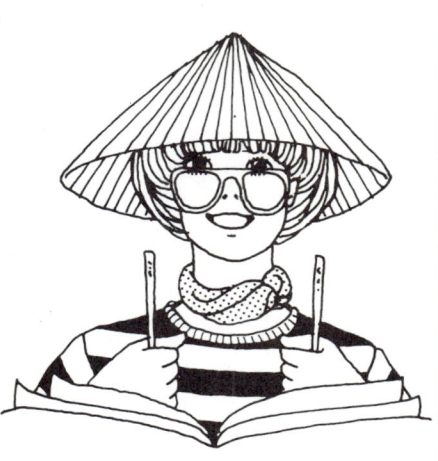

● **appetizers**

Hot and sour soup is a gently spiced, tart mixture of broth, mushrooms, bamboo shoots, and ribbons of egg and pork. The flavor is delicate but tangy.

Spring rolls are sophisticated egg rolls with thinner crusts and more varied fillings.

● **main dishes**

Moo Shu Pork is a delectable dish of eggs, pork, and assorted vegetables scrambled together and served with thin pancakes. You spoon the pork mixture onto the pancakes, roll them up, and eat them with your fingers.

Moo Goo Gai Pan is sliced chicken with button mushrooms in a light sauce.

Shrimp with sizzling rice is shrimp in a light tomato sauce, served with rice that's been cooked until it's very hot and almost crisp. When the hot sauce hits it, it actually sizzles. You can order many meat dishes with sizzling rice.

● **sauces for main dishes**

Hoisin sauce is brown and spicy-sweet. Order it with shrimp or almost any meat.

Black bean sauce is pungent and salty. Lobster with black bean sauce is a favorite combination.

● **desserts**

Chinese traditionally eat fresh fruit for dessert, but popular restaurant choices are tart kumquats, sugary lichees or loquats (similar to apricots), or candied fruits.

chopsticks
Oriental dining etiquette

There's more to eating with chopsticks than just trying to master the pencil grip without getting a writer's cramp by the end of the meal. Chopstick etiquette reflects an Oriental culture that emphasizes unity, balance, and symmetry in the arts, plus compatibility with nature in all aspects of life, including cooking and eating. Many connoisseurs of Oriental food will use only bamboo chopsticks, insisting that a metal fork or spoon ruins the natural balance and taste of the food. However, some people prefer ivory or even plastic, and more elegant table settings have included jade, amber, or silver chopsticks.

Carefully prepared and seasoned by the chef, Oriental food is meant to be relished and eaten morsel by morsel with kuai-tsi (chopsticks in Chinese), which sounds like the Chinese words for "quick little boys." It is the Chinese custom to eat community-style, with numerous dishes for everyone to share instead of one dish per person. In Hong Kong, the lazy Susan is the focal point of the dining table.

Here are some Chinese customs to help you feast the native way and maybe even spur you on to a new style of eating:

● Rice should be pushed directly into the mouth, using chopsticks, from the bowl held in your hand; it should not be picked up.

● When getting food from dishes at the center of the table, it's good manners to pick up the piece that is closest to you, instead of reaching over the plate for that far piece of chicken drumstick you really want.

● Use the top end of your chopsticks when passing food to another person. (One way you can get that drumstick is if someone sitting opposite you knows your tastes.)

● Eating Chinese style is a continuous motion—you should serve yourself food one piece at a time (as it is eaten) instead of filling your plate all at once.

● If the pair of chopsticks at your place setting are unequal in length, it can mean you'll miss a plane, train, or the like.

● Dropping chopsticks can bring bad luck, and some Chinese respond with a phrase comparable to saying "God bless you" when someone sneezes.

● Placing your chopsticks together neatly across your rice bowl is a gesture indicating that you've finished your meal.

Hold one chopstick as you would a pencil, see right, about two thirds of the way up. Slide the other chopstick between your thumb and index finger, directly below.

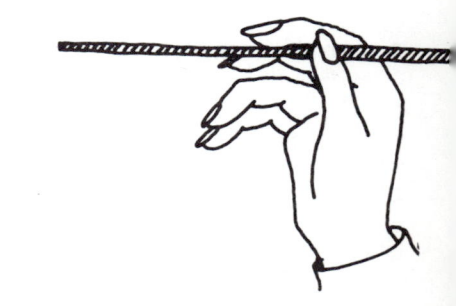

Some people, of course, vary this basic grip slightly—but it's important in all cases to keep the bottom chopstick stationary.

To pick up food, move the top chopstick up and down by bending index and middle fingers to meet the stationary bottom chopstick.

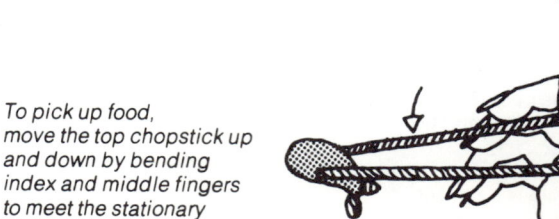

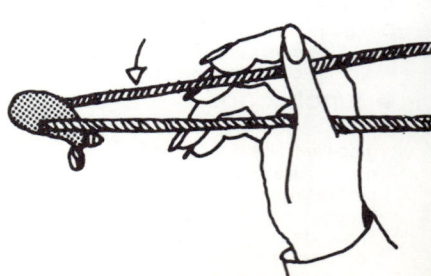

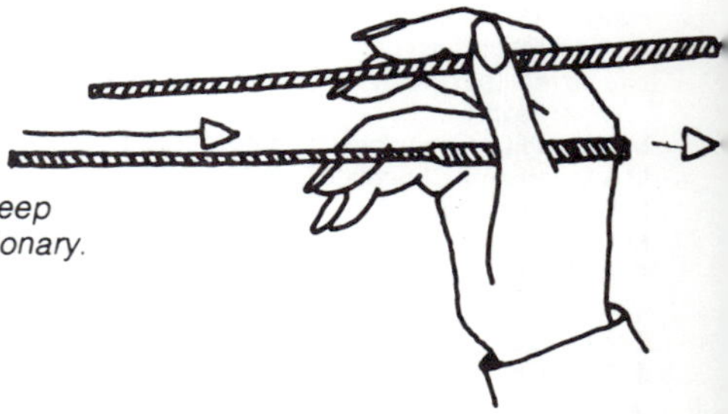

… dining out

French menu
a guide to reading a French menu

If one look at a French menu makes you wish you were ordering a Big Mac instead of trying to translate "foies de volaille à la Bordelaise," check the guide below. It will trim this and other elaborate descriptions down to basics—which, for any French dish, are simply the words that translate the main ingredient, its sauce or garnish, plus the way it's all prepared.

- **how is the food prepared?**
- Key words often give clues (see following tips), but don't be put off if you can't translate a dish. Descriptive words such as *à la maison* describe how a particular restaurant fixes the dish. It may not be duplicated anywhere else. If you're stumped, ask. Even in France, part of the fun is a certain amount of discussion about how a dish is prepared.
- You're off to a good start if you know the food is *rôti* (roasted); *grillé* (grilled); *poché* (poached); *bouilli* (boiled); *frit* (deep-fried); or *sauté* (quick-fried).
- Stew or casseroles are often tagged *ragoût, navarin, daube,* or *blanquette*—as in *blanquette de veau* (veal stew) or *navarin agneau* (lamb stew). Also worth remembering are traditional *bouillabaisse* (a seafood stew) and *cassoulet* (a beans-and-meat casserole).
- For hamburger diehards, *haché* or *fricadelle* spell "ground meat" French-style. You'll find at least one *pâté* or *terrine* on every menu. They're blends of ground meat, fat, herbs, spices, and liqueur. (*Pâté de foie gras,* from goose liver, is probably most famous.)
- Other tip-offs are *farci* (stuffed); *en croûte* (baked in a pastry shell); *en gelée* (in aspic); *en brochette* (cooked on a skewer like shish kebab); *gratinée* (browned in oven or broiler, usually with bread crumbs on top); and *flambé* (flaming).
- **what's the sauce or garnish?**
Half the trick to identifying a French specialty is knowing its sauce.
- White sauces are light and creamy. *Bercy, Bonne Femme, Mornay* (with cheese), *Aurore* (with tomato purée), and *Chaud-Froid* (a gelatin) are just a few.
- *Hollandaise* is a rich egg yolk, butter, and lemon juice mixture. Two variations you'll see often are *Mousseline* and *Bèarnaise.*
- Brown sauces are heartier blends of stock or essence of whatever meat is used, with butter, flour, tomato paste, and wine; e.g., *Bordelaise, Chateâubriand, Bigarade, Robert, Chasseur* (with mushrooms), *Diable,* or *Diane.*
- Tomato sauces are indicated by the terms *Portugaise, Basquaise, Provençale,* or *Italienne;* a butter sauce is *beurre à la meunière* (parsley butter). *Vinaigrette sauce* is oil and vinegar with spices.
- Other clues are *amandine* (with almonds); *Florentine* (with spinach); *Dieppoise* (garnished with mussels and shrimp); *Bretonne* or *jardinière* (with mixed vegetables).
- **what's the backbone of the meal?**
- Soups: *Potage* (usually thick vegetable purée); *consommé* (clear).
- Meats: *Agneau* (lamb); *biftek* (steak); *boeuf* (beef); *foie* (liver); *jambon* (ham); *veau* (veal).
- Fowl: *Vollaille* (barnyard fowl in general); *coq, poulet* (chicken); *canard, caneton* (duck); *oie* (goose).
- Seafood, fish: *Coquilles St. Jacques* (scallops); *crevettes* (shrimp); *escargots* (snails); *homard* (lobster); *langoustines* (crayfish); *moules* (mussels); *truit* (trout).
- Vegetables: *Aubergines* (eggplant); *champignons* (mushrooms); *haricots verts* (string beans); *marrons* (chestnuts); *pois* (peas); *pommes de terre* (potatoes).
- Desserts: *Glace* (ice cream); *melba glacée, bombe* (variations); *clafouti, flan, crème caramel* (custards); *tarte* (fruit pie); *crêpe* (thin pancake); *gâteau, biscuit, galett, génoise* (cakes).
- Fruits: *Ananas* (pineapple); *framboises* (raspberries); *pêche* (peach); *poire* (pear); *pomme* (apple); *fraises* (strawberries); *cerises* (cherries).

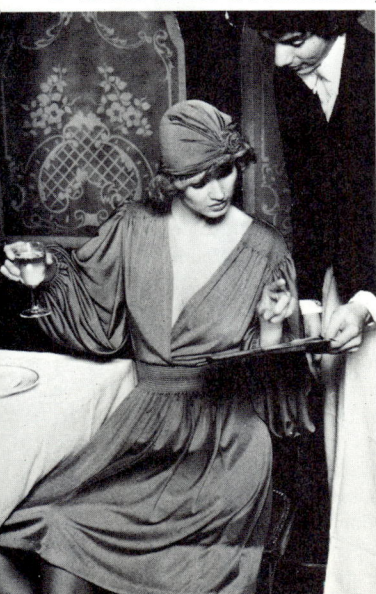

Italian menu
ordering something other than the same old lasagna or ravioli from an Italian menu

Italian food goes beyond spaghetti, lasagna, and ravioli, so put an end to ordering the same old standbys and try something exotic.

- **first courses**

In Italy pasta is generally the first course, with a meat dish following. If that sounds like a diet disaster to you, order one portion of pasta and split it with a dinner companion. This is common in Italy and in Italian restaurants anywhere. Just tell the waiter what you want to do. Instead of the usual tomato, or *marinara,* sauce, try *pesto,* a delicate and delicious green sauce flavored with fresh basil and garlic. A white sauce with Parmesan cheese, heavy cream, and butter is called *a la panna.* Favorite pastas to try with any of these sauces are *tagliatelle* or fettucine, both flat noodles. *Fettucine alfredo* is fettuccine in a rich cream sauce.

- **main courses**

Veal dishes are probably the most common. Veal scallopine are small, extra-thin slices usually served with various sauces—including *Marsala,* made with Marsala wine, or *piccata,* a lemon and butter sauce. *Vitello tonnato* is cold roasted veal in a wonderfully creamy tuna sauce.

You can order all kinds of seafood. Some of the most common are: *scampi,* shrimp with butter and garlic; *calamari,* squid served deep-fried or with a tomato sauce; *scunghili,* conch, served with tomato sauce or fried.

- **desserts**

Gelato is ice cream. *Zabaglione* is a light and delicious wine-flavored cream; *zuppa inglese* is worth every calorie—rum-soaked cake with custard. *Cannoli* are cream-filled pastries.

restaurant
how to pick one from the outside

Here's a rundown of things to watch for:
- If the menu is posted, check it out carefully. Interesting and seasonal dishes are a good sign but beware of menus that are loaded with superlatives, such as "succulent," "mouth-watering," and "scrumptious." Look over prices: Are they à la carte (if so, add up before you go in); do they seem in keeping with other restaurants in the area (too high or too low are both danger signals); are side dishes (vegetables, potato, salad) included with the price of the entrée or must you pay extra? If no prices are listed, be prepared—they may be very high. Too many choices or entrées can be a bad sign, especially if the restaurant is small. It may indicate that the food is not fresh or homemade.
- A restaurant that doesn't accept credit cards usually hasn't been "discovered" yet, so the prices are often a bargain. It may also be a

57

d dining out

sign that credit cards are not needed to attract business. If cards are accepted, their emblems are usually posted on the door.
- "Bring your own wine" on the posted menu means a real saving to you. Also, a restaurant that doesn't have a liquor license may choose to concentrate on food, not drinks, and that's a good sign, too.
- A restaurant that's dark as night—or one you can barely see into—isn't likely to be an appealing place to eat. Phony bricks, fake paneling, and plastic plants are a sign that the same "phony" thinking may go into the food.
- Peek in the window. Fresh flowers, tables placed far enough apart, a pleasant atmosphere, linen napkins, a good number of diners are all positives. Waiters and waitresses in outlandish costumes leave some doubt about the overall taste level.
- If the place is ethnic (Mexican, Chinese, Indian), look for people of that nationality dining there. If they aren't, the food may not be authentic.
- When the name of the owner is given, consider it a plus. It indicates that he or she takes pride in the establishment.
- In general, restaurants in shopping areas or malls or those with big advertisements of "specials" plastered all over their windows are poor bets.

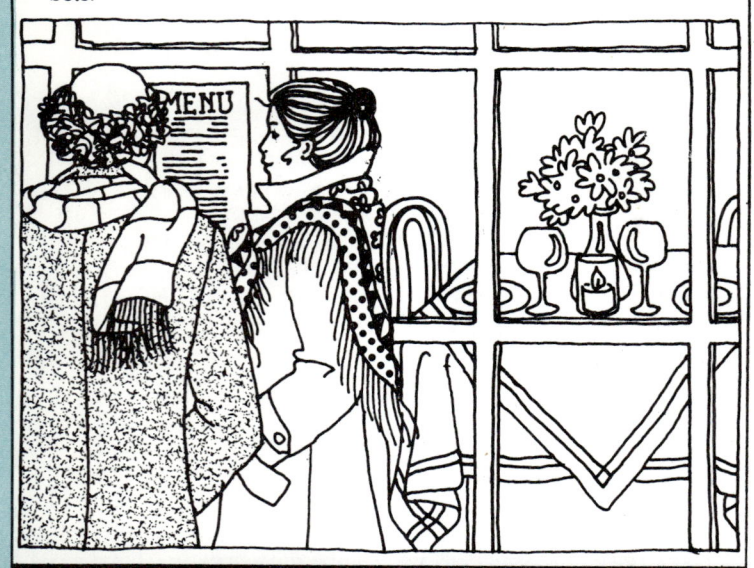

drinks

alcohol
know your facts about drinking

- **drinkers' fact sheet test**

True or False:
1. The ability to "hold your liquor" or "drink someone else under the table" is all in your head.
2. Wine and beer are absorbed less rapidly than hard liquor.
3. A small amount of alcohol in the bloodstream has a mildly tranquilizing effect.
4. Diluting a drink with water or lots of ice slows down the absorption.
5. Mixing drinks will make you drunker than if you stay with one kind.
6. Alcohol has little nutritional value.
7. A hangover is more likely to occur if you drink when you are tired or under stress.

Medical authorities claim that alcohol affects everyone differently. The answers we've given point to some general patterns in its effect, but remember that it would be impossible to cite every variable in every case—and how liquor affects you might not be the same as it does others.

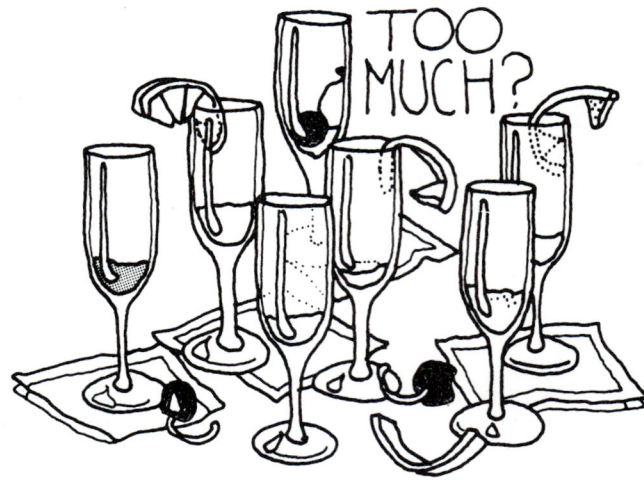

1. *False*—Since liquor affects everyone differently, some people do have a greater physical tolerance to liquor than others. One reason is that your weight determines how fast alcohol takes effect in your body. The same amount of alcohol can have a greater effect on a 100-pound person than on a 220-pound person, since alcohol is quickly distributed uniformly within the circulatory system. This means that the heavier person will have smaller concentrations throughout his bloodstream than will the lighter-weight individual. Other physical factors include whether your stomach is empty or full, since food coats the stomach and slows the rate of alcohol absorption; and how fast you drink, since your body can burn up only ½ ounce of alcohol per hour, and more than that will remain in your bloodstream. Also, a habitual drinker tends to build up a greater tolerance than an occasional drinker.
2. *True*—Wine and beer contain small amounts of nonalcoholic substances that slow down absorption.
3. *True*—Alcohol is a depressant; it relaxes the nerves that make you uptight. Thus the amount of alcohol you'd get from say, one drink, has a slightly tranquilizing effect. However, it may feel at first like a stimulant because it initially affects the parts of the brain where learned behavior patterns, such as self-control, are located. After a few drinks these learned behavior patterns may be temporarily weakened, leaving you less inhibited.
4. *True*—Diluting liquor with water can slow the absorption rate, by reducing the amount of alcohol you get with each sip. But mixing liquor with carbonated beverages speeds up the rate, so a Scotch and water would be absorbed more slowly than a Scotch and soda.
5. *False*—Switching drinks won't make you drunker since your degree of intoxication is determined by the total amount of alcohol absorbed, not by the flavor of the drink. In other words, 1 ounce of most vodkas, gins, whiskeys, or rums contains about ½ ounce of pure alcohol. So you won't get drunk faster by having one of each drink than you would by having four of the same kind. However, mixing drinks may make you sicker in the end than would sticking to one kind.
6. *True*—Alcohol is technically a food because it has calories. Thus, it does have nutritional value. However, it cannot substitute for food because it can't repair body tissues as only protein can do.
7. *True*—Alcohol can have a stronger impact when you're tired, or less than relaxed. For example, if you are sitting comfortably, quietly talking with a friend, alcohol will have less effect than if you are standing at a cocktail party. Although doctors don't entirely understand why this is true, they speculate that the physiological effects of stress—such as the release of certain hormones—are intensified when combined with alcohol.

drinks

drugs
why — if you mix alcohol and drugs — you may get more of a trip than you expected

Drugs that give you a high—or a low—can be risky when taken alone. But mixed with alcohol, their effects are even more unpredictable. "So if you drug, don't drink. If you drink, don't drug. And if you do both, be prepared to look for a lawyer, doctor, or even an undertaker," warns Dr. Richard Phillipson, associate director for clinical patient care at the National Institute on Drug Abuse.

"Alcohol taken with many psychoactive drugs—from barbiturates and methaqualone [like Sopors and Quaaludes] to amphetamines, cocaine, and marijuana—acts synergistically," says Dr. Phillipson. This means, for example, that if you smoked marijuana or were on a downer while you drank a small glass of Scotch, you'd get more of a "high" from each substance—in combination—than you'd get from either one taken alone. (One dangerous consequence of this "one plus one equals more than two" situation is that even moderate drinking could make you a drunken menace on the road.)

This synergistic effect might make for a bad trip if you combine alcohol with amphetamines, which are stronger stimulants than marijuana. Alcohol plus barbiturates or tranquilizers—depressants that slow down your breathing mechanism—can be fatal. You could take them hours apart and still feel adverse effects, since the downers stay in your system longer than does the booze—which means that they're not necessarily out of your system even though you took them yesterday.

But what if you have taken one alcohol-drug combination and gotten away with it? You might be surprised next time, because people respond differently to various drugs and even the same person can't count on the same reaction every time.

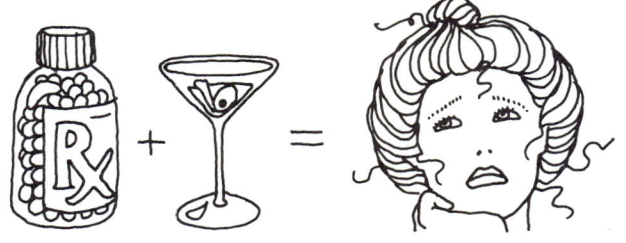

hangovers
do you know enough about them to prevent one the morning after?

Some of us could name five hangover remedies that friends swear by but that don't work for us or other friends. We asked Dr. Michael Schmerin of The New York Hospital–Cornell Medical College to answer true or false to some of the most popular ideas about cure and prevention.

● *If you know how to do it, you can drink as much as you want without getting a hangover.*
False. If you drink a lot, you'll have a hangover. There are things you can do to lessen the effects of the hangover (more about this later), but you can't completely prevent it.
● *Coating your stomach with milk before drinking will help keep you sober and prevent stomach irritation.*
False. This old wive's tale conjures up the image of your stomach receiving a special lining for a night of indulgence. It just doesn't work that way. One or even two glasses of milk won't do much to stop the absorption of alcohol through the walls of the stomach—thus keeping you sober longer—nor is it a good acid neutralizer. You'd have to drink more milk than is practical to neutralize irritating stomach acids. If you're prone to a queasy stomach the morning after, take a good, over-the-counter antacid made specifically to neutralize excess stomach acids (Maalox or Gelusil) before and after you drink.
● *It's better to drink on a full stomach than on an empty one.*
True. Food in your stomach helps slow down the absorption of alcohol into your bloodstream and keeps you from getting intoxicated as quickly as you might when drinking on an empty stomach. Food also helps keep the alcohol from irritating the stomach lining but does not totally prevent it.
● *A few cups of coffee when you get home will sober you right up.*
False. There's no known drug that will hasten the breakdown of alcohol in your body, nor is there anything you can take that will counteract its effects. About the only thing the coffee will do is intensify that shaky, jittery feeling that accompanies a hangover.
● *"A hair of the dog that bit you" will make you feel better.*
True and False. This old adage suggests that having a breakfast drink made with alcohol will alleviate the symptoms of a hangover to some extent. Since alcohol temporarily stimulates you, you may feel better briefly. In the long run, the drink just delays your symptoms for a half hour or so. Since alcohol can leave you with a feeling of depression, you may feel worse than ever an hour after having that drink.
● *Taking vitamin B1 before, during, or after drinking helps a hangover.*
False. Chronic alcoholics tend to develop severe vitamin deficiencies and are often treated with thiamin to control the DT's, but there's no solid evidence that vitamin B1 (thiamin) prevents or helps a hangover.
● *Aspirin at bedtime will keep your head from pounding the next morning.*
True, at least partly. If you take the aspirin before bed, it will be working on your pain center while you sleep. Two more aspirin when you wake up will help even more. You may want to accompany the aspirin with an antacid, since the aspirin may irritate an already tender stomach. If you have drunk a lot, however, you're bound to have some headache and hangover symptoms, no matter what you take. Alcohol actually seems to make brain tissue and linings swell slightly, thus the pain and that feeling of a "big head." Time is the only thing that will cure these symptoms completely.

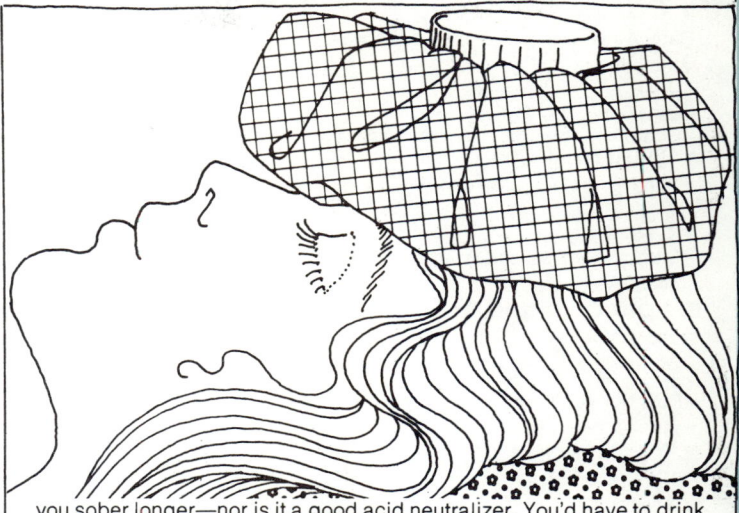

light
try drinking light at the party

If you're tired of the usual cocktail-hour drinks, or if you're looking for something light, try some of the following drink recipes. Most are considered aperitifs, the light refreshing drinks served almost exclusively at cocktail time in Europe. You'll find them a welcome change of pace, easy on the calories and on your budget.

59

d drinks

● **Campari and soda**
(Campari is a rich, red bittersweet aperitif with a taste comparable to vermouth.)
1 generous jigger Campari
Soda to taste (about 6 oz.)
  Combine ingredients in a tall glass over ice. Serves 1.

● **Lillet and soda**
(Lillet is another aperitif with a dry, vermouthlike taste.)
1 generous jigger Lillet
Soda to taste (about 6 oz.)
  Combine ingredients in a tall glass over ice. Garnish with an orange slice. Serves 1.

● **vermouth and cassis**
3 oz. dry vermouth
½ oz. Crème de Cassis (currant liqueur)
Soda to taste
  Pour vermouth and cassis into a highball glass with ice cubes; fill glass with club soda. Serves 1.

● **frozen eggnog**
3 egg yolks
½ c. sugar
1 qt. cream
¼ tsp. nutmeg
½ c. rum
½ c. brandy
  Beat egg yolks and sugar until light and airy. Add cream and nutmeg and beat a few more times. Freeze. When the mixture is firm but not hard, add the rum and brandy. Stir mixture to blend. Serve in small glasses with spoons. Makes about 2 quarts, depending on how much air you beat into it. This one is not for dieters.

● **spiced wine**
2 lemon slices
Whole cloves
2 T. superfine sugar
2 cinnamon sticks
2 c. claret or Burgundy wine
  Stud the lemon slices with cloves and combine them with the sugar and cinnamon sticks in a quart saucepan. Place over moderate heat, stirring with a wooden spoon until sugar melts. Add the wine and continue to stir until wine has almost reached the boiling point. Remove from heat, discard lemon and cinnamon sticks, and pour into two mugs.

● **wine and cassis**
6 oz. dry white wine
½ oz. Crème de Cassis
Lemon peel
  Pour ingredients over ice. Serves 1.

● **currant fizz**
1 to 2 T. (2 makes it sweeter) Crème de Cassis
Juice of 1 lime
Soda to taste
  Pour cassis and lime juice over crushed ice in a large wine glass; add a splash of club soda. Serves 1.

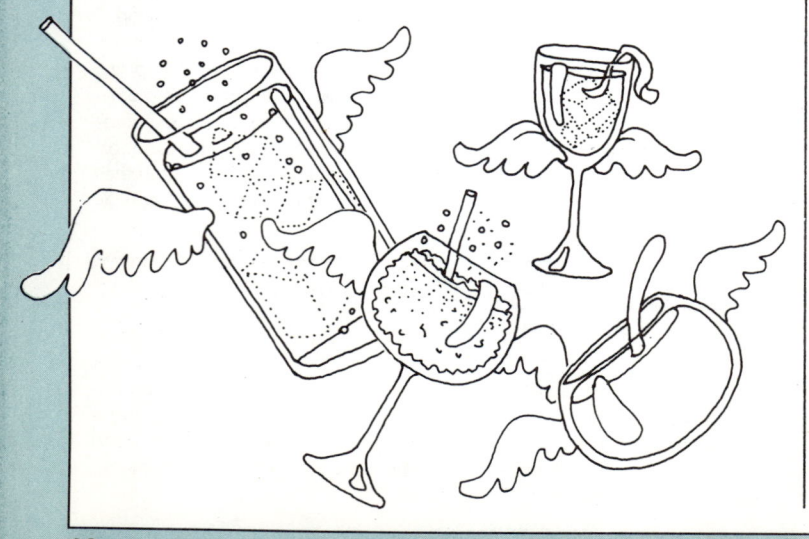

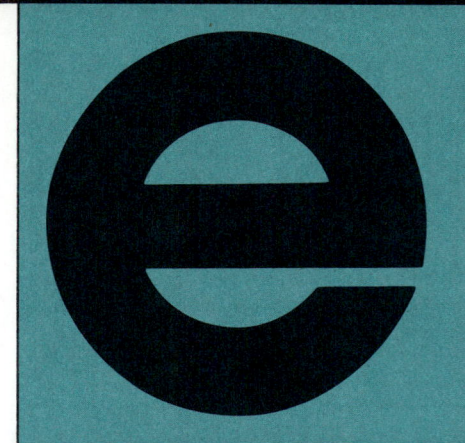

e exercises

bathtub
exercises: 4 easy ways to shape up feet and legs

Anyone who considers a bath simply a place to get clean may be missing out on some of its best benefits. The bath is also an ideal private place to let your mind unwind after a day of nonstop shopping or working—and to energize your tired feet and legs. Larry Lorence of Gala Fitness Studios (expert at getting anything into shape) suggests these quick leg and foot exercises:

Support yourself for all exercises by placing your elbows on the bottom of the tub, if it's wide enough, or on the sides (see sketch).

1. Hold legs together and straighten them, pushing your heels against the front of the tub until your feet are perpendicular to the bottom. Repeat 10 times. (You'll feel the stretch mainly in your thighs but it's good for calves, too.)

2. With legs straight, bring them to the surface of the water (see sketch). Make small circles, first inward, then outward, with both feet. You'll be creating small whirlpools each time—good for ankles and tired feet.

3. If your tub has a removable stopper, try to pull it out with your toes, using first one foot and then the other. (Good for tired feet, also strengthens arches.)

4. Sitting up straight, bring one knee up to your shoulder. Keep your knee in place, straighten your leg as much as possible. Do the same with the opposite leg. Repeat 5 times.

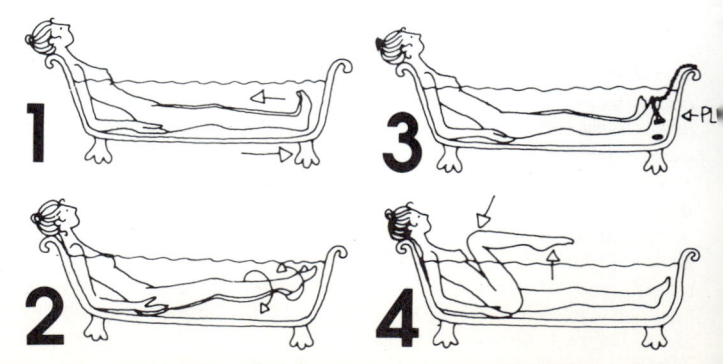

exercises

cast
exercises for people in a cast

If your arm or leg is in a cast, the doctor may not have stressed the benefits of exercising while your body heals. Here are some exercises recommended by Dr. Willibald Nagler, chief of Physical Medicine and Rehabilitation at New York Hospital–Cornell Medical College. Before you try any of these, however, you should check with your own doctor.

● **leg cast**
For broken ankle, the most common fracture: It's important that you keep your thigh muscles strong so that when the cast comes off your ankle, you'll be able to walk steadily.
1. Lie on your back on the floor, legs straight out. Tighten the knee of the leg with the cast. Without touching the knee, push it down toward the floor. Hold 5 seconds, rest 3. Repeat 15 times.
2. Sit comfortably in a chair with a pillow under the thigh of the leg with the cast. Lift leg and straighten it out in front of you. Hold 5 seconds, rest 3. Do 15 times. (You should also do these exercises with the good leg, using 3- or 4-lb. weights, available at a sporting goods store, wrapped around the ankle.)
    With a cast on your leg, you've probably been limping around, and you should therefore keep your abdominal muscles toned up to avoid back pain.
3. Lie on your back on the floor and push the small of your back toward the floor, breathing out as you push. Hold 5 seconds, rest 3. Repeat 10 or 15 times.
    If you're on crutches, don't worry about exercising arms and legs. They're getting enough of a workout.

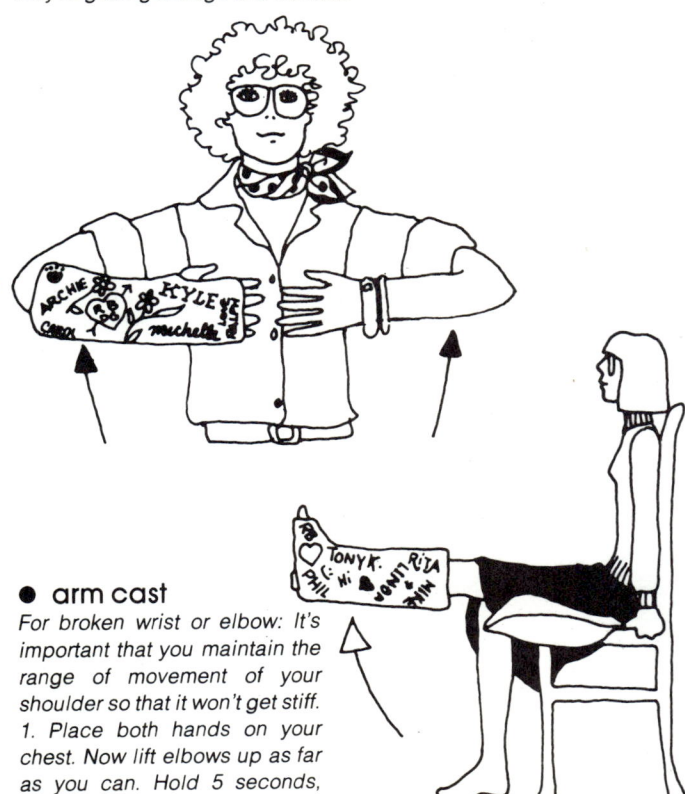

● **arm cast**
For broken wrist or elbow: It's important that you maintain the range of movement of your shoulder so that it won't get stiff.
1. Place both hands on your chest. Now lift elbows up as far as you can. Hold 5 seconds, rest 3. Do 15 times.
2. Put arms out straight and place the arm without cast over other arm. With palms down, fingers entwined, grip the hand of the bad arm with the hand of the good arm and lift over your head. Hold 5 seconds, rest 3. Repeat 15 times.
    Keep legs in shape with plenty of walking and jogging (be careful not to fall).

cramps
exercises to help relieve menstrual pain

Some kind of physical discomfort before or during menstrual periods is one of the most common problems women have. One informal survey at a women's college showed that more than half of the new women signing up for physical education classes felt some degree of discomfort every month. Many women, though, have cramps between the ages of fifteen and twenty-five and usually not later because pregnancy and childbirth apparently clear up discomfort, as do birth control pills. If the pain is persistent, a doctor must be consulted.
    In many cases, exercise can help relieve the pressure, tension, and dull cramps. The ones following should be done daily (except where noted) for several months to see real improvement. They are also good overall figure toners, so the benefits are doubled.

● **for dull cramps or pain**
1. Lie on your back, knees bent, hands at sides. Pull in your tummy muscles as you inhale deeply; slowly exhale. Do this several times and then push your upper abdomen toward the ceiling, hold, and relax. Your chest should lift as your lower abdomen remains flat. Repeat the sequence 10 times. When you synchronize this routine with the onset of a cramp, the rhythm of the breathing helps to relax you, thus reducing the pain.
2. Lie on your back, knees bent, hands at sides. Push the air low in your chest and push out your tummy as you inhale. Holding your breath, flatten your tummy, then exhale rapidly. Relax, breathe normally for a moment or two, then repeat. Do this 10 times, but not when the menstrual flow is heavy as it can increase the discharge, causing discomfort.
3. Get on your hands and knees, with arms shoulder-width apart, knees several inches apart and directly below the hips (see sketch). Raise your head slowly and bend arms, lowering your chest directly toward the floor. Bring your body back toward the knees until your buttocks rest on your heels. Pull in your abdominal muscles, round the lower back, and drop your head to your chest. Do this daily between periods.
    Weak back muscles and/or poor posture can contribute to your discomfort. So can a lack of hip-joint mobility, which may produce leg aches. Here are two exercises to help (they also loosen tight lower-back ligaments).
1. Stand with your hands at your sides (see sketch). Slowly move your arms forward and up, as you move your right leg backward as far as possible. Your toes should not leave the floor. Hold and return to start. Alternate legs; do this 10 times.
2. Stand sideways about 18–24 inches from a wall (see sketch). Place the elbow, forearm, and hand of the arm nearest the wall against it at shoulder level. Place the heel of the other hand on the hollow of your hip. Pull in your abdominal muscles and press your buttocks together so that your pelvis is tilted upward. Then firmly move the pelvis diagonally forward toward the wall. Hold for a count of 3, relax. Do this 3 times on each side. Your heels must stay on the floor and the hip should *not* touch the wall. This must be done faithfully for several months to be effective.

exercises

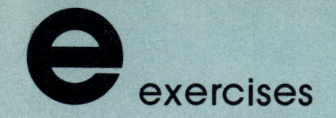

5 minutes a day
to tone up your whole body

Getting your whole body in shape can be as easy as spending five minutes a day on these quick exercises. Fitness expert Victoria Schatz of the Pretty Body salon in New York City has worked out six routines for her clientele that can tone and firm the muscles of your body in the time it takes to shower or perk coffee.

1. *To stretch and warm up your body, tone back of legs, sides.* Stand with feet apart and back straight. Using first one arm and then the other, reach as high as you can for 8 counts, then lean forward and bob for 8 counts. Try to get head between knees. Repeat.

2. *For thighs, buttocks, calves, and posture.* Stand with legs and feet turned out, keeping your back as straight as possible, with shoulders relaxed. Clasp arms in front of you and count to 4 as you lower your torso to a sitting position. Count slowly to 4 as you come back up to a standing position. Do 8 times, and on the last, hold your sitting position to a count of 4, or as long as you can, before you raise yourself back up.

3. *For legs and buttocks.* Lying on your back with legs together, clasp your right knee to your chest for 4 counts. Then extend your leg as straight as possible, with toes pointed, and again pull toward you for 4 counts. Flex your foot and pull it as close to the floor as possible for 4 counts. Do 4 times with each leg.

4. *For stomach and inner thighs.* Lie on back with legs raised, then spread into as wide a V as possible. Swing each leg in a half circle till legs come together about six inches from floor. Without touching floor, raise legs to first position. Do 8 times.

5. *For hips, waist, and buttocks.* On hands and knees, extend your right leg straight out to the side. Make 8 forward circles. Bring leg back into place. Extend leg again; make 8 backward circles. Repeat series with same leg. Then do entire exercise with left leg.

6. *To relax your whole body, especially back and neck.* Make circular motions with your shoulders, one at a time and then together. Then drop your head to your chest and roll it around like a rag doll's. This is actually a free-form exercise to make you as loose and floppy as possible—so improvise if you like.

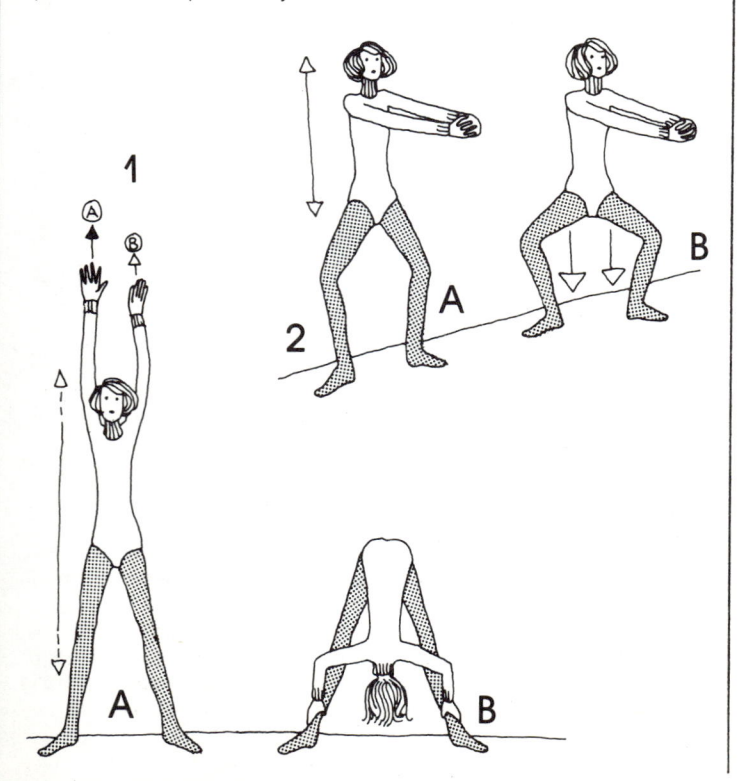

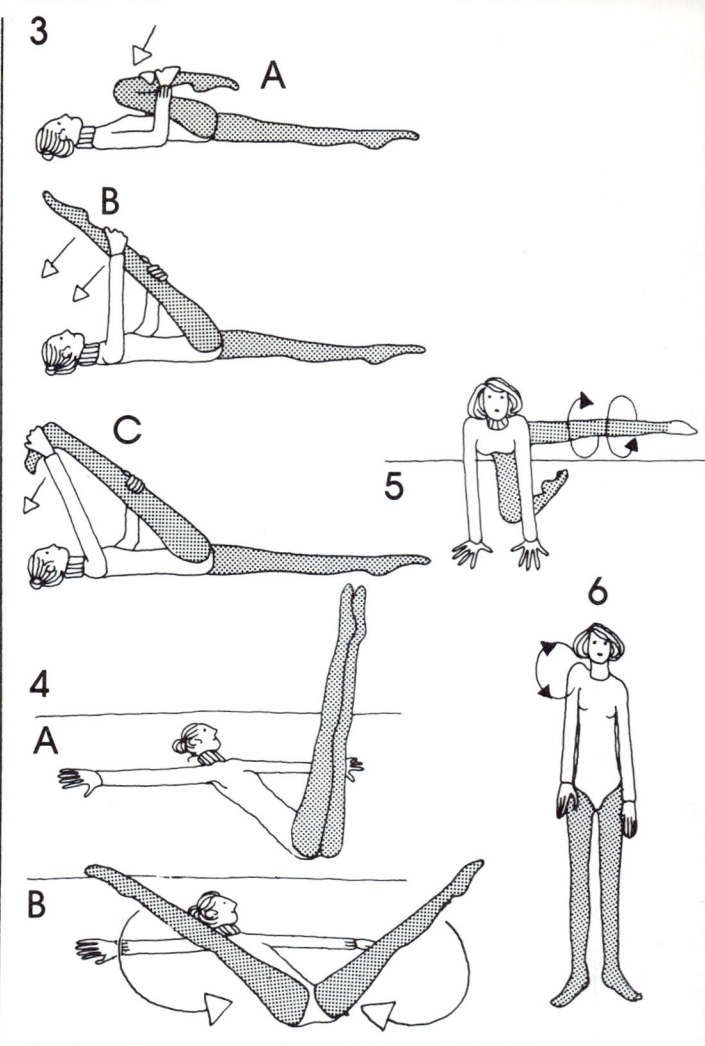

headaches
exercises that can help ease— or even prevent— tension headaches

Anyone who can't think "headache" without thinking "aspirin" may be surprised to learn that there's another remedy for simple tension headaches: exercise.

"Sufferers from 'tension' headache are afflicted with neck, scalp, or facial muscles that are in a state of sustained contraction," say Drs. Arnold P. Friedman and Shervert H. Frazier, Jr. in The Headache Book. "There is not only a psychic 'uptightness,' but a physical 'uptightness' as well."

As one remedy for such headaches, the doctors (both specialists in psychiatry and neurology) suggest that you take a class or consult with a fitness expert whose exercises are designed to relax taut muscles. We spoke with the staff of the Lotte Berk Method, Inc., whose exercises have been relaxing uptight New Yorkers for years, and found, happily, that you don't even have to take a class to benefit from a few that they advise. The Lotte Berk experts say you can do the following exercises almost any time you have or feel a headache coming on, or when you feel tense. Do each one five or six times, they suggest—the slower the better. And try doing them, if you can, with your eyes closed (but not squeezed tight); this helps you to zero in on tight muscles that need loosening up. (They are also good before-bed relaxers for anyone who

exercises

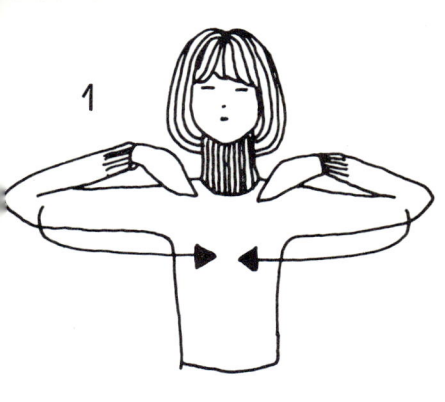

has trouble sleeping after a tense day.)

1. Sit or stand with your feet slightly apart. Put your hands loosely on your shoulders, with your elbows out to each side like wings, as in sketch. Slowly bring elbows together on top of your bust and try to touch them together. This exercise is even more effective in a warm-to-hot shower with the nozzle aimed just below neck.

2. Standing in the final position of the first exercise (feet slightly apart, elbows together on your bust), drop your chin gently toward your chest. Then make circles with head, rotating it across your chest, over to one shoulder, around to the back, over your other shoulder, and then down on your chest again. Be sure to hang loose and drop your head as far down on your chest as you can.

3. Stand with your feet slightly apart and your arms straight out at your sides, with fists loosely clenched. Roll your shoulders forward first, then backward without moving your arms. (You might think of trying to touch your shoulder blades together without moving your arms.)

4. Stand straight with your arms at your sides and feet together. Make big circles with your shoulders, as if you are shrugging first backward, then forward.

5. Lean forward from the waist, with your arms outstretched, back straight until it's parallel to the floor. Then bob down like a rag doll, dropping your arms between your legs and your head as close to your knees as you can get it.

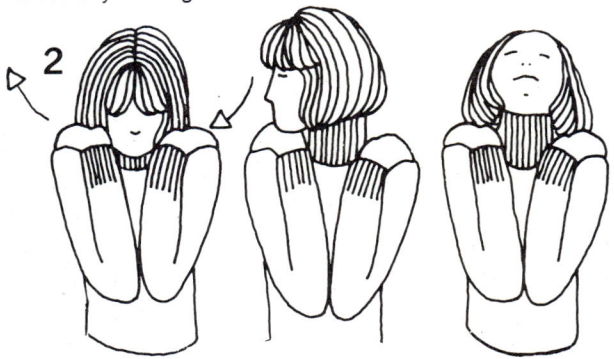

new mother
shape up your figure after baby

If you're anxious to get back to your favorite regular clothes again—and what new mother isn't—these exercises will help you reclaim your prepregnancy contours quickly and safely. Remember to get your doctor's approval before you start exercising. Unless you're nursing, you can usually begin exercising soon after you're home from the hospital. If you're eager to begin and have your doctor's OK, go ahead, but remember that you won't see earthshaking results until after you've had your first menstrual period. The reason for this is that the pelvic muscles have become relaxed in preparation for the baby's birth. It takes about five weeks for the body's hormones to send out all the signals to tighten up these muscles and connective tissue in the pelvic area again. The onset of the first postbirth menstrual period is the sign that all this has taken place and you have nature's cooperation in making exercise work.

● **for stomach**

Lie on the floor on your back, arms at sides. Raise your upper torso to a half-sitting position, your palms and elbows on floor for support. Slowly raise one leg a few inches off floor while you bend the other and bring it as close to your chest as possible. Return to original position. Breathe deeply as you do this and repeat about eight times in all.

Lie on the floor on your back, arms at sides. Slowly raise legs, keeping knees straight. Try to lift legs at least a foot off floor. Slowly lower them to floor again. Repeat about six times. Another version of this exercise: Crisscross legs together in air in a scissorlike kick. Repeat about ten times if you can do it without straining.

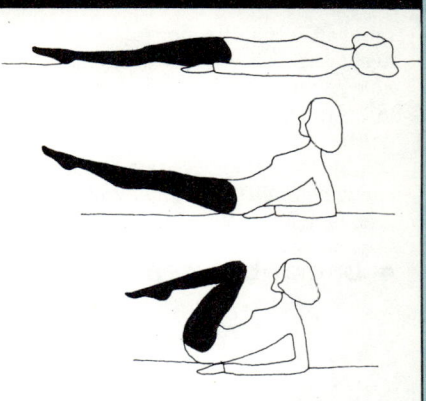

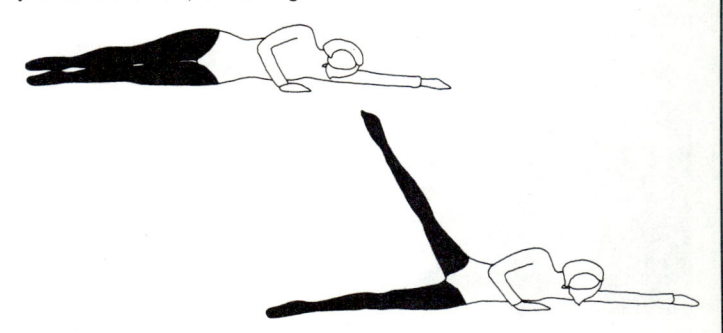

● **for outer thighs**

Because connective tissue in the pelvis and upper thighs gets slack and loose in the last months of pregnancy, many women notice a change in their upper thigh measurement. This exercise will help trim and firm these muscles. Lie on floor on one side, one arm out straight and your head resting on it, the other arm in front of your chest for support. Raise top leg slowly as high as you can and then lower it, but don't let it touch the floor. Repeat slowly about four times. Change sides. Remember to move slowly and to breathe deeply as you do it.

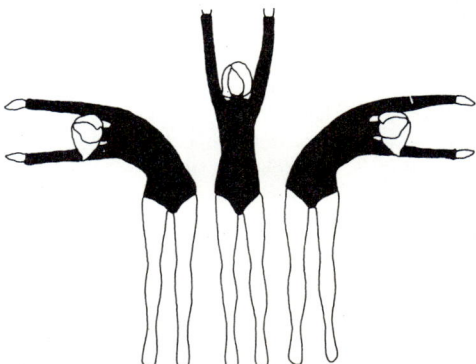

● **for waist**

Stand with feet about a foot apart, hands over head. Stretch arms up as high as possible and then bend to the right, from the waist only, and as far as you can. Return to original position. Repeat, bending to left. Do this slowly and repeat about six times.

pregnancy exercises
to help you look and feel better

If you're used to doing fifteen minutes of thigh lifts or hip rolls every day, do you have to give them up once you're pregnant? Many obstetricians feel you usually don't, and one of them is Dr. Sheldon H. Cherry, a New York obstetrician and author of *Understanding Pregnancy and Childbirth*.

Dr. Cherry thinks a woman can exercise moderately throughout

63

exercises

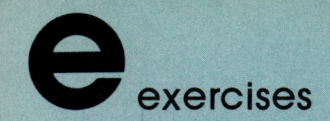

pregnancy, if it's her normal life-style; for example, if she plays tennis every week, she can continue until the ninth month—if she's comfortable and has informed her obstetrician. He also suggests calisthenics to build and tone muscles—"training for work involved in labor and delivery." While any pregnant woman should consult her doctor first, Dr. Cherry says most healthy women can do these exercises to strengthen parts of the body involved in labor and also to alleviate pregnancy discomforts—lower backache, leg cramps, abdominal heaviness. Continue these exercises as long as you're comfortable.

● **back, abdomen**

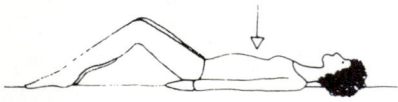

Lie flat on the floor, arms at sides, knees bent. Slowly flatten the curve of your back by pressing the entire length of your spine against the floor. As you do this, consciously tighten your abdominal muscles, pulling them in. Your pelvis should be tilting upward, your buttocks resting on the floor (see sketch). Then, as you relax your abdomen, your pelvis will tilt to its relaxed position and your back will regain its natural curve. Repeat five times daily.

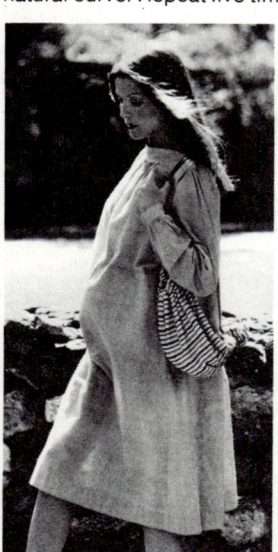

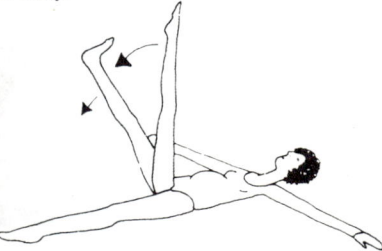

● **legs**

Lie flat on the floor, extend arms at right angles to body. Inhale slowly, point toes, raise right leg vertically. Flex the ankle and lower the leg as far to the right as possible, as you exhale. Don't allow the left buttock or hip to lift off the floor (see sketch). Point toes and inhale as you raise the right leg back to the vertical position; flex ankle and exhale as you lower it to the floor. Repeat with left leg. The following exercise for back and legs is suggested by the Gala Fitness Studio in New York: Lying flat on floor, arms down at sides and knees bent, raise hips off floor, as in Sketch 1. Lift right leg to vertical position, as in Sketch 2; lower it to horizontal position, keeping hips up, as in Sketch 3. Lift and lower again. Repeat with left leg.

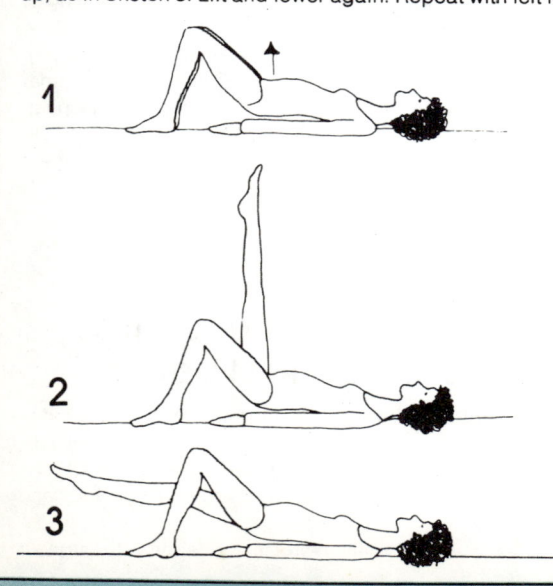

trouble spots

exercises for trouble spots

The classic exercises here are all soundly designed to focus on specific figure faults—flabby thighs and hips, tummy bulges, and bosoms and bottoms that need firming.

● **thighs, hips**

Sit on floor, holding a large towel under arches (1). In a smooth motion, straighten legs, holding towel (2). Hold 10 seconds. Do 10 times. Get down on all fours and extend one leg (3). Bring leg to one side (4). Keep hip straight and flutter-kick 15 times, without touching floor. Do 2 times with each leg, work up to 5.

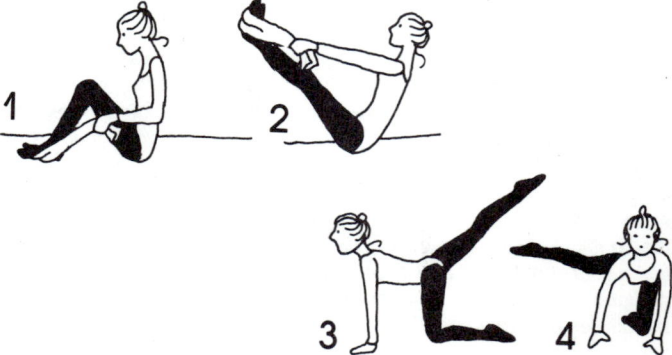

● **bottom, hips**

Sit in a chair, both feet in front of you. Contract all the muscles in buttocks as hard as you can. Hold for 10 seconds. Relax. Repeat as often as you can.

● **stomach**

Lie flat on floor (5). In one motion, assume position 6. Repeat 8 times. Now sit in position 7. Extend legs straight in front, keeping them off floor (8). Resume position 7 without feet touching floor. Repeat 5 times.

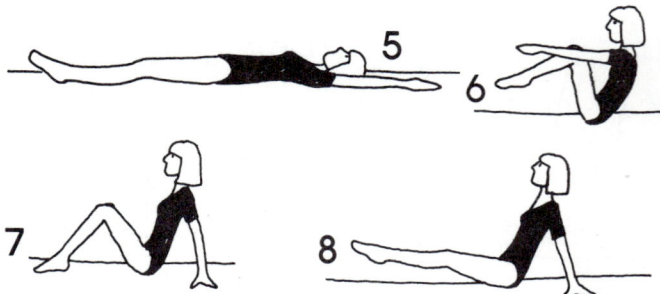

● **bosom**

Clasp wrists (9). Squeeze arms toward each other so that you feel pressure in chest muscles. Hold 10 seconds. Work up to 15 times. Assume position 10. Touch elbows together and squeeze (11). Repeat 5 times.

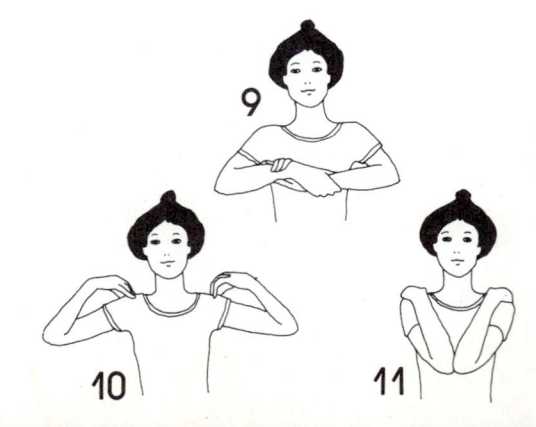

64

fashion

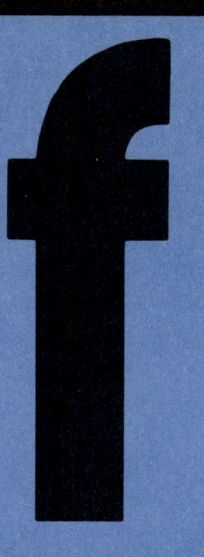

fashion
flowers
food
foreign
	languages

fashion

bras how to look more or less bosomy

Ask any woman if she's satisfied with the size of her bosom and she'll probably say no. Actually you can have pretty much the *look* you want, if not the measurement.
- *To look more bosomy:* Try a bra with no cup delineation; it molds a small figure well. Always pick a bra with a fiberfill cup to help fill out your figure. Watch your strap adjustment on any bra. If it's too loose, the top half of your cup will collapse. If it's too tight, you'll look artificial and high.
- *To look less bosomy:* A crisscross strap in front gives good support and separation to an ample bosom. A bra with minimal seaming helps round and flatten a too-large bosom. Underwiring is another feature to look for if you feel too bosomy. Stay away from stretch bras or stretch straps—they don't give enough support. And no matter what size you are, stay away from old-fashioned bras that make you look unnatural.
- *To go without a bra:* Women who are a bit too small or a little too large to go braless but want to try the look can use this tape trick (see sketch).

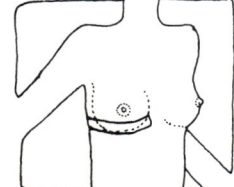

Cut a length of surgical adhesive tape—use either the 1" or 1½" width—long enough to reach from under your arm to the center of your chest. Stick tape down at underarm and press around under breasts, lifting them and using tape for support.

coats read this before you buy a coat

No woman—regardless of her shape, size, and tastes—wants to settle for anything less than her dream coat. To help you find it, check this list. You might also ask a friend to shop with you to lend an objective eye and some advice.
- **what to look for and what to avoid if you have any of these figure problems**
- Broad shoulders—stay away from padded, extended, epauletted, or caped shoulders and coats that are very fitted from the armhole to the waist. These extremely fitted and cinched-in waist shapes will accentuate too-broad shoulders. Avoid heavy wide collars. Pick a very simple shoulder and arm-hole line, or try a cape. Sometimes a prominent set of shoulders is just what a cape needs.
- Heavy all over—choose a tailored, classic-shaped coat, a blazer, or a reefer. Dark solid colors in flat, not furry or plushy, fabrics are more slimming. Be wary of plaids—especially large ones in bright contrasting colors. A cape might work for you, but on a very heavy woman, it sometimes calls attention to exactly what she's trying to minimize; it depends on just how heavy she is. Use your own judgment.
- Big bosom—avoid anything double-breasted, with a big collar or capelet. You'll look better proportioned in a coat that doesn't cinch in tightly over the rib cage and waist, and that has a flare or fullness to the skirt to balance your top. Try a blazer, reefer, or cape.
- Bottom-heavy, big hips—the coat with a circular or flared skirt, perhaps a blazer or riding jacket look, helps conceal the hips. A cape is another solution. Anything belted is likely to call attention to hips.
- Too skinny—add some volume by wearing a smock coat. Or you might pick a trench or wrap in a fabric that offers some depth, such as a pile lining.
- Short-legged—too long a coat will shorten your legs more, so look for a length just below the knee.
- Too long-legged—try a length between the knees and midcalf to give the illusion of shorter legs.
- **what to look for if you need one good-looking, all-around coat**

If you live in a very cold climate—try a bonded, double-knit jersey coat with pile inside (some are reversible), or maybe an inexpensive fake fur. Be sure the arms on any coat you choose aren't too wide, or they'll let in a lot of wind. Look for some kind of front closing to keep your coat from flapping in the wind while you're exposed and shivering.

If you live in a moderate-to-mild climate—try an unlined but double-faced wool wrap coat, or any of the lightly lined wools. Or consider an unlined double knit or a knitted sweater-coat. If only one or two months hit freezing, maybe a zip-out lining of pile or fur, or a wool melton cape is your answer.

Solid colors in classic shapes adapt easily from casual to dress.
- **how to tell if a coat is all-weather—for cold, rain, and snow**

It will usually have several layers, probably a rubberized poplin or canvas outside, an interlining, and a fake or real fur inner lining.
- **what about suede and leather?**

They look gorgeous but are not always practical. Suede isn't very warm even when it's lined; leather is a little more so. Unlined, they fit close and appealingly to the body, but in cold weather you freeze, and in fall you swelter. To own a suede or leather coat, you have to love it and be willing to suffer the limitations. If you can buy only one coat, put your leather or suede yearnings into a jacket or skirt.

65

fashion

colors
what colors do you wear?
what do they say about you?

If red is your favorite color, are you an extrovert—or just insecure? If you always reach for gray, is it because that's the color of your personality? The relationships between the colors you like to wear and your personality aren't that clear-cut, but according to color psychologist Dr. Deborah Sharpe in her book, The Psychology of Color and Design, there is a correlation between personality type and the choice of color one chooses to wear.

Many researchers have done work on personality and clothes colors, and according to Dr. Sharpe, the results generally show that more emotionally secure people tend to favor cool or neutral colors while more insecure people favor warm, bright colors. There's also evidence that as you get older, your preferences tend to change from warm brights to cool neutrals, relating to the emotional security that accompanies maturity.

Psychiatrist Dr. Wilbert Sykes reports that many of his depressed, negative patients habitually express their emotion by wearing gray, black, or other somber colors.

Dr. Sharpe points out the strong cultural influence in our clothes colors. For example, women who wear lots of pink are often perennial little girls who marry men who like perennial little girls. Wearers of brown tend to be down-to-earth, solid types; orange lovers are highly sociable, good mixers.

All of us use color to express our moods and emotions. So next time you reach for something in your closet, you may discover that your choice is more significant than you think.

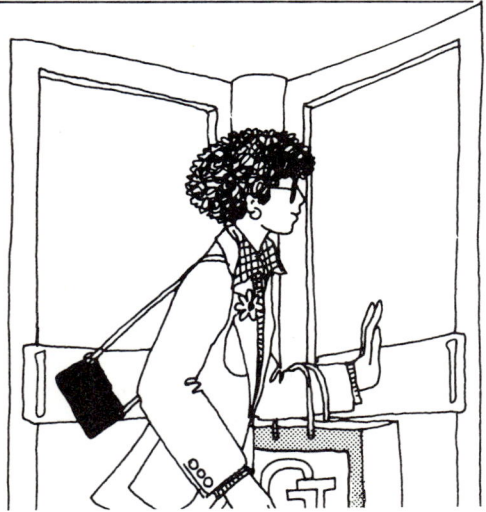

dime store
how to dress like a million-dollar baby on a dime-store budget

It's easy, especially in the summer. Simply roam the aisles of a dime store, where, to your surprise, you can put together almost a whole new wardrobe. Here are some items to shop for in a dime store—treat yourself to good quality, good looks, and great prices.

- *Shirts:* T-shirts of all kinds and colors are real bargains. You'll find pop T's, jazzed up with comic strip characters or messages, or classic, simple types in a rainbow of colors.
- *Tops:* Dime stores are bursting with great little halter tops, striped or printed ones that tie at the neck and waist, some hung from a thin gold or silver choker at the neck. You might also find elasticized, strapless tube tops or peasant blouses.
- *Pants:* Shorts are probably the best buy, as most five-and-ten emporiums have lots at low prices. Many also carry jeans or sturdy khaki pants of good quality. Dressier pants of first-rate cut and fit are usually not to be found.
- *Skirts:* Denim, khaki, or very sporty skirts are the finds in most dime stores. Many have wrap-around features or elastic waists to give you an easy fit.
- *Hats:* The dime store may be the best possible place to buy fun hats —jersey turbans, scarf caps, big brimmy straws, a sou'wester, little visor caps, the works.
- *Shoes:* In this category, of course, there are the usual sneakers and tennis shoes, but you'll find some snappy sandals, too: canvas sandals, cork-soled platforms, clogs, and, of course, the ubiquitous rubber-thong sandal.
- *Jewelry:* Summer is the time for dime-store jewelry shopping. You'll find a huge selection of terrific-looking earrings in all the bright summer colors. You can come away with armloads of plastic bangle bracelets and strings of bright-colored plastic or glass beads to wind around your neck—and waist.
- *Scarves:* Pick up a cotton bandanna scarf to protect your hair at the beach—it won't slip, slide, or blow off as easily as others. A few dog owners have even dressed up their pet with a scarf around the neck! You'll find silky scarves to fill in the neckline, too; just don't expect to find the most luxurious sizes.
- *Miscellaneous:* It may never have occurred to you to shop for lingerie in a dime store, but try it. There are super bikini underpants, some good bras, and little half- or full-slips. You can also find all kinds of buttons to give old clothes a face-lift, a wide assortment of hair ornaments, socks, terry beach robes and towels, bathing caps, and so on. Inveterate dime-store shoppers say there are also great buys in children's and infants' clothes.

fall looks
how to look great in early fall without buying anything new

Early fall can be a problem time as far as fashion goes. It's too hot for most winter clothes, yet summer outfits don't seem right either. Try reshuffling your clothes thoughts a bit and you can come up with some fresh-spirited fall looks without buying anything new and without being over- or underdressed.

- *Layer some of your cotton T-shirts over long-sleeved shirts. If you live in an area where this kind of layered dressing is still too hot for early fall, try a dickey set with a shirt collar and cuffs for the same kind of look. Consider wearing short-sleeved T-shirts or those with dolman sleeves over some of your long, full-sleeved shirts for a really super look.*
- *Wear a cotton shirt as a jacket over a lightweight sweater or T-shirt.*
- *Try slipping a knit vest over a summer shirtdress.*
- *Don't stow away all your halter sweaters. They make wonderful toppings for shirts. So do the bare, strappy tank tops.*
- *Turn your summer smock dresses into tops for pants. If the style permits, you might also wear a lightweight turtleneck under the smock.*
- *Summer sandals can go into fall when worn with colored opaque pantyhose in all sorts of colors.*
- *Take advantage of accessory changing to revamp the look of a dress or pants combination. Switch from espadrilles or other summer footwear to sturdy leather walking shoes, and exchange straw or hemp belts for leather ones. Crisp scarves in deep-toned foulards or checks add a colorful touch to T-shirts or sweaters.*
- *Remember, fabrics like corduroy, cotton gabardine, velour, and denim are seasonless—as suitable for August as they are for December.*

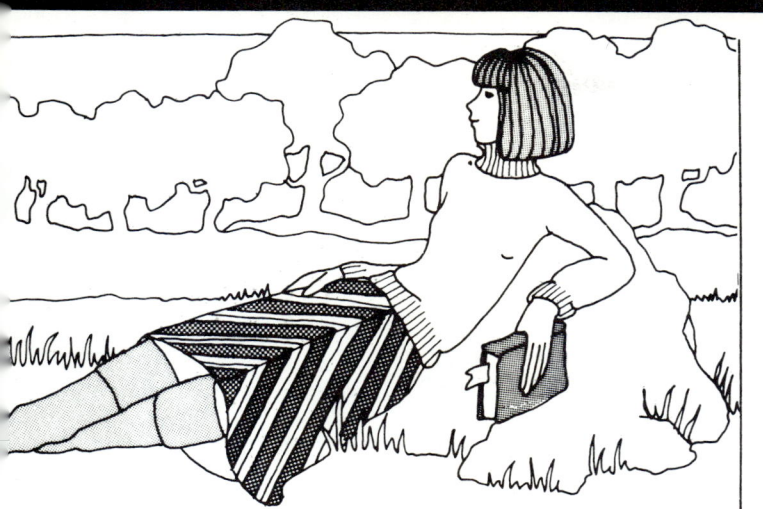

fashion

fall update
make big changes in your wardrobe for little money in the fall

You can update the fall clothes you own now by adding a few little touches that won't make much of a dent in your budget. Here are some suggestions:

Try new ways of wearing any long scarves you have tucked away in a drawer. Open a shirt neckline wide and then tie a long scarf in a full bow at the neckline. Or tie it in a half bow and wear it with a crew or V-neck sweater. Loop it once around your neck and let one long end trail down the front, the other down your back. Or just pull it under the collar of a jacket and let the ends blow freely in front.

Consider buying a little hat in a rich fall color—rust, dusky green, burgundy. Try one shaped like a little brimmed tennis hat or consider a small cuffed knit cap.

Invest in a bulky sweater of a versatile color to wear over all your shirts and skirts or pants until the weather gets too cold.

If you've been wearing mostly pants lately, think about buying one classic skirt of good quality.

If you're buying new shoes, look for a classic pump or moccasin type with a well-shaped heel.

Think about adding a couple of pairs of sheer pantyhose in tones that match the skirts or dresses you own.

figure
how to dress in summer for your figure

There are many cool and pretty looks for summer—the soft pants with drawstrings, front pleating, or gathers, the pant lengths, and a wide variety of bare looks from sundresses to little bare tops. And, of course, almost everyone buys a bathing suit and needs to do a little planning to get just the right look. If you are lucky enough to be perfectly proportioned, you won't need the guide here, but if you're like most of us, with certain problem areas, read on.

● **pear-shaped figure—narrow shoulders, wide hips**
GOOD IDEAS TO TRY
Bare looks: Chemise-type sundresses with thin straps and fullness starting under the bosom; apron wraps with A-line skirts; narrow halter-strapped dresses or tops. Strapless tops or sundresses will work if you avoid the fullest skirts.
Pants: Straight cuts with no fullness in front. Midcalf clam diggers or pedal pushers if you're not too hippy.
Swimwear: A bikini with a high-cut (French-cut) leg and a softly gathered top; a one-piece maillot with French-cut leg.
Sportswear: Classic A-line skirts and T-shirts are good. Look for a soft, natural shoulder line, nothing exaggerated.
WHAT TO STAY AWAY FROM
Bare looks: Anything with wide-set or wide shoulder straps—they emphasize narrow shoulders.
Pants: Drawstring or pleat-front pants; short shorts, Bermuda and Jamaica lengths.
Swimwear: Avoid little boy shorts or skirts.
Sportswear: Any very gathered or full skirt. Exaggerated shoulder lines, either dropped or cut out.

● **broad shoulders, narrow hips**
GOOD IDEAS TO TRY
Bare looks: Anything with wide-set or wide shoulder straps; a butcher-apron wrap.
Pants: Drawstring or pleated styles are great. You can wear most pant lengths if the proportion looks right to you. If you're very tall or short, see the following sections.
Swimwear: A classic maillot or a bikini with wide-set straps and fairly brief bottom.
WHAT TO STAY AWAY FROM
Bare looks: Spaghetti-strap looks—your shoulders will seem monumental; avoid totally strapless looks for the same reason.
Pants: The straightest cuts will accentuate narrow hips.
Swimwear: There's no particular style to avoid; trust your eye to tell whether the proportion between your hips and shoulders looks right.

● **short figure**
GOOD IDEAS TO TRY
Bare looks: Anything cut close to the body; an A-line butcher wrap.
Pants: Straight cut; drawstring or pleat-front styles will work if the fullness is not exaggerated; short shorts.
Swimwear: One-piece maillot in a dark color will give a sleek line. A fairly brief bikini is another good idea.
Sportswear: Aim for one continuous line; don't break colors at the waist; tone-on-tone or monotones are best. A slim jumpsuit is great.
WHAT TO STAY AWAY FROM
Bare looks: Anything with lots of fullness or gathers, avoid the fussy, "little girl" look.
Pants: Full drawstring or pleated styles; Jamaica, Bermuda, or pedal-pusher lengths will emphasize your smallness.
Swimwear: Large prints will overpower your size.

● **tall figure**
GOOD IDEAS TO TRY
Bare looks: You can wear almost any style. If you're very thin, make sure the neckline doesn't make you look bony.
Pants: Pleat-front or drawstring styles; Jamaicas, clam diggers, pedal pushers.
Swimwear: A bikini in a bold print or a sleek maillot will work.
Sportswear: If you break the color scheme at the waist, your height will be less obvious. Wide waistbands and belts are good. Jumpsuits, especially with a drawstring or elasticized waist, are great for you.
WHAT TO STAY AWAY FROM
Bare looks: Anything too fussy or "little girl."
Pants: Straight string-bean cuts.
Swimwear: No particular style to avoid.

● **large-bosomed figure**
GOOD IDEAS TO TRY
Bare looks: Moderately bare halter or wrap tops or dresses; butcher-apron wraps.
Sportswear: The looser T-shirts with boat necks and dropped shoulders; classic shirts; shirt jackets; any wrap top or dress.
Swimwear: A classic maillot is your best bet. A bikini with an underwire top or with a wide band under the bosom will work. Look for a suit with bra-sized cups.
WHAT TO STAY AWAY FROM
Bare looks: Anything will fullness starting just under the bust or anything that's very bare; strapless or peasant tops.
Sportswear: Tight T-shirts, ribbed knit tops, smocks, or bosom-gathered styles.
Swimwear: Any nonsupportive bare style.

67

fashion

fur coat
giving an old fur coat a new look

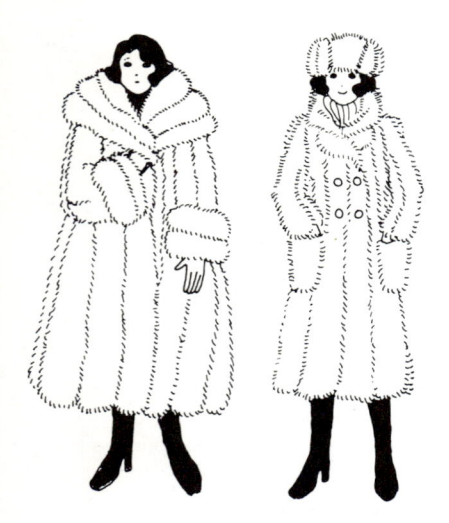

If you own or have inherited an outdated fur coat, it may be possible to turn it into a super-looking wrap. Here are some ideas:
- First, make sure the fur is worth the money you'll invest in the alterations. A good furrier will be able to assess its value and estimate its worth after the restyling (a free service). Then, check prices for new coats and figure out if you'd be saving a worthwhile amount.
- Comparison shop. Get price estimates from private furriers as well as those in department and specialty stores. Look over their models to see their work. Choose a furrier who designs a model very similar to the style you want, because once you start making changes on the basic model, the price—and the chance of mistakes—go up.
- Don't be tempted by the most contemporary styles. Simple classic shapes like wraps, reefers, or chesterfields are best.
- Make sure any extra fur that's cut off will be returned to you. It could be used to make a hat (or to trim one), to line a wool jersey scarf, or to make a fur vest. You could even use scraps of fur to cover pillows or buttons.
- Although your furrier will make suggestions about alterations, it's smart to have some of your own. Do you want to have cuffs removed, a collar made smaller, armholes cut higher? Full coats look much better once some of the width is removed. If the coat is too short, have it altered to a chubby or hip-length wrap or, great for inexpensive furs, a blouson shape with knitted bottom and cuffs.

holiday glitter
update your clothes with holiday glitter

You don't have to go out and buy new clothes or accessories to glitter your way through the holidays. You can add lots of special touches to things you already own—if fact, you can probably make use of some things you thought you'd never use again! Here are some suggestions:

Buy glitter appliqués—sequined fruit, cars, and so forth—from notions departments. Many have self-adhesive backings so you don't even have to sew them on.

Add a silver or gold edging of metallic crochet thread around the neck or cuffs of a sweater; just chain-stitch it right on the sweater.

Metallic piping or decorative braid looks great on any jacket. You can also stitch piping or giant silver or gold rickrack (available in dime stores) on the outside leg seams of your pants or jeans.

With some metallic embroidery thread, embroider an animal, fruit, or other design on a sweater or T-shirt.

Change the buttons on a silky shirt. Buy some rhinestones or gold or silver buttons to add a festive touch to a pretty skirt.

Edge a shirt collar and cuffs with rhinestone studs.

Spray an old pair of sandals or pumps gold or silver for a jazzy new look.

Buy containers of metallic sparkle dust in a dime store. Spread a little white glue wherever you want to glitter, then drop dust on the glue. Cover plastic earrings, bangles, the heels and/or platforms of shoes, belt buckles, and so on.

Glitter old jewelry by wrapping a bangle or cuff bracelet with metallic thread, brushing lightly with white glue as you wrap. Or wind a rope of bugle beads around a cuff bracelet, also securing with glue.

long dress
summertime question... what to wear over a long dress

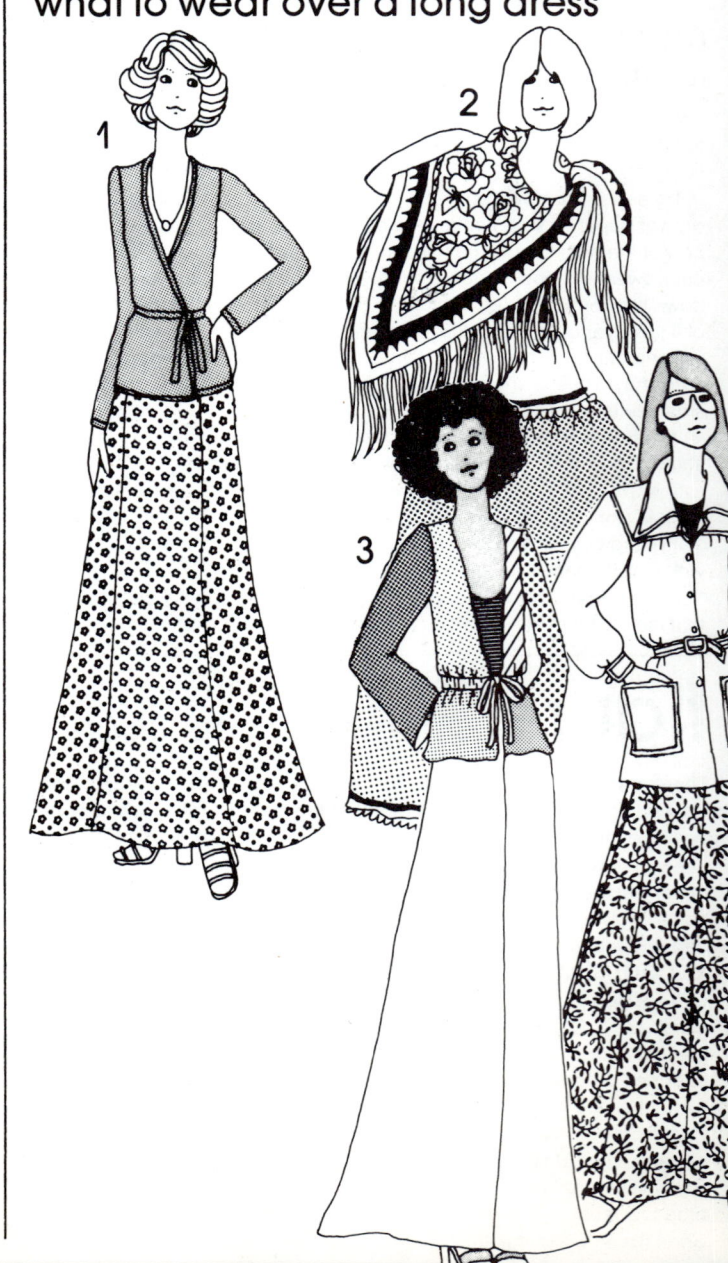

fashion

The right top to wear over a long dress or skirt should be something light—just warm enough to fend off air conditioning or an evening breeze. Here are some ideas:
1. A wrap sweater is so popular that nearly everyone owns one. Try wearing it over a long skinny dress or a long slinky skirt and blouse.
2. Probably the most classic coverup is a shawl. Your best bet is a pretty, peasant-embroidered one or a plain one with long fringe. Wear it over a full or peasant-looking skirt like the one shown here.
3. Another good coverup is a drawstring top. Pop it over a tank top and long skirt and you have a super look.
4. A shirt jacket looks terrific over a casual or sporty long dress or skirt. If your outfit is more dressy, wear a sheer chiffon shirt over it as a fancier coverup.

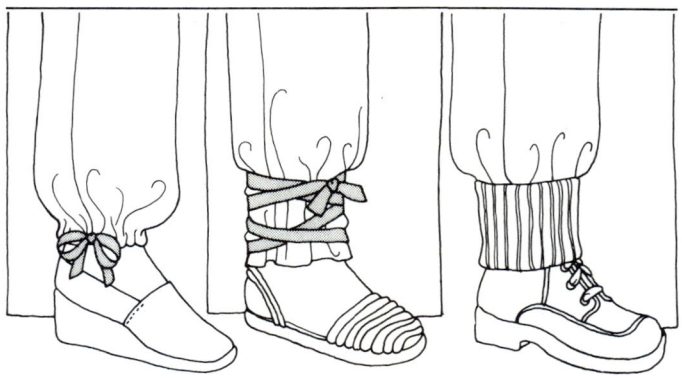

pants
tie up a new look for your old pants

Ankle-tied pants are an interesting look you can have without buying anything new—except maybe a piece of pretty ribbon. You'll get the best results with soft pants, but any pants, even jeans, will work. For full-legged pants of a fairly stiff fabric, make a pleat in the bottom of pant leg (see sketch). Secure pleat by tying a ribbon around the ankle. Be sure you ease pant hem up around your ankle when you tie the ribbon so you'll have enough fullness in the leg to allow you to bend your knees comfortably.

If you're wearing soft pants, like cotton gauze or another lightweight fabric, you might want to run a drawstring through the leg hem and tie them this way (see sketch). Just make a tiny slit in the front of a side seam of the hem through which to pass the ribbon. This way, you can always pull the ribbon out if you don't wear the pants tied at the ankle.

Another nifty idea to try involves a little sewing, but the effect is worth the trouble. Buy a yard of knit ribbing in a notions department, and sew the ribbing to the bottom of your pants (see sketch). To determine size of ribbing, measure your ankle and add an inch to allow for a seam. You can wear the pants at the ankle or push them up to midcalf for a knickers look.

If you have espadrilles with long laces, you might try lacing the espadrilles up over the pant legs for another great look.

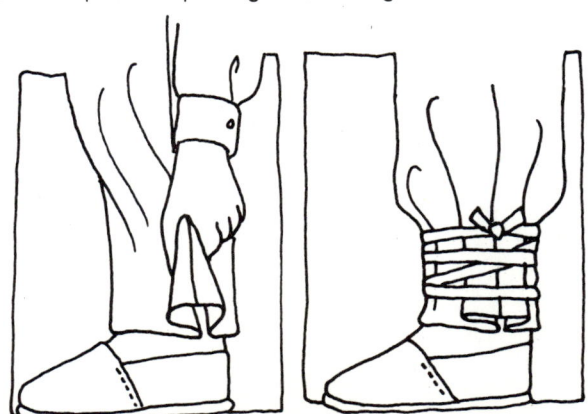

pants
the right pants for your figure

Whether you're carrying too many pounds or too few, your waist is long or short, or whatever else your figure faults may be, they can *look* like less of a problem in the right pants. And what you wear with the pants can be just as important as the pants themselves in giving you a sleek total look.

If hips and thighs are the biggest part of you, look for simply cut pants with either a straight, slightly flared, or wider leg. Stay with sturdy, no-cling fabrics in deep colors. Avoid pleat-front pants or high waistbands—they both tend to emphasize the bulk below your waist. Smock tops and loose jackets—like safari jackets—are concealing. If you do tuck a shirt into your pants, wear low-cut hip-riding pants to help lengthen and slim your torso.

If a thick waist is your problem, look for pants that close at the natural waist or below. Hip-huggers are a good choice because their low cut gives the illusion of a longer, slimmer waist. A well-cut, not-too-clingy bodyshirt is a good choice with pants, or an easy-fitting sweater or T-shirt worn outside the pants and belted low.

If you're fighting a tummy bulge, low-cut, hip-riding pants are flattering because they give such a long, slim line. Pleat-front pants or any high-waistband pants make a tummy bulge seem worse than ever. Wearing sweaters or T-shirts on the outside of pants is more flattering for you.

If you're too thin, pleat-front pants are made for you. The extra fullness in front and the ample legs are both flattering. Pick pants in fabrics with some bulk; steer clear of clingy soft fabrics that make you look bony. Layered tops are super for you—little sleeveless vests over shirts or a layering of T-shirts (short-sleeved over long). Wear soft blouses instead of clingy bodyshirts.

If you're on the short-waisted side, hip-huggers give the illusion of a long, slim middle. You can also wear pants that hit at the natural waist. Don't get involved with high-waisted pleat-fronts or pants with any sort of waistband—both will cut your figure. Unless you're wearing hip-huggers, a top worn outside your pants will look better than something tucked in.

If you feel you're too long waisted, pants with a waistband will help cut the long line at the waist. Try high-waisted, pleat-front pants or a bodyshirt tucked into pants. A sweater or T-shirt worn outside and belted at the natural waist will also work. Stay away from hip-huggers; they tend to emphasize your problem.

No matter what your figure, you can spoil the overall look by wearing your pants too short. A good general rule to follow is to wear pants that

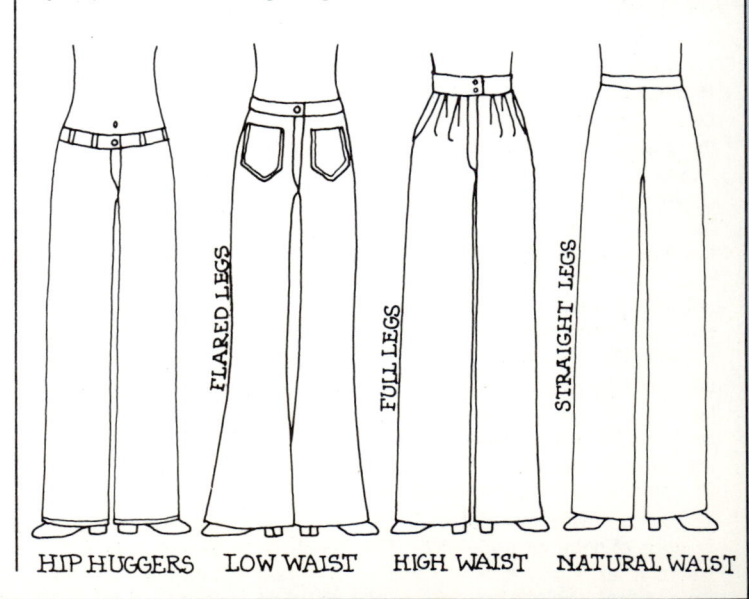

HIP HUGGERS   LOW WAIST   HIGH WAIST   NATURAL WAIST

FLARED LEGS   FULL LEGS   STRAIGHT LEGS

69

fashion

fall (in back) at the spot where your shoe heel joins the shoe and (in front) just brush the shoe without breaking or buckling. Of course, heel heights and platforms determine the length of your pants. Don't assume that because a pair of pants is right with one pair of shoes, it will be right with all your shoes.

Another thing that contributes to a sleek look for dressier pants is a crisp crease down the front. If you can't press it in at home with your iron, have the cleaner steam one in. Very casual and full evening pants are, of course, an exception.

party looks
how to decorate yourself for a special party or holiday

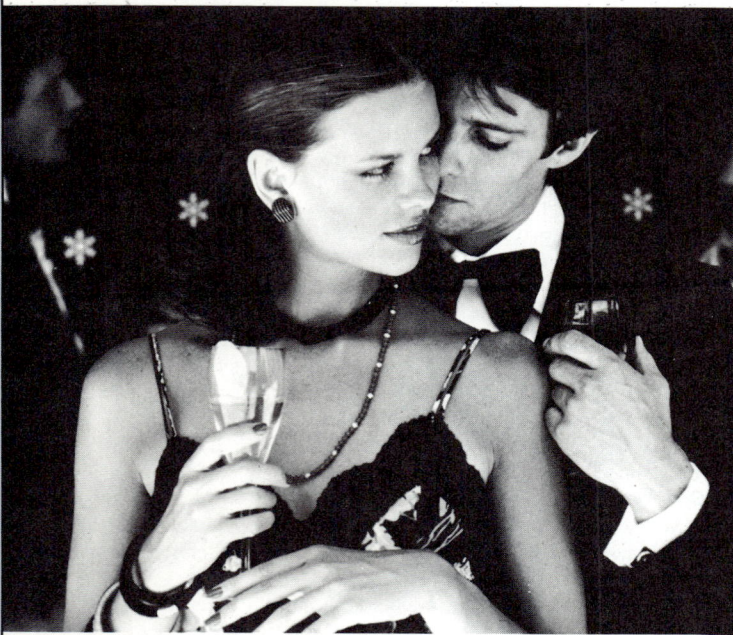

The most smashing looks are often the result of small money and big imaginations. Here is a collection of ideas that will add dazzle—inexpensively—to any party look.

- **rhinestone a sweater**
You can buy rhinestones in strips—by the yard—to circle the neck of a sweater or a pair of velvety espadrilles. Or try outlining the collar and front of a blazer with them. (Rhinestones by the yard are available in notions and trimmings departments.)

- **rickrack and ribbon flowers**
Design flowers to decorate your hair, the neck of a dress, or even use this pretty, easy-to-make "bud" as the buckle on a belt. All you need is a package of bright rickrack—for all-out dazzle, gold or silver metallic rickrack. To make a small rose, cut off about ¾ yard of rickrack. Fold in half and interlock the V's of the rickrack together as if you were braiding. Fold the raw edge in and begin rolling the rickrack to form the center bud of the flower. Continue until bud looks full. Tack lower edges with needle and thread to secure the bud. Then, with the same thread, run tiny basting stitches along lower edge of remaining rickrack. Pull thread together slightly and curve rickrack loosely around the bud to form petals. Tack petals in place. You can use the same technique to make ribbon flowers too. Use ribbon at least 2" wide and fold in half to give the flower more body. Form the flower exactly as you did with the rickrack.

- **appliqué a neckline**
You'll find rows of tiny embroidered flowers, medallions, and designs in strips of decorative trim, available in notions departments or dime stores. It takes only minutes to tack the flowers around the neck and sleeves of a sweater to get a fresh, flower-garden effect. Or you might prefer one big beautiful appliqué—like a bright red quilted rose—for the front of a sweater.

- **shine up your waist**
A gold or silver mesh belt can light up a whole dress. You can make one yourself by buying a yard of the mesh, either 2" or 3" wide, then cutting it to size and attaching a pretty buckle.

- **dust your collarbone with sparkle**
Give a party look to cutout necklines or bare shoulders. Buy a container of colored glitter in a dime store—you'll find all colors, including gold and silver. Smooth on a little eyelash adhesive where you want the glitter, then just sprinkle it on.

- **stud your hair with jewels**
If your hair is long, pull it into a chignon and add your biggest single rhinestone stud in the center of the chignon (some rhinestones are sold in strips; others are sold separately as studs). A bobby pin or hairpin will hold the stud in place. Or you might pull your hair into a ponytail, then attach one or more lengths of the rhinestones (cut to the same length as your ponytail) to the base of the ponytail. Twist the ponytail and the rhinestones all together and make a soft, plump knot at the nape of your neck. Another idea—glue a few individual rhinestone studs on a barrette or comb and wear in your hair.

- **surprise gilding**
Dust a bit of gold eye shadow in your cleavage if you're wearing a very low-cut neckline. Try dusting gold shadow over your blusher to gild your cheeks.

- **silver- or gold-spray your clogs**
All it takes is a can of gold or silver spray paint and you're ready to go. Use masking tape to color sections or when using two colors for a combination. Let paint dry completely before you remove tape. A skinny leather belt, a bag, a pair of sandals all can be sprayed to give a festive holiday look.

scarves
new tie-ups for scarves

If all you can do with a scarf is tie it around your neck à la John Wayne, don't give up. Here's a rundown of great scarf ties that are guaranteed to work for "all thumbs" types.

1. *The dog collar:* Fold square scarf into an oblong. Place around neck with ends in back. Cross ends and bring around to front. Tie a square knot and fluff out ends. (You'll need at least a 22" square.)
2. *Girl Scout tie:* Fold a 27" or 36" square scarf in half to form a triangle. Place center point in back. Tie front ends together in a low square knot or turn scarf sideways so the triangle lies over your shoulder.
3. *Necklace tie:* Place a small chiffon scarf around neck, tying in back. Tuck loose ends into collar.
4. *The muffler:* Place a long oblong scarf around neck, crossing in back, and bring ends forward to hang in front.
5. *The loop-through:* Fold a 72" oblong scarf in half (so it's 36" long) and place around neck. Pull ends through loop the fold has made; let ends dangle in front or throw one over shoulder.
6. *The easy tie:* Fold a

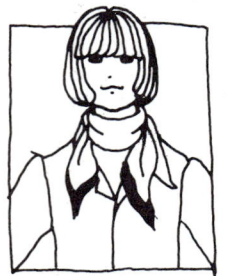

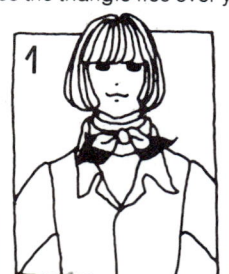

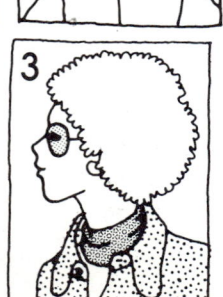

fashion

square scarf into an oblong, wrap around neck, and tie into a loose, fat knot in front. Wear one end over shoulder, the other in front, off-center.

7. *The twist:* For a variation of the muffler, twist two coordinating scarves together, then wrap around neck in muffler-style.

Tips: To fold a square scarf into an oblong, spread open scarf and bring up one corner a few inches beyond center of scarf. Fold opposite corner down over this. Then keep folding the two opposite sides of scarf toward center until you get desired width. This gives the scarf more ease. To make a square knot, take left end of scarf and tie over right; then take right end and tie over left, shaping knot into a square shape.

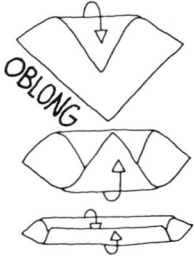

scarves
tie up a great summer look — scarf top

Need a pretty summer top to wear with long summer skirts? This one's made from a scarf, takes no stitching at all, and even shows off a tan. To make it, all you need is a square scarf at least 45" × 45" (an Indian cotton gauze scarf is a good choice). Fold scarf into a triangle and hold both ends in both hands. Center point in front of your body and wrap scarf around torso, crisscrossing in the back at about shoulder level. Bring ends to front and tie at your neck (see sketch). For a finishing touch, wrap another coordinating scarf around your waist.

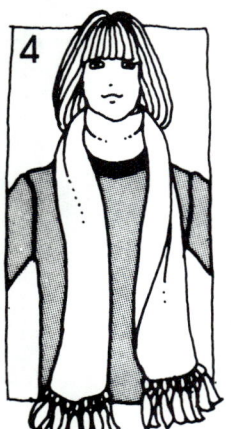

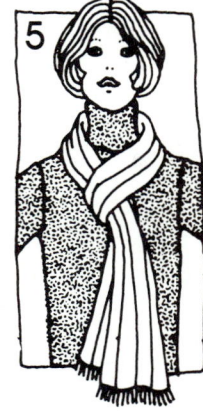

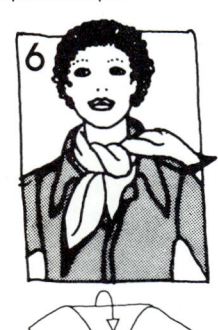

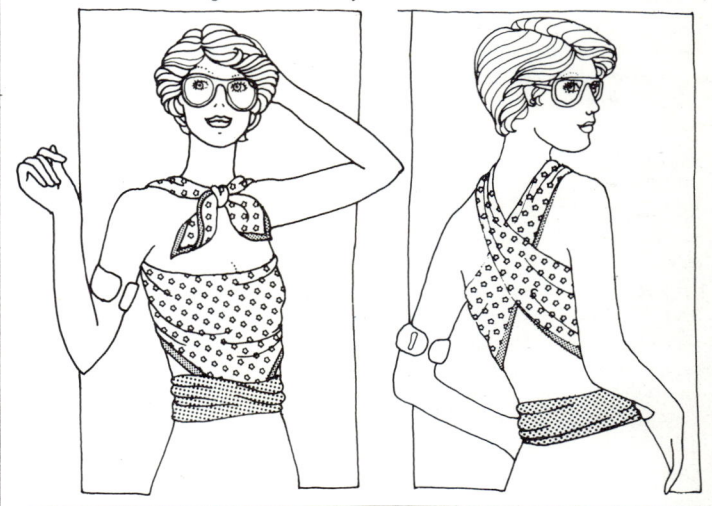

scarves
waist scarves and how to tie them

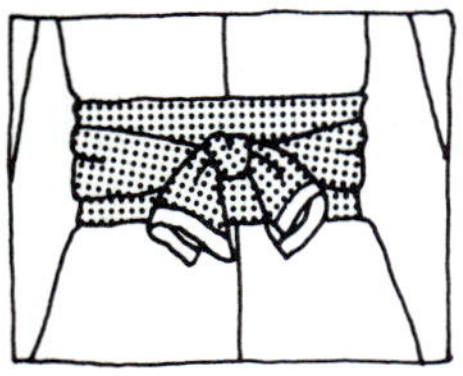

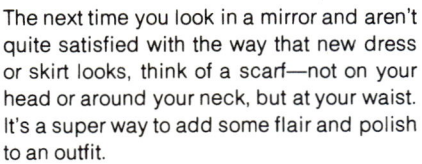

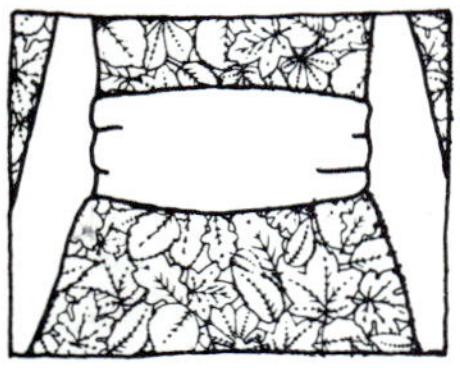

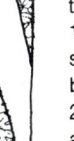

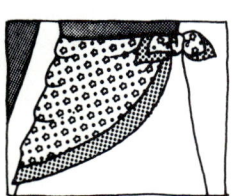

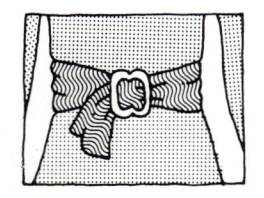

The next time you look in a mirror and aren't quite satisfied with the way that new dress or skirt looks, think of a scarf—not on your head or around your neck, but at your waist. It's a super way to add some flair and polish to an outfit.

1. *The cummerbund:* Place a 72" oblong scarf around your waist, cross in back, and bring around to front, tying at side or center.
2. *The sash:* For a 48" oblong, wrap scarf around waist, knotting at side. Or wrap and tie the scarf around waist with ends in back. Tuck ends into skirt waistband or pin in place. You can also take another scarf and place it over the first, knotting in front (as in cummerbund) for a pattern-on-pattern look.
3. *The gypsy:* Take a large square scarf (challis scarves are especially pretty), fold into a triangle, and place around waist, tying in a square knot. Wear point in back or at side.
4. *The belt:* If you have a beautiful belt buckle, pull a scarf through it. First pin one end of scarf around the center bar of buckle, then wrap scarf around waist as you would a belt, pulling opposite end through belt buckle. Pin in place or let hang.

shopping
strange places to hunt down fashion finds

Fashion lives in strange places—like hardware stores or sporting goods shops, even fishing tackle stores. And when you shop this off-beat route, you often end up saving dollars as well as finding something indeed unique. Here are some tips to broaden your fashion horizons:

Most any hardware store carries shiny metal chains that can be made into handsome belts, necklaces, shoulder straps, or handles for bags. The uncut blanks for keys make good-looking ornaments to hang on a chain; so do some of the unusual nuts and bolts.

Fishing tackle shops turn up beautiful brass tackles to use in jewelry making. You'll find an assortment of feathery flies—great for jewelry—and leather or canvas bags to sub for handbags. Hunting stores also sell unusual pouches.

Sporting goods shops house an assortment of pants, shirts, shorts, and T-shirts that will amaze you—with both their styling and their low price tags. A T-shirt with a giant number on it teamed with satiny athletic shorts is just one possible combination.

Army-Navy stores are famous by now for inexpensive shirts, pants, and jeans.

Try the kitchen shop of department stores for a big wrap-around butcher's apron, usually sold as a man's barbecue apron. They look great with T-shirts or as sundresses in summer.

Even a pet shop is not devoid of fashion. Chain "choker collars" can be wrapped around the waist and look smashing as belts.

The notions or trimming department in a large store is resplendent with fringe, sequins, appliqués, tassels—all just begging to be turned into jewelry.

71

fashion

shopping
thrift-shop fashion—how to find it, take care of it, make it fit

Buying in thrift shops turns up not only fashion bargains but some beautiful party clothes in intriguing styles as well. The shopping tips below came from two thrift-shop proprietors, Harriet and Lewis Winter, who got so involved with the mystique of antique clothes and fine workmanship that they closed their thrift shop and started a wholesale fashion business called Yesterday's News. Their creations are inspired by the look and quality of antique clothes.

Autumn is usually a good time to thrift shop. Outdoor sales have particularly inexpensive merchandise. Look for garage sales, church sales, tag sales, and flea markets and check local papers and bulletin boards for sale notices. The Salvation Army and charity shops are also good bargain sources.

Before you buy a garment, it's a good idea to first check it out carefully—there's no point to buying a dress that won't survive even one cleaning or washing. Check underarms, around neck, and down back for signs of wear and perspiration. Don't buy a garment with excessive odor, because although dry cleaning or washing will remove it temporarily, your own perspiration will immediately revive the original odor. Check seams for signs of rot. Give them a gentle pull and see if they withstand it. Be especially suspicious of pure silk, as it has a tendency to rot quicker than other fabrics. Hold up any wool, knit, or jersey to a light and check for tiny holes—especially in garage sales where things may have been stored in mothy barns.

Generally, it's best to have a garment dry cleaned (tell the cleaner it's antique and needs special care), though you can always get it clean by washing. Silk and wool can both be washed with a cold-water soap. Rayon, especially rayon crepe, shrinks terribly, so be careful; better yet, have it dry cleaned.

To shrink wool sweaters, wash them with cold-water soap, then put them in a hot clothes dryer. When they're almost dry, remove them, block, and allow to finish drying. You can also take a sweater in by sewing it. Turn it inside out and follow the shape of original seaming, but take it in the necessary amount. Run up two seams about a quarter of an inch apart, then cut off excess. You might also like to try dyeing a sweater. You can get wonderful effects by dyeing old wool with ordinary fabric dyes.

Whenever you need to take in an antique garment, do so before you rip the original seam. Ripping the seam may tear the garment and ruin it. In fact, it's a good idea to just take it in and leave the old seam intact.

Finally, don't forget to consider buying thrift shop garments for just their buttons or trim.

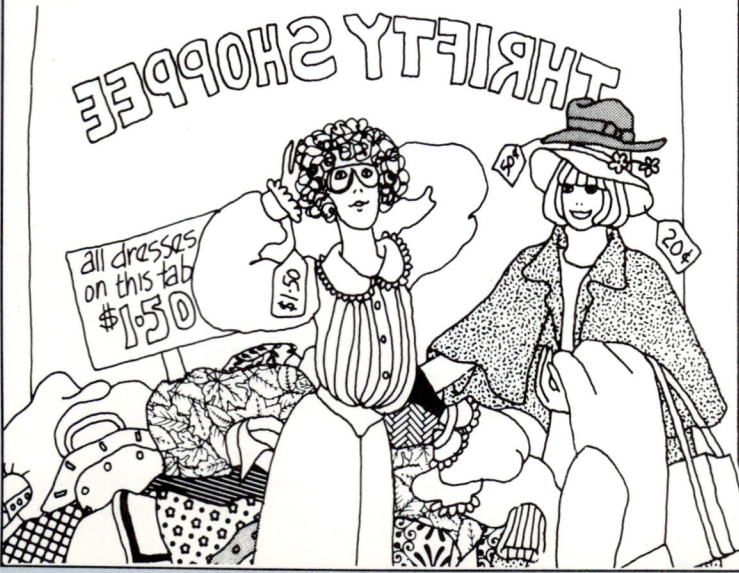

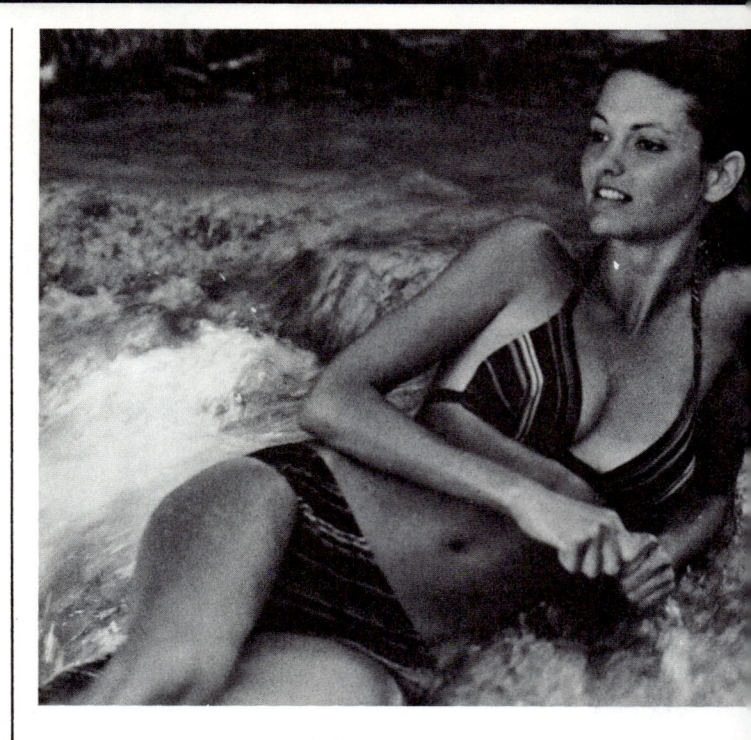

swimsuit
how to find the best-fitting swimsuit you've ever worn

Finding a swimsuit that makes the best of the worst of you is easier now than it's ever been—if you know what to look for. Here are some tips:

If a small bosom is your problem, buy a suit that makes the most of your best feature—like a sexy back. But if you are self-conscious about your bosom, buy a suit with a well-shaped bra top in a substantial fabric that will hold its shape. Look for a one- or two-piece suit with a fiberfill bra top. There are also suits that are "one-size-fits-all," which can work if you're not too small. Just be sure the stretch action lifts the bosom instead of flattening it. Or consider a bikini style with a different size top and bottom.

If your problem is a full bosom, don't feel compelled to buy a suit that's all covered up on top. A good idea is one of the bikini styles with separately purchased tops and bottoms. Try to find an underwired cup or one that's shaped so that it doesn't push all the fullness to the center and cause a bulge. Straps that button or snap to the back are more supportive than those that tie behind the neck. Or pick a one-piece suit that has bra-sized cups and a soft, naturally shaped cup.

If a thick waist is your problem, a one-piece suit in a dark color is one solution. A dark suit belted in a bright color is good, too. Cutouts through the waist of a one-piece suit can give the illusion of a curve. A dark bikini with a bottom that starts well below the waist can be flattering.

If you're fighting heavy thighs, you may be able to find a semibikini—one with a low waist but a shorts leg. A very high cutout leg, usually called a "French" leg, is the most flattering of all. It gives the illusion of a slim curve.

If you're overweight in general, a slim one-piece suit in any dark color is the best choice. If you're just a few pounds overweight, a stretchy suit will help smooth your figure—one with a supportive bra and a shorts leg. Always sit down in any suit you're considering to be sure it doesn't bulge unattractively.

If you're slender, don't buy the barest suit and expose all your bones. Look for suits that give the illusion of curves—maybe one with cutouts at the waist, a deep curvy back. The high-cut French leg is good for you.

tops
a quick quiz to help you pick the best tops for your figure

Tops—like figures—come in all shapes and sizes, but some look better on certain figures than others. We've sketched some of the most common shapes. Pick the ones you think work best for your figure, then check to see if your opinion agrees with ours. This doesn't mean you shouldn't wear tops not listed in your category—there are exceptions to every rule. But in general, the ones listed for you will be most flattering. These are the figure problems we worked with: short waist, long waist, small bosom, large bosom, broad shoulders, narrow shoulders, generally thin, or generally overweight. If you feel you have more than one of these problems, pick your most troublesome one or compare the listings.

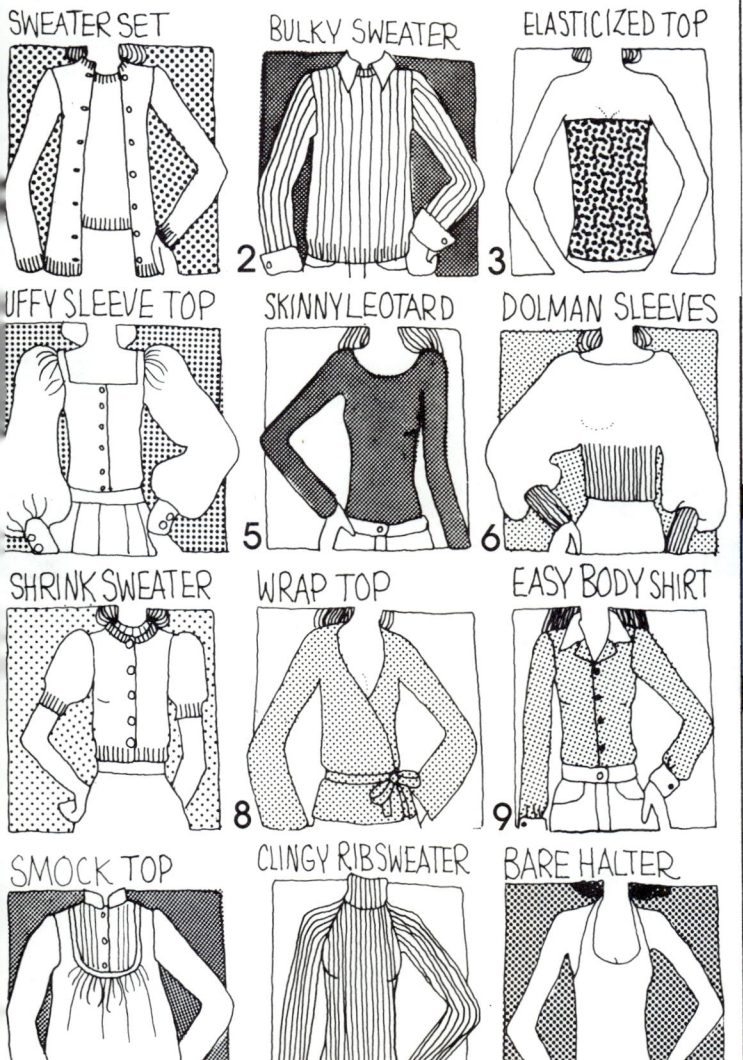

1. SWEATER SET
2. BULKY SWEATER
3. ELASTICIZED TOP
4. [P]UFFY SLEEVE TOP
5. SKINNY LEOTARD
6. DOLMAN SLEEVES
7. SHRINK SWEATER
8. WRAP TOP
9. EASY BODY SHIRT
10. SMOCK TOP
11. CLINGY RIB SWEATER
12. BARE HALTER

● **figure types**

Short waist: 1, 2, 3, 5, 8, 9, 10, 11, 12
Long waist: 1, 2, 3, 4, 6, 7, 8, 9, 10, 12
Small bosom: 1, 2, 4, 6, 7, 8, 9, 10
Large bosom: 1, 2, 3, 9, 10
Broad shoulders: 1, 2, 8, 9, 10
Narrow shoulders: 1, 2, 4, 7, 8, 10
Generally thin: 1, 2, 4, 6, 7, 8, 10
Generally overweight: 1, 8, 9, 10

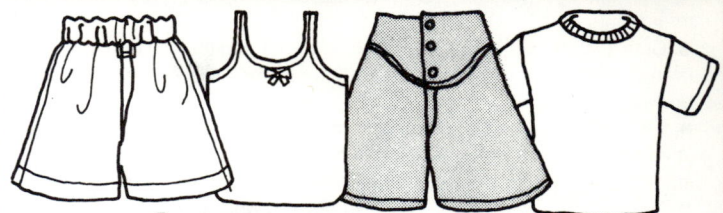

underwear
good reasons to wear underwear out on top

The best reason for wearing "underwear" as outerwear is that it can sometimes be considerably cheaper and better-looking than what it's substituting for. Aside from that, it's fun to know you're being a little more adventuresome and inventive than the next person. Just for fun, try . . .

● Little boy's white boxer shorts on the tennis court. They're light and roomy (get a small boy's size or a slim-cut men's size). You can close the fly with a few snaps or stitches. They look amazingly like tennis shorts.

● At your nearest Army surplus outlet, ask for a pair of olive drab Army-issue boxer shorts. They're great-looking short shorts that button down the front.

● Some nightgowns can double for party dresses. If you pick an opaque floral, a bright color, black or white (stay away from pastels), no one will be the wiser. Add bracelets, a bag, maybe a shawl, and your sexy secret is safe.

● A pair of slinky pajamas could make your next cocktail party. Oriental ones, some with pretty brocade jackets, are fabulous looking.

● A camisole top can pretty up any summer bottom—pants or a skirt. Often sold as outerwear, they're not quite as inexpensive as many underwear items, but so romantic!

flowers

arrangements
11 ways to make a $1 bunch of flowers look like more

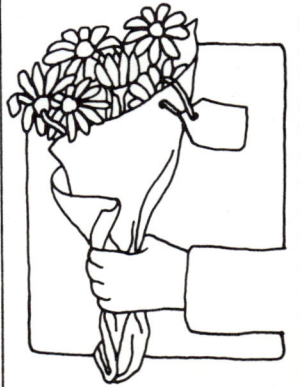

Sometimes the only flowers many of us can afford are the nice-but-skimpy bunches available for $1 from street vendors or florists. There are some easy ways to make them look like more than they really are.

● Place individual flowers in tiny wine carafes. Daisies, anemones, or small pink or purple asters look especially attractive displayed this way, maybe with one to a place setting at a dinner party. The carafes themselves are inexpensive and can be used again and again.

● Instead of using carafes, you might place individual flowers in dark green soda bottles. Fresca and 7-Up bottles look so amusing when used in this way that even restaurants often use them. Wine half bottles also make nice vases, with or without

73

f flowers

their labels.
- Cut the stem of a single flower to ¼" long. Float the flower in a small brandy snifter half filled with water. Or use small white china or glass bowls.
- Cluster a group of flowers in an empty mustard or cheese crock, or in a creamer. One woman created a charming centerpiece by clustering petunias, with lots of green leaves, in a white ironstone gravy boat.
- In a more traditional vase, fill out your flowers with evergreens or other leaves. You also might try mixing real and fake flowers or leaves, particularly silk leaves, with real flowers. This is a common practice in Europe.

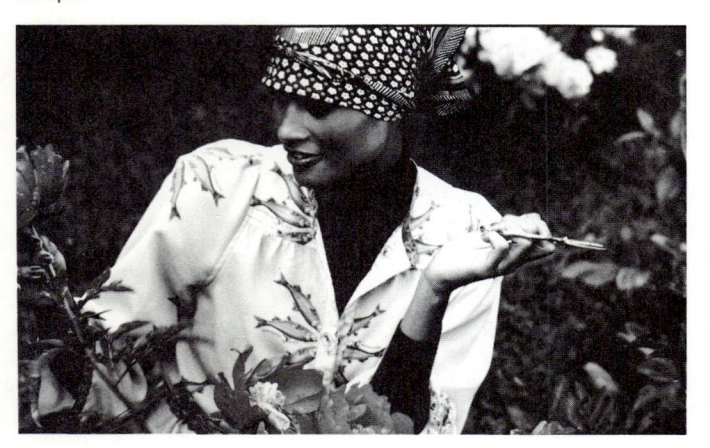

cut what florists do to make cut flowers last longer

Roses or chrysanthemums especially respond to a few special tricks that make the most of their vase life. Cut rose stems, but leave on thorns unless you're expert at removing them without damaging the stem. Mums absorb water best if you first scrape stems with a paring knife and break off, rather than cut, to the length you want. Next, place roses or mums in any deep pail filled with hot water (don't cover blooms); soak them one to two hours. Then, put regular tap water in your vases, adding a floral life extender (available at florists' or dime stores). Arrange flowers so there is breathing room and no leaves below water line. In three to four days, if any blooms wilt, make a fresh cut of stems or break 2" to 3" from the bottom and put them into hot water again for a good soak till the blooms perk up. Other tips: Tulips need plenty of water; a tablespoon of sugar per quart of water helps, and so does tossing in about five copper pennies. Gladioli bloom best if you nip off the top bud right away. Stock absorbs water more efficiently if you pound the stem ends flat. When you buy other flowers, always ask your florist what methods to use.

drying how to get the best results when you're drying cut or wild flowers

If you've tried to dry flowers but wound up with crumbling flakes, the steps below can make a difference next time you try. They not only work really well on many wild flowers including daisies, pinks, asters, and Queen Anne's lace, but also give beautiful results with cut flowers such as mums, roses, and zinnias.

If you are drying wild or garden flowers, pick them on a sunny day—not after a rain or heavy dew, which may have trapped moisture within the flower. Try to pick them at the height of bloom, and dry soon after cutting. (This helps preserve color and luster.) Remember, too, that clear, light, or medium colors—such as bright pinks and blues—dry better than, say, dark reds, which may turn black in the drying process.

Pour 1" to 2" of a drying medium into the bottom of a shoebox, cookie tin, or other container with a top. (The more airtight, the better.) Commercial drying mediums containing silica gel work best—but you can also use a mixture of ⅔ borax and ⅓ fine sand or kitty litter.

Cut flower stems to 2" and place flowers in the container so they're not touching. Sprinkle more of your medium over them until they're completely covered, then seal the container all the way around with masking tape.

Put the container away for seven to eight days in a spot where it will not be disturbed or exposed to bright, direct sunlight.

Later remove flowers from container and attach each short flower stem to medium-weight florist's wire by spiral-wrapping it with green florist's tape.

Select a vase or crock with a design that doesn't compete with your flowers. (Soft colors and matte textures are usually good.) Arrange flowers; hold in place, if need be, with clay, builder's sand, or styrofoam blocks.

Keep flowers away from direct sun to retain their color and texture for years. *Note:* Several field flowers—particularly yarrow, goldenrod, and coxscomb—can be dried simply by banding them together and hanging upside down in a dark, dry place for about ten days. If you have extra flowers, try this method first. If you don't like the results, use the drying method described above.

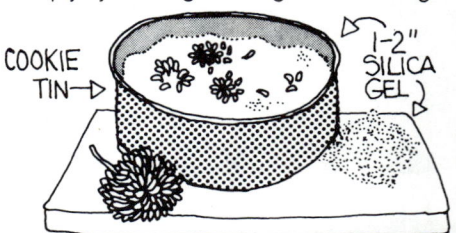

food

avocado a quick avocado guide

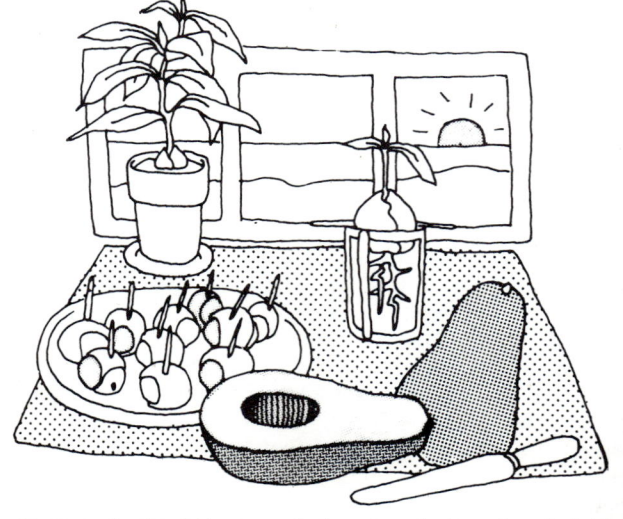

An avocado should be served when ripe, that is, when it yields a little to gentle pressure on its skin. However, most avocados sold in stores are usually hard and unripe; you can allow them to ripen at room temperature for three to ten days, depending on how ripe they are when you buy them. Ripe avocados will keep for several days if stored,

uncovered, in the refrigerator.
- To hasten an avocado's ripening by a few days, you can wrap it in a brown paper bag and store at room temperature until soft.
- Avocados are in season all year long. In winter you'll see mostly the tight-skinned bright green variety; from May through October, a summer fruit with pebbly skin in shades from deep green to black. Both have the same creamy fruit inside. And both have roughly the same nutritional content: one half of an average-size avocado has about 135 calories, two grams of protein, no cholesterol (but it has about 19 grams fat), and hefty doses of vitamins A and E. (An avocado, by the way, is a fruit—not a vegetable—even though it is often used as the latter.)

And, finally, here are some avocado combinations:
- *For an appetizer*—Make avocado balls, using a melon baller; serve with any fresh vegetable dip. Or wrap avocado balls in prosciutto and spear with toothpicks.
- *For a sandwich*—Spread a soft avocado, like butter, on rye toast; crumble a slice of crisp, fried bacon over it.
- *For a salad*—Add one diced avocado to a salad made with four cups raw spinach, three cups iceberg lettuce, one and a half cups orange sections, and one thinly sliced Bermuda onion. Serve with French or Italian dressing.

birthday cakes
for dieters, health-food fans, nonsweet lovers, or anyone at all

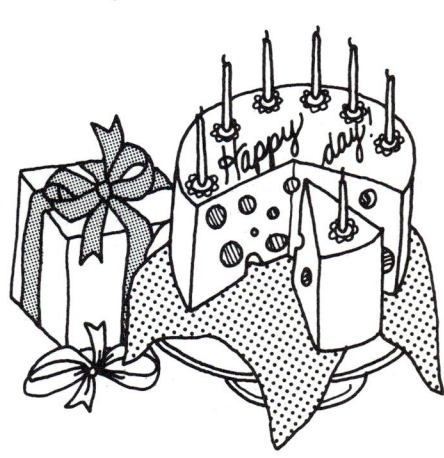

If thinking of the perfect birthday present can be hard, then thinking of the perfect birthday cake can be even harder, especially when it's for a dieter, health-food fan, or just someone who dislikes sweets. Giving any of *them* a traditional cake is like giving a vegetarian a lamb chop; however, these ideas may let friends have their cake and diet too.

- *For a dieter*—Stud a small wheel or brick of cheese with candles and surround with luscious fresh fruits and a pile of unusual crackers.
- *For a health-food fan*—Bake a beautiful, moist carrot cake and don't frost it. Or bake or buy a loaf of banana, honey, yogurt, or other preservative-free bread or cake; drizzle honey across the top and write "Healthy Birthday," using nuts.
- *For someone who doesn't like sweets*—Write "Happy Birthday" on a pizza using thin strips of green pepper. Or use a quiche Lorraine and a strip of letters purchased at a dime store that spells "Happy Birthday."
- *For an astrology buff*—Draw his or her sign on the cake using a ready-mixed, cake-decorating tube, or attach a picture of the sign with toothpicks.
- *For anyone*—Give a "cocktail birthday cake"—tiny candles in slices of orange or lemon floating in punch or sangria. You might also have a cake that will have special significance because it reflects something in a person's background. For example, if he or she is in love with all things French or has just returned from a year of study in Paris, buy several individual *baba au rhum* cakes and put a candle in each.

convenience foods
which ones are the bargains?

In a study of 162 convenience-food products, the U.S. Department of Agriculture found that 36 percent had a cost-per-serving *advantage* over their home-prepared or fresh counterparts. Here's a brief rundown of the results:

- **mixes**

Better than half of the products made from a complete mix were less expensive than their start-from-scratch counterparts. Bargains included mixes for brownies, corn muffins, yellow cake, devil's food cake, chocolate and white frosting, and complete mixes (those that required milk or water but no eggs) for pancakes and waffles. However, nearly all of the frozen, chilled, or ready-to-serve baked goods, desserts, and candies studied were more expensive than preparing them from recipes *or* mixes.

- **fruits**

The study turned up two super buys here: bottled lemon juice and reconstituted frozen orange juice concentrate—regardless of the season. But for the most part, the best buys in strawberries, peaches, grapefruit, etc., are probably during their season and at your fresh-fruit stand.

- **vegetables**

A number of frozen and canned vegetables actually cost less than fresh—green peas, lima beans, beets, spinach, and french fried potatoes. Some that were more expensive, however, were broccoli spears, whole boiled potatoes, and canned carrots. Remember that fresh vegetables are more apt to be money savers during their particular seasons. Also, when comparing a convenience-vegetable product that has some kind of embellishment—potatoes au gratin, broccoli with hollandaise sauce—with its fresh counterpart, you will save money by doing the embellishment right in your own kitchen.

- **main dishes**

Here's where convenience can cost you. Most convenience beef, chicken, turkey, pork, and fish products were more costly than fresh—including beef patties, lasagne, chicken à la king, sweet and sour pork, and tuna-noodle casserole. (While frozen and chilled cheese pizzas cost about 60 percent more than home prepared, the packaged-mix combination cheese pizzas cost about the same.)

Although the study didn't say so, do consider that from your point of view, small-size convenience-food dishes may save money in the long run if you're cooking for only one or two. You don't waste portions with them—so your garbage can doesn't end up being just another mouth to feed.

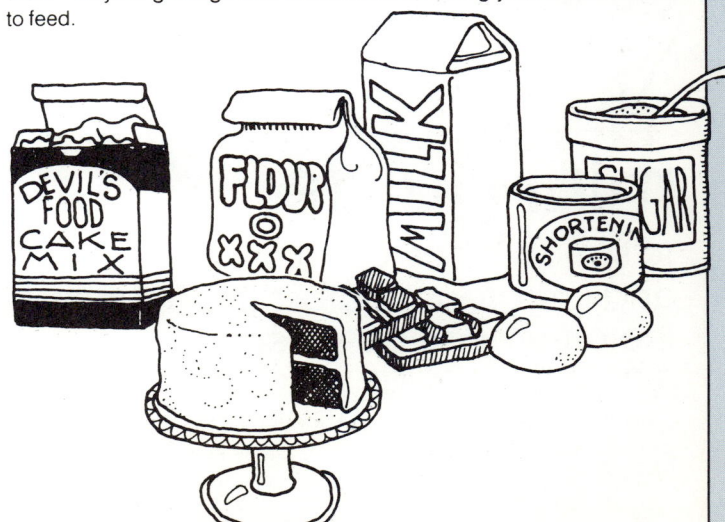

f food

fruits & vegetables
how to pick the best

If you squeeze the tomatoes, sample the grapes, exasperate the vegetable-store owner, and still come up with less than tasty, fresh produce—take heart! Here are super tips for using your fingers, eyes, nose, even ears to track down great fruits and vegetables. They were suggested by Joseph Doria, a partner in Balducci's, the fabulous landmark greengrocer shop in New York City.

- Melons—*Persians, casabas, and other summer melons are ripe if they smell sweet and feel a bit soft when you press their ends. They're usually better when average size, not small, and more likely to ripen at home if skin color isn't pale. A cantaloupe with rough webbing is sweeter than one with smooth webbing.*
- Berries—*Raspberries should be packed loosely; crammed wet, they can burn in hot weather. Pick red, round strawberries over pale, long ones.*
- Tomatoes—*Roll them in palms to check firmness without bruising. Red color is important but brown marks don't affect taste.*
- Apples, pears—*A fresh, tight-skinned apple squeaks when rubbed. A pear that's tender near its stem is ripe all the way down.*
- Eggplant—*Be a female chauvinist and pick females (with larger "bellybutton" dents on top) over males, which have too many seeds.*
- String beans—*Run your hand through the bin. If it feels velvety smooth, you're in luck.*
- Roots—*Fresh carrots keep about three days before the ends go soft. Buy them plastic-wrapped if you plan to store them longer. Turnips, parsnips, and black radishes should feel heavy and firm—soft or shriveled means old.*
- Squash—*Check firmness: For example, zucchini that's soft at its rounder end is old and will taste sour when cooked.*
- Salad greens—*Escarole is more tender if it has some white heart. For spinach-and-mushroom salads, look for spinach with big, crispy, wrinkled leaves and not much stem. A fresh green pepper has a hard stem.*
- Asparagus—*The season starts in October. Cut waste by looking for stalks that are green almost to the bottom. And listen: stems squeak if they're fresh.*

mini-guide
to sandwiches, soda, and ice cream across the country— the difference between a hoagie, wedge, and sub

You don't have to be from another country to be confused by American food—another state is far enough. Different regions have different names for the same thing and to make some sense out of it all, we polled the whole *GLAMOUR* staff—a good cross-section of the U.S.A.—and came up with the following:

- *Sandwiches*—Large sandwiches made with Italian or French bread and almost any kind of filler from ham, cheese, lettuce, and tomatoes to meatballs are called *heroes* in lots of places all across the country, *wedges* in parts of New England, *submarines* in the Washington, D.C. area and West Coast states, *hoagies* in the Mid-Atlantic region, and *grinders* (usually longer than the others) in Rhode Island. If you go to New Orleans, you'd better ask for a *poor boy*. Other kinds of sandwiches you may discover are: *Tex-Mex*, which is a *taco* (a thin, crisp cornmeal pancake) filled with lettuce and ground beef; a *smörrebrøt* (big in Minnesota), a Scandinavian open-faced sandwich made with shrimp or liverwurst and cucumber on whole wheat bread; or a *muffuletta*, an Italian version that's a combination of salami, cheese, and ham with a minced garlic and olive oil dressing. While hamburgers are hamburgers from coast to coast, did you know that a hot dog is called a *tube steak* in some Eastern resort areas?
- *Beverages*—Of course, to go with your sandwich, you need something to drink. But that can be a problem because *soda* on the East Coast means *ice cream soda* in the Midwest. And to get a *soda* in places like Seattle, Virginia, and the Midwest, say *pop*. In L.A., though, they're very specific and say *soda pop* so there's no confusion. To get a *milkshake* in Massachusetts, order a *frappe*.
- *Desserts*—If it's ice cream you crave, you'll probably make yourself understood anywhere, but keep in mind that *ice cream pops* are often called *eskimo pies* in the Midwest, *Good Humors* in the East. If someone mentions a *DQ*, that's short for New Jersey's Dairy Queen, a soft-ice-cream chain similar to Carvel in New York, Tastee Freeze in Virginia, or Foster Freeze in California. To wash all this down, you might want a slug of water, available at any water cooler, water fountain, or *bubbler* if you're out Wisconsin way.

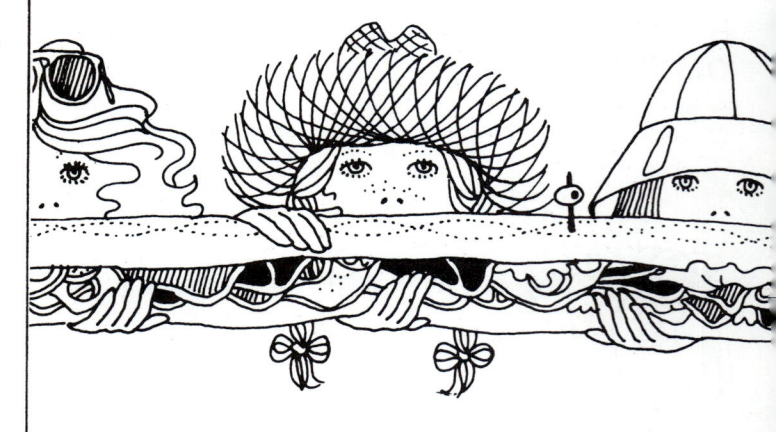

peanut butter
gourmet peanut butter sandwiches— too good for the peanut-butter set

If you think peanut butter sandwiches are simply a matter of picking your jelly and declaring for creamy smooth or crunchy, think again. The peanut butter sandwich has grown up out of its old kid-stuff rank. If you don't believe us, just try serving any of the following variations at a pre-game party, a tailgate picnic, or a brunch. All you need is your favorite kind of bread and peanut butter to combine with each of the following selections for fifteen different gourmet peanut butter sandwiches.

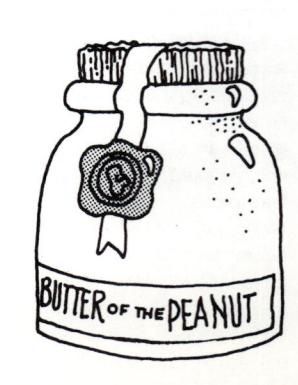

Bread, peanut butter, and
- Sliced leftover London broil or steak and Swiss cheese (mayonnaise or butter optional)
- Curry powder and raisins
- Bacon and sliced Bermuda onion
- Butter and sliced bananas
- Cream cheese and olives
- Sliced cucumbers
- Fresh chives with or without butter
- Fresh apple slices and butter
- Butter and crumbled milk chocolate
- Sliced bananas and India relish
- Cream cheese and India relish
- Garlic-salted watercress and mayonnaise
- Sliced leftover roast lamb and mint jelly
- Ginger preserves and butter or cream cheese

And don't forget that a few classics such as "the fluffer nutter" sandwich—peanut butter and marshmallow fluff—are still tasty.

picnics
4 gourmet picnics for anyone in a potato salad rut

Have a Parisian tailgate picnic with baskets of *charcuterie* (Spanish, Italian, French, and German sausages, liverwurst, bologna, salami), different cheeses, fresh French bread, and *vin chaud*—hot mulled wine—in insulated bottles.

Offer an assortment of Danish open-faced sandwiches, halved and layered with curried egg salad, anchovy, and tomato on pumpernickel; cream cheese, sardines, and olives on white; ham, Swiss cheese, and asparagus on rye. Serve with pea soup sprinkled with croutons, paper cups of cinnamon-flavored applesauce, and homemade gingerbread for dessert.

For health-food enthusiasts, carry the food in wicker or raffia baskets (use them later to hold plants). Fill with health foods like yogurt, sunflower seeds, carrot cake, and granola-bread sandwiches filled with honey or organic peanut butter.

If it's just a snack you want, slice and fill the round, flat, Middle Eastern *pita* bread with several very thin slices of cold roast beef and Greek salad—a mixture of shredded lettuce, chopped onions, chopped parsley, black olives, and *feta* cheese (optional) tossed in oil and lemon dressing.

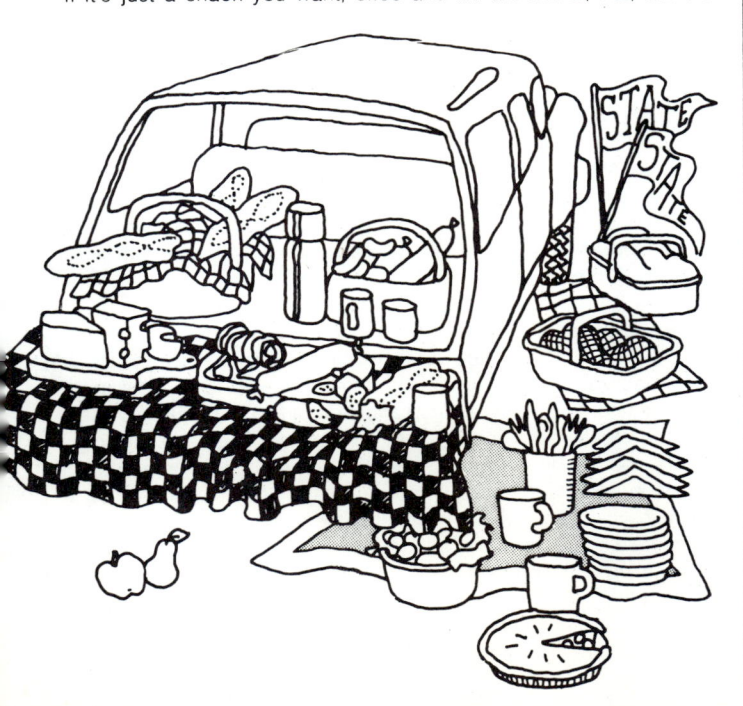

salad
a beautiful salad you can take anywhere — even to the office or beach

This salad will keep fresh in a beach basket, picnic hamper, or even an office lunch bag. You can make it on individual plates or in a large bowl for everyone. If you plan to take it to the beach or elsewhere, arrange in a foil pie plate, chill for a few hours, and wrap with foil before you leave. It's best to use an insulated tote to keep the salad cool, but salad won't wilt in an uninsulated tote that's well shaded from the sun.

As we've sketched the ingredients, the salad has less than 225 calories for an individual serving. (The substitute ingredients may add a few more.)

Arrange ingredients, according to sketch, on top of a bed of lettuce. Sprinkle with crumbled blue cheese, and chill until serving. Make a dressing of equal parts salad oil and red-wine vinegar, salt and pepper to taste, plus a pinch of each of these: dill, oregano, parsley, paprika, and minced green onion. Put into a jar. Toss into salad just before serving.

Substitute ingredients: diced pimiento, artichoke hearts, tuna, mushroom slices, sliced potato, water chestnuts, or green pepper.

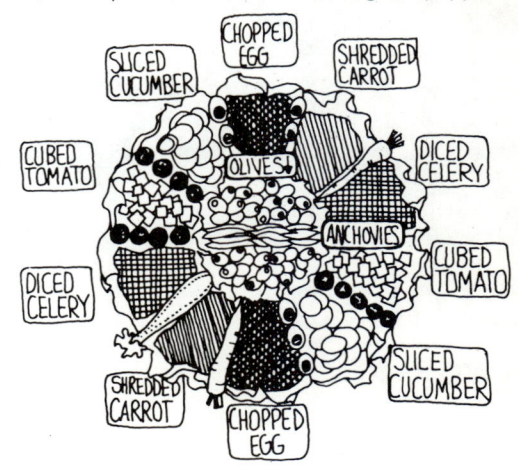

wine, cheese, and fruit
some ideas on what to serve with what

Next to "a jug of wine, a loaf of bread—and thou," wine with fruit and cheese is probably the most famous food combination there is. Autumn is one of the best times to enjoy them, with so many fresh fruits at their peak of ripeness, so here are some ideas:

Most wine books say that fruits don't actually require any special wine, but they do call for a relatively good one. Somehow fruits tend to show up faults in a thin or poor-quality wine more than other foods. If you're serving a basket of assorted fruits, avoid citrus fruits—oranges, grapefruit—or pineapple, which are too acidic to mix well with wine.

f food

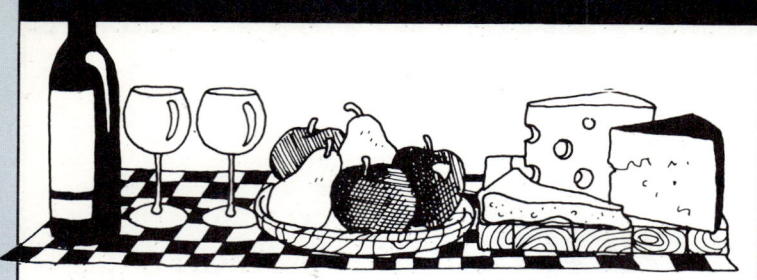

You should also try to serve more than one cheese since some varieties are particularly savory with certain fruits. For example, pears, especially the little, firm sickle pears, are delicious with Gorgonzola or any not-too-strong blue cheese. Pears are also good with Brie or Camembert. Apples mix well with the same cheeses pears do, so they are fine fruits to serve together. If you include peaches in your assortment, be sure you have a smooth cheese that won't overpower their flavor, like Bel Paese, Brie, or Camembert. A Swiss-type cheese such as Gruyère or Emmenthaler is also a good all-round cheese.

As to the particular wine, your own taste preference is, of course, important, but some choices might be a good-quality Burgundy or Bordeaux. Either has an exceptional affinity to pears and cheese, also peaches. In fact, either wine is a good standard choice with most fruit-cheese combinations. A lightly chilled Beaujolais or Valpolicella is excellent with blue cheese, apples, and pears.

foreign languages

learning
3 fast ways to learn the language you'll be hearing on this summer's trip

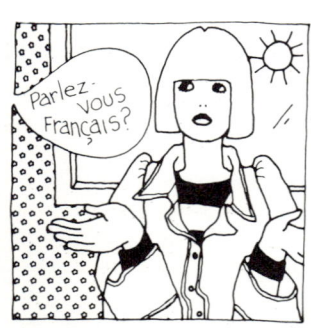

The trouble with toting an armload of phrase books to Europe is that they can be cumbersome—and may lack the very phrases you most want to know. If you are planning a trip abroad, you might prefer to consider the sources of foreign language instruction described below. The prices, methods, and results will vary from school to school, but all will provide you with the ability to maneuver through most travel situations—airports, shops, restaurants, and hotels.

- *Berlitz* offers a do-it-yourself "Basic Cassette Course" in French, Italian, and German. The course consists of three tapes and two study manuals for $34.95, available in book and department stores.
- *The Alliance Française*, a combination language-cultural center, offers courses of varying lengths and costs in French, in New York City; Larchmont, NY; Washington, D.C.; Boston; San Francisco; Los Angeles; and Houston. In New York City, for example, a seven-week, five-hour-a-week course costs $120. Alliance Française uses the audio-visual method: you watch a filmstrip, then with the help of a professor, practice with cassettes and recorder in a language-lab setting. This method combines conversation with grammar.
- *Linguaphone Institute* (79 Madison Ave., New York, NY 10016), a division of Westinghouse Learning Corporation, offers home-study courses in 22 languages. Some courses are made up of 30 lessons, each taking about an hour to do. The cost is $179.50 (you can pay on the installment plan), which includes an illustrated textbook with its lessons recorded on 4 cassettes or 21 records, a student handbook with extremely thorough explanations in English, a book of exercises that you correct yourself, and written assignments that Linguaphone corrects and returns to you.

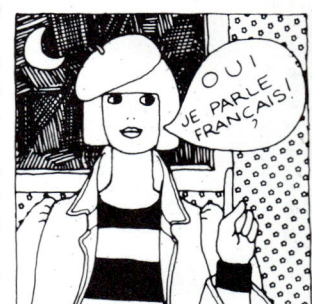

natives
talk to the natives when you can't speak the language

If you are planning a trip abroad and are worried because foreigners won't speak English and you speak nothing else, don't clutch. There are three solutions to your problem.

One is to take a cram course in the language of your choice. Unless, however, you are an atypically American linguistic genius, this probably won't work very effectively. (Besides, you can't cram nine languages for a nine-country tour.)

The second solution is to carry a phrase book or books, but this has some drawbacks, too. One popular Greek phrase book, for example, lists the sentence "I should like to send a telegram" in its section on what to say in the post office. The phonetic spelling of the translation given is: "Thah EE-thella nah STEE-llo ENNah teeleh-GHRAffeemma." Now, even if you do manage this mouthful, chances are you won't say it the way a Greek would, and the telegraph operator won't understand. Phrase books are also a bit impractical at times. A Spanish phrase book, in its "train travel" section, lists the question "At what time does the train leave for Acapulco?" Terrific! But there are no trains leaving for Acapulco and there never have been—from *anywhere*.

Which brings us to the third and best solution: common sense. If you have ever studied any European language, you should be able to work out your own quick version of Esperanto (defined here as "saying it in one language if you can't say it in another"; Webster defines it as "an artificial international language based . . . on words common to the chief European languages"). The point is that certain words—some English, some not—are understood internationally. The ones that describe your most basic needs are, happily, English: hotel, restaurant, toilet, taxi, airport, and Coca-Cola. (But don't say "Coke"—that's not international.) Other such words are *agua* (water), *autobus* (bus), *tram* (streetcar), *cuanto?* (how much?), and *merci* (thank you).

Concentrate on such key words. If you ask a waiter in a Paris restaurant, "Can you please tell me the way to the nearest ladies' room?" you'll get nowhere—just a shrug and a grunt in return. But if you sensibly and clearly say "Toilet?" with questioning voice and raised eyebrows, you will be quickly pointed on your way. Eyebrows and hands are often important. They can convey a sort of helplessness that will usually evoke sympathetic interest. In the case of the aforementioned post office, the key word is "telegraph."

Applying common sense should enable you to get around without much difficulty, but if it doesn't, relax. Two women we know met the cordial male population of Dijon when their mysterious French rental car conked out on the main street and they didn't know the French word for "starter."

games

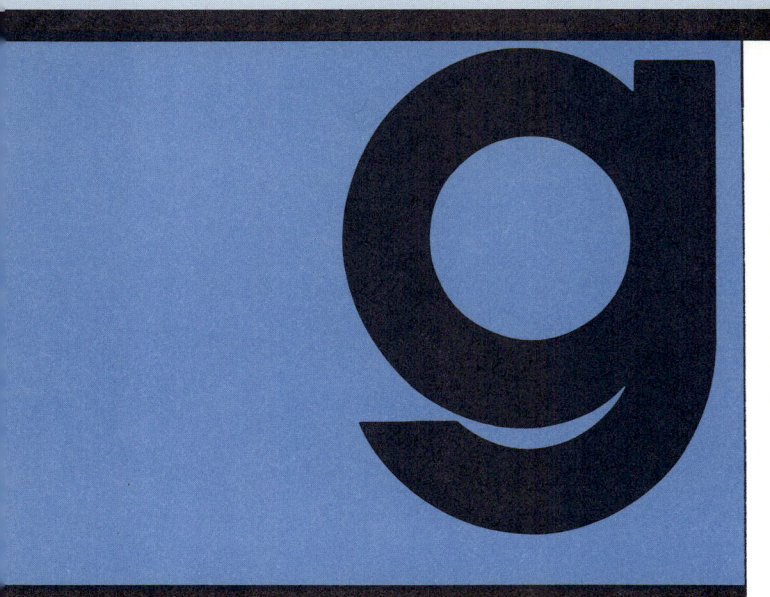

games glasses

crossword
how to do crossword puzzles

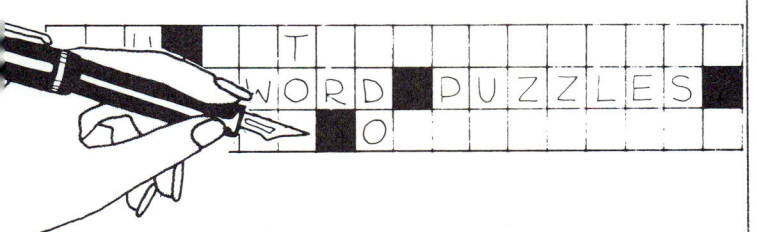

The true crossword-puzzle addict is easy to identify. She seems to sit perpetually with pencil in hand, newspaper neatly folded in quarters, and brow furrowed. If you ask, she can instantly tell you the name of a "Philippine tree" (*dao* or *ypil*), the "Egyptian sun god" (*ra*), or an "East Indian nurse" (*amah*). In fact, those—to her—are the *easy* ones.

To Jack Luzzatto, a professional crossword-puzzle constructor, it makes sense. "The more puzzles you do, the better you'll get at it," says Mr. Luzzatto, whose puzzles have appeared in *GLAMOUR*, *The New York Times*, the *Nation*, and *Time*. "There are certain words that crop up again and again, words like *epi*, a 'roof finial,' or *oca*, an 'edible tuber.' After a while, you'll get to know them."

He suggests beginning with simpler puzzles, such as those syndicated in newspapers, and perhaps working up to the puzzle in *The Sunday Times of London*, generally acknowledged to be the world's most difficult crossword puzzle. He also suggests noting the author of a puzzle and sticking with one or two, since each puzzle constructor has a style—including pet words, phrases, and gimmicks—with which you'll become familiar after a while.

What if you always get so discouraged you can never finish one puzzle, let alone a string of them? Then, he suggests, you might take just a *peek* at the answers (just for a word or two) "to break the ice." He also recommends the occasional use of a good "cheater's" dictionary. As another idea, you might try to stick with themed puzzles in an area you know well (cooking, baseball greats), learn a foreign language such as Latin or French, and try to read more fiction (for general vocabulary building).

Above all, *don't* do crossword puzzles just before bed. It is almost universally agreed that there is *no* torment like the insomnia that results from knowing you could finish that maddening puzzle if only you knew a three-letter word for "Yangtze tributary."

Monopoly
be a Monopoly champ

Along with the Davis Cup, the Heisman Trophy, and the Olympic Gold Medal, there is now the Charles B. Darrow Cup for the Monopoly Champion of the World.

If you think you are, or could become, good enough to compete for the title, you'll first have to win one of the regional championships in the U.S. or Canada. The winners compete for the national title, and that winner competes for the world champion title. For more information, write to the Marketing Department (Monopoly), Parker Bros., 190 Bridge St., Salem, MA 01970. To brush up on your game technique, you might also check out The Monopoly Book *by Maxine Brady.*

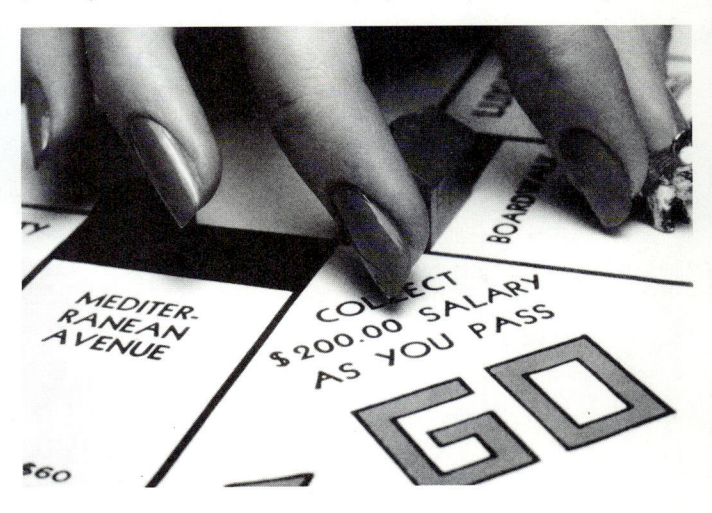

Scrabble® win at Scrabble® without cheating

The words below will help you play a super game of SCRABBLE®, whether you know what they mean or not. They're all listed in *Funk & Wagnalls Standard College Dictionary*, used at SCRABBLE® tournaments, and in the *SCRABBLE® Word Guide*. Rules allow all words listed as parts of speech (even foreign, archaic, slang, English/foreign alphabet letters if they're spelled out—like "c" as "cee"). You can't use hyphenated, apostrophed, capitalized, or abbreviated words.
- **handy two-letter words**

aa, ad, ae, ba, de, ea, ha, ja, jo, ka, li, lo, mu, na, nu, od, os, si, ut, xi
- **words for high-point tiles**

that you love to get but sometimes can't get rid of:

J—haj, jee, jus, raj, juba, soja, jinn

Q—qua, fique, quean, toque, squal, torque

X—kex, pyx, xis, axil, ilex, moxa, sext

Z—azo, zax, zoa, fuze, zero, foozle, kazoo

79

games

- **words with lots of vowels**
  boo, oii, agee, agio, aseo, aalii, cooee, inia, raia, unau, inion
- **three great words to remember**
  setter, retina, and satire

The six letters of each word—put in different order—can combine with most other letters to form a seven-letter "Bingo" word. Bingos give you a 50-point bonus plus their regular score and they're not as impossible to come up with as you may think. For example, add these letters to "retina" and get: C—certain; D—trained; E—trainee; F—fainter; G—granite, ingrate, and so on.

For other pointers you might join SCRABBLE® Players, 200 Fifth Ave., New York, NY 10010. For $7.50 a year, you'll get a strategy handbook, a bimonthly newsletter with items of interest to SCRABBLE® buffs and a handy word list. You can also get information about entering or starting a tournament or a club.

glasses

makeup
for your eyes behind glasses

Any woman who wears glasses knows that some glasses require more emphatic makeup to keep eyes from getting lost. Try these tips:
- *Eyebrows*—Brows should be neat and natural. Tweeze regularly, and follow your natural arch. If your brows are too heavy, too dark, or too exaggerated in shape, they'll only fight your eyes for attention. It's a good idea to check for strays every morning and pluck them out, because lenses magnify small flaws.
- *Eyelashes*—One of the biggest helps to eyes behind glasses is an eyelash curler. Use it before applying mascara to open up and emphasize eyes. As for mascara, apply several coats, but use a clean brush in between to prevent any clumping together of lashes. Plenty of dark mascara gives your eyes the depth that glasses tend to take away.
- *Eyeshadow*—The color shadow you choose is up to you, but in general, stay away from very dark browns and greens; they tend to look murky behind glass. Your best bet is a soft color contrast—warm brown shadow for blue eyes, muted green for brown, subtle violet for hazel. Avoid shadows that are very frosted. Medium-intensity tones work better. Cover entire upper lid with shadow, then bring a bit of it around and under the outer corners. If you want to use a darker color in the crease or a highlighter on the brow bone, blend only slightly—some contrast between the shades gives the extra definition needed behind glasses.
- *Eyeliner*—You might try a very thin line of dark brown or black drawn close to the upper lashes. Or use a brown, gray, or navy eyeliner pencil, and line upper lid and lower lid from center to outer corner, then smudge to soften. You can outline in combination with shadow. Choose eyeliner pencil a few shades deeper to define and emphasize your eyes.
- *Frames*—If you are too nearsighted to put makeup on without your glasses, try flip-down-lens glasses. In general, you should choose frames that work within your wardrobe, but the following colors will also complement your hair coloring: coppers and tortoise-toned frames for redheads; pales and beiges for blondes; shades of grays and blues for gray hair; and an open choice of colors for brunettes.

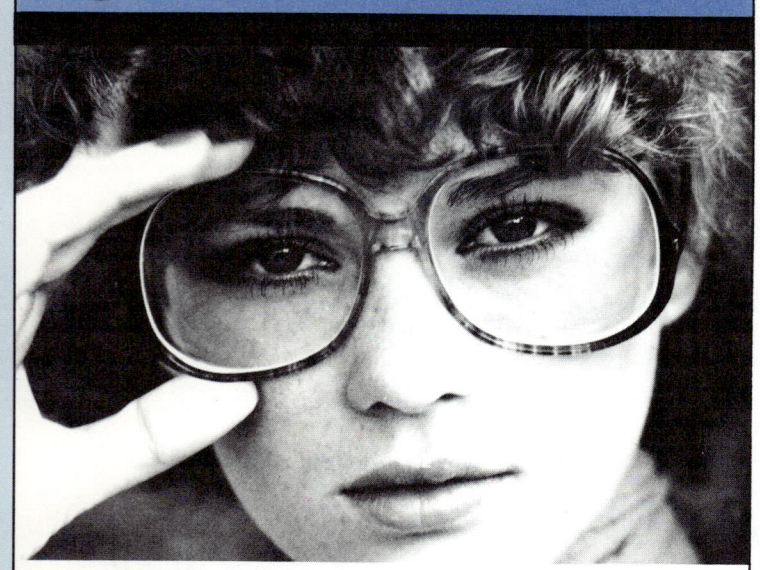

mistakes don't make costly mistakes when you buy eyeglasses

The tips here should help you find a pair of glasses that give you maximum performance at minimal cost. They are from Frances Shapiro, who runs one of New York's most well known eye centers.
- *Frames—Plastic or metal is really a matter of personal preference. Be aware that many fashionable plastic frames are made with hidden hinges that cannot be repaired. If you pick plastic, make certain the temples are reinforced by a metal strip inside. Metal frames are less likely to have hidden hinges than plastic ones, but some metal frames—like the popular aviator style—bend easily and require more care when worn, handled, and stored.*
- *Lenses—You have a choice of plastic or glass lenses. Both are shatterproof, as required by Federal law, but plastic is harder to break. Plastic lenses cost about one third more than glass in most shops, are lighter weight, and practical (especially when your prescription requires a thick lens), but get scratched more easily. When scratched, plastic lenses are also harder to see through than scratched glass lenses.*

If the frames are large, and many of the jazzy new ones are, you'll need oversized lenses, which cost more. Figure on 20 percent more for glass lenses, 30 percent more for plastic. If you plan to have your lenses tinted, that adds another $6 to $10 to the lens price. The flattery can be worth it, however. To save a few dollars, you might ask to see the standard tinted lenses. You will have less choice of color in the standard tints, but you might find something you like. Most experts say not to worry about wearing tinted lenses indoors as long as the tint isn't extremely dark. Too dark a tint can affect your eyes' reaction to light if worn indoors for long periods of time. Anyone with an outdoor job or who's outside a lot might find investing in a pair of light-sensitive (glass only) glasses worthwhile. The tint in these glasses is sun sensitive, darkening with the degree of the sun. You can wear them indoors or out. They're not recommended for indoor wear only.

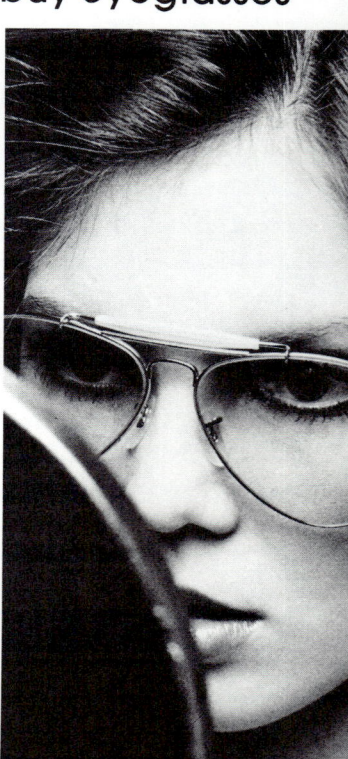

h hair

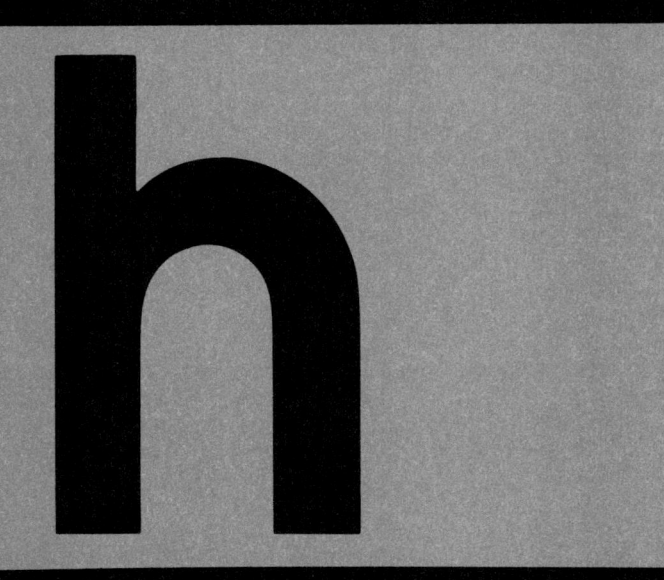

hair
Halloween
health
home furnishings

hair

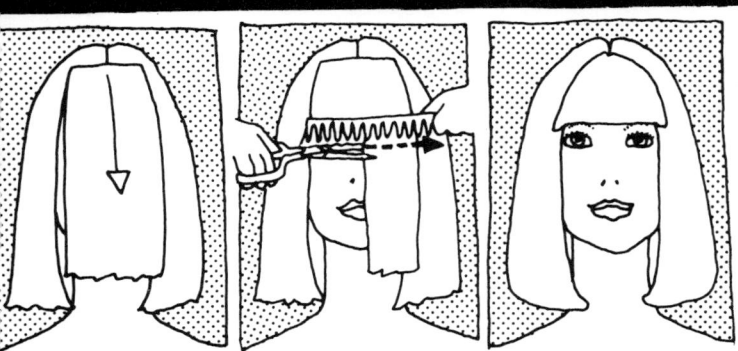

bangs
how to cut your own bangs

If you're tired of looking into the mirror at the same old hairstyle, think bangs. They can give you a sleek new look, and it's fairly easy to cut them yourself. Just follow these tips:
- Wash hair and towel dry. Comb out tangles and part in middle.
- Make a horizontal part across the center part, about 1½" back from front hairline. Comb this hair forward. This section will form your bangs. Depending on thickness of hair, however, you may have to vary the 1½" measurement. In general, thick hair doesn't need as deep a bang as fine hair does.
- Comb through this section, spreading it across forehead as you do.
- Using bottom of comb as a straightedge, cut hair with small, sharp scissors straight across to a length that hits bridge of nose. Stop just past outer corners of eyebrows.
- Check mirror to see if you have the right shape. You may want to extend bangs a bit at the sides.
- Now trim bangs to correct length. When dry, they should sit just covering arch of eyebrows, so that no skin shows between bangs and eyebrows.
- dos and don'ts for bangs
- DO allow for shrinkage when cutting bangs. Wet hair will dry to a slightly shorter length.
- DON'T cut bangs if you have very wavy or curly hair.
- DON'T worry too much about bangs being exactly straight. No one will notice if a few hairs are out of line.

black women
hair tips for black women

To get the answers to some of the most-asked questions black women have about their hair problems, we talked to hairstylist James Farabee, an expert on black hair care. Following is a rundown of solutions we got from him.
- One fabulous look for black hair is a headful of touchable curls, softer and curlier than an Afro. The base length for this look is 3" to 6" all around. Do have hair trimmed before you switch to this style since the right cut makes hair work with the curl, not against it. To get the curls, set hair wet on small or medium-sized rollers whenever you shampoo.
- To get the best set, always roll hair while it is still damp, and use end papers. Besides giving additional pressing (straightening action), end papers distribute the moisture more evenly and result in a smoother look. A good trick you might want to try is setting hair with a diluted body conditioner (use two parts water to one part instant or deep conditioner). Comb through hair, then apply your regular setting gel or lotion. This way you get holding power plus manageability.
- Have your hair cut when it is at its straightest, shortly after it's been pressed or chemically straightened. If your hair is too curly or kinky at the time of the cut, it can throw off the style.
- If you have an Afro, always style it when wet or at least damp. Use tortoise, rubber, or plastic combs. Metal combs can cut and damage hair.
- Don't try to trim your own Afro. This is a style where the cut counts for everything, and you can't trim at the right angle when doing it yourself.
- After having hair chemically straightened, use a neutralizing or hair repair shampoo—found in some drugstores and most beauty supply stores—for your first shampooing after the straightening process. This will help restore hair to its natural chemical balance, yet won't affect the straightening. For the second washing, go back to your regular shampoo.
- If you want a subtle color change, a shampoo-in hair color or rinse close to your own shade will accent highlights and make hair look richer. Anything other than a slight lightening or "warming" of your natural color should be done at a salon.

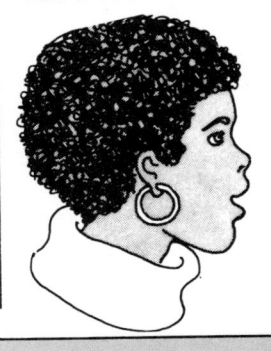

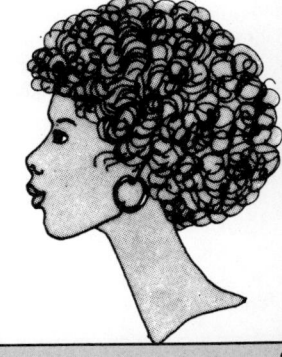

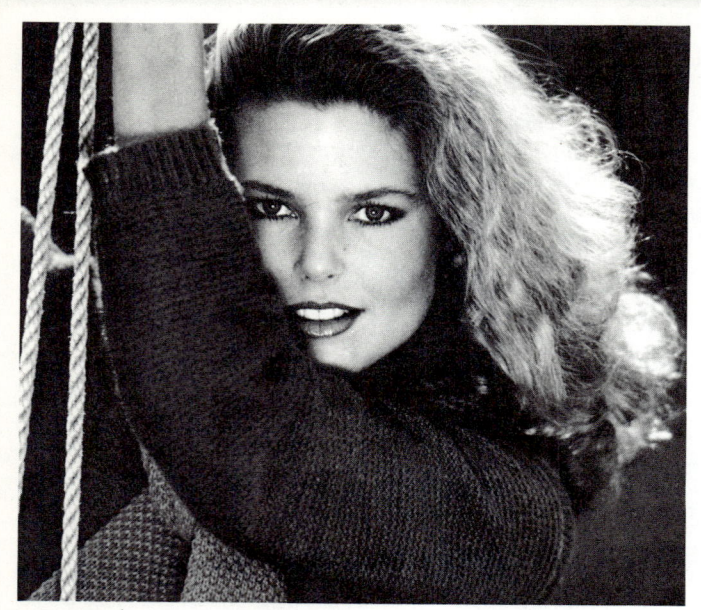

hair

blonding
dos and don'ts for at-home blonding

Going blonde at home can be done if you know what you're doing. Constance, the extraordinary colorist at Louis Guy D' Salon in New York City, has some dos and don'ts that will help you get the best do-it-yourself results.

- DO know the difference between single- and double-process blonding. A "double-process" job means that the hair is prebleached to an exact shade, and then a toner is applied to the bleached hair to give it the finished color. "Single-process" blonding means that the bleaching and toning are all done with a single product. This kind of coloring is much easier on hair because the chemicals are only applied once instead of twice every time you color. Also, many of the single-process home products are the shampoo-in type, which helps eliminate most of the problem of retouching. You just shampoo with the product when you have enough growth to color. Hair that's quite dark cannot be made pale with a single-process product, although any woman with light- to medium-brown hair can get a good blonde color with a single-process product. Darker hair needs a double-process product to get the lightest shades of blonde.
- DO pick one of the *warm* blonde colors; look for shade names that imply honey or warm toasty colors. Avoid ash tones. They can be tricky to do well and are not as flattering to most skin tones.
- DO ask for the manufacturer's color chart when you buy. It gives a good idea of how the color will turn out.
- DON'T buy your blonding products piecemeal. Read the package directions while you're still in the store and you won't get halfway through the job at home and discover you didn't buy everything.
- DO follow the timing instructions with your product *to the letter*. The biggest cause for unsuccessful results, Constance says, is improper timing.
- DO be sure you make the patch test all directions call for. Although most people aren't sensitive to hair colors, you may be one of those who are.
- DO try what Constance calls the "preview color." Test to see how your own hair reacts to the shade you've picked. Cut off a small strand of hair from underneath in back and tape it to a piece of cardboard. Then make a "strand test" according to product directions so that you'll know how your new color will look.
- DO consider using a nonperoxide toner for double-process blonde coloring. This eliminates some of the wear and tear on your hair. Or, if you can't find the color you want in this kind of product, pick a 10- or 15-minute toner instead of a 30-minute one. The toner package will indicate whether it is a nonperoxide product or a 10- or 15-minute one.
- DO use a three-way mirror or one that gives you a rear view, especially if you're doing retouch work. You can't do a good job if you can't see what is happening.
- DON'T stop at the coloring. A big part of its success is keeping your hair in good, healthy condition. If you color your hair, you *must* condition it regularly. Use a deep-penetrating conditioner once or twice a month and, in addition, consider using one of the products made especially to condition hair while it's being bleached. It is put on the ends when you bleach the roots.
- DO consider exchanging hair coloring jobs with a friend. You can do hers; she can do yours. This makes it easier for you both, especially when you're retouching roots in a double-process blonding. It's very important that you apply the bleach to new growth only. This is hard to do, especially in back if you're doing your own hair.

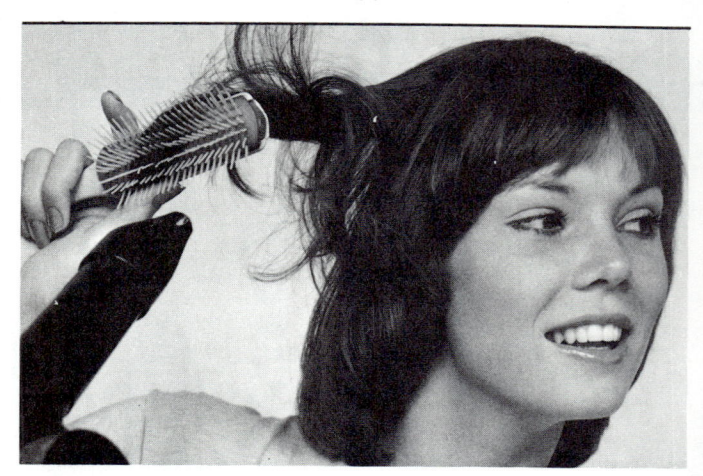

blow dryers
how to pick the right blow dryer for your hair—and his

The right blow dryer for you depends on several things, including your budget, experience, and deftness with using one. Blow dryers fall into three main groups.

- The simple *hand-held dryer* just dries your hair as you brush it with your usual hairbrush. To get any kind of styling contour with this dryer, you have to be handy with your own hair, curving it with the brush in one hand while you're holding the dryer with the other. These are often called mini-dryers, and they usually cost the least.
- The *styling dryer* is often larger and may have as many as five different attachments to help style your hair as it dries. These might include a brush, comb, and wide-tooth detangling comb, among other gear, that snap in and out.
- The *styling comb*, which tends to be long and narrow, is used on dry hair to tame unruly spots or to add fullness. Many of these combs have built-in sprayers that spray a mist of water, and in some cases, conditioners, as you use them.

The wattage of any blow dryer you buy is important. On both types of dryers used on wet hair, this ranges from 200 to 1,000 watts, although the hand-held dryers usually have lower wattages than styling dryers. The higher the wattage, the shorter the drying time. To dry long, thick hair quickly, you need at least 800 watts. Short, fine hair, and most men's hair unless it is long and thick, can usually be dried quickly using lower wattages.

Air flow or the amount of air released also affects drying time, but this is harder to measure than wattage. A strong rather than mild gust of air obviously will cover more hair area and thus dry the whole head

hair

faster, especially when it's teamed with high wattage and temperature. The easiest dryers to handle are those that have two air-flow settings, which may simply be labeled "dry" and "style."

Consider also the temperature of the air released by any dryer. A hair dryer with alternate hot and cool settings assures maximum drying comfort, especially on dryers with air heated to 220° F. or above. Air this hot can be uncomfortable to ears and scalp and damaging to hair when dryer isn't kept moving briskly.

Dryers that shut off automatically when they begin to overheat are your best bet against unintentional damage. Some dryers have a thermostat device that shuts them off automatically when the heat goes too high, then starts them running again when they cool off. Others shut off automatically but will not start up again unless a trained repairman replaces the fuse. The instructions should say whether or not yours will reheat automatically. In either case, you should be able to prevent overheating by not blocking the air outlet with your hand—and not letting strands of hair get caught in it—as you're drying. Read carefully the instructions about this element on your dryer.

Other points to check: how comfortable the dryer is to hold; how long the cord is; and whether or not it has a dual voltage (110/220) setting for European currents, if you plan to travel with it.

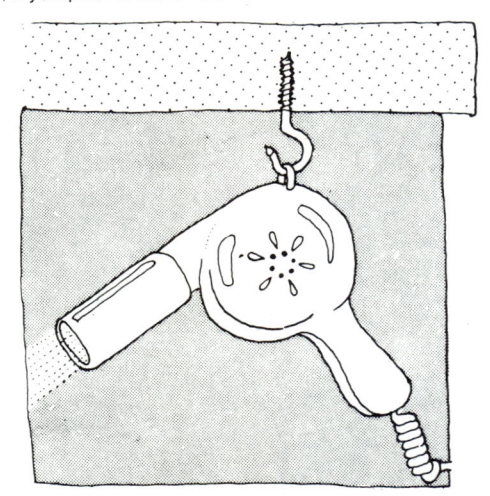

blow dryers
improve your blow-drying skills

Almost everyone has tried blow drying by now, but even the pros like to keep adding to and perfecting techniques, so we thought you might like a quick refresher course, including some updating.
- *DON'T hold the dryer too close to your hair. Keep it at least 6" away to protect hair and scalp.*
- *DO dry hair almost all the way before you begin styling it by rolling the ends around your brush.*
- *DON'T use a flat-backed hairbrush to style. It will give you a flat curl. Instead, use one with a rounded back or bristles all around.*
- *DO start drying hair at the nape of the neck first and work up the back, then do sides and front. The drying process will go faster this way because the top layer of hair starts drying while you're working on the underneath part.*
- *DO let hair dry naturally as much as possible when you have the time. You'll be exposing your hair to heat and brushes less and helping it to stay in better condition.*
- *DON'T forget that regular conditioning is part of the blow-dry routine if you want shiny, healthy hair. Deep-condition hair once a month if it's healthy, twice a month if it's dry or damaged.*
- *DO look for the new conditioning products made especially for women who blow dry their hair.*

brushes
is the hairbrush you're using the right one for you?

The right brush can make styling your hair easier, improve its condition, and be easier to use. Here are some things to look for when you buy:
- *Bristles*—The type of bristle you need depends on the texture of your hair. In general, the heavier or coarser your hair, the stiffer the bristles should be. Natural bristles, although available in various stiffnesses, tend to be softer than synthetic bristles and are often too gentle for coarse or thick hair. On the pro side, they remove more dirt than synthetic bristles, and are quite good at smoothing and styling hair. In general, synthetic brushes clutch the hair well, are lower priced, and are easier to care for than natural bristles. Some synthetics don't actually have bristles at all, but rows of rounded flexible teeth made of rubber or another synthetic set into a cushioned rubber pad. These brushes are excellent for wet or fragile hair on which a bristle brush should not be used, so they're great for blow drying. They're also great for curly or permed hair because they slide easily through the hair without pulling or tearing it. Oily hair benefits from these, too, because they aerate better than bristles and move less oil down the hair shaft. For exactly this reason, however, they're a bad choice for dry hair, which needs lubricating.
- *Shape*—Shapes are geared primarily to the way you brush. Flat-backed brushes are meant for straight front-to-back or up-and-down brushing—good for long hair. A brush with a slightly curved back is for people who brush with a flick of the wrist (the way most people with medium to short hair brush). The curved shape is practical because the turning, flicking motion would only wear down the side bristles of a flat brush. A full, round brush, with bristles all around, works for wrist-flickers too, but its biggest asset is for blow-dry styling. Hair brushed around this shape takes on curves and shape in the final blow-dry stages.

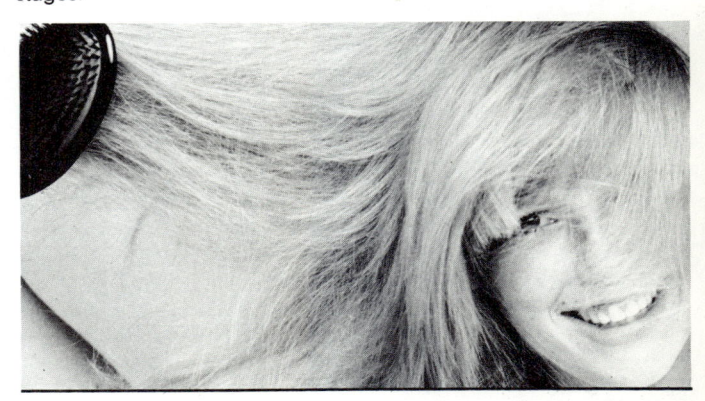

care products
what are you getting from hair care products?

Hair care may have gotten simpler in the past few years, but the terms that describe all these "quick and easy" methods seem to get more and more complicated. So that you'll be an informed consumer, read this brief rundown of which hair products actually do what.
- *Protein shampoo coats hair to give strength, pliability, and manageability.*
- *Instant shampoo (also called dry shampoo) is a spray-on or brush-on product that removes soil and oil from hair without water.*
- *Deep-conditioner helps put back some of the oils and moisture that*

83

h hair

hair loses from sun, weather, chemical, and heat processing. It is left on 10 to 30 minutes, depending on the product.
- *Instant conditioner* replaces some of the oils and moisture hair loses but not as thoroughly as a deep-conditioner. It is left on the hair for only a minute or so.
- *Creme rinse* (sometimes called a detangler) coats hair with a waxy or creamy substance to make it easier to comb when wet. It is not good for oily or fine hair.
- *A permanent* chemically changes the hair structure to curl it.
- *A body wave* gives the hair less curl than a permanent, usually just a bend.
- *A straightener* chemically uncurls naturally curly hair. It cannot be used to "undo" a permanent.
- *Frosting and streaking* are two terms generally used interchangeably and refer to the bleaching of selected strands of hair to give a blonde glow.
- *Highlighting* is similar to frosting and streaking, but more subtle and natural since fewer hairs are bleached.
- *Hair painting* is a new method of giving a subtle blonde look to brown hair. Bleach is actually painted with a brush onto a fairly wide band of hair, generally around the face.

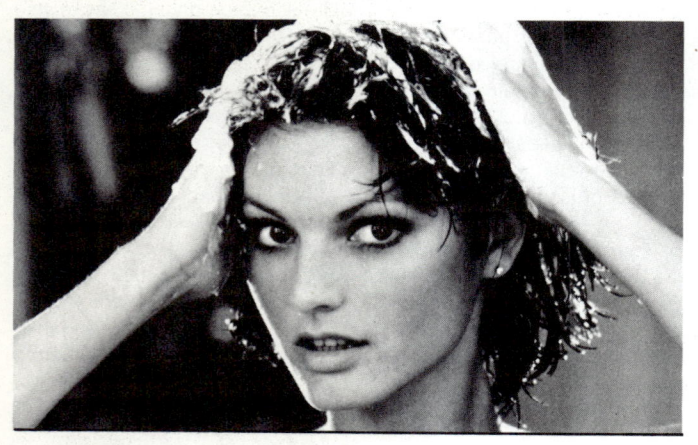

coloring
guide to hair coloring products

Faced with the incredible array of tints, toners, cream developers, single- and double-process blonding kits, how is a poor "mouse brown" woman to know what will give her just a hint of blonde highlights or what will turn her into a genuine Jean Harlow? Following is a rundown of the most common terms for hair-coloring products. Becoming familiar with them should spare you any unpleasant surprises later on.
- *Permanent hair color*—This color won't wash out. You're stuck with it for better or worse until it grows out, or you cut it off.
- *Temporary rinse*—This is a color highlighting product that lasts from shampoo to shampoo. It will not dramatically alter hair color; it just adds a hint of color.
- *Semi-permanent color*—This is color that lasts through several shampoos. The color gradually fades after repeated washings and leaves no line of demarcation between colored hair and new growth. These products are used most commonly on hair that's graying.
- *One-process color (or single-process)*—This is permanent color that lightens or darkens hair within certain limits. For example, a medium-brown-haired woman can become a dark blonde with single-process color. But a brunette can't become a platinum blonde.
- *Double-process color*—This means that there are two steps involved in changing the color of hair. First a bleach is applied to remove color. A toner is then applied to give the hair a new, blonde color. A brunette can become a light blonde with double-process products; this is the only way such an extreme change can be made.

- *Lighteners or bleaches*—Products that remove the natural pigment, usually used with a toner. A toner is used *only* on prelightened or bleached hair to give it a new color.
- *Shampoo-in color*—This is permanent color that's incorporated with shampoo. While you wash your hair, the color change takes place. Although these products aren't usually used for a dramatic change in color, they will lighten or darken several shades and give natural-looking results. To color new hair growth, you just shampoo again. There's no sectioning and parting as there is with all other permanent hair-coloring products.
- *Frosting and tipping*—This is a process in which selected small strands of hair are lightened to give the effect of blonde highlights or the illusion of total blondness depending on how many strands are lightened.
- *Drabber*—Drabbers are used to get rid of brassy red tones in lightened hair. If not used correctly, they can give hair a greenish tinge, so always follow directions carefully.

cut how to get a good hairdresser

When you want to make a major change in your hairstyle, common sense tells you to go to the best hairdresser around. Here are some tips to find the best for *you*:

When you see someone with the same kind of hair as yours in a style you like, ask who cuts or styles it for her. Beware of going to someone who's good with curly hair if your hair is straight, or vice versa.

Be aware that some salons are known for a specialty—like streaking or coloring—or that give great permanents or haircuts. Take advantage of what the salon is known for; go somewhere else for another service.

If you've heard of a good hairdresser from friends, try to find out if his or her specialty is the kind of look you want—long smooth cuts, short ones, whatever.
- Salon shop. Don't be afraid to wander into a salon and look over the heads that are coming out and the photographs in the salon. If you like what you see, make a date; if not, try somewhere else.
- Make a consultation date. If you've found a hairdresser you *think* may work out, make an appointment for a consultation. If you're not simpatico, go somewhere else. The money you spend may save you a lot of trouble later.

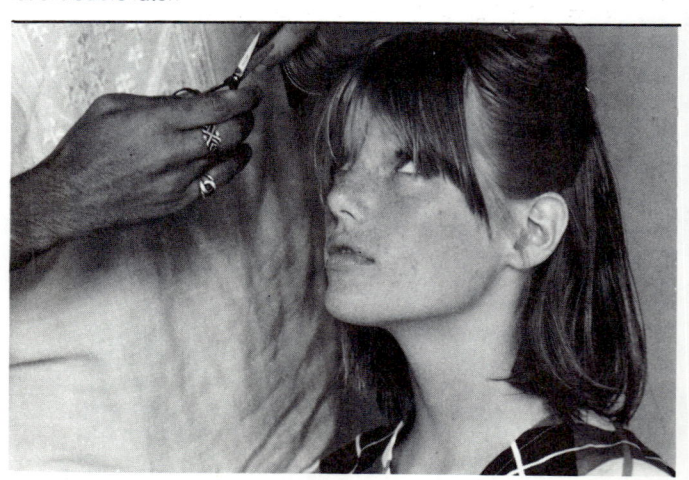

cut find the right haircut for you

To determine your haircut and style needs, ask and answer the following six questions. (Our consultant on these questions was famous hairdresser Kenneth Battelle of the Kenneth Salon in New York City.)
1. What texture is my hair—fine, medium, or coarse?
- *Fine hair* has the texture of silk thread, tends to be flyaway, and

hair

doesn't hold a set well. It's usually thin and shouldn't be longer than chin length to look its best. It should be blunt cut and is usually easier to live with if it's one length. Layering presents problems.
- *Medium hair* is more like cotton thread, holds a set, and behaves itself. It can take almost any kind of styling.
- *Coarse hair* has the texture of darning thread, is sometimes unruly and hard to curl. A long blunt cut is often the best bet. Length tends to weigh it down; blunt ends hold it in place.
- *Curly hair*, no matter what its texture and bulk, shouldn't be cut supershort—unless you want a natural. Curly hair tends to curl up tightly in humid weather and you'll end up looking like a skinhead.

2. How much time can I spend on my hair?
If the answer is not much, choose either a straightish blunt cut if you have no curl, or a layered one that you can wash and blow dry (for this cut, it doesn't matter whether your hair is moderately curly or straight, although a little wave helps).

3. Am I handy with my hair?
Some women just aren't. If that's you, tell the hairdresser that you want a style that requires a minimum of fussing.

4. Do I get bored with one look?
Long hair tends to be more versatile than short. You can wear it up or down and change the look by parting it differently.

5. What climate do I live in?
If you live in a muggy, tropical climate or a cold, damp one, curly hair can become bushy, straight hair can go limp. In either of these climates, the more natural and basic the style, the better it will hold.

6. What things have I tried in the past that didn't work?
Bangs? Layered hair? Very short hair? If you're going to try any of these again, be sure you have a good reason for believing they'll work this time.

- **four basic cuts**

Here are the four best cuts for most heads. None is so extreme that it will be out of date in a few months; they're all good solid classics.

1. Hair is blunt-cut to one length all around the head. It can be any length from chin to shoulder or longer, varied with bangs, a side or center part.
2. Hair is blunt-cut with the back slightly shorter than the sides. It could be very short, hugging the nape of the neck in back and chin length or even shorter in front. Or, if you want longer hair, the front could be anywhere between chin length to just above the shoulder with the back cut a bit shorter.
3. The sides are cut shorter than the back. The front and side pieces might be chin length while the back is left just short of shoulder length. Part of the front section could be cut like long bangs, about eye level, and the rest cut shoulder length or left long.
4. The cut here is similar to the preceding description, but the angle of the front hair is more extreme. The very top hair is quite short, almost like bangs, the rest of the hair getting gradually longer. The ends are shaped to flip back, not under, as in Sketch 3.

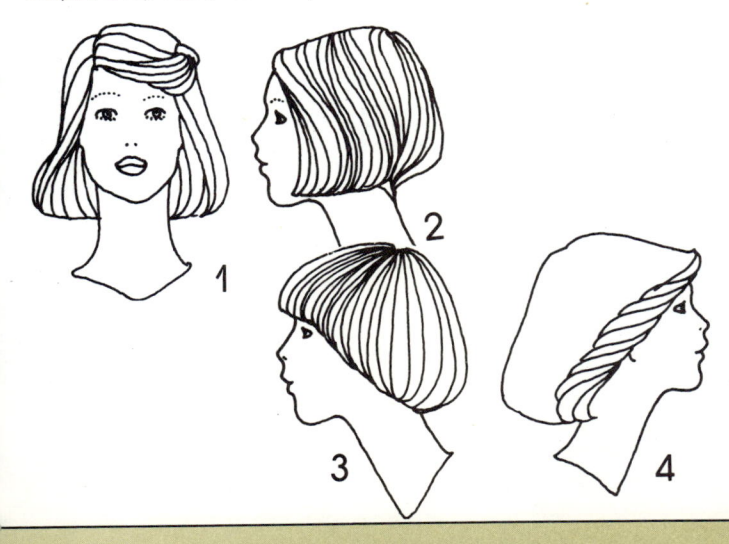

cut risk a great haircut—free!

If you want a new haircut without a great big price tag, you can get it, and get it free! But before you rush in, here are a few things you should know, including how to find a "free cut" salon.

In almost any city of medium size or larger, you'll find a beauty school, usually several. Their students need heads to practice on and will do cuts free or for a minimal cost. This can be a good deal if you follow a few tips. Before you go, be sure you know what kind of haircut you want, and be strong enough not to let the student talk you into something else. A picture is especially helpful. You should also have relatively easy-to-cope-with hair—problem types with super curly, fine, or difficult hair should avoid this route.

To find a beauty school, check the Yellow Pages of your phone book and call a few to see what their procedures are. Some take you by appointment; others make you come and wait your turn.

Another way to get a free cut, and sometimes at one of the best salons in town, is to find a shop that has a training program for stylists. With the big trend to "wash and wear hair," many shops are finding themselves shorthanded on hairdressers who are pros at this technique—so they give their stylists lessons. You can benefit by getting a free cut as they learn on your hair. The classes are usually held on certain days of the week only, often after the shop is officially closed. You may hear about them through word of mouth from a friend or you can call a few large salons and ask if they have such a service, or if they know of a salon that does. Salons in large department stores are likely choices. This is a relatively safe way to get a free cut for most types of hair because the cutting is usually done under the supervision of fully trained hairdressers who are interested in keeping up with the latest techniques. Unless you have a unique hair problem, you can relax here, but do plan to spend some time. Service is often first come, first served.

henna rinse
give yourself a henna rinse for added color or more body

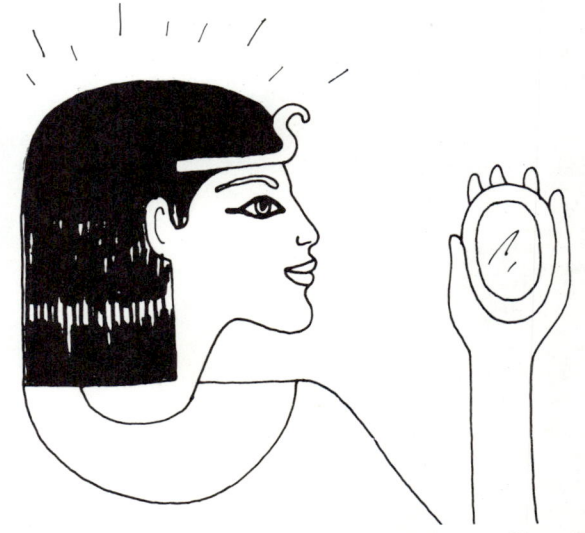

Henna is one of the oldest cosmetics around; even Cleopatra used it to make her dark hair glisten. You can use it to give your hair more body and a very special shine. Most people think of henna as having a reddish-brown color. Actually, red is only one color; there's also black, brown, and natural henna.

The following directions should be appropriate for all hennas and were given to us by Constance, the colorist at Louis Guy D' Salon in

h hair

New York City. Constance explains that henna once had a reputation for being difficult to use, primarily because people tried to turn blonde or light brown hair red by using it—with disastrous results. The charm of henna is its subtlety, and used on dark brown or black hair, red henna adds glorious auburn highlights. The brown or black hennas will add wonderful depth and shine to their corresponding hair colors. Colorless henna gives hair color more body and a wonderful shine. Don't use the colored hennas on natural blonde or very light brown hair. If you use red henna, don't redo for four to six months. Don't use henna on hair that is colored, permanented, straightened, or damaged. It should be used only on healthy, unprocessed hair. The directions are as follows:

1. Buy henna powder in drugstores or beauty supply stores.
2. Mix henna with water to form a paste the consistency of thick shampoo.
3. Apply the henna to clean, dry hair. If you're using colored henna, protect your hands with plastic or rubber gloves. Cover entire head with henna and comb through hair to distribute it evenly. Wrap head with a plastic bag or plastic kitchen wrap.
4. Sit under a dryer (you can use a hand dryer, just keep it moving over your entire head) for about 30 minutes.
5. Rinse hair thoroughly and style in usual manner. The sensational results will last from three to six months.

The red henna can be used to create beautiful auburn streaks on dark hair. Mix red henna and water to form a paste the consistency of toothpaste. Apply mixture to sections of hair all around your face and through the crown of your head. You can pick up fairly big sections, about ½" wide and ½" deep. Apply the mixture with a toothbrush and wrap each streak with aluminum foil. Sit under a dryer for about a half hour. Rinse hair well and style.

removal how to get rid of hair your bikini exposes... and in other places you don't want it

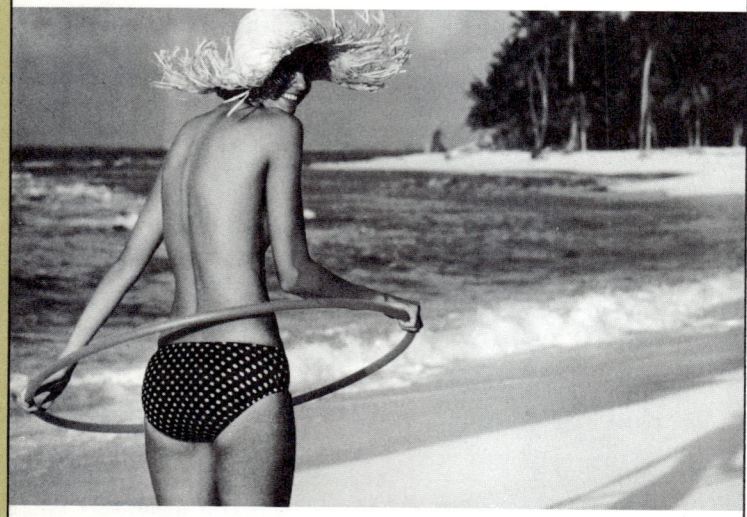

Here is a rundown of the effective and practical means of removing or making less visible facial and body hair, plus information on what methods are best for which problems. Since the methods are effective but different, read about all the possibilities of help before you decide to use any one.

- *Plucking* with tweezers is a sound method for removing scattered hairs on the face and breast, but obviously impractical if the hair is dense. Although some women find it uncomfortable, it has no adverse effects. Anyone who finds the discomfort acute might consider clipping breast hairs close with a sharp, small scissors, but the regrowth will be quicker than from plucking.
- *Shaving* is a very efficient way to remove excess hair from legs. It causes no change in the texture or growth of hair. Shaving is not a satisfactory solution for hair on arms or face, where regrowth presents more of a problem.

Some women with coarse, curly hair complain of ingrown hair as a result of shaving. The best way to handle this is not to shave as closely as you ordinarily would and try never to pull or stretch the skin. Use an electric razor to shave hair in some hidden places like the upper thigh and armpit—a good way to cut down on the itching that usually results from blade shaving. Using a medicated powder, or moisturizer if itching is a problem, afterward should help, too.
- *Bleaching* is a most satisfactory way to make hair on the arms, face (except eyebrows), tummy, and inner upper thighs appear less conspicuous. You can buy a commercial bleach made for facial hair.
- *Depilation* is another effective hair-removal method for arms, legs, and bikini-exposed hair on tummy and thighs. Follow the directions on the label carefully, but remember that if your hair is coarse, the time needed for the depilatory to work may be a disadvantage, especially since it has to be done about as often as shaving. The regrowth of hair after a depilatory is used tends not to feel stubby. Depilatories should never be used on the face unless the directions specifically state that it is safe for this kind of use.
- *Waxing* is also a fairly common way of removing excess hair from arms, legs, tummy, upper inner thighs, and small areas of the face—upper lip, sides of cheeks (where hair is apt to be fine so regrowth is not so noticeable). The wax is first heated and then applied in strips. A cloth is pressed against the wax, and when dry, is pulled off with the cloth against the direction the hair grows.

The advantages of waxing: It lasts longer than depilation or shaving, since the hair is removed below the surface of the skin and the regrowth is not particularly stubby. Disadvantages: It is uncomfortable; there is the risk of getting the wax too hot; and because the hair must be fairly long to be waxed successfully, you have to endure a period of hairiness before rewaxing is possible. Women who are prone to ingrown hair may have more of a problem with waxing. If there is an increase in the ingrown hair, bleaching is probably a better solution than waxing.
- *Electrolysis* can be considered if you are really self-conscious about body hair and feel you have a great deal of it. But it involves time. Clearing large areas on arms and legs can take a couple of years of weekly or twice-weekly sessions. There's also the expense. Fees vary, but you can expect to spend about $5 for 15 minutes or $10 for a half hour in most cities. There are also certain risks to electrolysis. Even the most skilled technician can't guarantee that there won't be some regrowth. Although electrolysis is permanent, it sometimes takes more than one treatment to completely destroy a hair. There is also the risk of scarring, depending on the area to be treated. A good technician is your best insurance against this, but certain areas of the face—the upper lip, for example—carry more risk no matter how good the technician is. Finally, electrolysis is somewhat uncomfortable, especially if you're undergoing prolonged treatment to clear large areas.

split ends
what you can do for split ends

Split ends are one of the biggest hair bugaboos, especially in summer, and they can make the prettiest hair look ragged and unhealthy. To help you cure your hair of the "splits," have a look at the dos and don'ts that follow.

- DON'T think that anything is going to bind that poor old split end together again. (The best thing is not to let it split in the first place.) The only real remedy for a split end is to cut it off, before it has a chance to split further along the hair shaft.
- DO have the ends of your hair trimmed regularly—every six to eight weeks—to prevent dry split ends from appearing.

hair

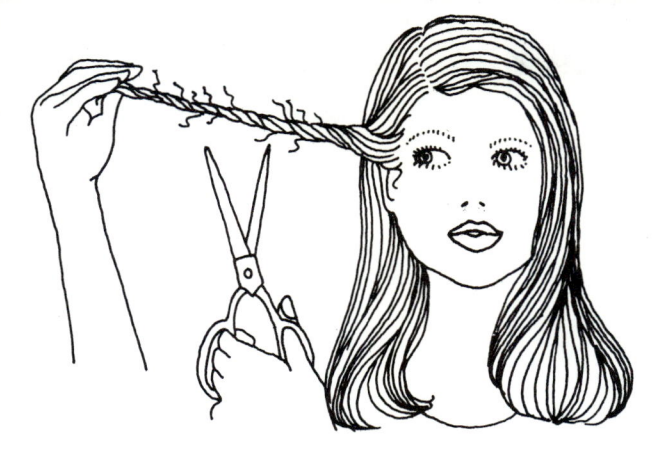

- DO try this little trick to get rid of a few occasional split ends between trims. Twist a length of hair about the thickness of a pencil. As you twist it, the split, broken hairs will pop out away from the rest of the hair so that you can cut them off.
- DON'T forget to condition your hair regularly, even if it's oily. The ends of even the oiliest hair usually don't receive enough nourishment unless hair is very short.
- DO use heated rollers to perk up your set, but don't overdo it. Used two or three times a week, they're great, but used more often, they can dry out your hair and cause it to split or break.
- DO use end papers when you set your hair. They help keep ends smooth, even if there are a few splits here and there. They prevent splits from getting worse.
- DO use hairspray to hold stray hairs in place, but don't douse your hair with it needlessly. The alcohol most sprays contain is drying if used in excess.
- DON'T backcomb or tease your hair. This encourages split ends. If you want some lift to your hairstyle, try this idea instead of teasing: Lean over and let your hair fall forward. Start at the nape of the neck and gently stroke forward with your brush. Continue for about half a minute. Then throw your head back and arrange hair.
- DO have a bodywave to give fine, limp hair a boost. But don't have more than one every eight weeks. Overprocessing your hair chemically can cause split ends.
- DON'T overcolor or overbleach your hair. Always follow manufacturer's instructions if you're doing it yourself. Get the help of a professional at the first sign of trouble. If you're doing tricky coloring like bleaching and then toning, you should talk to a good colorist before tackling the job yourself. It may be more than you can do successfully.

streaking
10 things you should know about having your hair streaked

The one thing you probably already know about hair streaking is that tawny blonde highlights are one of the prettiest things you can put next to your face. In addition to this, there are a few other things to consider so you're sure to get the kind of results you want. Here are some tips from famous colorist Constance at the Louis Guy D' Salon.

1. Start with just a few streaks. Don't feel you need a whole headful to get pretty effects. The fewer streaks you have to start, the less you'll notice the regrowth of new hair and the less frequently you'll need touchups.
2. Ask your hairdresser about the possibility of leaving the hairline out of the streaking. Streaks can be done in a halo effect just behind the hairline. This way, you'll barely notice the regrowth since it won't be right around your face.
3. Ask for the finest possible streaks. This gives the most natural effect.
4. Talk to your hairdresser about the method of streaking he or she uses. The cap method, in which hair is pulled through tiny holes in a plastic cap, is fine for a first-time streaking, but it does present problems for retouches. The foil method, in which tiny strands of hair are covered with bleach and wrapped in foil paper, is much easier to control. Your hairdresser can see just which strands of hair he or she is picking up because they're not covered by a cap.
5. Don't ask for the lightest blonde streaks—unless your hair is very light. Streaks that are too light will give you a gray effect. For most brown hair, tawny blonde streaks are the most natural looking—ask for gold-toned. If your hair is dark brown, ask for tortoise-shell-colored streaks.
6. Don't present yourself for a touchup the minute you see new hair growth. Most hairdressers say that a six-month interval between streakings is the least damaging to hair. But depending on its length and the way you wear it, this ideal period may have to be shortened. As a rule, it should never be done more often than every three months if you want to keep your hair in good healthy condition.
7. If you have been straightening or curling your hair with chemical solutions, you'll have to make a choice between streaks and the straightening or waving. Doing both will damage your hair.
8. Be prepared to condition streaked hair more often. Bleaching dries hair to some extent, and a deep-penetrating conditioner is the only way to compensate.
9. It's not a good idea to expose any hair to much sun, but this is especially true of streaked hair. Don't sit for hours on the beach without something covering your hair.
10. When you have streaks, brush or comb wet hair very gently to prevent hair from breaking or splitting.

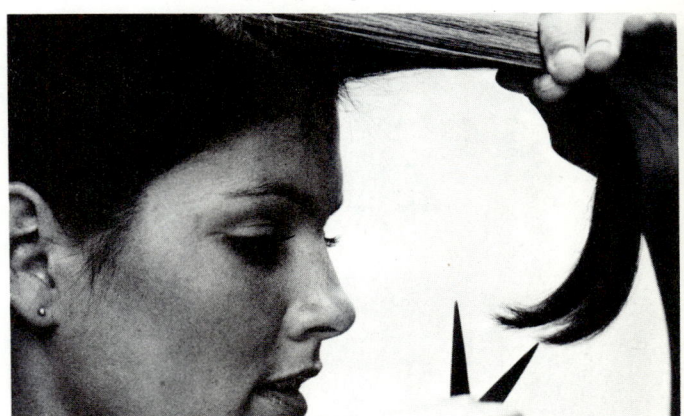

style pick a new hairstyle you'll really love

There is absolutely nothing like a new hairstyle to give you a lift, but before you go under the scissors, here are some tips to consider, adapted from *How to Cut Your Own or Anybody Else's Hair* by Bob Bent and Jack Bozzi.

Go over all the hairstyles you've had that you liked and felt good in. Then look through a few fashion magazines to see what's new and incorporate features of those successful styles—bangs, a side or center part, whatever. Next, check through the following guidelines.

If you have a tendency to be overweight, don't cut your hair too short. It can make you look bottom-heavy. Pick a longer version of a style you like.

As a rule, fine, straight hair should not be layered. A one-length, shortish blunt cut is the best idea for this kind of hair.

Keep thin, sparse hair fairly short to give the illusion of more body and fullness.

Very curly or very thick hair should not be blunt cut or worn below the shoulders; it looks wild and unruly. You can get a good degree of

h hair

control with a layer cut, not exaggerated layers—that's old-fashioned —but a gentle layering to control the bulk.

Take your ideas to a first-rate hairdresser and discuss them with him or her. Listen to professional advice, but don't be talked into the latest thing if you don't want it or don't feel it's right for you.

wet sets
that look as great as their comb-outs

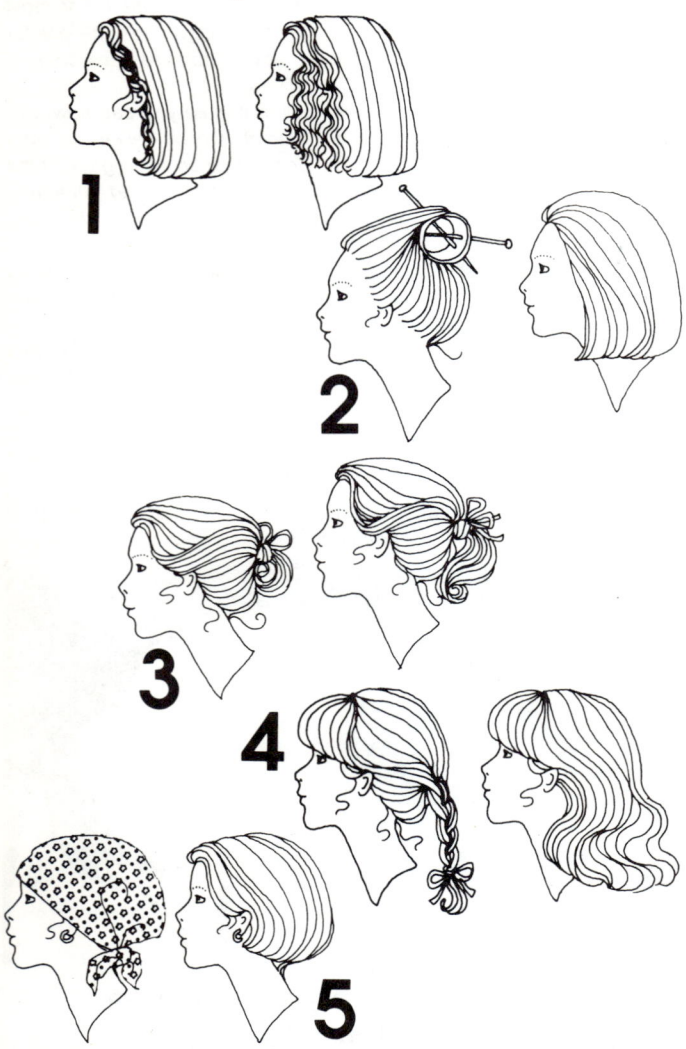

1

2

3

4

5

To have hair that looks pretty wet and dries as if it had been set, see sketches above. For all, comb in a strong body-building setting lotion. For the crinkly look, Sketch 1, pull one small section of front hair into a braid on each side of center part. Fasten. Put ends behind ears with hidden bobby pins. Comb back hair under. Comb when dry. For long hair, Sketch 2, make a roller about 5" in diameter and 2" long out of cardboard tube. Spray it a color; punch four holes in it. Comb hair smoothly up and over roll. Secure with short knitting needles. When hair is dry, comb it out and under. To get the look in Sketch 3, comb hair into ponytail. Roll ends under, secure with bobby pins in one big, rolled curl. Then comb it out when dry. For Sketch 4, simply comb wet hair smoothly back and braid into one long, thick tail. Fasten with a covered elastic band or ribbon. When hair is dry, the braided part will be wavy, the rest smooth. For Sketch 5, comb hair back from brow, behind ears, except for squiggles above ear. Turn hair ends under in one roll, fasten with pins. Tie triangle-folded square tight, ends slightly to one side. Put dab of setting lotion on squiggles and wind into corkscrews. Comb when dry.

Halloween

costumes
easy-to-make surprise ideas

This Halloween, instead of dressing your child as the same old ghost, try something different. A crayon maybe. Or a playing card. Or let your kid be a striker for something he or she wants—like staying up late, eating more hot dogs, etc. The ideas here are easy, inexpensive, and nonsexist to boot.

● *The crayon*—Buy oaktag* in the shade of your child's favorite crayon. Wrap around the child's body like a tube, cutting holes for arms, and staple it closed down the back. Use another piece of oaktag to make a cone shape to fit over the child's head, cutting holes for eyes and mouth. Fasten to body tube with staples. Write the word "Crayon" and the name of the color with paint or a felt-tipped marker.

● *The shark*—If your child wants something scary and wicked, try a shark. Buy a piece of gray oaktag and make a cone to fit over head. Cut out a big mouth, and paint on eyes and teeth. For the body, dye a sheet gray, cut a hole in the middle, and place over head. Wrap tubelike around body, cut holes for arms, and pin in place. Stitch up the back and staple to the cone "head." Add fins made from oaktag to back.

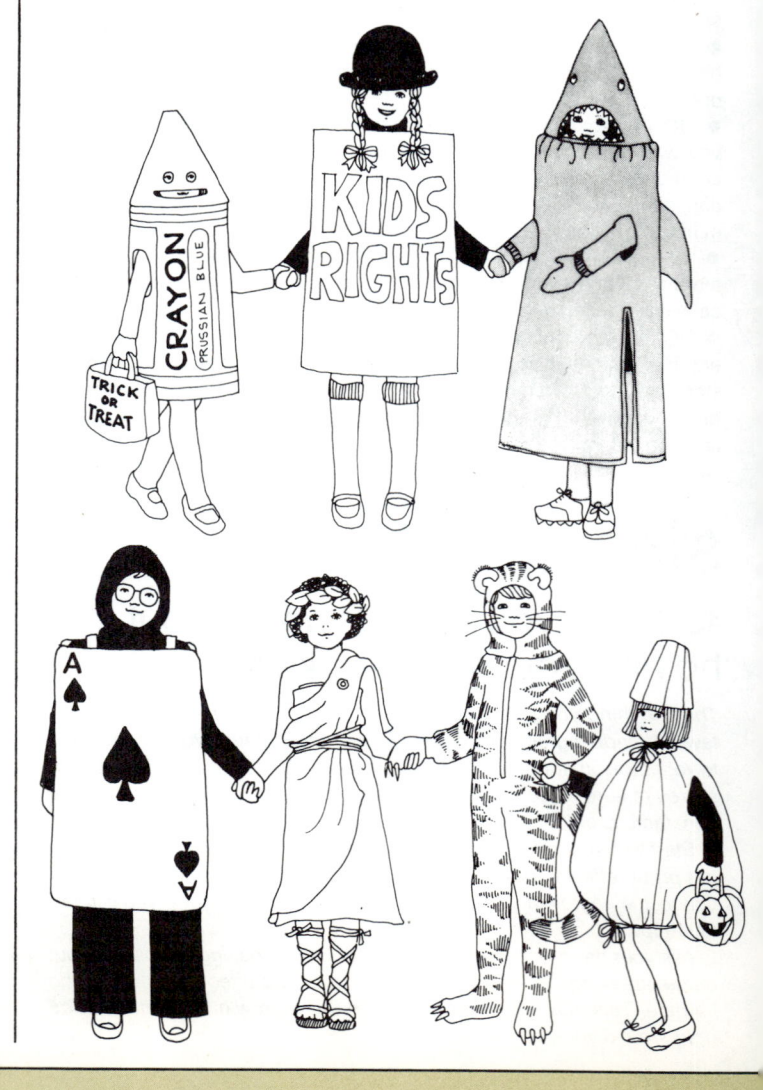

- *The striker*—Make two sandwich boards from illustration board*, attach with cord, and hang over child's shoulders. Let child write on his main gripe or even a campaign slogan, and illustrate it any way he or she wants.
- *Playing card*—Make sandwich boards from illustration board and draw card suits. Choose something simple like the ace of spades. Dress child in either black or red turtleneck and pants, depending on the color card, and top off with a matching hood made of felt.
- *The pumpkin*—Buy a bright orange sheet (or dye a white one) and cut to fit your child's body from neck to mid-thigh. Make a casing at top and bottom edges and run a piece of cord through each. Stitch other two edges together. Then tie two bed pillows around child's body (this will plump out the pumpkin). Put sheet over child, pulling the two cords closed like a drawstring. Cut out holes for arms. Make a green cone hat from oaktag for the stem and use green tights for legs.
- *Dr. Denton animals*—Dr. Denton pajamas are perfect for turning into rabbits, tigers, etc. Just pick the appropriate pajamas (or dye a pair), make a hood to match, and attach ears, tails, whatever. For spotted animals like leopards, just draw on spots with felt-tipped markers or fabric paint. Use mittens for paws.
- *A "toga'd" Roman*—Holding a sheet lengthwise, fold it to fit the length of the body. Then, starting at the left front of body (near armpit), wrap neatly around body from left to right. After first wrap, pin in place. Continue, bringing end of sheet up over left shoulder. Finish off with a piece of cord tied as a belt, and add sandals. (For a very small child, a "crib sheet" will be less bulky.)

*Oaktag is a very heavy-duty-type paper. Illustration board is even heavier, thicker, and nonflexible. Art supply stores carry both.

pumpkin
5 new faces to put on pumpkins

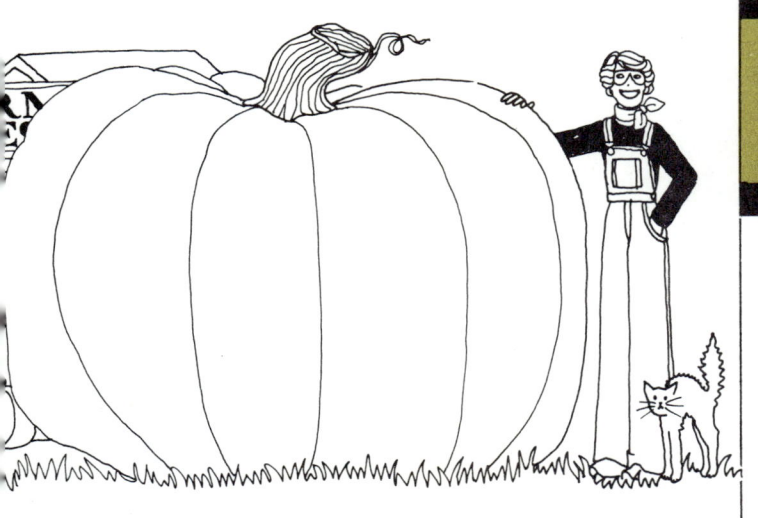

If you can't think of Halloween without pumpkins—and a toothy jack-o'-lantern seems old hat—why not try one of the alternatives below? The life span of an average pumpkin is a week if it's intact and three days if cut, so don't carve your pumpkin too far in advance of using it; the same day is best.

- A scooped-out pumpkin—with a burlap bow off to the side— makes a great Halloween flower holder, suggests The Gazebo, a gift shop in New York City. Flowers should be roughly 1½ to 2 times the pumpkin's height. You'll need to hide a vase to hold fresh flowers—like bronze and yellow chrysanthemums and pompoms. Green styrofoam fitted into the pumpkin can anchor a dried arrangement of wheat, baby's breath, and strawflowers—also in yellow and bronze.
- Candlelight shining from a carved pumpkin can take on extra spar-

kle if you carve out something more original than a toothy grin—like your class year or a scattering of moon and stars. You can also cluster together three small but different-sized pumpkins, each carved with its own geometric shape—circles for one, squares, triangles, or diamonds for the other two.
- You can reverse the lighting effect by placing candles next to your pumpkin instead of inside it. Leaving the pumpkin uncut, decorate its surface with a design made from attractive hardware: for example, aluminum or colored pushpins or studs. You can also glue on a glitter-and-sequin face.
- If you're having just a few friends over for Halloween, try spray painting tiny pumpkins (they can come about 4" in diameter and cost under $1 apiece) an unexpected color—like ghost white—then stenciling them with your friends' names or initials, using a felt-tipped marker. The pumpkins can serve as place cards for your table. Or scoop out several small pumpkins and use as candle holders. Your florist might sell or recommend spray enamels suitable for the waxy pumpkin surface—like Accent Designer Sprays by Illinois Bronze.
- As a treat your favorite toddler is sure to remember for years, The Gazebo also suggests that you draw a face with a felt-tipped marker and use yarn for a wig. Secure skeins of yarn with straight hairpins stuck down and some glue. Let the ends hang loose or braid into pigtails and add a fringe of bangs. You can use a carrot for the nose and a bright gingham bow tie or hair bow as an extra ornament.

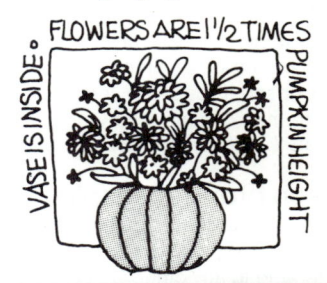

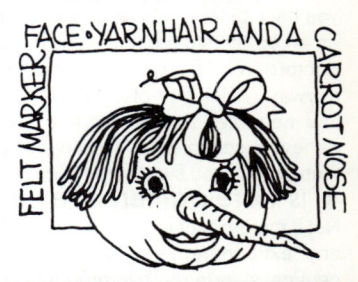

health

aspirin
what you need to know about aspirin

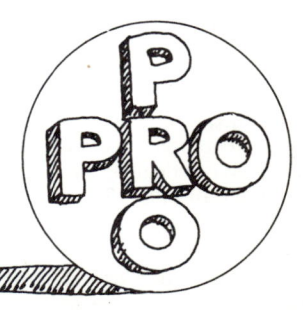

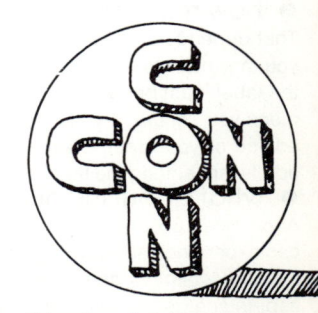

Doctors know nothing beats aspirin for mild-pain relief, but they know very little about how it works. Here's what they do know about it.

- **what does aspirin do?**

Aspirin is an analgesic, which means it relieves pain. It also reduces fever. But aspirin doesn't "cure" anything. If it makes you feel more

h health

comfortable, it doesn't eliminate the *cause* of your discomfort—a headache, cold, etc. That's why you should always consult your doctor if symptoms persist.

● **does aspirin end the "blahs" or ease tension?**
Advertisements claim some products will. Doctors tend to disagree with them. One official of the American Pharmaceutical Association testified before the Senate that there is no evidence that the "blahs," nervous tension, and insomnia can be treated with over-the-counter analgesic products. A professor of pharmacology added, "There is no evidence that these products have any tranquilizing, hypnotic, or antidepressant activity."

Tension and pain have a chicken-and-egg relationship, a Food and Drug Administration spokesman said. If your tension grows out of pain, aspirin may relieve it for that reason and no other.

See your doctor if you need a tranquilizer; don't expect aspirin to be one.

● **does aspirin help you to sleep?**
No, unless pain keeps you from getting to sleep. "Aspirin isn't a sleep-producing drug," the FDA official said. On the contrary, some aspirin-combination drugs that contain caffeine can keep you awake because caffeine is a mild stimulant. Check the label of your product for its ingredients.

● **what effect does aspirin have on your stomach?**
Aspirin tends to irritate the lining for some people. Don't take aspirin if you have ulcers, or even if you suspect you do. Try not to take aspirin on an empty stomach if your stomach is generally "sensitive." (Many doctors feel it's a good idea not to take aspirin on an empty stomach anyway.) Drink half of a glassful of milk or some soup first, then swallow the tablet. Follow with the rest of the milk or soup. Many doctors believe a seltzer-type aspirin that you drink irritates the stomach less than aspirin you swallow whole.

● **is there a difference between brands of aspirin?**
Not if the product is labeled simply "aspirin" and doesn't claim to have any "extra ingredients." *All* aspirin, by law, must meet certain pharmaceutical standards. "No product is preferable to any other," according to *The Complete Home Medical Encyclopedia*.

". . . all aspirin powder manufactured in the United States comes from six sources . . . therefore patients should buy the least expensive aspirin tablets, without prescription," says Dr. Richard Burack in *The New Handbook of Prescription Drugs*.

● **what about "buffered" aspirin and those that claim to be "stronger"?**
Buffered aspirin is said to be less irritating to the stomach than plain aspirin, but not everyone agrees. If a product claims to have extra strength, it may have other pain relievers besides aspirin, or it may contain more aspirin in one tablet. Ask your doctor or pharmacist to explain the contents of the aspirin you take.

● **can aspirin cause any side effects?**
Yes—it's caused a spectrum of reactions ranging from rashes to shock to gastrointestinal bleeding in people with a tendency to ulcers. Consult your doctor immediately if you have any symptoms.

● **how much aspirin is too much?**
That depends on your physical makeup and involves any tendencies you may have to ulcers, allergies, etc. Always follow the directions on the label. Just because it says you *can* take eight in one day, doesn't mean you *should*. If you're taking aspirin in any quantity, do so on the advice of your doctor. Aspirin overdoses, among both children and adults, are among the main causes of accidental poisoning in the U.S.

● **what about the nonaspirin pain relievers?**
Aspirin can upset some people's stomachs and allergy-prone people can experience allergic reactions as a result of taking it. If you'd like to try the *acetaminophen* products (the technical name for a kind of nonaspirin analgesic), keep in mind that they are as effective in relieving minor pain as aspirin. Aspirin has an anti-inflammatory property that the acetaminophen has not. Aspirin and nonaspirin are also competitively priced.

breasts
how and why you should do a thorough breast exam once a month

Doctors say that 95 percent of breast cancers are discovered by women themselves. They also point out that breast cancer is one of the easiest to find and diagnose. But to help ensure the earliest possible detection, doctors advise that you examine your own breasts once a month after your menstrual period for the lumps and thickenings that are cancer's early-warning signals. Then, if you do find a lump, see your doctor right away, since only a physician can determine what needs to be done next. (Lumps may simply be noncancerous cysts.)

Here's how the American Cancer Society recommends that you do the check: (1) Lie down, as in Sketch 1. Put one hand behind your head. With the other hand, fingers flattened, gently feel your breast. Press lightly, beginning where you see the A in Sketch 2. Follow the arrows, feeling gently for a lump or thickening. *Remember to feel all parts of the breast.* (2) Now repeat the same procedure sitting or standing up, with your hand still behind your head, as in Sketch 3. (3) While you are sitting or standing in front of a mirror, you should also relax your arms at your sides and look for changes in the size, shape, and contour of your breasts and nipples. Gently press each nipple to see if any discharge occurs, and tell your doctor if there is any.

The American Cancer Society says it's especially helpful to do this check after a bath or shower while your skin is still wet, since the fact that your skin is slippery makes it easier to feel for a lump or thickening.

Your own doctor may prefer a slightly different method of examination, so ask how he or she wants you to do it.

Copies of the pamphlet, "How to Examine Your Breasts," are available free from your local American Cancer Society.

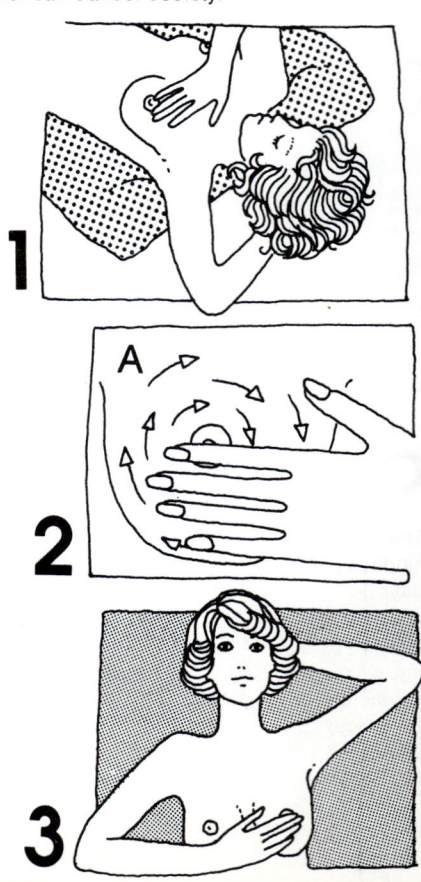

health

clubs
6 things to know before you join a health club

Joining a health club can cost a lot of money, so before you put your money down, here are some things to consider:

● Don't be dazzled by the jargon used in ads and brochures. Many ads try to glamorize very basic facilities, things you may even have in your own house. For example, a needlepoint shower is simply a shower with heavy water pressure.

● A good health club will offer you a tour or even a trial day for free or minimal charge ($5 to $7). If a club doesn't offer such options, you might ask yourself, "What have they got to hide?" Be sure to check out several different places to see what each offers for the price. (The New York City Department of Consumer Affairs recommends that you visit a club at the time of day when you'll most likely be using it if you join; an exercise room that looks spacious at 10 A.M. may be like a packed can of sardines at lunch hour.)

● On your trial day, take along the club brochure and check off the facilities you think you'll use regularly. If you'll use only the pool and exercise class, you might be better off at a Y.W.C.A. that offers the same things for much less.

● Remember that certain services may cost you an additional fee every time you use them—lockers, massages, manicures, facials.

● If you're interested in joining a club but not sure you'll stay dedicated, look for one that offers a three- or six-month membership. Also be wary of any club that suggests a special deal "only for you."

● Read the contract carefully before you sign. If you pay on an installment plan, there may be a high interest rate. If you make one payment and then decide to quit, you're still liable for all the money you owe for your original membership plan.

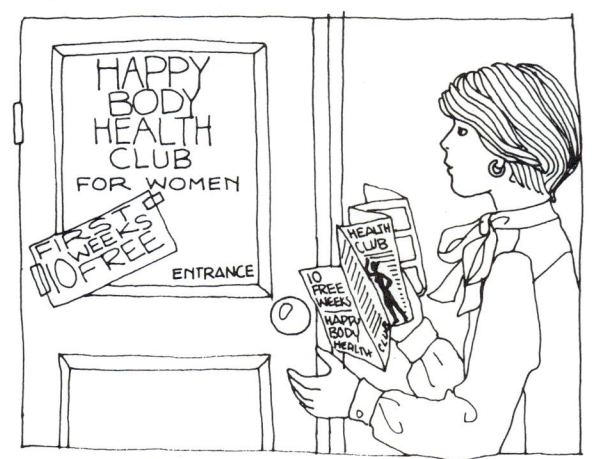

colds
what to do for a friend with a cold

The best prescription for almost any cold is an extra dose of a friend's kindness. Most mid-winter sniffles will run their course in a week to ten days, so *what* to do for a friend usually isn't as important as *that* you do it. Some people love to be soothed, coddled, and fussed over, while others—particularly men—may resist anything that smacks of mothering. So do, but don't overdo, and ask, "Would you rather I stay around or just leave you alone?" The most important thing is to let the person know you care that he or she has a cold. When you'd like to show that you do care, try one or more of the following. (We've referred to the friend as a "he," but any suggestions would be equally soothing for a female friend.)

● Give your friend a gift of legwork. Volunteer to have his prescriptions filled, return or pick up library books, move his car, or drop something off at the cleaner's. If you're both students in one of the same classes, put a piece of carbon paper under class notes as you take them; it's an instant duplicate for him.

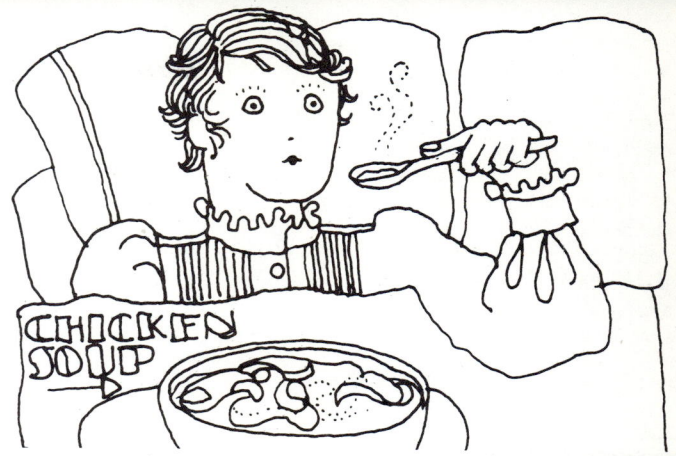

● Bring him a plant that won't mind a few days' neglect. Good bets in this category are agalonema, aspidistra, dracaena, philodendron, and snake plants.

● Let him snuggle up in bed while you read a great short mystery story, such as any one by Agatha Christie, Dashiell Hammett, Ross MacDonald, or John Dixon Carr. If he's feeling a little glum, cheer him up by reading a funny short story, such as any one from *Getting Even* by Woody Allen or *Welcome to the Monkey House* by Kurt Vonnegut, Jr.

● Give him a baby powder or warm-alcohol back rub just because it feels nice.

● Listen to a "nostalgia radio" program together. Many stations have begun to run revivals of such classic shows as "Sherlock Holmes," "The Green Hornet," and "Fibber McGee and Molly."

● Buy him the ultimate crossword-puzzle book, like the collection of *The New York Times*'s greatest hits, *The Sunday Times Crossword Omnibus* by Margaret Farrar.

● Brew up a steaming herbal tea. You might check gourmet food shops for an assortment of peppermint, camomile, sage, yarrow, and others. While you're at it, fix up this yummy cocoa toast suggested by the *Munchies Eatbook* by Alice and Eliot Hess: Melt 4 T. butter in pan. Add 6 T. cocoa and 5 T. sugar. Spread on toast or muffin, sprinkling on a little cinnamon if desired.

● Make him a "six pack" of different juices, from cranberry to apricot nectar, in individual cans.

● And last, but certainly not least, warm his heart and stomach with:

1. *Hot toddy*—Put 1 cube of sugar in a mug and add enough water to dissolve. Add a single or double shot of bourbon, rye, or Scotch; then fill up with boiling water and stir. Decorate with a slice of clove-studded lemon and a stick of cinnamon.

2. *Chicken soup*—Place in saucepan: 2 whole chicken breasts, 5 peppercorns, 2 sliced carrots, 2 stalks celery with tops and 2 small onions cut in large pieces, and salt to taste. Cover with water. Bring to a boil, then simmer for 30 to 45 minutes, skimming as necessary. Strain soup into another container. Skin and bone chicken; shred meat into small pieces. Return meat and vegetables to soup. Refrigerate. Before serving, skim fat from top, add cooked noodles or rice, and reheat.

colds
how to look pretty when you have a cold

The only thing more dreary than suffering through a cold is the way you look when you have one—that pallor, red nose, lips like cardboard. Here are some tips on how to look better, even though you don't feel that way.

● Ignore the old wives' tale that claims you shouldn't take a bath or wash your hair when you have a cold. Doing both will probably make

health

you feel as well as look better. If you aren't up to washing your hair, try a dry shampoo and then add body with electric rollers or a curling iron.
- If you've been neglecting your skin-care routine, give your complexion a pick-me-up with a face mask—you can nap while it dries. Then protect the chapped area around your nose with a moisturizer (reapply each time you blow nose) and dab lightly with waterproof foundation to cover the red. To put the bloom back in your cheeks, try an allover face-color wash or gel in addition to your usual blusher.
- For chapped lips, smooth on a healing, lubricating pomade. It will soothe your lips and make them look shiny and pretty.
- The best thing to do for watery, itchy eyes is to keep your hands away. Soothe them by rinsing with cool, clean water. Avoid eye shadow and mascara, but if you'd like to add a touch of color without irritation, dust deep-toned powder blush or pearly highlighter just under the outer portion of your brows.
- Throw away that wad of shredded tissues and carry a nice cotton handkerchief (they were made for runny noses).
- No matter how loudly people are clamoring for your return, don't push yourself too hard. According to the Center for Disease Control in Atlanta, Georgia, the best thing for a cold is "to do as the spirit moves you." If you feel low, stay in bed and rest, drink lots of liquids, and give your body a chance to recover.

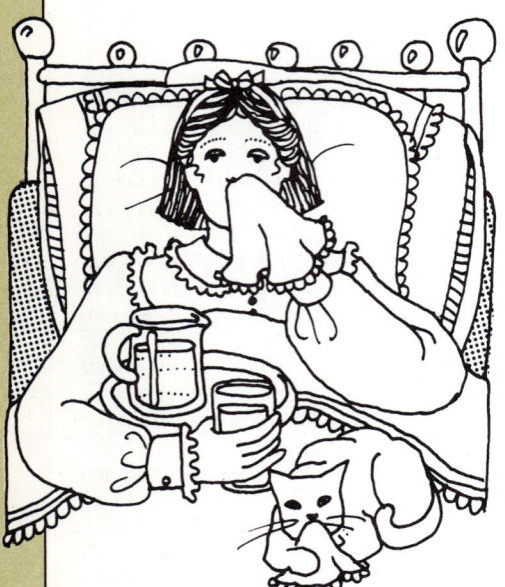

colds should you call a doctor about your cold or cough?

● the cold

How can you tell if your cold is just a classic case of the sniffles or something more serious that requires a doctor? A cold is usually caused by a virus, and as long as it lasts only a couple of days and is confined to a runny nose, stuffiness, scratchy throat, cough and little or no fever, you can nurse it away by adding extra liquids and rest to your normal routine.

However, the more serious troubles usually start when bacteria gain a foothold in the parts of the body that have been weakened by the virus. Then colds can trigger off infection of the sinuses or the middle ear, inflammation of the pharynx or the trachea, bronchitis, laryngitis, tonsilitis, influenza (a common precondition for pneumonia), diphtheria, respiratory allergies, an infected postnasal drip, and asthma. If your cold is accompanied by any of these symptoms, *check with your doctor:*
- Persistence of fever
- Persistent or severe headache
- Earache
- Swollen glands
- Difficulty in swallowing
- Incapacitating aching (difficulty in moving or concentrating)
- Disabling fatigue (difficulty in getting out of bed or keeping awake)
- Chills
- Chest pains
- Difficulty in breathing through mouth when nose is stopped up; shortness of breath
- Persistent and severe cough

● the cough

The cough is a protective reflex that helps keep the breathing passages clear. As long as it merely clears out mucus and relieves throat or chest irritation, don't worry about it; under these circumstances, it is helping you to maintain or regain health (for instance, if you have a cold). However, you should *see a doctor if:*
- Any cough drags on indefinitely, even after a cold.
- There is persistent hoarseness or huskiness in your voice for more than two weeks.
- A cough has a dry, hacking quality and you are continually clearing your throat.
- You spit up blood, pus, or bad-smelling, discolored semisolid secretions when you cough.

Any of these symptoms is a warning that some abnormal respiratory condition—from bronchitis to tuberculosis—*may* possibly exist. Remember, though, that any of these conditions is remediable in the early stages but may be irreversible if ignored.

drugs don't mix these drugs

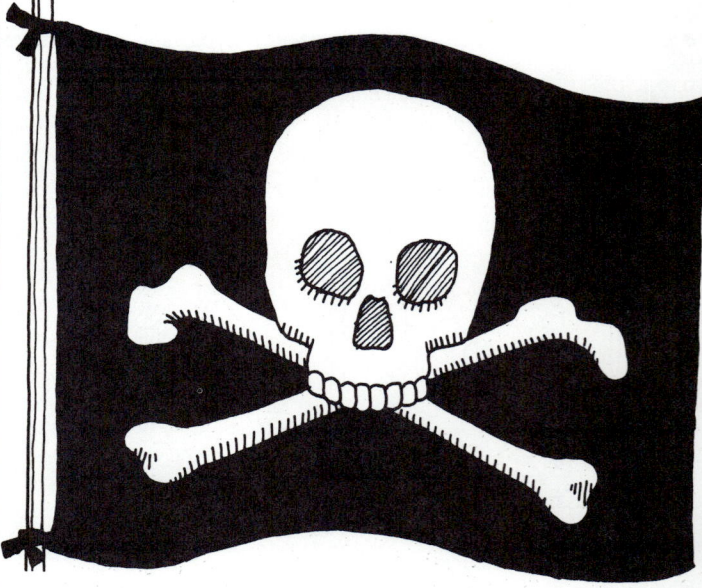

Let's say you are taking an antihistamine drug for hay fever, an amphetamine for weight loss, an antibiotic for acne, and a pain killer for menstrual cramps. Your prescriptions may come from three doctors, none of whom knows the others' orders. You may be in trouble.

Pharmacologists no longer believe that a drug is a drug is a drug. They now know that one medicine a patient takes can alter the action of another. When the two have similar effects, a combination may change from a mild to a whambang reaction. If their effects are opposite, they may cancel out each other. A drug that slows down metabolism may make another more toxic. If it speeds up metabolism, it may make a second drug practically ineffective.

What happens when you mix-match your pills is often unpredictable. It depends on your heredity, body weight, sensitivity, the size of the dose, and your current emotional or physical status. If you've skipped meals or sleep, if you're tense, a drug combination that never bothered you may become toxic. Consider this checklist:

Pep pills—These are amphetamines prescribed for weight reduction or mild depression, bootlegged as bennies, dexies, speed. Amphetamine-type drugs are also present in many over-the-counter remedies for colds or coughs. Pep pills stimulate the central nervous system—overstimulate it if you inadvertently take two or more drugs of this or

health

related families. Suppose you're staying up late to write a term paper. You take your diet pill, swallow a dexie, add a handful of No-Doz (an over-the-counter pill containing caffeine, a mild stimulant), and drink several cups of coffee (also containing caffeine). The result—you may be too high to sit at a typewriter.

If you're taking a thyroid drug for weight reduction and mix it with an amphetamine, you're also likely to get the jitters. It's possible, if you're depressed, that a psychiatrist might prescribe a drug in the tricyclic antidepressant family (trade names: Elavil, Aventyl, Tofranil, among others). Don't mix these with an amphetamine or your blood pressure may shoot up to a dangerous level.

Sedatives—Drugs that sedate fall into two groups: barbiturates (goof balls, downers) that also induce sleep and tranquilizers that quiet the nerves without making you drowsy. Both drugs depress the central nervous system. If used with each other or with other drugs that slow down motor function, a temporary blackout could result. The most dangerous combination is a sedative with a couple of alcoholic drinks. (Liquor also depresses the function of the central nervous system.) If you take a phenobarbital (a barbiturate) or Miltown (a tranquilizer) before a party, even one cocktail may make you reeling drunk. An alcoholic evening topped off with a handful of sedatives could put you to sleep—permanently.

Antihistamines—You may be taking Benadryl or Chlor-Trimeton for hay fever or Dramamine for motion sickness. These are antihistamines, which are also present in just about any product you buy over the counter for a cold or cough. Like the sedatives, they have a depressive effect on brain function and should not be combined with a barbiturate, a tranquilizer, and particularly with alcohol.

Drugs that fight infection—Some antibiotics not only fight infection but fight each other. You may, for example, be taking tetracycline (Aureomycin, Terramycin) for acne and then develop a strep throat for which penicillin is prescribed. The tetracycline will make the penicillin less effective. This problem occurs with several different antibiotic combinations.

If you sunbathe while you're taking some of the antibiotic or sulfa drugs, there's a chance of developing a rash or an unusually severe sunburn. An ultraviolet lamp will have the same effect. Several foods, particularly milk, may interfere with absorption of antibiotics. Make sure you follow prescription directions to take your pill well before or after mealtime.

A common vaginal infection called trichomoniasis is usually treated with Flagyl, a highly effective drug. If you're taking Flagyl, be sure not to drink liquor. The drink will taste peculiar; you may feel sick with cramps, vomiting, flushing.

Pain killers—Salicylates (aspirin) are a major ingredient in most over-the-counter pain killers, including those for menstrual cramps. They're also present in the majority of cold remedies. Remember this if you should develop back trouble or a muscle sprain for which your doctor prescribes an anti-inflammatory drug like Butazolidin or Indocin. Like aspirin, these pills can irritate the stomach lining. If either is prescribed, stop taking aspirin in any form. Gastrointestinal bleeding or ulceration of the stomach could result.

Drug interaction is a complex field. Be cautious and remember these tips:

● When a doctor prescribes a drug, be sure to tell him what other drugs you are taking. Don't forget such apparently innocuous items as aspirin, antacid pills, cough medicine.
● Always know what pill you're taking. The name of the drug should be on the prescription label.
● Patronize one druggist for all your prescriptions. He may notice a drug interaction problem the doctor has missed.
● Stop one drug when you start another for the same illness unless you have directions from your doctor to take both.
● If you've taken a drug that depresses brain action (sedative, antihistamine), don't drive a car unless you are absolutely certain that your reactions are still quick and sharp.
● If you suspect you're pregnant, stop taking all drugs until you check each one out with your gynecologist.

flu what to feed a flu victim

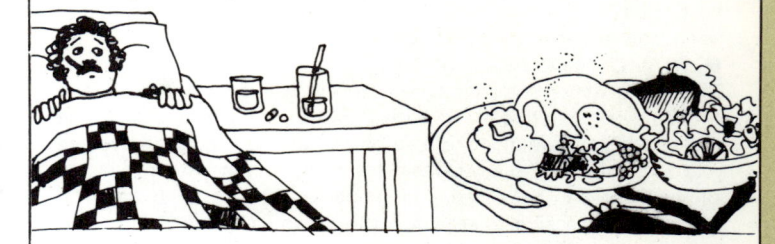

Few flu victims—with intestinal virus or any kind that makes you nauseous—think to ask their doctor what to eat during a bout of flu. Who's thinking of eating? But once they start to recover a bit, they're longing for nourishment; however, foods that are mouth-watering most times may be all wrong during recuperation.

While a person is in the acute stage, "the best thing to offer is a clear liquid or semisolid like tea, gelatin, and light bouillon—not Mama's fatty chicken soup," says Dr. Elliot Heller of Mount Sinai Hospital in New York. Sodas are great, too. Together they'll replenish fluids, sugar, and salts lost from bouts of vomiting or diarrhea. To spike up the menu you might also try juices—such as apple or tomato. But don't overdose with orange or grapefruit juice, whose acid can irritate an already upset stomach. Also stay clear of coffee, milk, or alcohol, and try not to serve any liquid ice cold.

Once the victim starts recuperating, you can ease into bland light solids—plain-cooked vegetables, bananas, boiled or poached eggs, broiled chicken, lean hamburger (but not hard-to-digest steak). You might serve yogurt, but otherwise keep avoiding milk and other milk products plus highly spiced or greasy foods. Save them for your "got well" party.

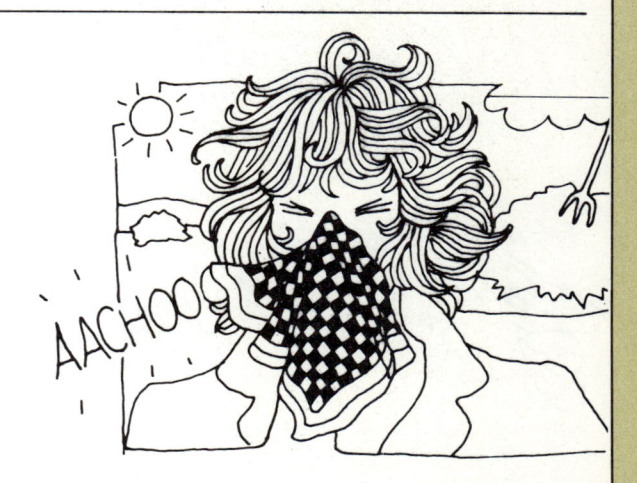

hay fever
what you should know about it

About 1 out of every 15 Americans suffers from hay fever, the most common allergic reaction in the U.S. today. And while the symptoms can be uncomfortable enough in themselves, untreated hay fever can lead to asthma or even more serious lung damage, according to the Allergy Foundation of America—which is why it shares these facts:

● **what causes hay fever?**
Hay fever is purely and simply an allergy to pollens that irritate the mucous membranes of the nose, eyes, and throat. It occurs during the pollinating periods of certain grasses, weeds, and trees such as elm or oak in spring. The main cause in this country is ragweed, and hay is *not* a cause.

health

- **when is hay fever most likely to occur?**
Its symptoms can appear at almost any time of the year, but the peak season for most areas of the country is from mid-August until the first frost, usually sometime in October. This eight-to-ten-week period is when ragweed pollination takes place.
- **how do you recognize it?**
The most common symptoms are sneezing spells; itchy, tearful, and swollen eyes; sore throat and nose. However, the variety of possible causes for such symptoms are so great that you should always see your doctor if you have any of them. He or she may then refer you to an allergist who can run a series of simple "scratch tests" (scratching your skin with possible allergens at one- to two-inch intervals) to determine those to which you react.
- **what can be done about it?**
A doctor will often prescribe an antihistamine to control some of the symptoms. However, hay fever sufferers usually have at least one series of "desensitizing" injections, which helps the body to build up antibodies to the specific pollens it's allergic to. Some people show great improvement after relatively few injections; others require as many as two or three injections per week for years. Sometimes air conditioning provides some relief, if the temperature is kept not more than 12 degrees lower than the temperature outside. In severe cases, some hay-fever sufferers must move to an area without high concentrations of the offending pollen in order to get relief.

pills
how to be a sensible pill taker

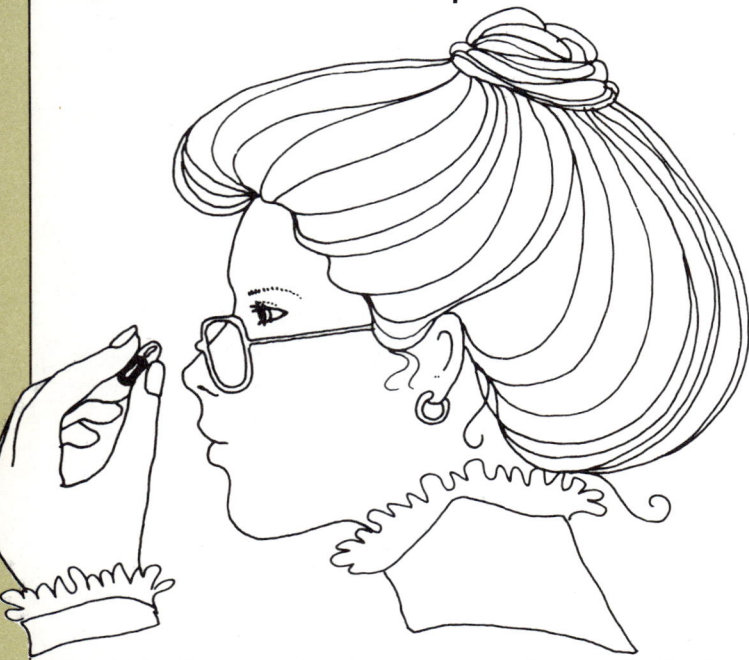

If you're like the average American woman, you take more pills than the average American man, according to Dr. David L. Rabin, Associate Chairman for Community Medicine and International Health, Georgetown University Medical Center, Washington, D.C. Dr. Rabin also points out that as a nation, the United States is one of the most pill-consuming in the world.

Researchers have speculated that women are culturally more conditioned to acknowledge illness or pain than men and that they may also have a slightly lower pain threshold. Reproductive-system differences also account for some pill-taking.

What could be dangerous in your pill-taking habits is the frequency with which pills or other drugs not really prescribed for a *current* illness are taken. If you feel sick and you—or a member of your family—has suffered similar symptoms before, the tendency is to take whatever medicine was taken then without really knowing whether it's appropriate for the new illness. This is an especially bad habit where antibiotics are involved. You may build up a tolerance that makes the antibiotic less effective when you need it most.

Dr. Rabin has these suggestions for sensible pill taking:
- Never take a medication that hasn't been prescribed for your current illness.
- Throw out all prescription drugs when you get well—unless your doctor specifically says to keep them and advises you on future use. Medications can get stale.
- Don't take pain killers unless you really need them. If you have a headache or similar symptoms, try to wait it out for a half hour. The condition may clear up without taking anything. Consider, too, that the headache may be caused by hunger or a stuffy room. Food or a little fresh air may be all you need.

VD guide to the facts and fiction about VD

Venereal disease is the most commonly reported communicable disease after flu in the U.S., but ignorance adds to the problems of bringing the epidemic under control. Here are the most common misconceptions health experts continually run into and the facts that counter them.

- *Fiction—You can pick up VD from glasses, bathing utensils, toilet seats.*
Fact—VD is caught only by sexual relations, intercourse, or oral contact with a female or male partner who has the infection. The use of condoms is a help but no guarantee of safety.
- *Fiction—Once you get VD, you're immune for life.*
Fact—There is no immunity developed by having gonorrhea. Reinfection is possible immediately after a course of treatment is over. Syphilis may sometimes cause immunity to reinfection, but don't depend on it.
- *Fiction—There's a magic one-shot treatment that takes care of VD every time, or you can take care of it yourself with home remedies.*
Fact—Gonorrhea is becoming resistant to treatment by penicillin and other antibiotics, while syphilis germs are easily killed by these. Current injections call for a much higher dosage of penicillin for both men and women than a decade ago for gonorrhea. Only a doctor can decide the right combination and amount of medicine needed.
- *Fiction—If you don't have a private physician or can't afford to pay, there's no place to go for VD treatment.*
Fact—Often the free treatments provided by local public-health clinics in every state are just as efficient and might be less embarrassing than your family physician. The public-health doctors also specialize in care without moralizing. If a clinic is not nearby, check phone listings for county health or district health services (a group of counties). As part of its regular family planning services, most local Planned Parenthood offices also provide VD tests. Fees are on a sliding scale, depending on ability to pay.
- *Fiction—Parents have to agree to VD treatment and sign permission papers.*
Fact—Most states have passed laws permitting minors to give their own consent for VD treatment.
- *Fiction—The public-health clinics have to give names to government authorities.*
Fact—Public-health clinics forward statistics, but never names, to Federal authorities. Confidentiality is vital to the clinic-patient relationship, so much so that treatment and subsequent visits are always arranged in person and no calls or messages reach a patient's home or school.
- *Fiction—You have to give the names of the sexual partner you caught it from and others you might have infected or they won't treat you.*
Fact—It's a favor to give someone's name who might be infected with

home furnishings

VD, but you won't be refused treatment if you don't. Part of the public-health-service practice, though, is sensitive interviewing of VD contacts. For everyone's protection against serious health damage, follow-ups on contacts are the only way to halt VD's spread. If you're too shaken up to tell a partner directly, the public-health service may do so without revealing your name.
- *Fiction*—VD marks you for life—you never can be completely cured. *Fact*—VD can be completely cured if caught in the early stages. Signs of syphilis develop from ten days to three weeks after sexual contact with an infected person, and usually consist of an open but painless sore on the genitals or mouth where the germs entered the body. Gonorrhea produces symptoms three to five days after infection: itching and burning, acute inflammation of genital and urinary tracts may develop. The accompanying discharge is easily noticeable in men but often goes undetected in women. Untended, both forms of VD can eventually cause sterility, heart disease, and other systemic damage. Because syphilis and gonorrhea are sometimes symptomless or move into a "silent" phase, the follow-up of contacts by the public-health service and their cooperation is vital—a blood test for syphilis or a culture test for gonorrhea is a small effort to make to be sure.

at high-wear spots—like fork tines. Reputable manufacturers guarantee that the silver won't rub off for a generation or they'll replate free.
  Both sterling and silverplate look best and need less polishing if used often. Constant use builds up a mellow luster or "patina." (Just rotate place settings so they get equal use and the same lived-with patina.)
- The best *stainless* is what's known as 18/8, or steel mixed with 18 percent chromium, 8 percent nickel. (Chromium makes it "stainless." Extra nickel brightens the shine and makes the stainless nonmagnetic —one way to tell 18/8 from cheaper grades, which are magnetic.)
  Quality stainless is durable, strong, and reinforced at high-stress spots. It's better at resisting tarnish, scratches, corrosion, and stains. (You just use stainless or copper cleaner to wipe off purple discoloration that may result from detergents or chemicals in local water. Never use these cleaners on silver.)
- *Pewter* is mostly tin with some antimony and copper added for hardness. But it's still too soft for rubbing or scraping, so "pewter" flatware just has a pewter handle attached to a stainless spoon, fork, or knife blade. Care is easy. Scratches on the handle just add to pewter's special patina. Dark stains caused by detergents or chemicals in local water can be wiped off with special pewter cleaners.

home furnishings

flatware
what to know about buying flatware

If you're ready to invest in quality stainless, pewter, silverplate, or sterling flatware, here are some tips:
- Well-made flatware has smooth edges. Each piece should feel balanced but not too heavy.
- Expect to pay more for elaborate patterns—and trust your instinct when choosing one. Narrow your choice to three, then see each one with the china and glassware you prefer. There are no hard-and-fast rules, so you might even mix patterns or metals; e.g., cut costs by buying silverplate serving pieces and sterling knives and forks.
- Your budget sets obvious limits. Even if you entertain moderately, you'll need about eight place settings. A good-quality, four-piece setting costs about $14 in stainless, $26 in silverplate, $30 in pewter, $132 in sterling. Here's a rundown of the different metals to choose from:
- *Sterling* is solid silver except for a bit of antimony and copper added for hardness and strength. Durable and lustrous, sterling adjusts instantly to temperature changes, so it won't clash with hot or cold foods. It's also one investment that keeps pace with inflation; as the world price for silver bullion rises, your flatware becomes that much more valuable. There are three sizes: dinner (largest and most costly), place (most versatile), and luncheon. Whatever you choose, some stores offer club plans that let you buy a minimum amount of sterling and pay for it over one to two years without extra charge. You can also add pieces later. Sterling manufacturers never destroy a die; they may "deactivate" a pattern, but usually once a year they fill orders.
- *Silverplate* is flatware with silver coated over a less expensive metal. Quality plate has a thicker silver coating all over and more of it

grass rug
how to buy a grass rug

"Grass" rugs made of sisal, coco fiber, hemp, straw, sea grass, maize, and rush are especially pretty teamed with other naturals—unpainted furniture, batik fabrics, pottery, baskets, and plants. Here are tips to consider:
- *Your best buys are area rugs rather than wall-to-wall "grass,"* since natural fiber rugs (except those made from 12" × 12" squares) are hard to cut and seam. You can buy a 9' × 12' area rug for about $75 to $225. Chinese rice straw, Haitian rush, and Indian coco matting are great budget choices. Sisal or Chinese rush/maize run $150 plus.
- *Consider the location for any rug before you buy.* Sisal and coco matting are extra durable and great for heavy traffic areas—like your den or enclosed porch. They're reversible, too. Maize, rush, sea grass, and straw are more fragile and work better in a bedroom or dining room.
- *You can choose from a range of neutral tones*—off-whites, creamy yellows, earth browns. Some rugs are solid matting in striped, waffle, or diamond weaves. Others are pieced together from 12" squares— each one in a tightly braided or lacy design (see sketches).
- *Most natural rugs go directly on your floor without backing,* but if you want padding it should be hair or hair-topped rubber to cut down on friction. Also keep in mind that sisal and coco matting tend to "walk"—that is, stretch a bit if the air is very moist, shrink if it's dry.
- *Don't just think floors.* You can use sisal or coco matting for added texture or to soundproof a room by running it up the wall (use a staple gun or some liquid latex-rubber glue). Or use rugs to cover cubes or platforms that will hold pillows.

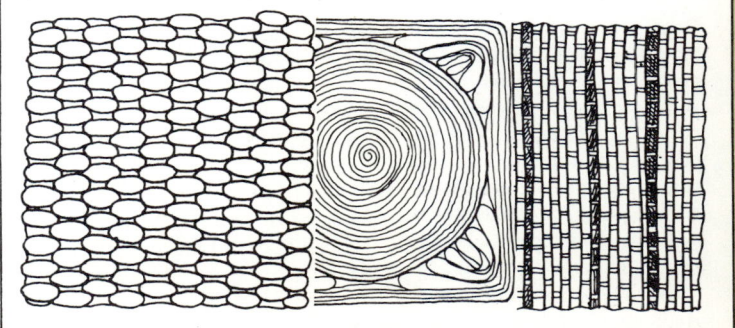

sisal   rush and straw   coco matting

95

home furnishings

Note: *Rugs can be professionally dry cleaned. For grease stains, you can sprinkle on dry cornmeal, let stand an hour, then vacuum. For spot cleaning of other dirt, use spray spot remover, or try a soft-bristle brush and mild detergent.*

mattress
dos and don'ts for choosing a mattress for one or two people

- DO buy the best mattress you can afford. Aim for a top-of-the-line model from a name manufacturer (like Simmons, Sealy, Serta, Eclipse, or Stearns and Foster). A reliable store's "house" line—made to its specifications by a top manufacturer—is a good bet, too.
- DO plan on spending $250 to $400 for a good-to-luxury, queen-size mattress plus box spring. You may save 20 percent or more if you look for sales, which can be held any time during the year, except, perhaps, November and December.

Life span for top mattresses is ten years or more (for poorer mattresses, five to seven years).

A box spring acts like shock absorbers in a car. If you put your mattress straight on a wood platform or the floor, it will break down faster. A new mattress on an old, saggy box spring will start to sag, too.

If you're saving money, don't skimp on quality construction, but cut down on frills, such as a damask cover.

- DO check out innerspring *and* foam mattresses. Innersprings make up over 85 percent of sales and come in a wider range of firmness. Quality largely depends on the center coil construction (thickness of steel, number of coils, how they're joined, insulations, etc.). Foam mattresses have a slightly different "feel." They're also nonallergenic, light, and bendable—a plus if you're moving a large mattress through cramped spaces.

There are natural foam rubber (latex) and synthetic polyurethane foam mattresses. Both can give equally good support and endurance, but the consumer has no way of judging the quality of the latex or polyurethane used. Your best bet is to assume that the higher the price, the better the quality may be.

- DON'T shop for a mattress late in the day when your back is tired. Test different models for comfort by lying down and turning on each one. Don't just tap them. You cause wear and tear on your back when you sink into a "swayback" position on a too-soft mattress. On the other hand, an inflexible mattress puts pressure on back muscles so you toss and turn.
- Buying a mattress for two? DO lie down on it together. If you can't compromise on firmness, pair up twin beds.
- DO consider queen or king sizes, because a double mattress gives you each just 27" to move in—about the width of a baby's crib.

sofa pick the right sofa for your room and budget

Fresh from the showroom or vintage Salvation Army, a sofa may be the most expensive piece in your home—so use these easy guidelines to avoid making mistakes when you buy.

- When shopping, take along your room dimensions, a swatch of curtain fabric, and a color sample of your wall paint. Shop with your husband or a friend, since a comfortable sofa for you may be short-seated for someone with longer legs.
- Size is an important choice, since sofas have anywhere from two to five seats. Small two-seaters (50" to 60" long) look great in small apartments; longer, 90" sofas are best in spacious rooms. Consider placing two small sofas at right angles; or try sectional sofas.
- Sit on any sofa in your favorite position before deciding it's "comfortable." Better yet, sit on one cushion and have a friend sit next to you; a sturdy sofa has springs that work independently and you won't be jostled.
- Check for cushions and back pillows with zip-on covers. They make the sofa much easier and cheaper to clean.
- Make sure sofa buttons are recessed, or they may come off or be uncomfortable.
- Look for arm caps (especially on light-colored sofas), which protect against wear and dirt buildup on arms.
- Sofa beds look great but may be heavier and harder to move than others. Because of the metal construction underneath, sofa beds tend to feel firmer than ordinary sofas. Day beds are great for casual lounging, but are sometimes too deep for people with short legs to sit on comfortably.

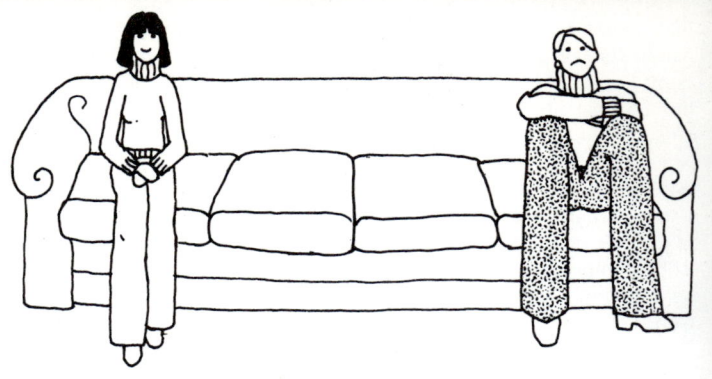

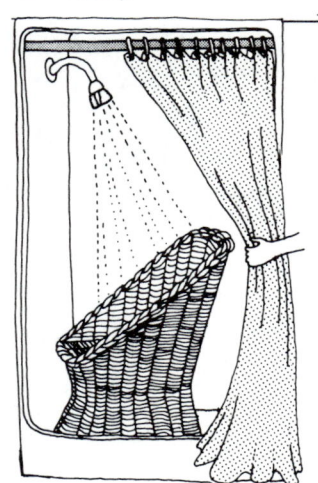

wicker why you should put wicker furniture in the shower—and other tips for its care and feeding

If you have wicker furniture that's in nonstop use, it needs to be wet down at least once or twice a year to stay supple. Wicker that hasn't been painted or varnished—and that has no wood or other trim—can simply be put in the shower or hosed down with a garden hose for about 15 to 20 seconds. Just allow it to dry out thoroughly—but not in the sun—before reusing it. Painted, varnished, or wood-trimmed wicker should be sponged down with water; use mild, soapy water if it needs cleaning. (If you have any questions about whether or not your wicker has been varnished, be sure to check with the store that sold it to you first.)

A can of spray paint or an "antique" finish can also brighten up a weary-looking wicker chair; or you might consider staining an unpainted wicker chair with a mahogany or pecan stain followed by a coat of varnish.

insurance

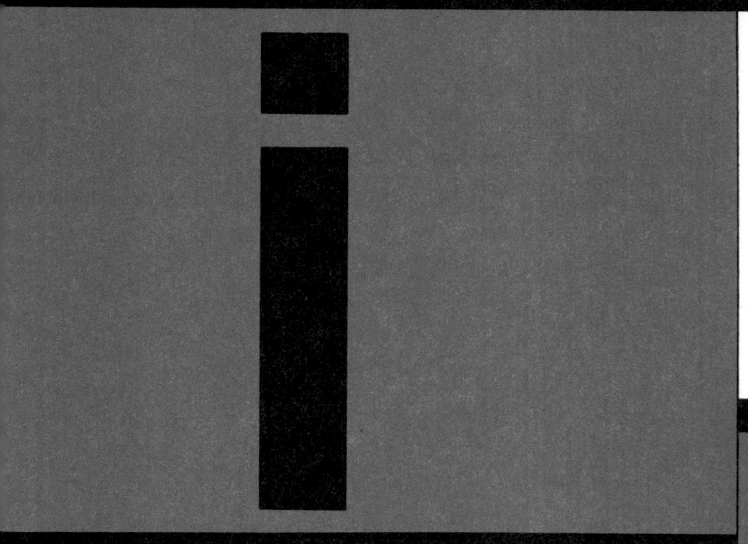

i

insomnia
insurance
italic writing

insomnia

how to beat insomnia before it leaves you beat

Most of us spend an occasional night tossing and turning in bed. The next time it happens, consider these causes and aids from Dr. Robert Van de Castle, director of the Sleep and Dream Laboratory of the Department of Psychiatry, University of Virginia.

- It's important to keep regular sleeping hours, getting to bed at roughly the same time each night. If you start shifting around your sleeping schedule too much, you disturb the natural rhythmic cycle of your body.
- However, don't be a slave to your schedule. One of the biggest obstructions to sleep is worrying about it. When you're not feeling particularly sleepy at night, get out of bed and read, crochet, or make your grocery-shopping list for tomorrow.
- Keep up a regular exercise routine to rid your body of tension that might impede sleep, but don't exercise strenuously right before bed. You're apt to be too stimulated to fall asleep quickly.
- Take a warm bath about a half hour before bed. It draws blood out to the periphery of the body, away from the brain, making you feel groggy. It also relaxes muscles.
- Fix yourself a glass of warm milk or Ovaltine before bed (cocoa isn't that helpful because it contains a small amount of caffeine), or perhaps something light to eat. The digestive process will also draw blood away from the brain.
- Try following a bedtime ritual—assume a certain sleeping position, punch your pillow a couple of times, listen to one side of a record album. Your body will come to associate the ritual with falling asleep.
- If the occasional night when you want to sleep but can't still occurs, it's probably because your brain is busy replaying all the day's ups and downs or working over a particular problem. Try this simple relaxing technique. Get comfortable in bed, lying stretched out on your stomach or back, whichever you prefer. Now tense up your whole body, hold a few seconds, and then relax. Repeat several times. Notice how heavy your body suddenly seems. Now concentrate on the toes of your right foot. If you concentrate hard enough you'll actually be able to feel your toes. Now the toes of your left foot, your feet, calves, thighs, buttocks, fingers, arms, chest, shoulders, right up to the features on your face. But you're likely to find yourself asleep even before you reach the tip of your nose.

insurance

newborn
a warning about family health insurance and your newborn

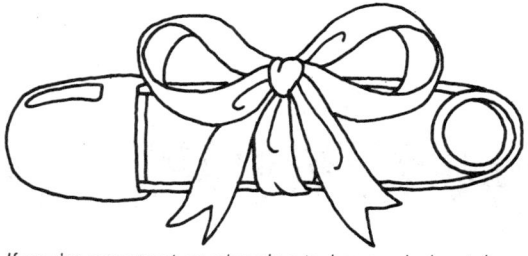

If you're pregnant or planning to have a baby, take a careful look at your family health-insurance policy. Many policies exclude newborns for 14 to 30 days after birth; some even refuse later coverage for problems that surfaced early.

For many parents, this has meant thousands of dollars of extra medical expense—often for complications due to prematurity (like hyaline-membrane disease) or early surgery to correct heart, kidney, or other birth defects.

The situation has improved, though. Some insurance companies voluntarily changed policy forms to include first-day coverage for newborns. During the past few years, 47 states, with the exception of New York, Rhode Island, and North Dakota, have passed laws requiring it. The hitch in states that have laws is that they apply to new policies; if yours was written before the law was enacted, your newborn may not be covered. Most insurance companies will add first-day coverage to your policy if you ask for it.

student how to insure your clothes, stereo, and just about anything you're taking to college

The fact that campus crime rates are soaring may not surprise you, but one way of protecting your valuables against theft probably will. Personal property insurance is available to students living on or off campus from National Student Services, Inc., whose coverage is underwritten by The American International Insurance Company. On-

insurance

campus and off-campus students can get $1,500 worth of insurance for about $25 a year ($25 deductible), or $20 a year ($50 deductible), or $15 a year ($100 deductible).

For both on- and off-campus students, rates are for an all-risk policy, which provides coverage for damages resulting from theft, fire, smoke, explosion, vandalism, riot, and other causes, according to NSSI. However, on a policy with a $25 deductible, for example, you pay the first $25 on any loss incurred, and wherever you live, you must report your loss to town or campus police within 24 hours after discovery. For more information, write to National Student Services, Inc. (Box 1240, Stillwater, OK 74074), which has provided more than 100,000 policies on 450 campuses in 48 states.

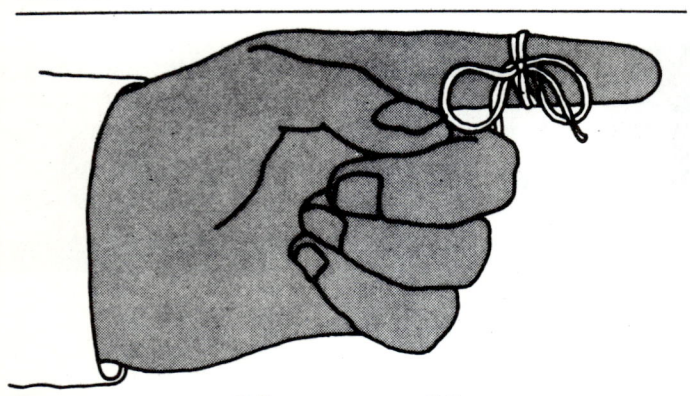

tenant's policy
what every woman should know

No matter how much money you don't have or what kind of building you live in, it's a good idea to have insurance on your personal belongings—your furniture, stereo, and clothes, for example. A "tenant's policy" can insure most things you own for loss or damage from such perils as theft, fire, collapse of any part of the building, certain types of accidental leakage, etc. Added benefits in most policies include coverage of up to $100 worth of cash whether it is destroyed in your home or stolen from you on the street, and $1,000 worth of off-premises insurance on your personal belongings.

To get an insurance agent, first ask your family or friends for the names of theirs. You can also try your employer or your company's personnel department for suggestions. Agents will advise you free of charge about coverage and rates. It is a good idea to consult several agents so that you can compare the policies and rates that different companies offer.

In most cities, insurance companies will not write a tenant's policy for less than $4,000, and in some places the minimum is higher; it may also vary from one company to another. To find if you need more coverage than the minimum, evaluate all your possessions on the basis of their replacement value; your agent will be able to help you. Insurance companies set maximum limits on the value of items in specific categories, such as $500 for all your jewelry and furs, and $500 for all art and antiques. If you live with one or more roommates, you may have difficulty getting a policy because of complications in writing up conditions and settling claims. You might also have difficulty if, for example, you live in a high-crime area or if your apartment is easily accessible through a fire escape. In that case, you might check into Federal Crime Insurance. Check with an insurance agent or write to the Safety Management Institute, Federal Crime Insurance, P.O. Box 41033, Washington, DC 20014. Or call them toll free at 800–638–8780 for more information.

Under a tenant's policy, there is usually at least a $50 deductible (often higher), which means that you must pay any loss less than $50. The cost of your policy is based on a number of things—amount of coverage and deductible, type of construction of your building, etc., and it also varies from city to city.

italic writing

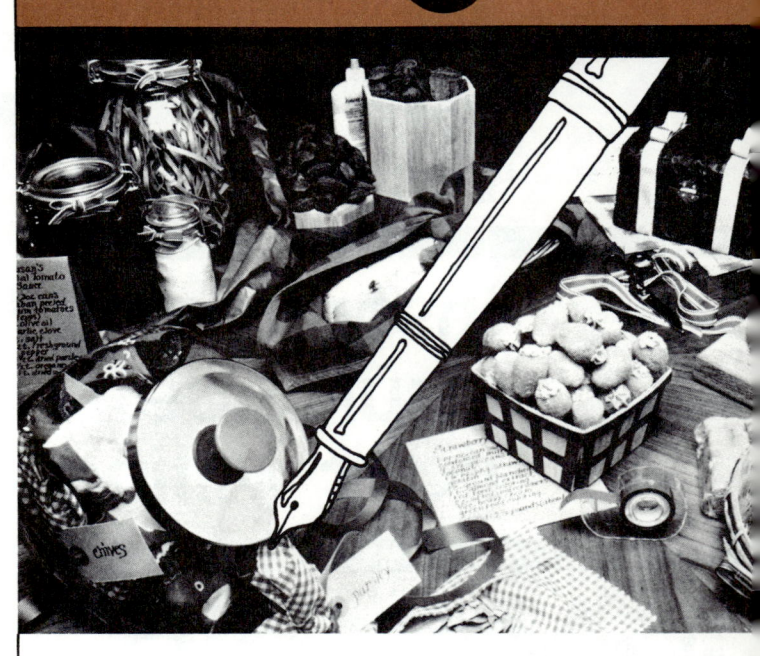

class up your cards and notes with italic writing

For a quick way to make even the plainest notes, cards, and gift tags special, think italics. With the right tools, italic lettering is easy to do. Keep in mind the following tips:

● For the best lettering, you'll need an italic nib (pen point with a square edge) and nib holder, or an italic pen set. Nib holders come in all lengths and widths (choose the size that fits your hand most comfortably). Buy a few different-size nibs to experiment with. A kit consisting of a holder plus around ten different nibs costs under $3 at art supply stores. An italic-pen kit is more expensive, about $7, but the pen is easier to use because it doesn't have to be dipped and it's designed for beginners. Most of these kits contain a fountain pen, several nibs, and an instruction booklet.

● If you buy a nib holder, look for one with a recess, called a "well," that will enable the nib to retain more ink at a time. If you buy an italic pen set, don't use waterproof India ink; it's too thick and will clog the pen. Use regular fountain-pen ink. Both types should be washed occasionally with lukewarm water.

● Once you have your tools, experiment a little. Hold the flat of the nib at a 45° angle to the paper, hold steadily, and letter.

● Allow enough spacing between letters—the size of a small letter o is a good guide.

● On rougher paper, use a blunter, wider point. A very delicate point gets stuck in the bumps.

● When using a nib and nib holder, wipe off surplus ink before you begin writing or you get spotty lettering.

● If you're left-handed, pass up the regular square-tipped italic nibs and choose an oblique one instead. It will be much easier to use.

● If the terms here leave you a bit dizzy, don't worry. An art supply store will know what you want and can give you even more tips.

jeans
jewelry

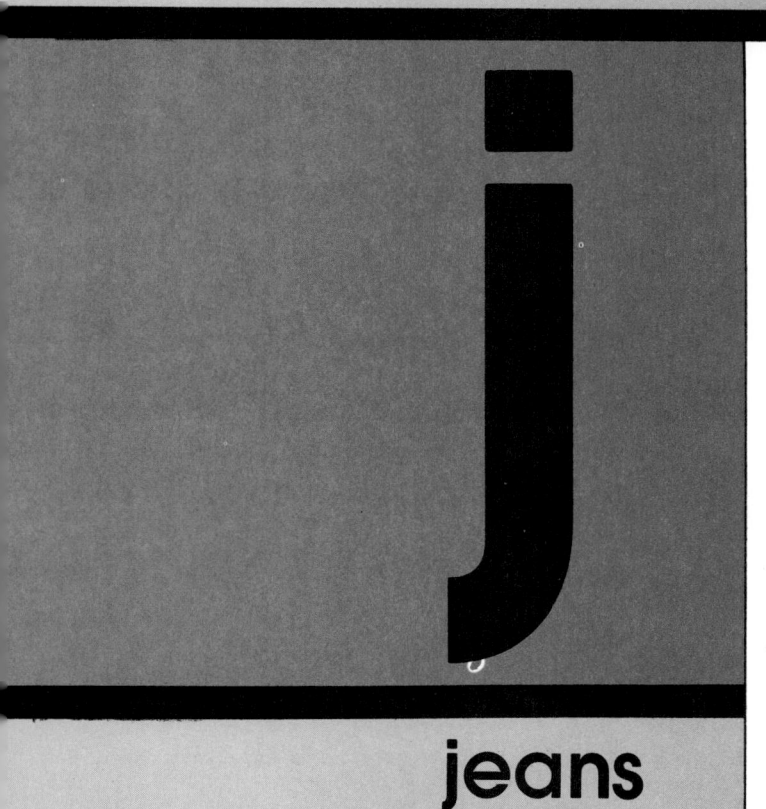

halter
make a halter from your old jeans

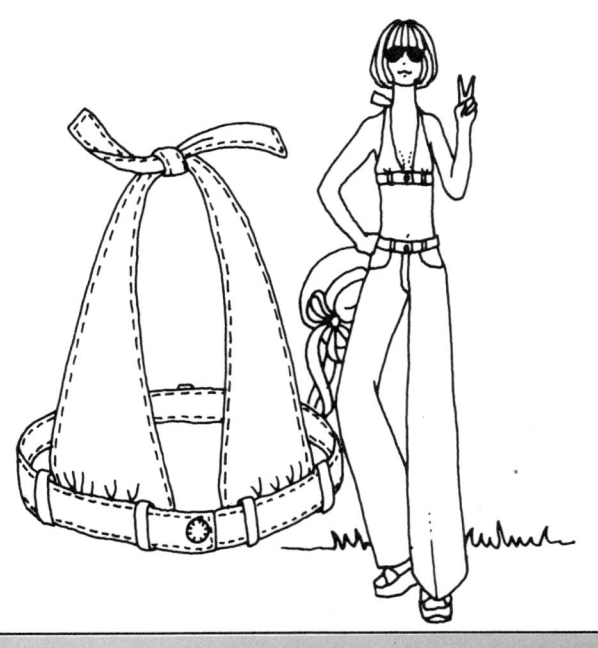

Don't throw out those old worn-out jeans! Instead, make a halter to wear in the summer.

Start by cutting off the waistband. If belt loops extend below band, either cut them off completely or tack the loose bottom and underneath waistband and leave on for the look. Next, cut two triangles of fabric from the jeans legs for the cups of the halter. The bottom edges should be from 8" to 10" wide, depending on how much fabric you can salvage. The triangles should be about 25" from tie ends to base. Turn under edges and topstitch two long sides. Then run a line of machine gathers through bottom edges and gather up to about 5" wide. Pin cups to inside top edge of waistband and try on to adjust fit. Use the original snap or button closing as a front closure for your halter. If waistband is too large for your rib cage, cut band open at center back and seam together to fit. Topstitch cups in place. Tie halter ends behind your neck when you wear it.

his how to shorten his jeans

The next time he needs a pair of jeans shortened (or some other casual pants), save him money by doing the job yourself. The trick is to make the back hang longer than the front. Follow these steps and you've got it made. You can do your pants the same way, too.

1. Have him put on the pants with the pair of shoes he plans to wear most often with them.
2. Fold under the front edge so that it just grazes the top of the shoe. Pin edge in place.
3. Fold the back edge under about ½" less than the front hem. Actual length depends on the width of the pants legs, individual preference, even the type of shoes. The back edge should be about ½" off the floor (or at the point where heel attaches to shoe).
4. Now have him take his pants off and pin up the sides, making sure both side seams are even. The hemline at the side seam should be exactly midway between front and back hem measurements. For example, if you've turned under the front hem 1" and the back hem ½", the width of the hem at the side seams should be ¾".
5. Check hemline pinnings to see that each hem is flat and neat all the way around.
6. If you have to take up more than 1½", cut off the extra fabric. A hem that's more than 1½" will be bulky, hard to work with, and will destroy the smooth line of the pants.
7. When sewing, split the fabric at the side seams to get a smoother hem.

knickers custom-tailor your jeans for this great look

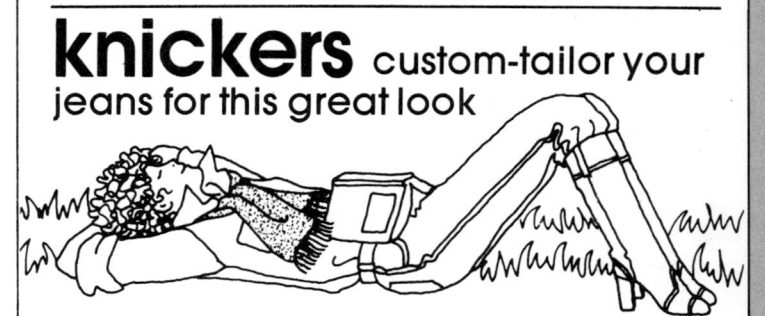

One of the niftiest fashion ideas around is the look of jeans tucked neatly into tall sleek boots. It's particularly great looking under smashing sweaters and tailored jackets. You can have the look without all that bulky fabric in your boots if you try this little trick. It's an especially good idea if you have a pair of jeans that are basically still good but are frayed or torn at the ankle.

Try on your jeans over boots. Have a friend measure your jeans 4" down from the top of your boots. Cut off jeans at this point. Sew a 1" hem by hand or machine in the bottom of jeans to form a casing for an elastic. Leave a small opening to insert a ¾" wide elastic of a length that will be snug but comfortable around your calf. Insert elastic into casing, stitch ends of elastic together, and close opening.

j jeans

tops
great summer jean tops

A fresh, casual look going in summer is the "Big Top"—a shirt, T-shirt, or smock top with big, luxurious proportions that, besides being great looking, are unbeatably cool. Look for anything that swings full at the hem, has deep, wide armholes and a soft, seductive way of sitting on the body. One of the easiest ways to give your favorite jeans a summer lift is to slip a Big Top over them. Here are five versions to show you the variations you can choose from:

1. The new version of a classic shirt—short-sleeved and cut with fuller, roomier proportions.
2. A soft Big Shirt top that looks terrific worn loose or belted, alone or over your favorite T-shirt.
3. The Big T-shirt, summer's snappiest look. This one has two nifty pockets and would look super popped over a bikini when it's not topping jeans.
4. Lace trim makes this the dressiest of the lot with a "period" mood about it. If the top isn't going the casual route, it could go over a long skirt for summer evening festivities.
5. The Big Top that has a "middy" feeling. Wear it over jeans or as a beach cover.

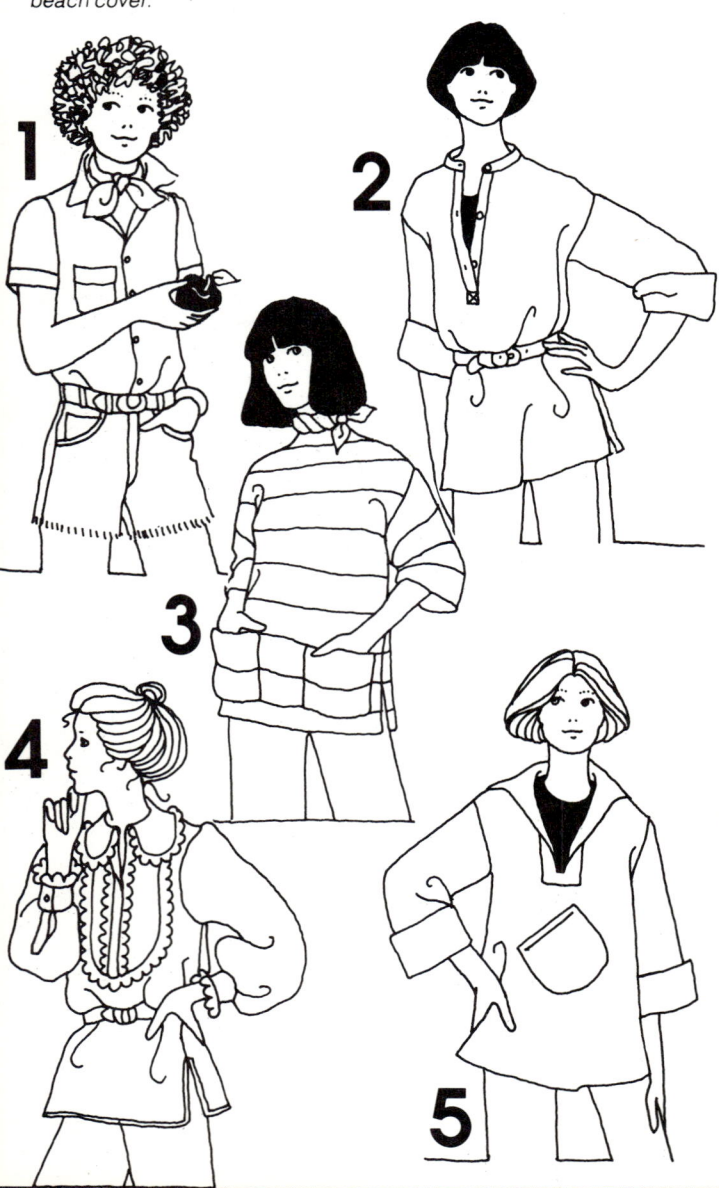

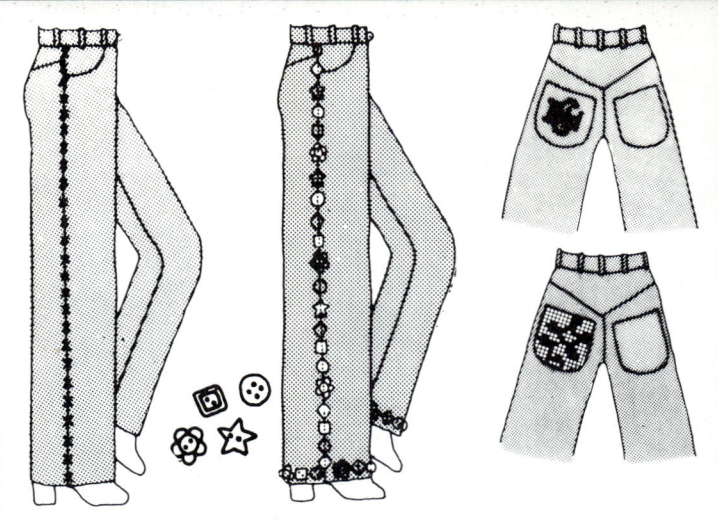

update
5 fresh looks for your jeans

Here are some snappy ways to liven up any pair of blue denims—old or new.

- *Cross-stitch* jeans with rainbow-colored embroidery thread. Sew along outside leg seam with even, 1/4" stitches.
- *Leather bind* pockets and bottom edges with 1" to 2" wide strips from a notions shop. Fold strip in half lengthwise and place over edge. Stitch or glue in place with rubber cement. (If you opt for rubber cement, always dry clean jeans.)
- *Monogram* a pocket. Many sewing machines have a monogram attachment that will do the job; otherwise, take the jeans to any place that does monogramming, such as the towel department of a large store or a notions shop that monograms. You can also buy monogram iron-on transfers from notions departments, and embroider over the transfers.
- *Needlepoint* a pocket. Buy a piece of needlepoint canvas and cut it 3/4" larger than your pocket. Trace a design on the canvas, work the needlepoint, then hand hem the canvas over the jeans pocket. If you can't make your own design, you can buy a small canvas with a design already on it. Once the pocket is in place, have jeans dry cleaned instead of washed to protect your work.
- *Button decorate* your jeans. The tiny plastic buttons shaped like dogs and cats, flowers, and so forth that many dime stores sell make great decorations. Sew them down the outside seam of the legs, around the pants hem, on pockets, wherever you like.

jewelry

beads
string your own—
it's easy!

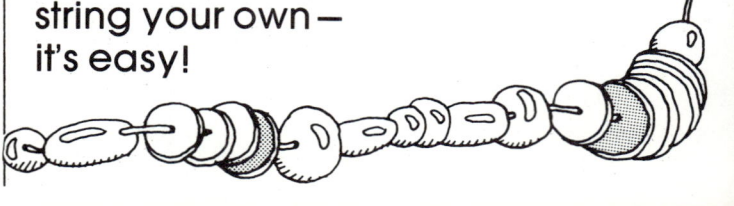

jewelry j

Some of the best-looking jewelry you own could be made by you. Glittery bead necklaces—with beads of different shapes, sizes, and colors—are fun and really a snap to make. Try stringing necklaces in beads that are tone-on-tone, too, for a nice, subtle effect. Here are some tips to start you out.

Most beads are best strung on *beading monofilament*, which is a clear nylon thread. Bead shops usually sell it in various weights, depending on what you're going to string on it. If in doubt, use the heaviest weight that will pass easily through the beads' holes. "Findings," or the little metal closings for your necklaces, are also sold at bead shops, usually in little packages holding several. Beads are not expensive so it can be fun to just stroll through the shop and buy whatever catches your eye plus some findings and monofilament. Then go home and put them together as you please.

Flat *African clam shells* that look like round buttons are very handsome mixed with pieces of *amber* or *carved ivory* beads. This kind of necklace looks terrific on spring and summer clothes. The clam shells are sold in long strings for about $10, but you can make many necklaces for a string by adding other beads.

To finish your necklace, tie a *knot* of monofilament around the loop of the closing and dot the knot with glue to be sure it holds.

If there's no bead shop near you, Sheru Beads, 49 West 38 St., New York, NY 10018, sells beads, findings, and beading monofilament by mail order. Send for their free price list.

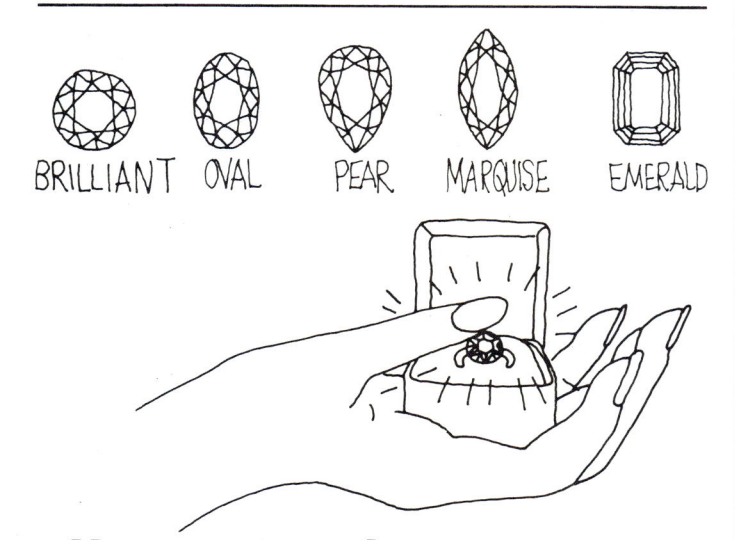

BRILLIANT OVAL PEAR MARQUISE EMERALD

diamonds
what you should know about a diamond before you buy one

Many people assume that size or carat alone determines the cost of a diamond, although its price tag actually reflects four factors: cut, clarity, color, and carat weight. Here are the important facts about diamonds.

● The most important factor is cut, since a poor cut will reduce the brilliance and value of even the finest stone. The best cuts have all of a diamond's facets angled exactly in their relationship to one another. When the "table" of the diamond, which is the flat top surface, is excessively large because the cutter did not cut it to its ideal proportions, the diamond has what's known as "spread." This is a kind of "padding" that makes a diamond look bigger but reduces its value and brilliance. However, an untrained eye usually can't detect this "spread," so it's best for you to talk with a trusted jeweler who won't want to endanger his reputation by giving evasive answers to your questions about it. A small, beautifully cut diamond is often a better value than many larger ones, and a good jeweler will point out these differences.

As long as a diamond is carefully cut, you can pick any shape you like; the sketches, below left, show the most common: brilliant, oval, pear, marquise, and emerald.

● Color will also influence the price of your diamond, because the closer a stone comes to being "colorless," the more expensive it is. The rarest and most costly are icy white, while others show a tinge of color under close inspection. You can test for color by looking at a diamond through its side against a white background, or with a jeweler's help.

● "Flawless" diamonds are rare and expensive—so don't panic if your jeweler uses the word "flaw." According to the Federal Trade Commission, a diamond can't be called "flawless" unless it keeps its clarity under ten-power magnification. Most stones will show tiny natural carbon spots or other imperfections if magnified highly enough.

● The weight of a diamond is measured in carats, with 100 points making one carat. Carat alone does not affect price, but the price tends to increase proportionately to the carat because large stones are much rarer than small ones. The typical engagement diamond is 1/2 to 2/3 of a carat. A general price range is: 1/4 carat, $160 to $250; 1/2 carat, $330 to $830; 1 carat, $1,150 to $3,900.

● Remember to have your jeweler check your diamond's setting every six months for loose prongs that may need tightening.

● Clean your diamond occasionally to remove dirt that dims the brilliance. A mild detergent solution and eyebrow brush work well.

family jewels
turn inherited uglies into jewelry you'd really like to wear

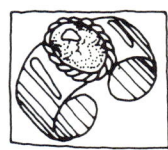

If some inherited "family jewels" are collecting dust in your drawer, pull them out, brush them off, and have them changed from dust catchers into eye catchers—something you'd really like to wear. Here are some ideas on how to have the job done.

Don't go to an ordinary jeweler unless you've got a very easy job—like lifting an old diamond out of a ring and putting it into another catalog-chosen setting. If you really want something *remade*, go to a goldsmith, someone who designs and makes jewelry. (Find one in the Yellow Pages.) The goldsmith can take a beautiful old brooch (if you don't wear brooches) and work it into a big silver bracelet or pendant.

First, ask the goldsmith to appraise the piece of jewelry you want remade to be sure it's worth the investment. Unless it has great sentimental value, setting glass in gold is not worth it.

Show whoever is redesigning for you some of your favorite jewelry pieces. Tell him or her a little about your clothes style. Point out things in the shop that you like and would feel comfortable wearing.

Make it clear from the start how much you want to spend—anywhere from $25 and up (way up when you're working with silver and especially gold). Consider bronze and copper if you're trying to keep costs down.

Ask to see a precise drawing of the piece you will be paying for, and initial it only with the projected cost attached. Be skeptical of a fast and foggy artist's rendering done while you're describing; often what the goldsmith envisions and what you see are two quite different things.

Finally, just to start you thinking: A carved-ivory pin could be made into a hair barrette; the stones from an antique wedding ring could be redesigned into double rings; tiny rubies and sapphires from an old fraternity pin could be remade into two pairs of earrings.

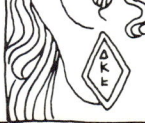

j
jewelry

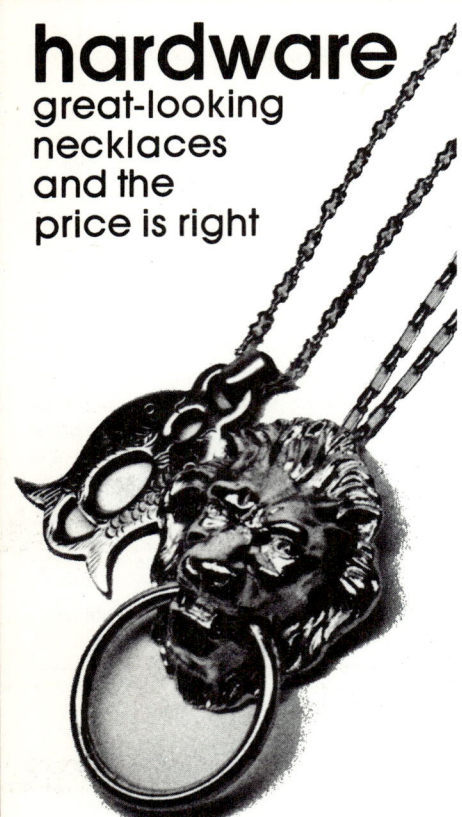

hardware
great-looking necklaces and the price is right

If necessity is really the mother of invention, the price of many beautiful pendant necklaces may send you to the hardware store to do a little inventing of your own. The handsome lion and fish pendants are actually brass drawer pulls hung on a chain. They make spectacular necklaces, fobs for a belt, or even a buckle. The two here cost only a few dollars and they're solid brass. Scout in any good hardware store for drawer pulls or other hardware in the shape of lion heads, fish, maybe zodiac signs, or just a big chunky brass bolt or screw.

The findings may have screw backs, a knob on top with a tunnel for a screw, or whatever. In most cases, you can tell just by looking at the item how to suspend it on a chain. This lion head has a screw tunnel on the back. We used a short, large-head screw and pushed it through the link of a chain, then screwed the screw and link tightly into the screw tunnel to hold the chain in place. A bit of fine brass picture wire will help your pendant hang straight. The fish had a knob on top with a screw tunnel. We simply filed it off, and the remaining loop gives it a nice finished look and is perfect for running a chain through. Ask the hardware store if they'll file off what you want or put in a hole. If not, you can usually do the job easily with a metal file from the tool chest. An ice pick used with care on thin pieces can make a hole large enough for a chain loop.

originals
you don't have to be rich to own originals

Is original jewelry something you have always wanted but never thought you could afford? Well, with a bit of imagination, some help from your local jeweler, and just a few dollars, you can start your own collection.

● *Necklaces*—Often the more simple a piece of jewelry is, the more "expensive" and real it looks. For an elegant but inexpensive necklace, take a plain gold or silver chain (available at a jeweler's for about $10 to $25) and hang from it a delicate trinket that you've found at a flea market or antique shop—for instance, an old lavaliere (about $35) can be worn tight around your neck on a choker-size chain, rather than a long one, for a more contemporary look; a little heart made of gold, silver, or a semiprecious stone (you can have a whole collection of hearts that you alternately wear on the same chain); gold coins from faraway countries (jewelers often carry standard "frames" in which to insert coins so they can be attached to chains). One really clever idea is to hunt around antique shops for the clasps from old necklaces—some are pretty-colored balls, others are paste diamonds, rhinestones, or plain gold (available for $10 to $15)—and wear the clasp on a chain.

If an item you find doesn't have a loop for stringing the chain through, your jeweler can solder one on.

● *Rings*—Find an interesting "stone"—perhaps a classic-looking earring that lost its mate years ago or a little animal head from an old-fashioned stickpin (from $25 to $35). Now shop around for a secondhand wedding band that's your size or a baby's ring ($10 to $15) that will fit on your pinky, and have your jeweler solder the two together (it will probably cost a minimum of $5).

● *Earrings*—You can put together your own original "antique" earrings by having your jeweler solder marvelous old buttons—made of rhinestone or cut glass—to standard earring posts or backs (you'll find many old buttons at secondhand stores or flea markets). You can also have a button or mateless earring soldered to a pin.

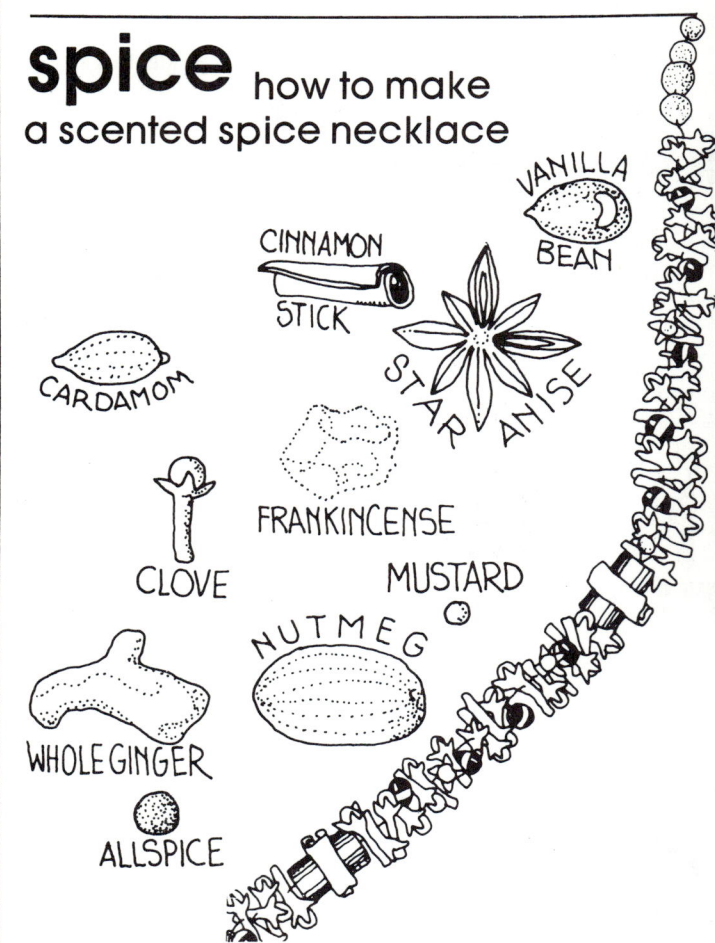

spice
how to make a scented spice necklace

Certain whole spices have such great shapes and colors that they look like beads and, once they're strung together, make very pretty necklaces. Your body heat will bring out the fragrance of the spices.

Decide what spices you want. Cloves, allspice, nutmeg, cinnamon sticks, cardamom, star anise (available at gourmet or Oriental grocery shops), frankincense, ginger, and vanilla beans are all great. Buy the standard-size boxes or jars and use extras for cooking. Soak the spices in water to make them more pliable. Then, thread monofilament thread (or fishing line) on a small needle. Heat the needle and pierce each spice one by one and string together. (For the harder spices, like nutmeg, star anise, frankincense, and ginger, you may have to heat the needle a few times.) For color, you might want to intersperse the spices with a bead or two. End by knotting the monofilament around a brass jewelry clasp (available at hobby shops and some dime stores). If you have a difficult time finding certain whole spices, you can order them from Country Gardens, 777 East Main Street, Branford, CT 06405. One-ounce packets of smaller spices (frankincense tears, allspice, cloves), cinnamon sticks, nutmeg, vanilla beans, and whole ginger are all moderately priced.

knives

it get taut again. "The idea is to keep enough tension on the line so that it doesn't tangle and you keep control of the kite," says Mr. Yolen.
- If the air seems too calm to get a rise out of anything, you might still coax your kite up by having a friend hold your kite vertically while you hold the flying line about 100 feet away. Your friend then tosses the kite up in the first breeze and you run with the kite against the breeze. Again, boost it by pumping.
- Once your kite is flying high—away from changeable ground winds—it's likely to catch a steady air current and soar. If it starts to dive, start pumping again. But don't run with any kite when its line is taut; you'll worsen the dive and may break the line.
- Keep these safety rules in mind. Don't kite near streets and highways; you might cause an auto accident. And definitely not near power lines or when the sky is filled with storm clouds; you might electrocute yourself. Wear gloves when it's very windy to protect your hands from being cut or bruised by the flying line. And don't fly a kite in extra-strong, tree-swaying winds (over 18 mph) or you'll lose control and the string may break.

kites knives

kites

how to get a kite up

"When you fly a kite, it's like having a living thing in your hand that keeps you in touch with the infinite," says Will Yolen, who claims a world's record for flying the largest number of kites—178—from a single line.

Basically, "all kites respond to the breeze in the same way and the technique for getting them into the air is the same," says Mr. Yolen. Here's how to fly a kite:
- Stand with your back to the wind and toss up the kite. Then boost it higher by pumping rapidly in short takes on the flying line—releasing a bit of line, then letting it get taut, then giving off more line, then letting

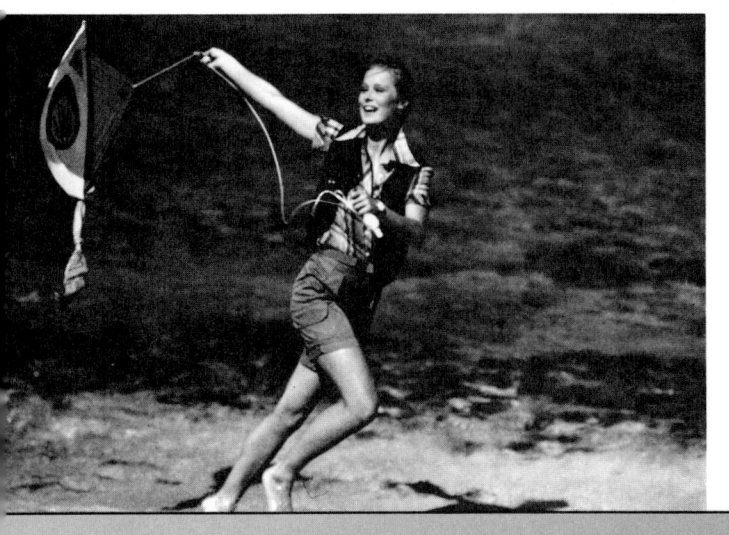

yes, you can sharpen your own knives

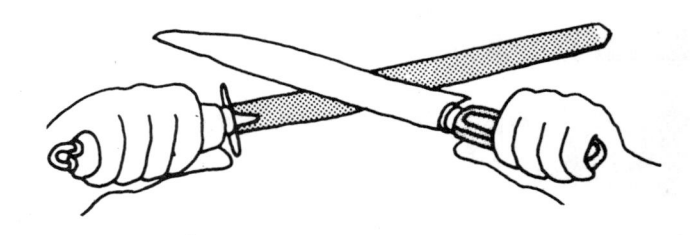

Sharpening knives—like carving roasts—is a job most women leave to men. But sharpening any knife is so simple, why not do it yourself? Just follow these easy dos and don'ts, suggested by Albert H. Stone, vice president of Hoffritz, the world's largest cutlery retailer.
- DO use a "sharpening steel" or a sharpening stone (i.e., a "hone") to tone up a dull edge. A steel is a rod-shaped file with handle and fingerguard (see sketch). One way to use it, if you're right-handed, is to hold knife in left hand (edge up) and steel in right at about a 20° angle to blade. Move the steel in one motion from base of blade to tip, first on one side, then the other until blade is sharp. Filings stick to the steel's magnetic tip where you wipe them off. With a sharpening stone, the same angle position and motion apply. Stones are coarse (for dull blades) or fine (for final sharpening). Rub stones with motor oil before use—so filings don't clog pores and ruin abrasiveness—then wipe clean.
- DON'T use electric sharpeners or gadgets that file off too much knife steel.
- DO sharpen serrated knives, but less often than smooth-edged ones. They're serrated only on one side, so always run the stone or steel over the flat side.
- DO have knives sharpened professionally about once every three years to smooth out the slight irregularities.
- DO cut on wood or plexiglass boards (harder surfaces dull blades). Store knives in their case or on special wall racks; you'll dull them by throwing together with other utensils in a drawer.

landlord/tenant

landlord/tenant
legal matters
lighting
living problems

landlord/tenant

leases
you've got to do more than read a lease before you sign it

The lease you sign is usually a standard form that doesn't necessarily contain all the provisions you and your new landlord have worked out verbally. In order to legally substantiate any agreements you've made, you must write them into the lease yourself—in the blank space above the signature line or on a separate sheet of paper to be attached—before you and the landlord sign your names.

According to Barbara Chocky of the New York State Tenants Coalition, it might be necessary for you to add clauses regarding such things as:

● Any equipment not presently in the apartment but which the landlord has promised to supply—for example, an air conditioner, a new refrigerator (the clause should read "The landlord agrees to provide immediately...").

● Services that the landlord claims are included with the rent, such as heat and/or utilities.

● Repairs or decorating changes that the landlord has promised to make—e.g., a new paint job, wall plastering.

● Major decorating changes that you plan to make with the landlord's permission, such as sanding and staining the floors, or any major structural changes, such as tearing down cabinets, exposing a brick wall.

● Use of certain facilities on the premises—garage, pool, tennis courts, recreation center—that the landlord has stated are available to you free.

● Your right to have a pet.

● Your right to have a roommate. If you're planning to live alone and sign the lease alone, you might wish to reserve the option of having a roommate—male or female—sometime.

There are also clauses in a standard lease that you may wish to ask the landlord to delete—for instance, one that gives the landlord the right to enter your apartment when you're not there other than in an emergency. Remember that no matter what's in the lease you sign, no one can throw you out on the street without first taking the case to court—where you have a chance to defend yourself.

rip-offs 4 ways landlords rip off young women

Not all landlords want or try to rip off their tenants, but those who do usually have no riper victims than young women who are so desperate to find an apartment that they will sign almost anything in order to get one. To avoid being had, know these rip-offs and what you can do about them.

● **failure to provide services you're entitled to**

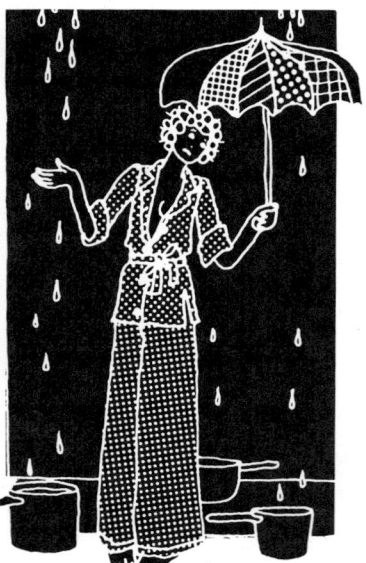

When your landlord won't fix a broken window, hire an exterminator, or paint your apartment, call your city housing authority to find out what local laws *require* him to do. That office, or its literature, can answer such specific questions as "How often is he required to paint?" Then, simply reminding him of his obligations may prod a landlord into action. If not, starting, or threatening to start, legal action should.

It's also a good idea to take photographs of damaged fixtures and in a furnished apartment, furniture, before you move in; be sure to obtain a dated receipt from whoever develops the film. These pictures may be helpful if a landlord tries to avoid fixing damages on the grounds that he didn't know about them—or worse, that *you* did the damage.

● **unfair or deceptive leases – and what you can do about them**

Your only sure protection against these is having a lawyer read yours before you sign it. If you don't, you'll provide *partial* protection by at least reading it yourself and paying special attention to any *riders* or *waivers* attached to the main body of the lease. Riders sometimes carry unexpected restrictions, such as bans on pet canaries or watching TV after 11 P.M. Waivers are clauses under which you relinquish a right legally due you. Since such provisions are often expressed in confusing "legalese," ask questions about any that seem unclear. If

legal matters

your landlord dismisses your question with "Oh, don't worry about that," take your lease to a lawyer. For information on what to watch out for in a lease, check *The Tenant Survival Book*, written by tenant lawyer Emily Jane Goodman.

● **refusal to return your security deposit**
If a landlord refuses to return all or part of the money you've given him for "security" (collateral) and you haven't damaged the apartment in any way, a letter from a lawyer may speed its return. You can also sue for its return in Small Claims Court.

● **harassment**
To a lawyer, "harassment" is any landlord action taken with the specific aim of forcing you to move out. It often includes such ploys as a refusal to provide heat or hot water for more than one tenant—and maybe even less obvious tactics, such as "renting nearby apartments to junkies" or "encouraging other tenants to play loud music at night or walk with heavy boots on," according to one rent official. When you suspect harassment, you'll get the best results by getting together with other tenants and protesting as a group, because landlords rarely single out only one person for such treatment.

legal matters

documents
how long to keep checks, tax returns, leases, and other records

Knowing how long and which financial and legal documents and records to keep, and which ones to throw away, can save you time, space, and possibly some costly headaches. Who hasn't lost or thrown away the very deposit slip the bank mixed up, or the canceled check you needed for your income-tax audit?

● *Permanently* keep your birth and baptismal certificates, naturalization papers, Social Security card, wills, diplomas, deeds, leases, mortgage papers, bills of sale for major purchases, marriage license, separation and divorce papers, all insurance policies (health, life, fire, etc.), record of securities, guarantees, employment records (so that you know exactly when you started and left each job you held), and a complete personal property inventory, including the serial numbers you find on your appliances (needed mainly in case of fire, robbery, etc.).

● *For six years* keep all records that pertain to income taxes, including *all* checks, bank statements, records of business expenses and charitable contributions, and duplicate copies of your income-tax returns.

● *For one year* keep receipts and duplicate deposit slips for your checking or savings account. If you pay for major purchases by check, the check is, of course, your receipt. But in many cases, having the actual store receipt for a purchase can be a big help when you'd like some kind of adjustment made, especially when it contains an order number, delivery date, or other similar information.

● *For at least sixty days* keep sales slips of small items; keep sales slips of valuable purchases longer.

divorce
what a good divorce lawyer should be like, and how to find one

It's not easy to find a good divorce lawyer. According to at least one young female divorce lawyer in Los Angeles, a lawyer may have all the right credentials, know all the legal tricks, but have no real sympathy or interest in *your* particular case. When a woman needs a divorce lawyer, she needs someone who sees her as a person rather than a business.

It's best to tap as many sources as you can for recommendations. You're looking for a mixture of specialties—a good negotiator, litigator, tax expert, and marital counselor—wrapped up in one paragon of a lawyer. Ask your friends, business associates, marriage counselor, psychiatrist, if you have one, or maybe your family doctor or minister for anyone they know who has skillfully and sensitively handled divorce actions.

You may find it takes time and some shopping around to locate a lawyer who suits you. While you can lose the price of a couple of consultation fees if recommended lawyers don't suit you (charges range from no fee at all to $100 an hour for the first consultation), you'll not only gain perspective about divorce attitudes, but feel surer when your reactions to a lawyer are positive.

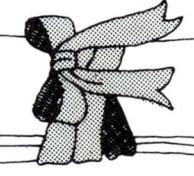

lawyer
need a lawyer who can give you simple legal advice?

If you need a lawyer, just call your local, county, or state bar association—sometimes listed in the phone book under "Bar Association"—and ask for its Legal Referral Service. A staff attorney for the LRS will talk to you briefly about your problem and put you in touch with someone who can help—a lawyer who has a general practice, or in some cases, a specialist such as a tenant lawyer. The fee for an initial half-hour consultation with the LRS lawyer usually ranges from $5 to $15, and you probably won't need more than that if you only want a minor service. However, if you do, the lawyer will probably take you on as a client. But don't bank on getting free *legal help that is available to some people under local legal aid or legal service programs. To qualify for either, you usually must have a poverty-level income—approximately $4,500 a year or less. While requirements may be flexible, it's highly unlikely that you'd be eligible unless you are, say, an impoverished college student who can prove that she has* no *financial support whatsoever.*

legal matters

small claims
how to sue in the people's court

People usually think that they have no recourse in situations where they feel taken except to hire a lawyer. And then either they don't think it's worth the money, or they haven't got the money. They've heard of the small-claims court but they don't investigate it or they think it's not for them. Don't think this way. Most states have a small-claims court that provides a simple, fast, and almost free way to reclaim at least part of your losses.

To start proceedings, it's best to go to the small-claims clerk's office (for address, look in the telephone book under small-claims court, city courts, or call your local bar association). You will be told if your case falls under the jurisdiction of the small-claims court. If it does, you must limit your claim to the maximum set by each state; amounts vary from about $150 to $3,000. If you are not old enough to vote in your state, you must take along a parent or legal guardian. You then file a claim, naming the person you are suing and the reason, and pay a small filing fee (usually under $5). The clerk will set a trial date, usually within two or three weeks (it may be at night), and notify the defendant. If necessary, you can get a subpoena to compel a witness to attend.

The hearing will be held before a judge or a lawyer acting as arbitrator; there is usually no jury. You will state your side of the story, and the person you're suing states his. Remember to bring any proof (bills or receipts) or any witnesses with you. If the defendant fails to show up, the judge may say you've won or ask you to tell your version—either way, you will know his decision within about 24 hours. If you've won, the court will order the defendant to pay you immediately; if he fails to, you will be advised as to the next step.

under arrest
what to do if you're arrested

It's unlikely that you'll ever see the inside of a jail cell, but mistakes do happen, points out Barbara Bigham, a former police officer turned writer from Phoenix, Arizona. Whether you make the mistake or the police do, here are a few dos and don'ts from Ms. Bigham that will help you through the ordeal.

- DON'T physically resist. Protest your innocence loud and clear, but keep it verbal. Police have the right, once you're under arrest, to search, fingerprint, and photograph you; physically resisting won't help.
- DO call a friend or member of your family. You'll be allowed to make at least one call, but it may be your only one so make it good. Don't try contacting a lawyer or bail bondsman yourself. A friend can make as many calls as are needed.
- DON'T make incriminating statements to police without legal advice. You may be led to believe it will help your case, but always wait for an attorney to advise you before making or signing confessions or other incriminating statements.
- DON'T take cigarettes into the cell with you. Other prisoners may have been without cigarettes for a long time and fights frequently break out over them.
- DO cooperate with police and jail personnel. It's not their fault you're in jail, but they are human and can make your stay very unpleasant if you antagonize them. They can likewise be helpful (extra phone calls, medication, information) if they choose.
- DON'T panic once the iron doors are shut. Local jails are usually not filled with hardened "criminal" types. There may be those, however, who are high on drugs or drink, or perhaps scared enough to be belligerent, so don't try to be overly friendly.
- DO give complete background information on your school, job, and family to arresting personnel since such information may be used to check your eligibility for release (on your own recognizance rather than cash bail). Such information is not related to the crime itself, but to your identity or reliability. You may hesitate to give this information for fear that others may find out about your arrest, but withholding information from the police won't ensure secrecy. Right now, your main goal is to get out quickly. If rumors start circulating around your school or office, you're in a much better position to stop them if you're back at your desk rather than sitting in a jail cell.
- DO return to court when assigned. Whether you're released or on bail, be sure to appear in court when scheduled or you may find yourself behind bars again.
- DO consult an attorney as soon as possible. The charges may seem trivial now, but they can affect you throughout your life. You need professional advice, and it will be money well spent if it helps keep your record clear.

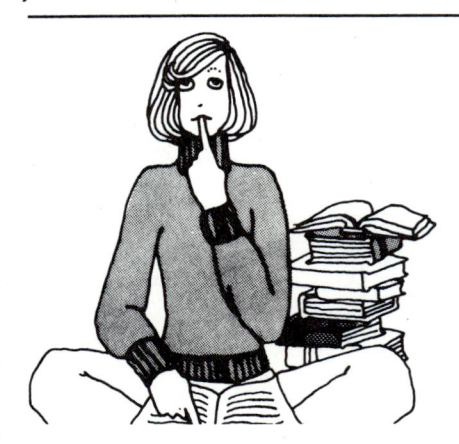

wills
facts any young woman should know about a will and why you need one

Drawing up a will usually isn't the complicated or tricky business you might expect it to be. Here are some facts you should know about a will:

- **who can draw one up?**
Anyone who meets his or her state's requirements for executing one. (In most places you need to be 21; in some 18.)
- **do you need a lawyer to make a will?**
No—the law recognizes any piece of paper that you have clearly labeled "will" and signed in the presence of two witnesses (who should not be beneficiaries of your will), provided you have complied with the statutory requirements of your state. However, the chances are slight that you would know these without a lawyer who can advise you also on such important matters as where to keep your will and who to tell about it. (A lawyer usually charges about $50 for a simple will.)
- **should a single woman have a will?**
Yes—if you own even a few possessions you consider "valuable." If you do not have a will, your property would go to your parents or next of kin. A will lets you leave things to your brother, sister, other relative, or friend—instead of relying on your parents' judgment as to who should get what. These distinctions can be especially important when, for example, your parents disapprove of your "liberated" lifestyle or haven't spoken to you since you joined a commune. Another advantage is that a will lets you name the executor of your "estate"—the person who would supervise the distribution of the assets of your estate in accordance with your will.
- **should a married woman have a will apart from her husband's?**
Yes—for similar reasons. You might prefer to set certain funds or possessions aside for your children or parents rather than letting your husband control their distribution.

lighting

fixtures 6 tricks to brighten up ugly overhead fixtures

1. Hang a paper parasol from your light fixture. Cut handle to desired length (keeping it long enough to allow room for ventilation). Drill hole in bottom of handle and put an "S" hook through it. Attach to fixture.
2. If your light has a glass fixture attached with a nut and screw through the center, substitute a basket for the glass by cutting a small hole in the basket's center. Screw on as before. Baskets dim light, so look for an open weave and use them where you don't need bright light. Or for more light, remove fixture, leaving overhead socket. Cut a small hole through bottom center of straw basket. Place base of a large globe light through hole and screw into socket. (Note: With any basket lamp, make sure bulb isn't too close to the straw; keep wattage at 60 or below.)
3. Try several small bulbs screwed into three-way sockets for a new look. Make a hanging arrangement by pushing two three-way sockets together, one on top of the other. Then attach three more three-way sockets to the open sides of the bottom socket (see sketch). Attach bulbs with socket plugs to all the remaining openings. Or make the flat arrangement with two sets of two three-way sockets. Attach bulbs with socket plugs to each set and join the two sets with a double lamp socket.
4. Suspend horizontally a large, bright paper kite from your overhead fixture with fishing line. Keep kite far enough from the bulb so it doesn't burn.
5. For a Mexican "tin can" light, take a can with a diameter that fits over your ceiling fixture and remove top and bottom lids. Punch holes through tin with can opener or awl in an attractive pattern. Punch three holes in top edge, string fishing line through and attach to ceiling with pushpins. (For maximum light, use a bulb almost as long as the can.)
6. Metal industrial reflector shades, available at hardware and electrical supply stores, are handsome and very inexpensive. They come in white enamel, plain metal, and sometimes color. To hang, buy a bulb and a long length of round wiring, attach to shade, and suspend from ceiling.

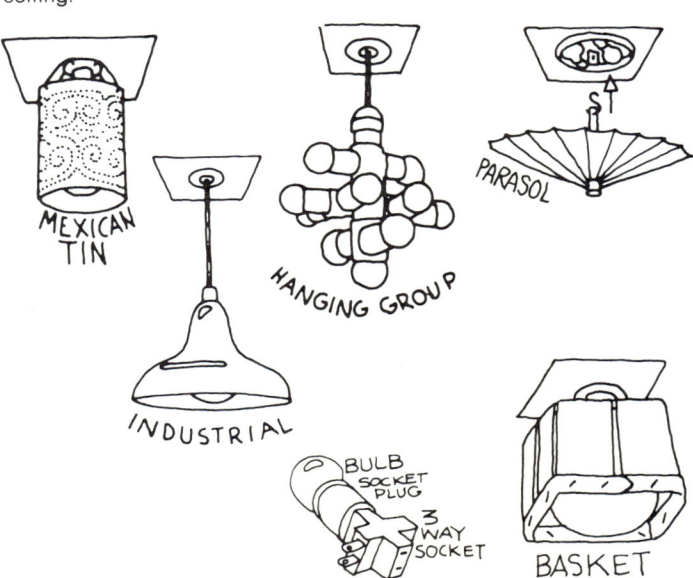

globe how to make a globe lamp for under $10

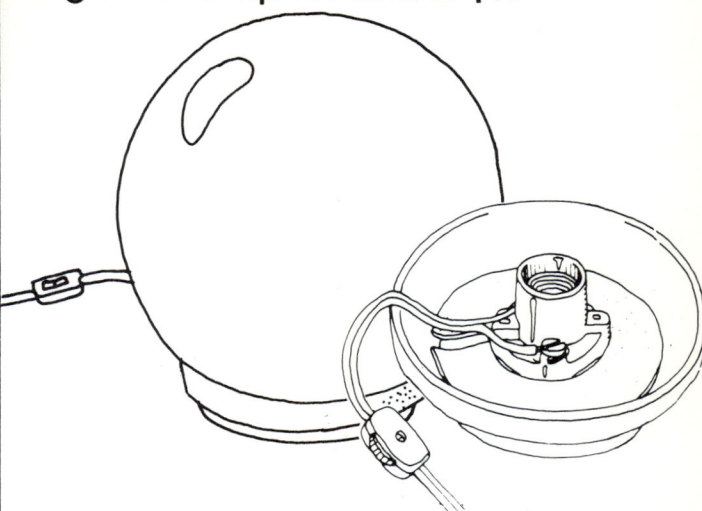

If you've been looking high and low for a good-looking, inexpensive lamp and have come up with absolutely nothing, why not make one? The globe light shown here is a cinch to make. You'll need: a glass globe (any size you want), a terra-cotta plant pot saucer to fit the base of the globe, some paint, a porcelain cleat socket, electrical cord with plug, a feed-through cord switch, a light bulb (we used 25 watts), a square foot of felt, and white glue. (Parts are available at dime stores and most hardware or electrical supply stores.) Paint the saucer any color you want, and glue some felt to the underside to prevent scratching. Glue the socket to the center of the saucer. Attach cord switch to the cord, following package directions. Split the end of cord in half with a razor and cut away about ½" of cord wrapping so that the wires are exposed. Twist half the wire around each screw of the socket. Cut felt to fit in saucer and around socket, leaving a slit for the cord to lay flat in. The felt should be as thick as the cord, so you may need a few layers. This helps the globe set firmly. Place globe over light bulb, resting firmly in saucer.

lampshade
cover a lampshade with fabric

You can give any room a quick change-of-season look by re-covering a lampshade with bright new fabric—maybe the same print used for your curtains or bedspread. Here are some cover-up tips:

● Choose an unpleated lampshade in a basic cylinder or cone shape with a plain covering; ours was solid white. A pattern might show through your new covering when the lamp is lit.

● Cotton, linen, burlap, or another not-too-sheer fabric all make fine coverups. Since you'll have a seam in back, avoid stripes or other patterns that don't match up well. Press any fabric perfectly smooth before using it.

● To cover the shade, first spray it with a mild spray adhesive. Wrap fabric around shade, smoothing out any wrinkles. Then cut off excess fabric from top and bottom. Finally, make a neat seam where the fabric overlaps in back by turning under and glueing down the bottom piece of material, then turning under and glueing down the top piece with white glue.

● Cover the raw edges of fabric by working contrasting colored plastic tape around the top and bottom rims of the shade, turning half the tape's width over to adhere to the inside of the shade. We used blue tape to set off bright yellow fabric. (See photograph on p. 108.)

lighting

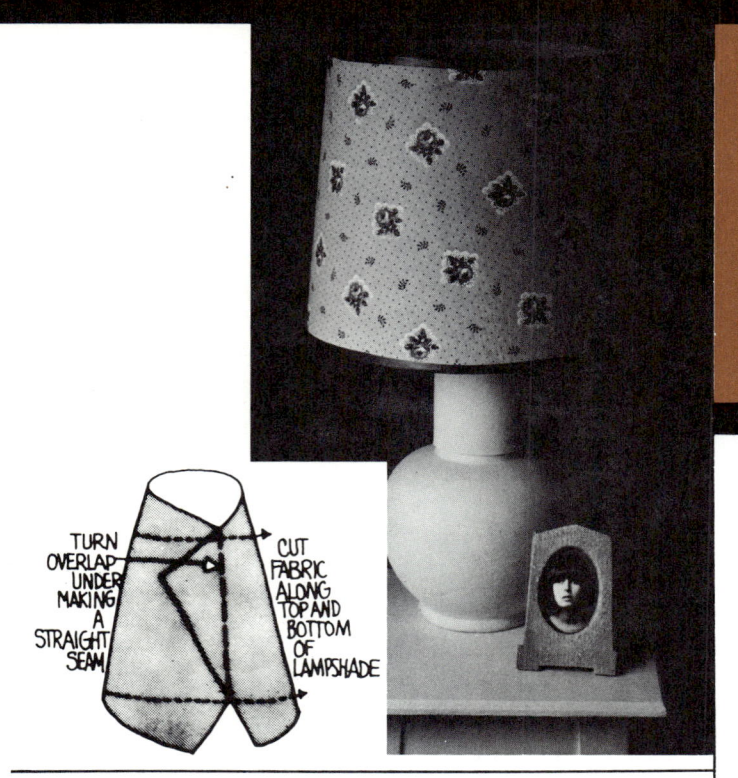

string make a ball of string transform an old lamp

Redoing a lamp with a ball of string may sound preposterous, but it works with results that are sensational. You can do either the entire lamp or only the shade. All you need is some white glue, spray adhesive if you're wrapping the base, and some string—bakery string, two-toned cord, hemp, twine, wrapping cord, even yarn. It depends on the look you want.

- *The shade*—Use an old shade or buy a plain, cheap new one at the dime store. Spread some glue over the top and bottom edges (this will help keep the string in place as you wrap). To start, place the string about halfway down the inside of the lampshade and glue in place. Then wrap vertically all around, covering the entire shade. If you want to vary colors and textures, just tie the new string to the last pieces of the old on the inside of the shade and continue wrapping. To finish, knot the end of the last piece to the previous wrap.
- *The base*—Wrapping the base is a little trickier, and you'll need a fairly simple shape—a perfect cylinder, ginger-jar, or squared-off shape works best. Spray with adhesive before you begin and wrap horizontally from top to bottom. If you want to switch colors, knot strings neatly. Plan the knots so they form part of the design—lots of knots placed randomly throughout give a wonderful nubby look. If your lamp has a flat platform-type base at the very bottom, leave it unwrapped for contrast, or cut pieces of string to fit over it vertically and glue in place.

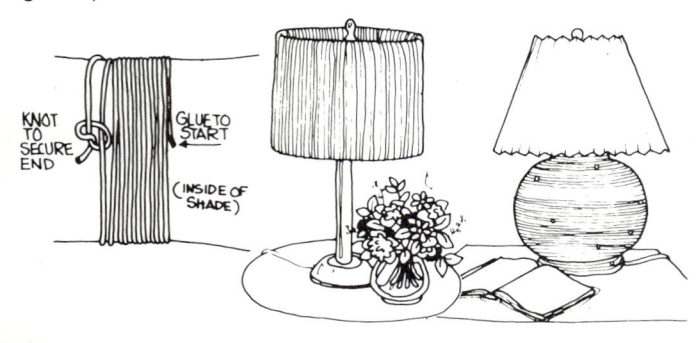

living problems

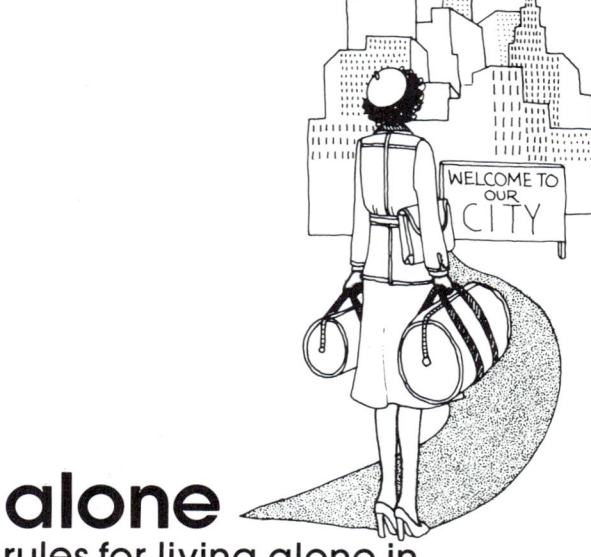

alone rules for living alone in big cities without getting mugged

Your mother probably told you nice girls don't get into trouble, that any girl who did had probably invited it. Well, she was wrong. Nice girls are too often robbed and mugged these days through no fault of their own. But there is a grain of truth in what mother says: There are accident-prone people who find accidents, and people who go around behaving like victims who find predators.

- **common-sense rules**

These are the usual common-sense rules for not inviting trouble: Don't open your door to strangers; install good locks on your doors and windows; don't walk alone late at night in deserted parts of the city. But beyond these rules, there is the shadowy area of human relations. In potentially dangerous situations, there are ways of behaving that tend to precipitate real trouble.

- **on the street**
- Walking past a group of rowdy men as though you're afraid of attack is a sure way to invite trouble. Do try to walk as though you are absolutely sure of yourself and where you're going.
- Don't be an appeaser. If someone approaches you on the street, being friendly or diffident won't disarm him. Ignore him and if he persists, tell him to get away or you'll call the police. Men who have to approach women this way usually have weak egos; they count on yours being weaker.

- **take a deep breath and . . . scream**
- Only the true victim doesn't scream. If someone grabs you, or your purse, yell as loud as you can. It takes an effort to undo the inhibitions against making a scene—but this is your life.

Being victimized is often a state of mind. If you can psych yourself into believing that no one would *dare* threaten *you*, your chances of living safely are much greater in today's risk-laden cities.

living problems

burglars
keep burglars away when you are

Coming home to a burglarized apartment certainly isn't the ideal finale to a great vacation. To help avoid it, follow these tips. They aren't the usual "lock your valuables in a safe-deposit box" or "buy a timer for your lights" kind, though we do recommend doing them, too. These tips are more off-beat, but equally as effective:

- Tape valuables under the toilet-tank lid, or hide a ring behind the switch plate of a light (clip it so it won't fall behind the wall; watch out for wires). Few thieves feel leisurely enough to unscrew things or check the plumbing. They take what's handy and run.
- If there's no garbage to be picked up in your driveway, it's a dead giveaway that you're away. Arrange with a neighbor to put something out in your spot every couple of days. If you live in an apartment, cancel deliveries (like newspapers, milk, etc.) that are left at your door for the time you'll be away. A pile of papers is another clue to burglars.
- Advertise how well protected you are. It won't cost much to have a little window sign printed up that says, "This property protected by electronically controlled alarm." There may not be a word of truth in it, but a would-be thief will probably think twice before ripping you off.
- You might be interested in looking into a property identification system called Identifax. For $9.95 (send to Identifax, 1370 Avenue of the Americas, New York, NY 10019), you get a kit that allows you to put a permanent stencil number on all your property—TV, stereo, bicycle. This number is registered in a computerized system that helps local police identify stolen property as yours. You also get decals saying, "All property is registered with Identifax."
- If you own a dog, don't kennel him. Instead, get a friend to walk and feed him. The dog's presence can be a big burglar deterrent.
- If you have a timer for your lights, consider another to turn on the television.
- Don't hide all your treasures in one easily accessible spot. A silver box here, another there, makes the burglar work harder—and miss some.
- Don't tell the neighborhood your vacation plans—and that includes publicity in the local gazette, church or school paper. The corner dry cleaner won't burglarize you if you blurt out that you're going away, but someone hanging around the shop might. Some burglars wait for just this kind of tipoff.
- Even if you want to get the earliest start in the morning, don't pack your car the night before unless it's in a locked garage.

crime
10 ways to protect yourself against crime

Protecting yourself from crime doesn't mean staying home behind locked doors or carrying mace in your handbag. Awareness and common sense are much wiser weapons, as you'll see from these ten tips, all from an excellent book, *How to Protect Yourself from Crime* by Ira A. Lipman.

● on the street
1. Whenever possible, walk toward oncoming traffic. This makes sneaking up behind you in a car—a common device—very difficult.
2. To protect your purse, walk near the building side of the street with your purse in the hand away from the street. Carry it against your body, clasp side next to you.
3. When you have to be out alone at night, do carry some money; an attacker can be vengeful if he gets nothing. About $15 to $25 would be reasonable.
4. If you're attacked, your best bet is to surrender your valuables and do it quickly. As you reach for your money, tell your assailant that you're getting your wallet so he won't think you're reaching for a weapon.
5. Don't carry mace, tear-gas guns, and the like; it's too easy for the mugger to grab them and use them against you. Instead, carry a traffic policeman's whistle. The noise of the whistle will attract attention—and help—and send the mugger running.
6. If you travel alone at night on subways or buses, avoid the door area, where a thief can easily grab your bag and run out of the door.

● at home
1. Know what kind of doors are most inviting to burglars. A patio, or sliding glass door, is not only easy to jimmy (locks are usually ineffective), it's also a show window to what's inside. Most burglars won't chance breaking the glass and making attention-getting noise, so you can foil them by cutting a broom handle to fit the track the door slides on. This keeps door from sliding even if it's unlocked.
2. Doors with glass panes in them should have double-cylinder locks. They require a key to open them from the inside as well as the outside, so a burglar can't remove a glass pane and open door by turning the handle.
3. Use a dead-bolt lock on solid-wood or metal doors rather than the conventional come-with-the-apartment type that's so easy to jimmy with a strip of celluloid. Dead-bolt locks usually have a square face and the lock drops a bolt through an open cylinder. To gain entrance, the lock or the door must be completely removed.
4. Windows that are secluded are particularly inviting to burglars. A large nail driven into the window track in a way that will prevent the window from being raised high enough to admit an intruder is a good safeguard.

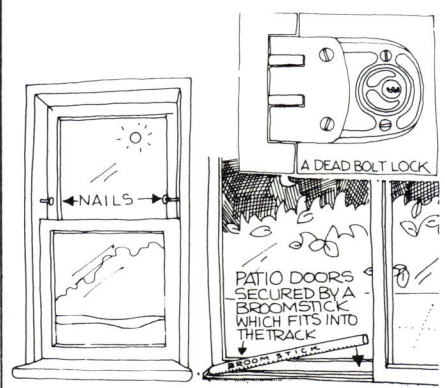

crime prevention with a neighborhood group

One good way to deter neighborhood crime is to form a neighborhood organization, according to Mike Dana, director of Citizen's Initiative Against Crime Program of the Law Enforcement Assistance Administration. A tenants' group lets you put the old safety-in-numbers theory to work against problems like muggings and burglaries. Here's how to get one started:

- *Organize a meeting of your neighbors to be held in a large apartment, a community room, or a nearby school. Photocopy an invitation and distribute by slipping it under doors or into mailboxes; post signs in the building lobbies.*
- *Have the group choose a committee of three or four people who will be in charge of coordinating future meetings and activities.*
- *At meetings, talk over neighborhood-crime problems and try to work out viable solutions with help from local service agencies and organizations—such as the mayor's community office or a city tenant association. Ask a representative of the police department to attend one of the meetings to discuss common crime patterns in the area and the best methods of security. In some cities, the police department offers special training courses in block watching for civilians and will teach any interested group such things as how to spot a crime being committed.*
- *Take measures to improve neighborhood safety conditions building*

109

living problems

by building. For instance, designate one entrance to each building and one route from the parking lot to be used by everyone coming in at night, thereby reducing people's chances of being alone and vulnerable after dark.

● At the meetings, you could also arrange for group activities, such as group jogging and dog walking, to help safeguard against muggings and other crimes that often occur when people are out alone early in the morning or late at night.

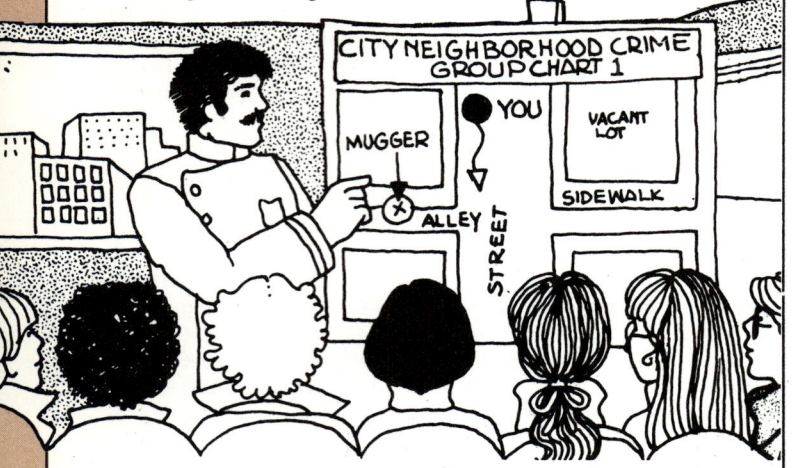

door
is your door as safe as it should be?

You've probably read about what kind of lock is the most burglarproof, but did you know some *doors* are safer than others? Here's why:

● Hinges can affect the safety of your door. A well-secured hinge protects against forced entry in two ways. First, secure hinges make it difficult to apply pressure on the hinge side and force the door in. Second, secure hinges make it hard for a burglar to push in the door, expose the hinge pins, and remove them—and the door—from its frame. Secure door hinges are made of heavy metal and well screwed into the frame by *several* strong, long screws.

● If possible, have your door open outward. It's more difficult to *pull* a door out of its frame than to push it in. One caution: A door that opens outward generally has its hinge pins on the outside where they're accessible. Be certain you buy hinge pins that aren't removable. If you're not certain, ask your hardware store to sell you the right kind, or check with a local locksmith.

● If you have a choice of doors, pick either a solid-core wood one or, best of all, a metal door. If you live in a risky area, it may be worth your while to buy a new door, preferably either one of the two above, and have it installed so that it opens outward for additional protection.

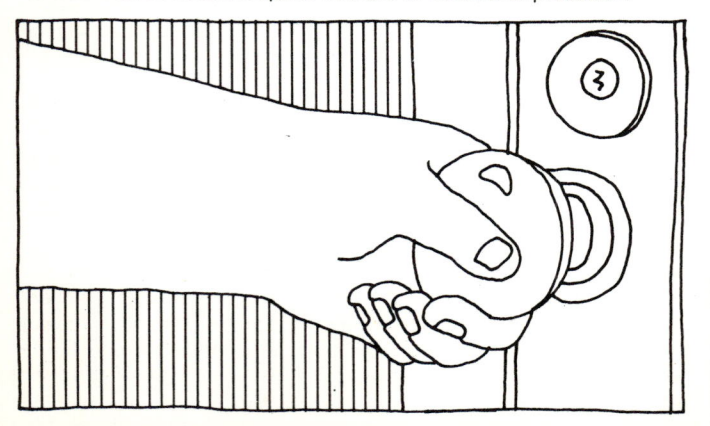

elderly
helping older people through the winter

Winter can be a lonely time for older people, who are frequently homebound by cold, stormy weather. If you have relatives and friends, or just know of elderly persons who live alone near you, do something special for them. It can give you a lot of pleasure, too.

● Ask if you can stop by for a cup of tea. Older people who live alone often go for days without seeing anyone. They like nothing better than company and conversation—and knowing they gave you something in return.

● Make a present of something good to eat. Not necessarily chocolate and cookies, but rather, a basket of fresh vegetables or fruit, a steak, a casserole.

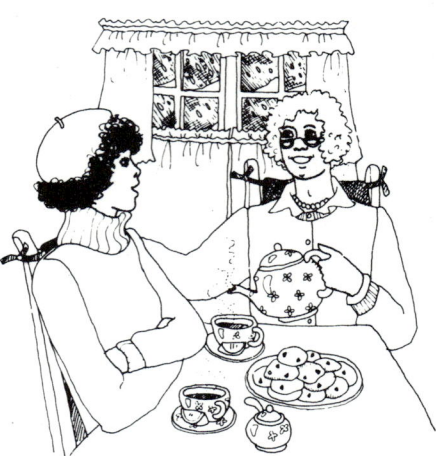

● Drop off the Sunday newspaper or give a subscription to the daily paper so they won't have to go out and get it. A magazine subscription is another idea.

● Undertake a small household chore like cleaning hard-to-reach places; do some shopping for them; take letters and packages to the post office.

● Telephone on a regular basis so they have the phone call to look forward to.

● Take them out on the town—to a movie or concert. Escort them to the doctor's office or to church.

garbage what to do with garbage when you're on vacation

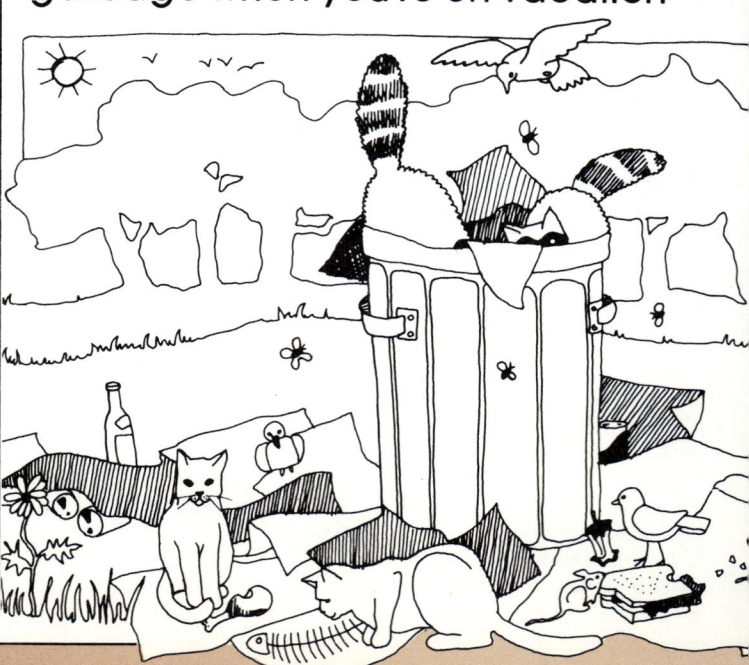

living problems

Getting rid of garbage can turn into a major engineering feat when you're vacationing in some resort areas and remote communities. To simplify the chore, here are some tips:

1. As soon as you arrive at a summer or weekend house, call the nearest municipal office or town hall to find out if the town has regular garbage collections and on which days. If not, check the Yellow Pages for private refuse-collection services. You may want to hire someone to cart your garbage away if you're staying for a couple of weeks or longer.
2. If there's neither public nor private collection, locate the town dump so you can dispose of garbage there. In some communities, Saturday afternoon at the dump marks a high point in the week's social calendar; people become friends while disposing of refuse.
3. Secure all of your garbage cans with more protection than a simple lid. Chain the lids to the cans, or fasten together with spring locks. To you it's garbage; to raccoons, stray dogs, and others, it's a feast. Try scattering mothballs through the garbage as a way of warding off raccoons.
4. Dispose of all garbage before you leave the house at the end of your vacation. If you can't get to a dump, pack all of your refuse into sturdy plastic bags, secure well, and drop into garbage cans in roadside picnic areas on the way home.

parents
how to survive moving back with your parents if you can't afford to live on your own

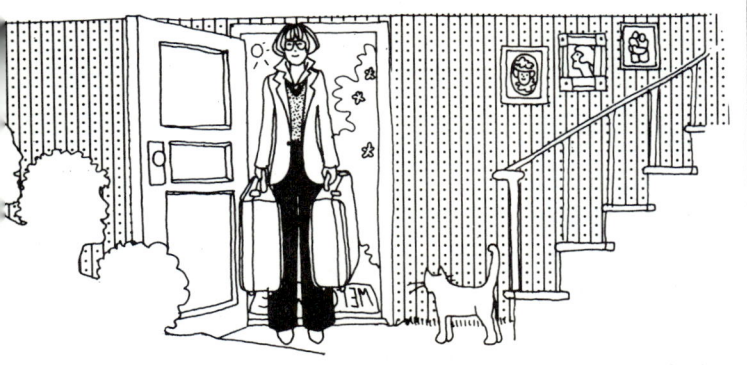

Hard-hit by the recession and the tough job market, many single women are saving money by moving back in with their parents—even after having lived on their own in a dorm or apartment. If you're considering such a move, it's worth thinking about problems you might face and possible ways of coping with them.

● **why are you moving back?**
"The first question to ask yourself is whether your motive for moving back is really financial or if that's just a red herring for some psychological reason," suggests Dr. Howard Halpern, codirector of the New York Student Consultation Center. There are times when it's perfectly healthy to touch home base for a while to cope with special stress and regain your strength.

But you may have less constructive motives. Independence can seem scary even if you've lived away at college, since that has some of the security of living at home. You may also be able to accept the idea of moving from home if it's toward a college or marriage, but find it hard to see leaving as valid in itself—as a step toward adulthood.

Parents may feel the same way or complicate the issue by wanting you close by to make them feel secure and useful, says Dr. Halpern. On the other hand, *you* might exaggerate *their* dependence. Many parents enjoy life more once their children have gone. Your parents may even resent your return but feel too guilty to say so.

● **what to do when you move home**
If you're definitely moving home, these tips might help:
● Try working out living arrangements ahead of time. Even if you're strapped for funds, Dr. Halpern thinks you'll be more independent if you pay something toward food, phone bills, etc., and if you share cooking and other chores.
● Freedom is trickier. Ideally, Dr. Halpern points out, you should be able to come home late, even go for a long weekend without giving your parents detailed explanations (just a courtesy warning not to worry). But many parents can't accept this casualness, and you may have to trade some independence for the convenience and financial savings of living at home.

There are other trade-offs, too. It's almost impossible to move home as an adult without regressing to some behavior patterns you had when you were younger—maybe refereeing your parents' arguments or placating a guilt-provoking parent. So even if you get along with your parents, it's probably worthwhile to set your finances in order and try to make it on your own.

● If living at home is clearly an interim solution, set a time limit and work toward it by saving money from part-time work, finding a permanent job, looking for roommates, etc. You'll get on better if you don't feel endlessly stuck. Also, if relations get strained, you can find a great apartment sooner than planned.

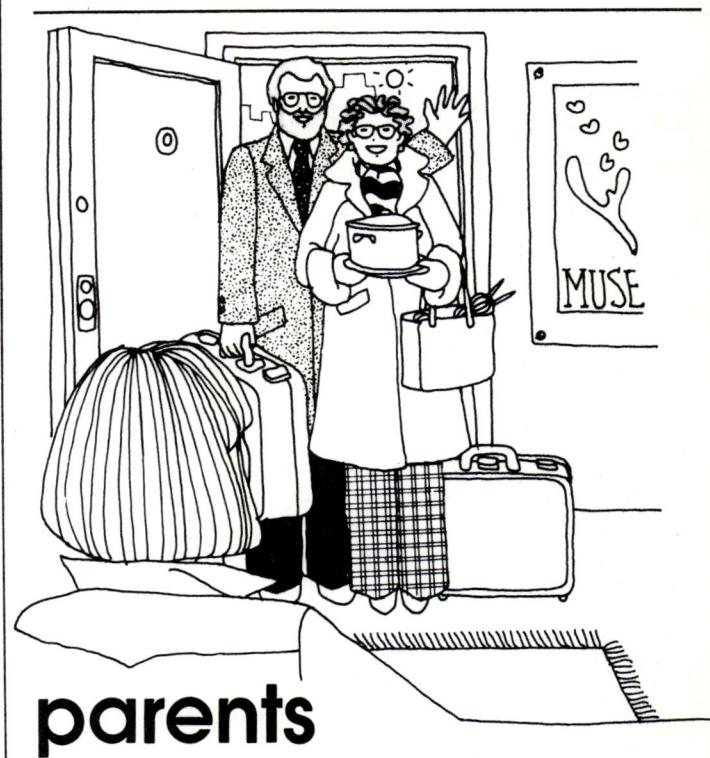

parents
making the most of a visit from your parents

If every time your parents or in-laws suggest visiting, you come down with a case of anxiety, depression, or hysteria, it's probably your mother's fault. The reason for fraught feelings is that you are really taking on the role she has held, offering hospitality, assuming responsibility for the emotional climate, managing independently without supervision. Here are a few dos and don'ts to help you overcome your worries:
● *DO have the actual dates of their stay understood between you. That way, you can decide whether you'll cope best with the parents on your premises or if they should stay in a nearby motel or hotel.*
● *DON'T try to clean everything in sight the day before they arrive. Better to have dirty windows than to work yourself into exhaustion and resentment.*

living problems

- DO keep menus natural and easy—the ones you're used to—and daily routines as streamlined as possible. You don't have to compete with your perfect older sister or measure up to your parents' standards of living. Presumably they are coming to see you—your very own self.
- DON'T be exploitive about their offers to help. If you plan to use them as babysitters for some special outing, let them know before they arrive and give them the choice of refusing.
- DO give some kind of party for introducing a few friends in a way that suits your style and that of your parents. Don't try to tie up every waking moment—they may want to take you to dinner or see a local event on their own. A few hours away from each other may help everybody.
- DO be flexible about what interests them most—more time with the grandchildren, less sightseeing, for instance.
- DO try to combine the realities of your personality and theirs, your new way of life, and what you know is theirs.

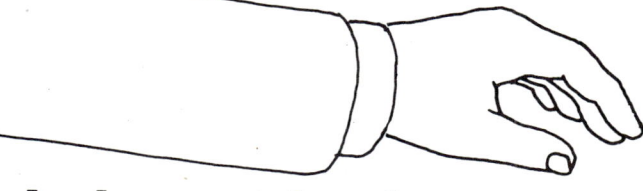

pickpocket
hangouts—and how to protect yourself when you're in one

Pickpockets, like everyone else, have their own special hangouts. So be on the lookout.
- Stay extra alert if you're near an open window or door on a bus or subway—or if you're waiting on a crowded bus line, where pickpockets often work in pairs (one causes a stir in front of you while the other rifles you from behind). Supermarkets, restaurants, and theaters are other places where it's easy to be distracted, so hold on to your bag; don't let it loose in a cart, on the floor, or looped over a chair. Watch out in restrooms; pros can whip bags off the floor in seconds. If you hang your purse on the door hook, hang your coat over it.
- Always tuck your wallet under other things in your purse, since pickpockets are looking for fast takes. Don't put all your valuables in one place; separate money, credit cards, keys, etc.
- Avoid single-strap handbags with clasps that can be knocked open. Double-strap bags with zipper closings are a better bet. Don't sling a shoulder bag behind you.
- If your purse is stolen, first ask the buildings-and-grounds security force to help you hunt for it, since thieves often take the cash and chuck the bag.
- If your bag is not found—and keys plus identification are in it—your apartment is wide open for burglary. Immediately call a locksmith to change the tumblers in your lock, and return home to keep guard (preferably with a friend) until he arrives.
- Don't leave if someone calls to say he's "found" your bag, warns Sgt. John Murphy of New York City's Pickpocket and Confidence Squad. A team of burglars could enter and go to work. Call the police.
- Report missing bank books, traveler's checks, driver's license, department store charge cards, and credit cards to the companies concerned. Send follow-up telegrams or certified letters and keep carbon copies plus receipts.
- Notify the police. Even if you can't describe the thief with certainty, a description of a suspicious-looking person who jostled you at the time of the robbery might be helpful.
- Finally, remember that you can claim personal theft losses worth over $100 as a deduction on your federal income tax.

roommates
coping with roommate problems

The best overall solution is to establish an atmosphere for clear communication. Otherwise, the "two people in four walls" situation may create a fifth wall that only parting ways will break down. Confront problems before they get out of hand. Honest discussion and experimentation can bring solutions to most of your gripes, but there will always be some things that get to you, like:
- You're more social and she's more sedentary. Take turns going out so the apartment can be shared in a solitary as well as a communal sense. Respect her early risings when you're creeping in at 3 A.M. Do talk to your roommate about how much, how often, and under what circumstances visitors, particularly boyfriends, are welcome at the apartment. Decide where overnight guests will sleep and what the "hosting" roommate is responsible for—food, towels, bedding, etc.
- She doesn't want to be your "best friend" or "buddy." Don't feel that just because you're roommates, you have to be each other's best friend. Finding your own niche—or helping her find hers—will help your relationship and avoid intrusion of each other's privacy.
- One of you is a borrower. Don't get into the habit of borrowing—even when your roommate isn't around. If you do, one of these days it may be your last roll of film that's gone. If your roommate is the borrower, be open and tell her you don't approve of constant borrowing. Try to come up with some compromises about mutual sharing, even split the cost of certain items—like a hair dryer, electric rollers, an iron, etc.
- One of you is super neat, the other very casual. If you dust the woodwork around your bed and her consistently unmade bed becomes a minor depressant, try to define a physical space for each of you and respect it. You don't have to set up a partition, but divide the space so you both have room to do what you like. Then deal frankly and rationally with individual problems as they come up.

weekend kit
a ready-for-anything kit for a weekend place

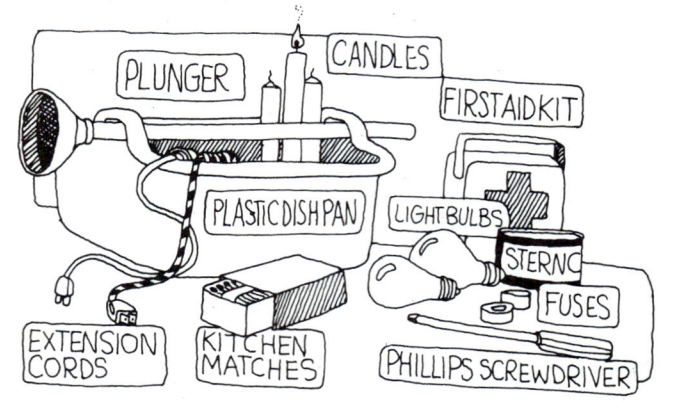

The best-laid plans for a weekend at a rented cottage, beach hut, fishing camp, or whatever sometimes fizzle because no one remembered to pack a screwdriver or flashlight. If you keep a small plastic dishpan stacked with all of the following—and don't forget it—you won't be left in a lurch when confronted by a blown fuse or other mini-disaster. Make sure you include: light bulbs; extension cords; plunger; fuses; Sterno cooking fuel; first-aid kit; kerosene lamp; flashlight; tools—wrench, hammer, regular and Phillips screwdrivers; heavy-duty cord or rope; matches—the longer "kitchen" type; and candles.

mail m

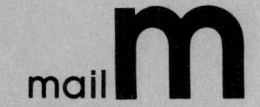

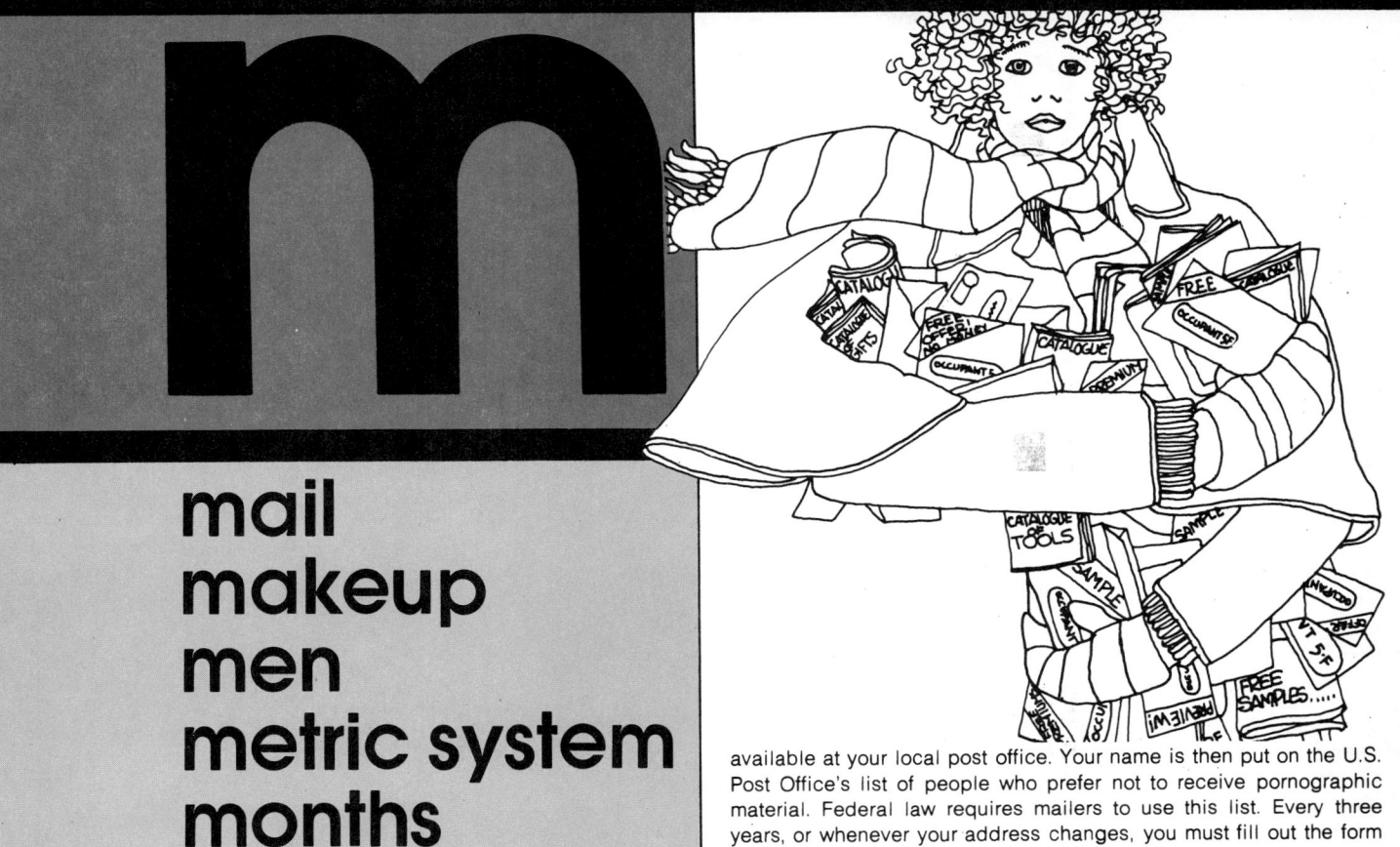

m

mail
makeup
men
metric system
months
movies
moving

mail

junk
what you can do about chain letters and other junk mail

Chain letters can promise you anything from a financial windfall to an international recipe collection to five hundred postcards in two weeks —*if* you send copies to 5 (or 20) friends. Some threaten bad luck or worse if you don't. Here's how to deal with this and other mail annoyances:

● Most chain letters are not illegal, according to the office of the U.S. Postal Consumer Advocate. Unless money or something of monetary value is involved, the only way to break a chain is simply not to answer. If money is involved, it's a case of mail fraud. For instance, it's illegal if you're asked to "send a dollar to five friends" and promised a much larger amount by mail. Complain to your local postmaster or inspector, and be prepared to supply him or her with all letters, envelopes, and other evidence of mail fraud.

● Discontinue unsolicited pornography by filling out Form 2201, available at your local post office. Your name is then put on the U.S. Post Office's list of people who prefer not to receive pornographic material. Federal law requires mailers to use this list. Every three years, or whenever your address changes, you must fill out the form again.

● Junk mail can be slowed by notifying the Direct Mail Marketing Association. It notifies big commercial mailers of your request and says that mailers sending about 65 percent of consumer junk mail will scratch your name. Their address is: Direct Mail Marketing Association, 6 East 43 St., New York, NY 10017.

● If your worst offenders persist, write them directly, enclosing their envelope or label showing your name and address as they mailed it to you. But don't expect immediate action, because most companies can only afford to go through their lists periodically.

travel
how to get mail from home when you're traveling

There's no problem getting mail from home if you have hotel reservations for every night of your vacation. All you have to do is leave a list of the hotels and their addresses with your friends. But if you plan a camping trip or don't want to be tied down to specific reservations, you might want to know about alternatives.

● In the United States, mail can be sent to you c/o General Delivery, City, State, Zip Code. All you will need to claim it at the Post Office is some identification.

● In Europe, mail can be sent to you c/o Poste Restante, City, Country. You'll need a passport for identification and may have to pay a small fee.

● If you have booked your travel arrangements through American Express, are an American Express card member, or have bought American Express traveler's checks, you may have your mail sent to any of American Express's six hundred offices and subsidiary or representative offices in the U.S. and around the world.

● In all cases, mail should be sent well in advance of your arrival date, with a return address, and your last name printed in capital letters so it is easier to file and find.

m makeup

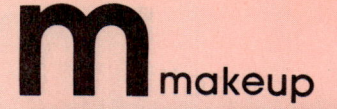

makeup

acne
makeup for acne or scarred skin

Today's natural look, done with sheer makeup, often presents problems for women with acne or acne scars. Sheer foundations don't cover like matte ones, so here are some hints to the rescue:

First off, don't make the mistake of reverting to a heavy, caky, matte makeup. This will actually call attention to problem skin by making you look more "made up."

If you have minor skin-breakout problems or scars left from acne, start your makeup with a water-based foundation in peachy, rosy, or tawny tones, whichever is the most complimentary to you. This type has no oil and some also contain oil-blotting agents. Since acne-prone skins are usually oily, you can see the benefit of the water base. If you have a few particularly bad breakouts from time to time or deep scars, try covering them with a cover stick blended under your foundation. This flesh-colored cover stick can't hide scars or breakouts completely, but it minimizes them by evening out any discolorations from them. When you buy your water-based makeup, be sure to ask for just that. Most cosmetic companies manufacture them but do not label them as such. Cover sticks give a light matte finish to the skin while evening out color.

You might want to choose your foundation from cosmetic lines that are especially designed for problem skin—like Allercreme, Almay, or Clinique. These are available in most drugstores and department stores.

If you have serious acne, you should see a dermatologist for treatment. Ask him or her to prescribe a medicated makeup base for you. The medication in the makeup helps keep infection from spreading and usually contains an ingredient that absorbs excess oils. Your dermatologist may prescribe one that blends with your own skin coloring or an untinted one to which some druggists could add color.

If you like powder, always use a good-quality loose one. Stay away from the pressed powders, as they tend to cake on oily skin. A fresh, bright blusher on your cheeks will help give a healthy glow to your skin. Choose from the powder blushers that you apply with a brush. Avoid creamy or gel blushers that add oil to your skin. They can clog the enlarged pores that frequently go with oily skin.

You can use any lipstick or eye makeup you like, but you may find that powder eye shadows stay on oily skin better than cream ones. Play up your eyes so that they, and not your skin, become the main focus of your face.

black women
makeup advice for black women

Many black women seem to have trouble solving these persistent beauty problems:

● *Finding the right foundation* is a problem that's getting easier to solve. In most cities, there are available very good lines of cosmetics made especially for black skin. Yellow, ruddy, olive, or gray undertones are the most common for black skin. For yellow undertones, a deep beige foundation is good. Ruddy tones also call for beige; avoid anything with pink or peach in it. Olive and gray undertones need brightening, so try a foundation with a bit of pink or peach.

Many black women also complain of uneven skin tone. Instead of trying to even it out with a deeper foundation, consider using a soft but bright blusher on your cheeks to provide a focus of attention. If your skin is oily, you'll probably find that a water-based foundation works best.

● *Finding lip colors* is another frequently heard complaint. One reason is that your lips may have a lot of deep-red pigment, so when you actually try the lip color, it may not look at all as you imagined. If there is a tester handy, put a dab on your finger first, then apply to your lips. Another solution is lip gloss. Most black women look sensational with just a slick of clear gloss over lips or one with the barest hint of color plus gloss. If you want to wear the deep-toned lipsticks but find they look too dark, use a yellow undercoat or a pink lipstick base which will make the lip color go on closer to the tube color.

blusher
how to apply blusher like a pro

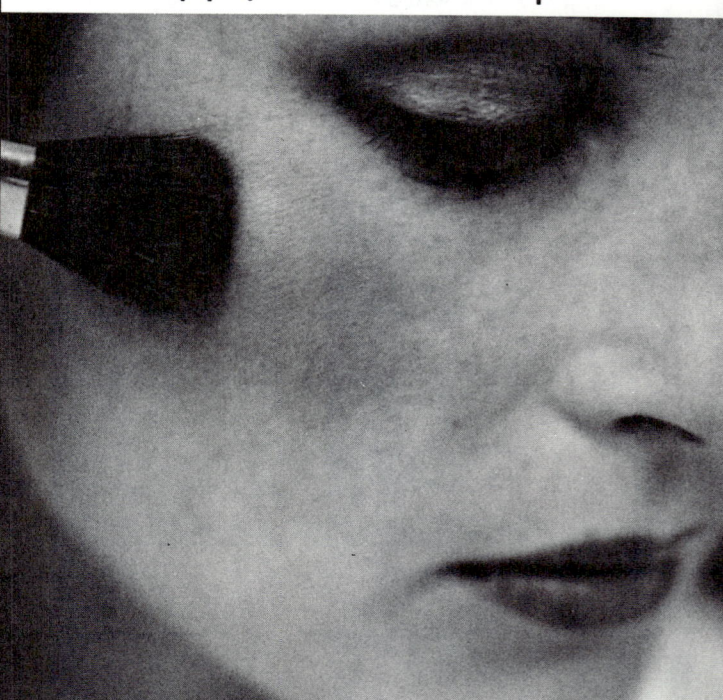

Even the prettiest blusher can fail to deliver all the beauty potential you expect if you don't apply it properly. Since nature's blush is often over the cheekbone, why not apply yours there? Put your index finger at the outer corner of your eye and move it down until you feel your cheekbone. Apply blusher here, then blend it upward to temple and downward to ear. Try not to get blusher below nostril level. Applied too low, it can make you look overly made up. You might also like to try blending just a touch of blush across the bridge of your nose for a sun-touched look and a bit more on forehead just below the hairline.

Oriental women
makeup tips for Oriental women

Here are tips on applying makeup for Oriental women from Fumiko Yokoyama, director of Japanese Beauty Artists for Shiseido Cosmetics.

Many Oriental women want to take away the slightly sallow tone their skin tends to have. To do this, Fumiko suggests using an under-

makeup

makeup color corrector—a sheer moisturizing liquid with a tinge of color in it. It is sold by most makeup houses and is easy to apply. A mint green will help minimize the sallow tone. If you follow this corrector with a medium-beige foundation, you will get a soft, fragile paleness that's very flattering. If you want a more rosy look with no trace of sallowness, try a pale blue under-makeup color followed by a slightly pink beige foundation.

Most Oriental women have broad cheeks with high cheekbones. To make the most of the lines, Fumiko suggests blusher blended in a high triangle from temple to cheek just under pupil of the eye, then back to earlobe. She finds pink or bronze tones most flattering to Oriental skin, with orange and brown the least becoming.

Eyes can look sensational if you'll follow these tips: (1) Try shading the lid with any medium-tone clear color that you like. Avoid muddy colors here. Blend color softly across the lid. (2) To give the eye depth, try blending a neutral brown or gray shadow in the crease. (3) If you like, you can use a pale, pale melon, mauve, or other soft shade blended just under the brow and just under bottom lashes at outside corners for highlight.

Lipstick should work with your blusher and what you're wearing, but wine colors are especially becoming to Oriental skin. Shiny glosses are also very pretty.

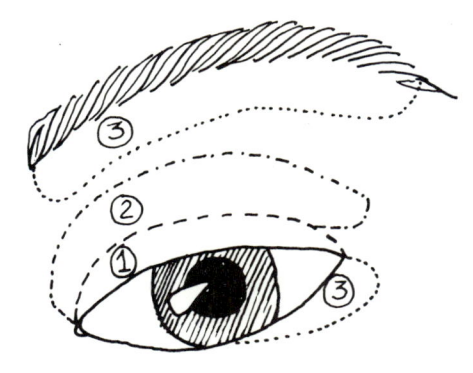

party
makeup for the morning after

There's bound to be at least one morning (and probably more) when your mirror tells you what you already know—you've had too much party the night before. To the rescue: soothing tea compresses for puffy eyes, a refreshing cucumber mask to put the glow back in your pale hung-over complexion, and a gleaming, fresh makeup idea to make you look as lively and healthy as you would after a day in the sun.

To make the tea compresses and the cucumber mask, put a large doubled piece of dampened gauze or cheesecloth into the refrigerator. While you wait, dampen two tea bags and chop one chilled cucumber, skin and all, into fine bits. Take the gauze out of the refrigerator, and cut two small squares to wrap around the tea bags. Cut two larger squares and fill each with half of the chopped cucumber. Fold gauze securely and seal ends with a bit of cellophane tape. Go back to bed with your compresses and gauze squares. Plop a tea bag compress over each eye, one cucumber-filled square on your forehead, the other over the rest of your face, leaving your nose out for air. Relax for 15 minutes.

Now for the makeup. Start with a peach or pink blushing gel, whichever color is best for your skin tone. Stroke it all around the outside of your face, blending gel close to the hairline. Then apply two coats of the same color to center of cheeks for a more intense glow. Finish with mascara and a bit of colored lip gloss.

party
keep your looks from drooping in the middle of the party

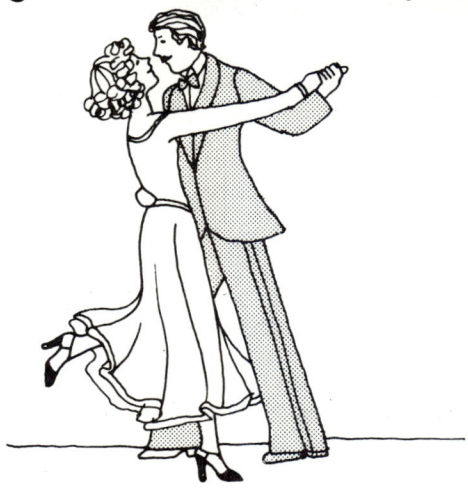

8 P.M. You look smashing. Your hair is clean and bouncy. Your makeup is perfect—not a trace of a blemish. Your dress is an absolute sensation and this is your night.

11 P.M. You don't look so great. Your hair has drooped. Your makeup has faded. Your nose is shiny. And you have perspiration stains.

If the scenario above sounds familiar, take heart. It happens to all of us. The combination of liquor, food, heat, and all the things that add up to a super party do a real killer act on party looks. But with a little planning, the next time *can* be your night. Look at the tips below:

● **hair**
- Make sure it's shiny clean. Oily hair usually looks best washed right before the party. If you have normal to dry hair, shampoo it the night before so it's clean but not too soft.
- This is not the time to try a new hairstyle. Stick to your usual, maybe dressing it up with a glittery clip. In general, the simpler the better.
- Give hair a *light* misting of hairspray—unscented—before you go out.
- If you have medium to long hair, take along a clip, a couple of combs, or a ribbon to pretty it up when it droops.

● **makeup**
- Before putting on any makeup, cleanse face thoroughly, then apply a toner (normal to dry skin) or an astringent or oil-blotting lotion (oily skin). Moisturize lightly, doing only under the eyes if your skin is very oily.
- If you have oily skin, use a water-based or oil-free foundation. You could also dab on oil-blotting lotion with cotton balls after makeup is on.
- Apply a little more blusher or a deeper shade than usual, but be sure to blend well. For oily skin, use powder blusher. For dry to normal, a cream or gel. Cream blushers stay put better if you dust lightly with powder before applying.
- For pretty eyes, line lower lashes with a mauve or navy blue pencil or eye-shadow stick. Use a powder shadow on lids—it has the best staying power. And give lashes a coating of baby powder for added thickness before putting on mascara.
- For lip color that lasts longer, first outline lips with a brush or pencil. Then use lipstick, or lipstick plus gloss. Gloss alone will fade quickly. You can also try this trick: apply lipstick color with a brush in up and down strokes, following the grain of your lips. Then go over with lipstick tube.
- Finish off your makeup with a light dusting of translucent or baby powder, especially nice when applied with a fluffy natural-bristle brush.

m makeup

- **personal touches**
- If parties always make you perspire, try a stronger antiperspirant cream. Apply an antiperspirant at least 15 minutes after your bath or shower at some calm moment, maybe when you're polishing your nails or before taking a catnap. This way your antiperspirant can start working before you get party nerves.
- Apply perfume 20 to 30 minutes before leaving to let the scent "mature."
- For extra scent power, bathe with bath oil or use body lotion.
- Brush teeth and use a mouthwash before leaving. You might bring along a pocket breath freshener for a pickup.
- **general tips**
- If you are going to be in bright light, stay away from deep, offbeat, or pastel-colored makeup; use earthy tones. In dim light, use brighter shades.
- Don't respray hair at the party. If it's going to fall, let it. More spray will only look sticky.
- If your skin is very oily, don't keep adding more color as makeup fades. Take along prepackaged, astringent-soaked pads to remove face makeup (leave eye makeup on), then apply makeup again.
- Heat intensifies scent, so don't drown yourself in fragrance. When applying, go lightly. And remember—you're not the only one who's drooping, but you are the one who knows how to cope.

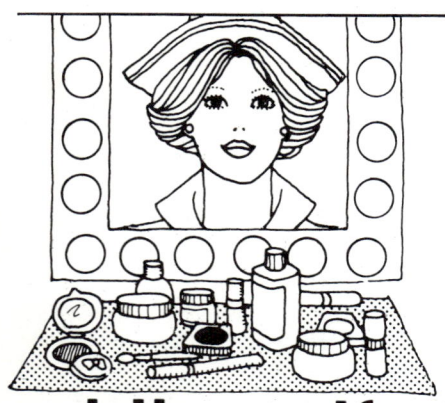

white uniforms
makeup tips for women who wear white uniforms

White might look great against a tan, but it can make even minimal makeup look obvious. Yet, if you wear no makeup, you're apt to look washed out. To solve the problem, follow these general tips:
- Use clear, not murky, colors and blend well.
- Aim for a see-through polish rather than coverage. Gels and glosses are generally the best way to achieve this minimal-makeup look.
- If you use a foundation, make sure it matches your skin tone and is not noticeably darker or lighter.
- Avoid powder, it tends to look heavy.
- Keep eye makeup very simple. Try using a dark brown, rather than black, mascara for a softer look, and use only a hint of shadow.
- Keep brows well-shaped to give added emphasis to eyes.
- A glint of earring or a pretty barrette or comb can also provide a color lift.
- For fair skin: An all-over color product (which gives a sheer wash of color to your face) is a good idea. Stay away from pale pink blushers and pale blue shadows. Try instead salmon or russet colors for cheeks and soft brown for eyes.
- For medium skin: Stick to clear earth tones; stay away from anything with an orange tint; it can make your skin look sallow.
- For dark skin: The big mistake here is using too much makeup. Let your natural coloring provide the contrast needed. Just pick it up with a blusher in the mulberry or wine family and a tinted lip gloss.

men

calendar
make a year-long present for the man you're in love with

Start by buying an attractive calendar or datebook. Then personalize it by writing or pasting in reminders of special (or ordinary) events—birthdays, big games you're planning to attend, a great day both of you spent last summer. You might include small cutouts from magazines or newspapers, quotes, photos, lines from your favorite movies or poems, your own sketches, individual cartoon frames (maybe for a series of Mondays, to brighten up blue ones). Just fill it with bits of humor or thoughts he'd never find in an ordinary calendar. The more personal it is, the more likely you're creating the first calendar he ever saved once the year ends.

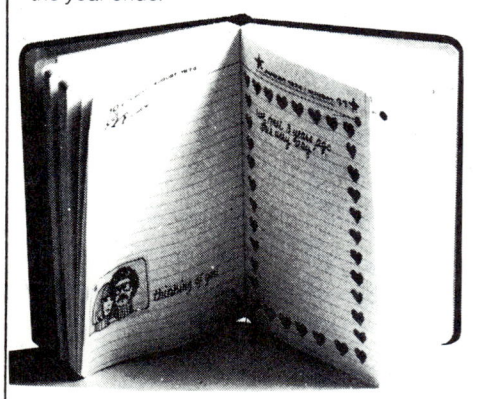

children
how to get along with his children

If the man in your life had a former life that included children, one essential in your relationship is rapport with them. Rapport can be a touchy business, but a rewarding one. Here are some sound ideas from Sally R. Warren, a *GLAMOUR* reader who has coped successfully:
- Never, never speak critically of their mother in the children's presence, even if they and/or their father do. This is the time to be diplomatic.
- Don't try to be an instant buddy or to convert his children into your fans. Transitions are very important, and if you want to build a lasting, growing relationship, you should proceed gradually.
- Handle embarrassing questions honestly and preferably without requiring their father to join in the explanations. Queries such as "Do you both sleep in this bed?" or "Are you going to marry my father?" are best handled by looking the questioner in the eye and giving a truthful,

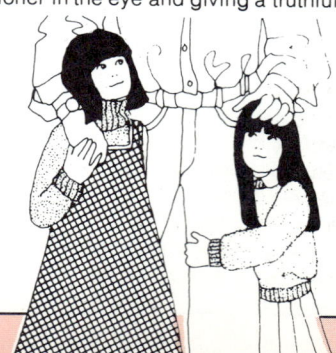

straightforward answer. Marriage questions can usually be put safely and candidly into the uncertain future.
- As you get to know the children, make it clear by your attitude and perhaps by casual comments that you are not trying to be their mother. The children *have* a mother; your role is as a companion to their father and, if it is the case, the idea can be subtly put forth that you may be a permanent factor in their lives.
- If it comes comfortably to you, establish a separate identity by expressing a style and interests that are different from the children's mother. If she's an outdoorsy type, you can be at home indoors, and vice versa.
- Don't try to buy the children's affection by buying them material things.
- Speak to the children's father about *your* needs in terms of his leisure time. If there isn't an established agreement on visitation, you may find yourself in the presence of the children for what seems like every leisure minute. If you need one weekend a month to be alone with him, tell him. It will be better for everyone to have this time understood and planned for.

gifts how to buy gifts for men to wear— without mistakes

Love alone won't keep you from making mistakes on gifts for men. No matter how well you know a man or his tastes, there are facts about male sizes, fit, and styles that most women don't think of before they buy. That's why we asked a lot of men to tell us the mistakes they found women made most often and how to select gifts that wind up on a man, not in his closet.
- Many women don't realize that *ties* come in long and extra-long lengths. Tall and wide-necked men generally need extra-long ties, as do men who prefer the fuller Windsor knot (it takes an extra 2½" of tie). A fairly light material, such as silk, as opposed to a more cumbersome fabric, is better for a Windsor.
- *Collar* styles affect how comfortable a shirt is and how well it looks on a man. A man with a wide face may prefer a longer, straighter collar (see Sketch 1) that tends to be thinner and flattering. A low, sloped collar (2) is usually more comfortable for a man with a short neck, while a long, thin neck can be minimized by a collar with more spread (3). If a shirt comes with removable stays, it's a good idea to ask for extras when buying them, since stays often disappear when accidentally sent to the laundry.

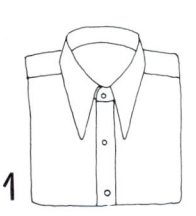

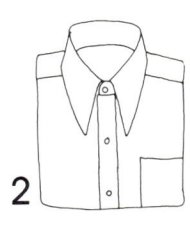

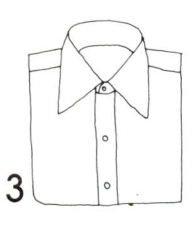

- In order to buy most *shirts*, obviously you need to know a man's collar or neck and sleeve sizes. You'll find these sewn or stamped into the collar or tail of a shirt he already owns, with the collar size first. For example, a label that reads 15/33 means it has a 15" neck and 33" sleeve.
- Most shirts are either 100 percent cotton or a blend of cotton and a synthetic such as polyester. Blended shirts tend to be cooler in winter and hotter in summer than pure cotton, which "breathes." For this reason, try to avoid highly synthetic shirts for a man who perspires heavily.
- Men's *sweater* sizes range from 38 to 46, or from small to extra large. A general rule is to buy a sweater one size above a man's chest measurement. For example, if he measures 36", buy size 38.

- The most common mistake that women—and sometimes men themselves—make in buying *belts* is to buy them too wide for the belt loops. It helps to measure the width of the loop, even when you think you know it.
- A man may have very specific opinions about the length and color his *socks* should be, despite their low visibility. Most men today wear over-the-calf stretch socks of the one-size-fits-all variety. Some prefer that their socks match their slacks or shoes; others like patterns and textures.
- Don't use a man's birthday or Father's Day to break him into some drastic color or style departure, such as a hot-orange tie if he lives in blue and gray. This ploy rarely works. If a man wouldn't buy something for himself, the chances are strong that he wouldn't wear it either.

haircut how to cut his hair

The next time he asks you to cut his hair, surprise him with a really good cut. This step-by-step how-to comes from experts at the men's division of Vidal Sassoon. First the outline cutting gives hair its outer shape, then comes the section-by-section inner cutting.

This cut works on curly or straight hair but looks different, as you see in Sketch 2 on straight hair, Sketch 3 on wavy hair, and Sketch 4 on very curly hair. Always keep curly hair pulled as taut as possible when cutting to avoid ragged ends. Cut very curly hair in 1½" lengths instead of 2" so it won't look bushy.

- **outline cutting**

Always cut hair while it's damp, after a shampoo and towel drying. Center part down the back. Comb hair toward the face from each side of part, front hair down over forehead from crown. With a good, sharp scissors 5" to 6" long (for better control when cutting), outline the basic shape by cutting the hair counter-clockwise all around the hairline. Start at nape of neck, leaving hair about 2" long, more if he wants it on the long side. Whatever length the nape hair is from the hairline, keep the side and front hair the same all around. The outline in Sketch 1 shows the shape to follow: straight across nape, straight up one side to outer corner of eye, straight across forehead. Avoid a rounded-bowl look.

- **section-by-section cutting**

Re-part hair down center back. The sketch shows how to divide the hair into sections, each one about 1½" apart on the scalp, extending from part to ear. Start at bottom back and work up. Use clips or bobby pins to keep top hair out of your way while cutting. Pick up one section at a time with a comb, holding section between your index and middle fingers with the hair at right angles to the head. Keeping hair taut, cut the ends straight across. Each 1½" section should be cut to the same length as the hairline hair. At the very crown, hair should be left slightly longer. For example, if you cut the back 2", the crown should be 3". When cutting curly hair, cut crown same length as rest of the hair.

After you've cut the back, section each side of the head according to the sketch. Divide each section to same 1½" depth as before. When the whole head is cut, check it out by picking up handfuls of hair at the back, about twice the depth of 1½" sections, and see if the ends are even with no long strays. When you're done, he should have one beautiful head.

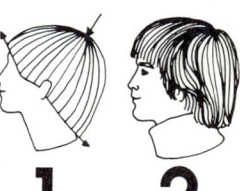

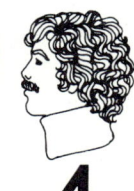

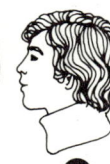

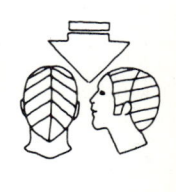

117

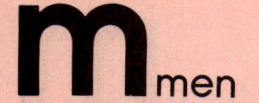

men

holding hands
make a mitten for holding hands

If you're in love—or falling in that direction—make a double mitten that the two of you can wear while walking hand in hand through the woods or sitting cozily at football games.

You'll need two sets of mittens, in two sizes—one for him and the other for yourself—and some matching or contrasting yarn. To make the double mitten, cut away the thumb from one right and one left mitten (be sure you use one mitten from each set), and slit that side about 3" (see sketch). Finish off the edges with matching thread or yarn, or machine stitch if you prefer, to prevent raveling. Then sew the two mittens together around the openings you've made.

Pull your mitten on next time it's too cold for handholding without gloves or mittens.

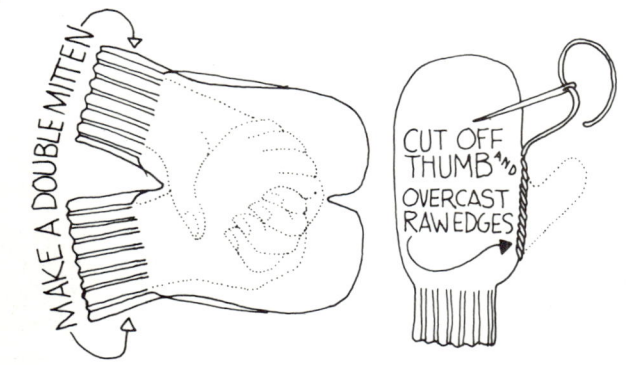

in-laws
how to get along with yours

If you're suffering from an in-law hangover because of home vacations or holidays, and wish you could take your in-laws better, here are a few brief ideas to help. Perhaps the best ground rule to apply to your relationship with in-laws is to try not so much to see them as his parents, but more as individuals, with their own personalities, likes, and dislikes.

Dr. Mary Jane Hungerford, Director of the American Institute of Family Relations in Santa Barbara, suggests the following to help warm up any relationship:

- Adopt a "you take care of your folks, I'll take care of mine" attitude. This ends up meaning that the partner best equipped to deal with each set of parents does so—usually you with yours, he with his.
- If in-laws try to meddle in your life, don't let them feel they're dividing you. Tell in-laws that you and your partner agree that you want to handle things your own way to prevent them from pitting the two of you against each other.
- On major holidays, take turns visiting in-laws: visit one set on one holiday, the other the next.
- Don't "use" in-laws—that is, turn them into constant babysitters or helpers. If possible, don't take favors or money from them.

Gloria T. Hirsch, a Los Angeles family counselor and Clinical Director of Friends of the Family, offers these additional suggestions:

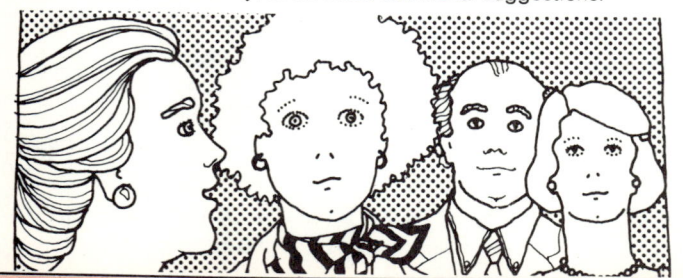

- Don't project what you see as faults in *your* parents onto in-laws. See in in-laws the qualities that make you love your spouse—*something* must have been transferred!
- Don't demand of your in-laws anything that would be unrealistic to demand of any other good friend. Try to put yourself in their place and see how you would feel.
- Try to see your in-laws as parents trying to adjust to a son or daughter's independent life.

living together
what are your rights?

Unmarried couples who live together don't have the same privileges married couples have. Before you move in together, know exactly what your rights are.

- *Is it legal?*—No: Living together unmarried is against the law in just about every state, but so is sex between unmarried people. However, enforcement of these laws is so rare that they are not likely to cause any problems.
- *Finances*—One of the trademarks of marriage is the joint checking account, but any two people can ask the bank for a joint checking or savings account. Be sure you completely trust anyone who has access to your earnings and savings.
- *Credit*—According to law, if a married person charges basic family expenses and then doesn't pay for them, the creditor has the right to collect from either spouse. If you're a couple living together but you maintain separate identities and independent credit, you are responsible for only your purchases and debts. However, banks and credit managers do allow someone other than a spouse to be a guarantor on a loan.
- *Discounts*—Married couples can often enjoy special discounts on travel, vacation plans, and club memberships; consorts can take advantage of some of these discounts, too. Organizations as diverse as the American Civil Liberties Union and the New York Health Club offer special membership rates to couples, yet both claim that a "couple" can be any two people who want to join together.
- *Income Tax*—Married couples do have the option of filing a joint-income tax return, which in some cases reduces the total amount of taxes paid. This option isn't available to consorts.
- *Crime*—By law a wife is not "competent" to testify in court against her husband and vice versa (there are some exceptions to this). This is supposed to preserve marital harmony, but consorts have no such privilege. A living-together relationship is not one that the law tries to preserve, so either consort can voluntarily or under subpoena testify against the other.

pre-marriage counseling
untie some of the knots before you tie the big one

Elaine and Ted have been happily engaged for six months when they're suddenly caught in a storm of arguments over whether they ought to have one or two checking accounts after they're married. Even though they rarely argue about other topics, both feel this disagreement is important to resolve. "It's not the bank account itself that bothers me," Elaine says, "it's why we can't seem to solve such a small problem."

Kate and Jim have dated steadily for a year, and Jim is now pressuring Kate to get married. Kate thinks she wants to but worries about "the institution of marriage itself." Jim says that's her hangup—while Kate feels his attitude toward marriage is "too idealistic."

men

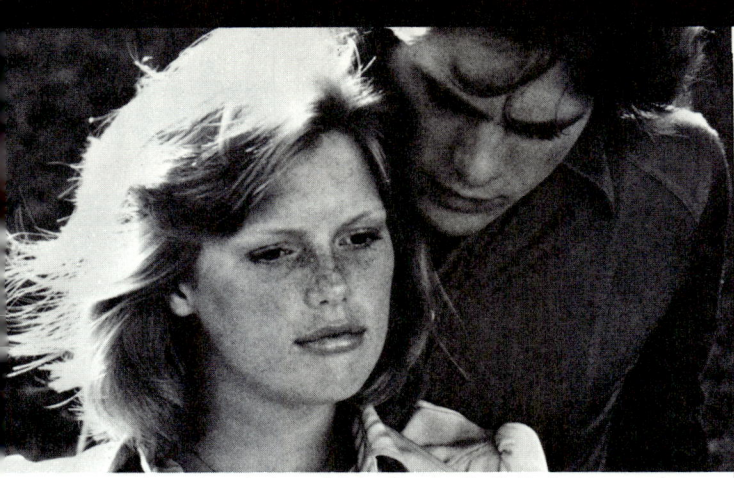

Two months before their wedding, Steve tells Sally that he wants to see a former girlfriend "one last time" for a reason he can't explain. Sally wants to postpone the wedding until he can.

Problems like these aren't new to engaged couples—nor are cold feet, the jitters, and just plain panic. But many soon-to-be marrieds have found a way to deal with them through pre-marriage counseling.

Psychologists, social workers, and clergymen report that increasing numbers of couples are trying to work out their anxieties about marriage through pre-marriage counseling or a series of sessions with a marriage and family counselor. He or she—and sometimes one counselor of each sex—may give both partners tests, invariably asking questions such as, "Who comes first, you or the one you love?" and "How much time do you feel you'll want to spend with your in-laws during the first year of marriage?" The goal of pre-marriage counseling, however, isn't to promote marriage; it's to help you understand yourself, your mate, and your feelings about your relationship. "We feel pre-marriage counseling has been successful when both people feel they've arrived at the best solution for them," says one marriage counselor. "But sometimes the best solution for them may not be marriage."

For the name of a counselor in your area, write to the American Association of Marriage and Family Counselors at 225 Yale Ave., Claremont, CA 91711; or the National Alliance for Family Life at 10642 Downey Ave., Downey, CA 90240. You can also call your clergyman, college counseling service, or your local affiliate of the Family Service Association of America. Be wary of finding a counselor through the phone book, since only a handful of states have minimum standards for a marriage counseling license. In the other states, many quacks practice.

reading aloud
rediscover the pleasure of reading aloud together

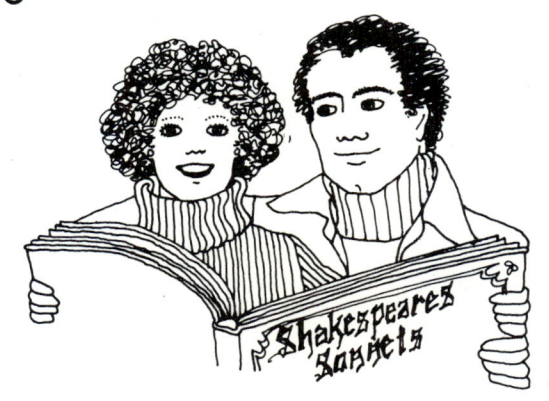

Reading aloud can be romantic when there are just the two of you, or party fun when there are more. You can even do it all alone on a cold or rainy evening. Here are some ideas to get you started:

- When the mood is romantic, read Shakespeare's Sonnet 116.
- Try Emily Dickinson's poems when your only company is a glass of wine and the house is dark and quiet. "I heard a fly buzz when I died" is strange and lovely.
- If you want to laugh and be challenged just to get the words out, try reading "The Jabberwocky" from Lewis Carroll's *Through the Looking-Glass*. It's more fun when there's a group of people. Another funny book is Don Marquis's series of letters from his typewriting companion, Archy, the cockroach. *Archy and Mehitabel* is the title. "Mehitabel Sings a Song" is a good letter to start with. Cat lovers—even cat haters—will be charmed by T. S. Eliot's poem "The Naming of Cats" from *Old Possum's Book of Practical Cats*. The Beatrix Potter books are also charming.
- If you want eerie, scary reading, try "The Great God Pan" from *The Strange World of Arthur Macken* by Arthur Macken. In the same vein, read "The Headless Horseman" from *The Legend of Sleepy Hollow* by Washington Irving.

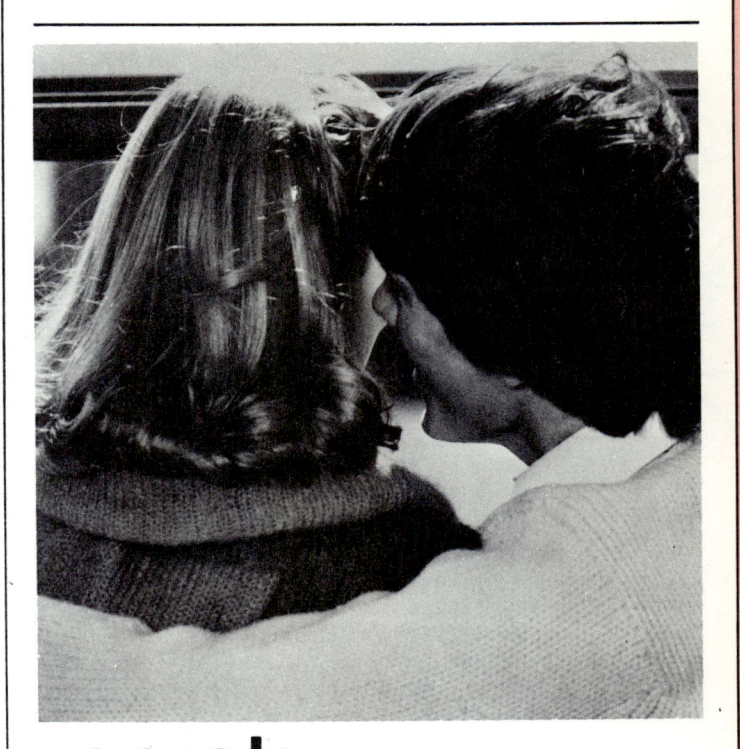

secrets
how to get a man to open up—and tell you what's bothering him

He's entitled to his share of secrets, silences, and skeletons in the closet, but the occasion may arise when he's got something he wants to talk about but just can't get it out. Here's how you can help him:

- If you sense he's preoccupied, unhappy, or anxious, try asking simple questions that show your sensitivity to him and your concern. "Something is bothering you, isn't it?" would be a good opener.
- Always listen to the whole answer. So often we hear only the first words of an answer which trigger in our own mind thoughts, ideas, ways to help, and I-can-top-that stories. We miss all the little clues that tell how a person really feels.
- Before you jump in with your response—wait. Give him some time to think over what he's just said. He may feel the need to elaborate and

men

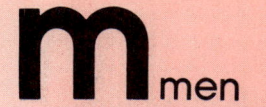

tell you even more.
- Don't constantly punctuate what he's saying with expressions that suggest skepticism like "Really!" "That's unbelievable!" "You've got to be kidding!"
- Avoid asking "Why?" too much; it can be very intimidating.
- Be careful about making nonverbal interruptions. You can lose his confidence as quickly as you won it by fidgeting, failing to maintain eye contact, and transmitting body signals that say "I'm getting restless."
- Listen to what he doesn't say. One well-known and often-interviewed person admitted that the most thought-provoking (and answer-provoking) question anyone ever asked him was, "Why don't you ever speak of your childhood?"

weekend date
how to spend a weekend with a new man— and still be talking on Sunday

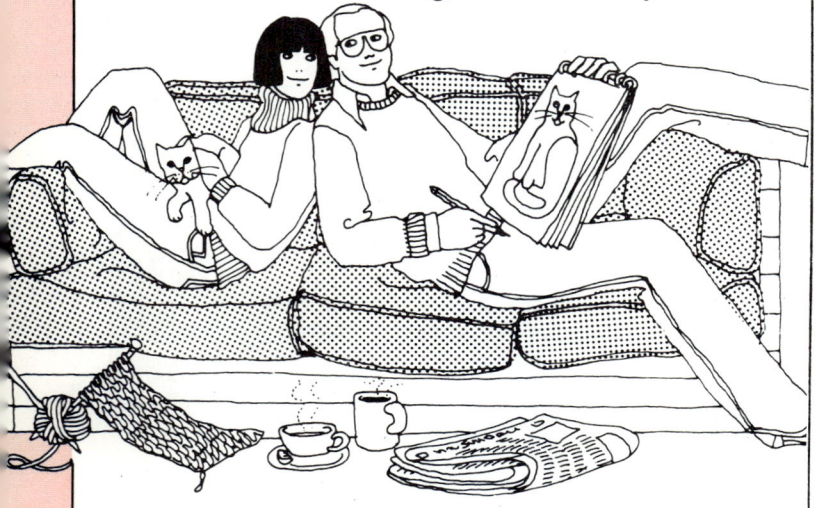

Spending a weekend with a new man in your life usually determines just how compatible the two of you are, but sometimes a romance that might have bloomed gets nipped in the bud because of misplanning. Here's how to avoid some common problems:
- First of all, don't head off into the Friday sunset together until you've learned to relax with each other and talk over your feelings honestly. When you're still in the early stages of a relationship, it's a good idea to hold off on invitations to visit his out-of-town old friends. Those weekends can be awkward, especially if you're the only one who wasn't in the football bleachers the day they beat State U.
- When you decide to go away, determine the sleeping arrangements in advance. If you don't share his bed now and don't intend to start this weekend, make that clear *before* you leave. You may wish to book separate room or hotel accommodations. If you're staying with friends, don't just accept "Oh, there'll be plenty of room" as an answer to your inquiry about sleeping arrangements.
- Don't mind the silences. If you're used to a steady conversational flow on your regular dates with him, those sudden quiet periods during the weekend may bother you, but they're normal when you're with the same person for an extended period of time. Think of the silences as something for the two of you to share and relax in.
- Give yourself some time alone. A sure way to kill a new relationship is overexposure—seeing too much of each other too soon.
- If things go badly, and it appears you're destined to incompatibility, don't pout, sulk, or wallow in misery. Talk over the problem, admit that there are problems, and then enjoy the rest of the weekend as "just friends."

metric system

metric system
do you know how many grams are in one pound or how many kilometers are in a mile?

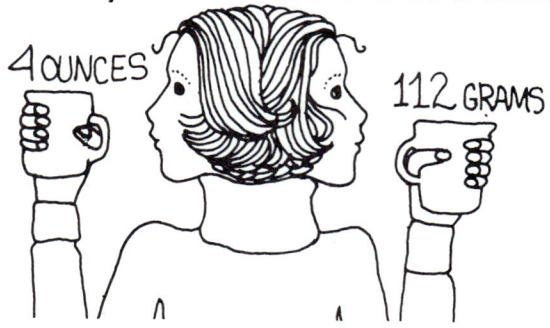

Have you ever tried to figure out how many calories are in six ounces of diet peaches when the can lists calories per hundred *grams*? If so, you've had your brushes with the metric system—and more are coming. So it's a good time to familiarize yourself with the metric system, which will replace ounces, inches, quarts, acres, and Fahrenheit degrees with their equivalents in grams, centimeters, liters, hectares, and centigrade degrees.

The metric system is actually simpler than ours because it's based on powers of 10. There are 10 millimeters in one centimeter, 100 centimeters in one meter, etc. So to figure out how many meters are in 6.2 kilometers, you simply multiply 6.2 by 1,000, or move the decimal point three places to the right.

Besides that knowledge, all you need to understand the metric system is the simple chart below, which should help you prepare for the day when your scale registers a gain of 2.25 kilograms instead of 5 pounds.

- **weight conversions**
1 *ounce*=28 grams
1 *pound*=0.45 kilogram
1 *quart*=0.9 liter
1 *ton*=0.9 megaton
1 *gram*=0.035 ounce
1 *kilogram*=2.2 pounds
1 *liter*=1.06 quart
1 *megaton*=1.1 tons

- **linear conversions**
1 *inch*=2.54 centimeters
1 *foot*=0.3 meter
1 *yard*=0.9 meter
1 *mile*=1.6 kilometers
1 *millimeter*=0.04 inch
1 *meter*=3.3 feet
1 *meter*=1.1 yards
1 *kilometer*=0.6 mile

- **square conversions**
1 *sq inch*=6.5 sq centimeters
1 *sq foot*=0.09 sq meter
1 *sq yard*=0.8 sq meter
1 *acre*=0.4 hectare
1 *sq centimeter*=0.16 sq inch
1 *sq meter*=11 sq feet
1 *sq meter*=1.2 sq yards
1 *hectare*=2.5 acres

- **volume conversions**
1 *cu inch*=16 cu centimeters
1 *cu foot*=0.03 cu meter
1 *cu yard*=0.8 cu meter
1 *gallon*=0.004 centimeter
1 *cu centimeter*=0.06 cu inch
1 *cu meter*=35 cu feet
1 *cu meter*=1.3 cu yards
1 *cu meter*=250 gallons

months

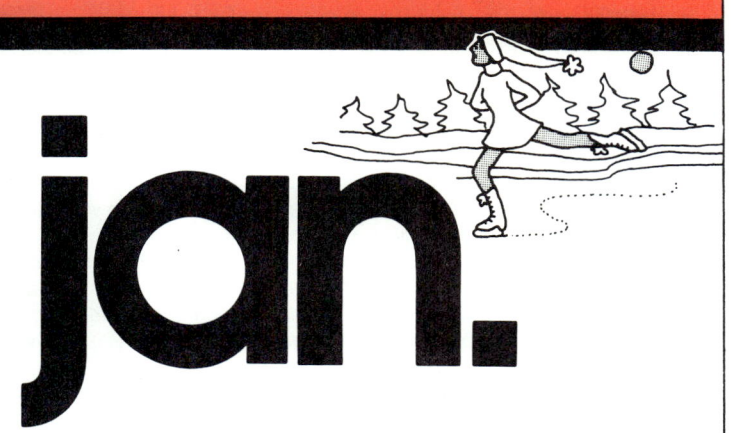

jan.

is a great month for . . .

- Starting a diary you'll really enjoy keeping. Don't tell yourself you have to write in it every day; even great diarists often went weeks without an entry, so why should you force yourself to do otherwise? Let "when-the-spirit-moves-me" be your guide; and for inspiration, pick up *Revelations: Diaries of Women*. It includes sections from the diaries of thirty-two women, including Virginia Woolf, Louisa May Alcott, George Sand, and Anaïs Nin.
- Counteracting winter weight gains with tap, modern, or belly dancing lessons—the theory being that music makes exercise more bearable. Also, any activity that keeps you away from the refrigerator is probably a good thing.
- Helping your plants take cold weather in stride. Keep them away from gusts of cold air from windows or hot air from heating units. Remember that a plant that got enough sun during long summer days may need a brighter spot in winter. In dry rooms, plants may need more frequent mistings. Overly dry air is a breeding ground for spider mites, among other plant disasters. If you can afford it, buy a humidifier—good for the plants and your sinuses.
- Sending for herb and seed catalogs to inspire spring plantings. Besides, there may be days ahead when even a photo of greenery will prove welcome.
- Starting a record of purchases and expenses that can be deducted from your income tax when you file next year. If you conscientiously keep a record, you may discover that you actually have more than the standard deduction. Save all receipts for such things as moving costs, medical expenses (including drugs and birth control), interest on revolving charge accounts, purchases that relate to your work but for which you aren't reimbursed by your company (travel, newspapers, magazines, a telephone answering machine), charity contributions, transportation to volunteer work. Mark all receipts with the date and category they apply to. Star the stubs of checks used.
- Spending a weekend or 24 hours alone with only your cat, gerbil, or whatever pet. No other human. Sitting down and really thinking out an attitude of yours you're not sure of, sewing or crafting, cooking yourself a special dish. Everyone needs a little self-love, selfishness, and privacy after the holiday crowds.
- Turning your big new wall calendar into an easy baby book if there's a new baby under the roof. Leave the calendar in a handy spot, such as the kitchen, and jot down notes about the progress of the child every day. It's a more complete record than occasional notes in a leather-bound album and less time-consuming than a daily diary.
- Not making hard and fast New Year's resolutions, but instead, flexible goals for yourself. Says Alan Lakein in *It's About Time & It's About Time*, "Goals should be written in sand, not in stone, and they should be updated once a month."

- *Filling your window with "hearts-entangled," a charming succulent (Ceropegia woodii) with small heart-shaped leaves. It has vines that can either drape for several feet over the edges of a pot or trail along the ground in a terrarium. Soil should be allowed to dry out between waterings, and with warmth and bright light, there'll be flowers come summer.*
- *Lifting your snow-and-slush spirits with a little something new and bright to wear, right off the sale racks—a red knit cap, yellow knee socks, a boldly striped sweater. It's a sure way to add some spunk to the winter clothes you feel like you've been wearing forever.*
- *Softening your winter-weary skin with real cocoa butter. You can buy inexpensive sticks and bars at your drugstore. Smooth on hands, lips, around eyes, all over a wind-burned face.*
- *Making up for too much sitting and too little exercise by taking a long bath, then trying one of these body massages: (1) Clench fists and knead your thighs in a slow, circular motion. (2) Grasp wrist and firmly twist and release, twist and release, working all the way to your shoulders and back down again. (3) Gently slap yourself all over to work up circulation. (You might first apply a body lotion.)*
- *Putting together a travel valentine for a friend who's often on the road—or with whom you're planning to spend a weekend. Take a bright red bath towel and sew on two face towels for patch pockets. Then fill each pocket with small surprises, like fragrant soap, a tin of pipe tobacco, road maps, and travel guides.*
- *Brushing up on these key winter sports terms:* slalom—*an obstacle-course ski race (*versus *downhill racing,* in which a skier speeds to the finish line); bobsledding—*a race down a high-walled, twisting course in a bobsled, a sled with runners;* tobogganing—*riding a flat-bottomed wood sled, or tobaggan;* luge—*a toboggan race;* school figures—*a figure-skating event in which skaters show off technical maneuvers, such as the figure eight;* free skating—*a skating event using school figures in a dance routine;* curling—*ice bowling with round flat stones.*
- *Ice skating . . . if you skate on an ice-topped pond, lake, or other natural "rink," stay on shallow-water areas close to shore and avoid night skating. Saw through ice to check its thickness (4" is a must), and beware of ice over springs, reservoirs, and other running water; it won't be uniformly thick. Darker color is also a tip-off to thin ice.*
- *Making Five-Minute Fudge for your valentine or your own sweet tooth. Combine 2 T. butter, ⅔ c. evaporated milk, 1⅔ c. sugar, and ½ tsp. salt in a saucepan over medium heat. Bring to boil and cook 4–5 minutes, stirring constantly. Remove from heat. Stir in 2 c. miniature marshmallows, 1½ c. semisweet chocolate pieces, 1 tsp. vanilla, and ½ c. chopped nuts. Stir for one minute, until marshmallows melt. Pour into buttered pan, cool, and cut into squares.*
- *Planning a June-in-February party with lots of bright flowers around, sunny yellow napkins, maybe even a small theatrical spotlight or two with amber filters (a marvelous way to simulate a warm sunlit day) focused on the table, and picnic box lunches for everyone.*

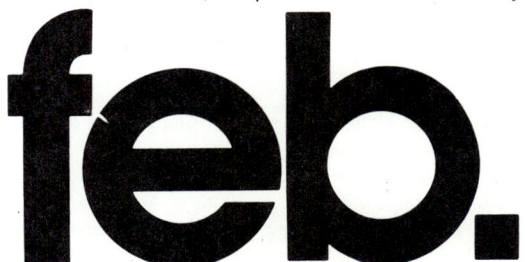

feb.

is a great month for . . .

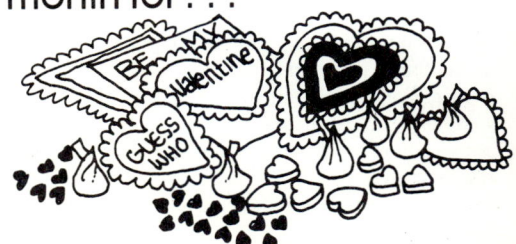

months

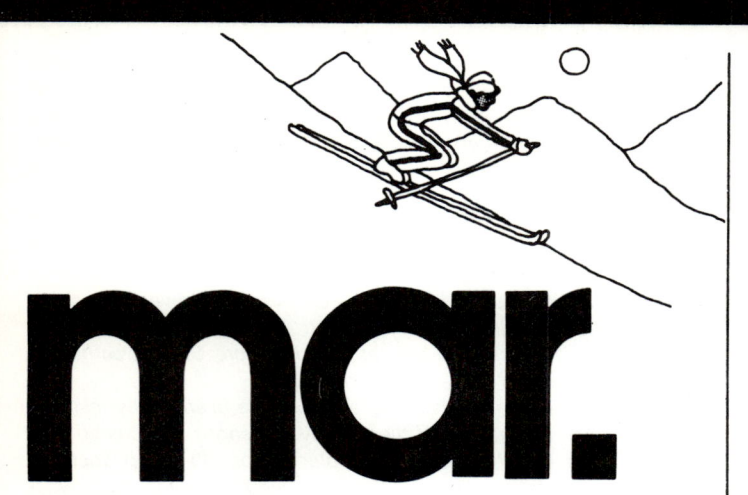

mar. is a great month for...

- Warming up your green thumb. March 17th is pea-planting day out in the country, but if you are stymied either because you're stuck in the city, or because the soil still hasn't thawed enough to be soft and crumbly, you can begin by starting seeds—peas, snapdragons, marigolds, and China asters—indoors.
- Getting a good haircut, having a professional manicure, giving yourself a pedicure, and otherwise catching up on beauty routines you may have missed during the winter.
- Limbering up for spring sports. Can't stick to exercise routines? Try jogging in place to music; the beat picks up where your motivation leaves off. Suggested music to jog by: a Bach Brandenburg Concerto, anything by the early Beatles, or your favorite show tunes.
- Beating winter weight gain with these in-season fruits and vegetables:
Artichoke (small, cooked)—44 calories
Asparagus (2/3 cup cooked)—20 calories
Honeydew (1/8 medium)—33 calories
Pineapple (3/4 cup)—52 calories
Rhubarb (3/4 cup cooked with artificial sweetener)—16 calories
- Remembering to give your plants a healthy dose of plant food once a month, from now through October. Most need it during their spring and summer growing spurts.
- Indulging a St. Patrick's Day sweet tooth with a cool, mint-green dessert called Grasshopper Parfait. To make it, melt 12 marshmallows in 1/2 c. milk in the top of a double boiler and cool. Add 1 to 2 oz. each of créme de menthe and creme de cacao. Fold the mixture into a pint of whipped cream and chill. Top with chocolate cookie crumbs.
- Not getting stranded at the airport over Easter vacation. Places like Bermuda, Jamaica, and the Bahamas don't require passports. But, regardless of what a travel agent may tell you, they do require proof of U.S. citizenship, which boils down to almost the same thing—a passport or birth certificate. So before you go, check with your local passport office.
- Picking up needed ski and skate gear, small appliances, or a sewing machine at the sales stores are having now.
- Getting your bike in shape for the longer trips you may be taking when the weather warms up. The Bicycle Institute of America warns you to park your bike in a dry place and keep its chain, gear apparatus, and other movable parts lightly oiled. Before riding, check that handlebars and saddle are secure, foot and hand brakes grip, accessories like reflectors are securely fastened, light batteries work, and the tire treads are free of glass or other particles that might cause a blowout.
- Starting a vacation account for a trip you'd like to take this summer or next. Two possibilities for your "Provence or Bust" fund: check into whether or not your company has a payroll savings plan you can join, or buy a time certificate (available for periods such as ninety days and one year) at a bank. The interest on a time certificate is higher than that on a regular savings account, and you won't be as tempted to withdraw from it.

- Learning a new sport. As long as it makes you feel great, you'll stick with it—and as a bonus, here are some of the calories you'll burn up in one hour of each of the following: biking—210; walking (slowly)—210; walking (briskly)—300; roller skating—350; tennis—420; squash and handball—600; running—900.
- Heading off the June passport office crunch by applying for a passport now. Even if you're not sure you'll be able to swing a trip during the summer, passports are good for five years.
- Planning a long May weekend in the U.S. or Caribbean. In the Caribbean, most hotel and other rates go down April 15. Plan now for the Memorial Day weekend. When you travel in May in the U.S.A., you miss the summer hordes, and hotels are busy sprucing up the premises and beefing up their staffs for the coming onslaught. So you can expect top-notch service and balmy weather.
- Switching from pie or cake desserts to festive fruit-based ones. Poires Hélène is a snap to make. Top one canned pear half with a scoop of vanilla ice cream, some chocolate sauce, and a dollop of Cointreau-flavored whipped cream—made from a half-pint of heavy cream plus about 2 T. Cointreau for four servings.
- Taking advantage of spring weather by walking a dog from your local pet shelter. Shelters need volunteers for other things, too—from showing puppies and kittens to prospective parents, to bathing animals and doing clerical work. Check the Yellow Pages for a shelter near you, or write for an address from the American Humane Association, 5351 South Rosyln, Englewood, CO 80110.
- Keeping your raincoat clean and ready for duty, which involves distinguishing between the terms water-repellent and waterproof. Repellent means chemically treated fabric, which should be dry cleaned and eventually re-treated. Waterproof fabric (with a rubberized or plastic finish) is impermeable and often can't be dry cleaned. Sponge it off with mild soap and water, or try a bit of abrasive household cleanser like Ajax on badly soiled areas. (Test this first on the inside hem and always rub gently.)
- Celebrating with someone who gets one of the college acceptances that pour in around April 15th. You might find out what city he or she will be in and give a gift of a newspaper or magazine subscription, or a gift certificate for a restaurant or department store.
- Planting at least one thing. April is the best time to start an avocado plant because during April, the seeds are naturally ready to germinate. You're practically guaranteed success if you use a green-skinned fruit. Chop off a bit at the top and bottom of the pit, and then suspend it in warm water, fat end down, by the toothpick method. Change water frequently and keep seed in warm place out of direct sunlight. In about six weeks, you'll see roots extending down into the water and green sprouts at the top. Now is the time to plant your pit, putting roots in potting soil in a clay pot. First, put a few stones or bits of an old broken pot in the bottom for drainage. Water with water from the jar the seed sprouted in so it doesn't get homesick at the beginning.
- Roller skating your way to class, to a friend's house, or just around the block for the fun of it. You can buy skates that clip on to just about any size shoe. There's nothing like their sound on well-worn sidewalks.
- Moving outdoors for the things you usually do indoors—like going to the season's first drive-in movies.

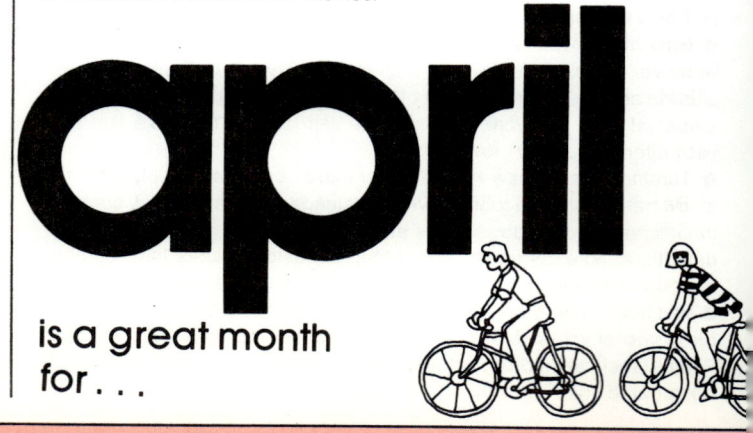

april is a great month for...

months **m**

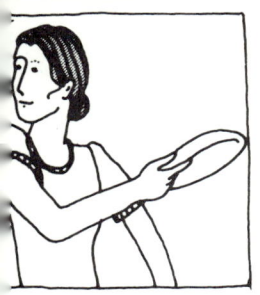

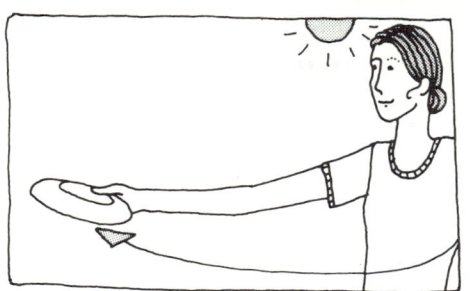

may
is a great month for...

- Throwing your Frisbee to the wind—but taking care not to develop a case of "Frisbee finger." Described in the *New England Journal of Medicine*, "Frisbee finger" is a blister or abrasion on the thumb side of the middle finger on the throwing hand, and abstinence is the only known cure. If you're forced to stop flinging, use the healing time to read up on the sport in *Frisbee* by Dr. Stancil E. Johnson.
- Celebrating Walpurgis Night. It's the eve of May 1 (which is the feast of St. Walpurgis) and according to old German folklore, a night much like Halloween when witches gather together. It's also a night for fantasizing, forgetting, and letting go of inhibitions without need of excuse.
- Planting a small tree in your yard or giving some loving care to a neglected one on a city street, maybe by watering it on dry spring and summer days or trimming weeds to keep it healthy. You'll boost the environment, because trees muffle noise, release fresh oxygen into the air, and help conserve energy by shading houses in summer and shielding them from cold winds in winter—cutting down the need for air conditioning and home heating.
- Perking up spring salads with seasonal vegetables such as fresh raw string beans or broad beans or some crunchy raw green peas. Toss with romaine lettuce and a mustard-based vinaigrette dressing.
- Checking with your local plant store to see which houseplants can or can't be safely moved outdoors later in May when it's warmer. For example, African violets are poor risks, but geraniums will thrive.
- Giving a May wine party with punch made from two bottles of May wine to one bottle of club soda, plus fresh strawberries and lemon sherbet to taste. May wine is a young German white wine that gets its spicy flavor and aroma from the addition of herbs, such as woodruff. It's also great served plain, accompanied by crackers and a bland cheese.
- Planning your strategy for Memorial Day weekend. Have your car checked for long-distance travel (tire pressure, for instance, may need to be changed). If your holiday traveling will take you away from your plants past the time they should be watered, you might find a florist or five-and-dime that sells small plant feeders or bulbs that release water to the plant over a period of days.
- Hunting for a bathing suit while stores still have lots to choose from.
- Beachcombing for shells and driftwood before crowds come.
- Shopping for shoes, jewelry, luggage, and indoor furniture, all of which go on sale in May, according to the National Retail Merchants Association. If you missed the January white sales, many stores have them again now.
- Taking any preschooler on a first visit to a florist or flower show. Around Memorial Day she'll stare saucer-eyed at the display—snapdragons, stock, iris, tulips, narcissus.

- Adding bright flowering plants to your collection of green ones. Fuchsia, golden marigolds, coral to magenta petunias, and paper white gardenias are just some varieties in bloom during June. They need plenty of sun and water (more than you'd provide for nonflowering potted plants) to stay alive and well all through summer.
- Swimming with a kickboard to get your legs in shape. Buy one at a sporting goods store for about $3 and use it to tone up muscles—kicking deep under water without making a big splash.
- Giving a really unusual wedding or graduation present: if you own a good cassette recorder, offer to tape all or part of the wedding or graduation ceremony (or the best man's toast).
- Understanding these professional moving terms if you're switching to a new home (June is a peak moving time): carrier—the moving company; shipper—you; tariff—mover's price list for services; accessorial services—extras you can ask for and will be charged for (like packing and unpacking, moving a piano up flights of stairs, preparing a refrigerator for the move); inventory—descriptive list of your goods and their condition; bill of lading—itemized receipt for your goods plus contract to move them; claim—your statement of goods lost or damaged.
- Marinating fresh pineapple slices in rum for a great summer dessert. Pineapples are in season; you can tell one's ripe if a spoke comes out easily when tugged. (The best pineapples are also heavy for their size and have a sweet fragrance.)
- Serving white and rosé wines instead of full-bodied red ones. They're lighter wines that go better with casual meals of fish or salad. And unlike red wines, which are usually served at room temperature, whites and rosés are chilled—so they're great summer coolers. If you prefer red wine, you might try mixing your favorite with an equal amount of chilled soda water, then adding a twist of fragrant lemon or lime peel.
- Changing perfumes to match the sheer, summer clothes you're wearing. You might want to select a lighter fragrance or the cologne of your regular perfume, since heat and perspiration tend to intensify scent. Also, as you spend more time in the sun, dab perfume on covered-up parts of your body only, says Dr. Arthur W. Glick, chief of dermatology at Mount Sinai Hospital in New York. This protects you from redness or brown spots that may appear on skin that's been rubbed with certain perfume oils, then exposed to sun.
- Keeping an eye peeled for sales on underthings and lingerie, panty stockings, sleepwear, shoes, and especially men's and boys' wear, perhaps in the nick of time for Father's Day. Many stores have sales on these now; a few may throw in bargains on bedding and floor coverings, too.
- Having a Midsummer Eve Party on June 21, the longest day of the year. Make it an all-night outdoor revel, as the northern countries do to break the tension of winter.

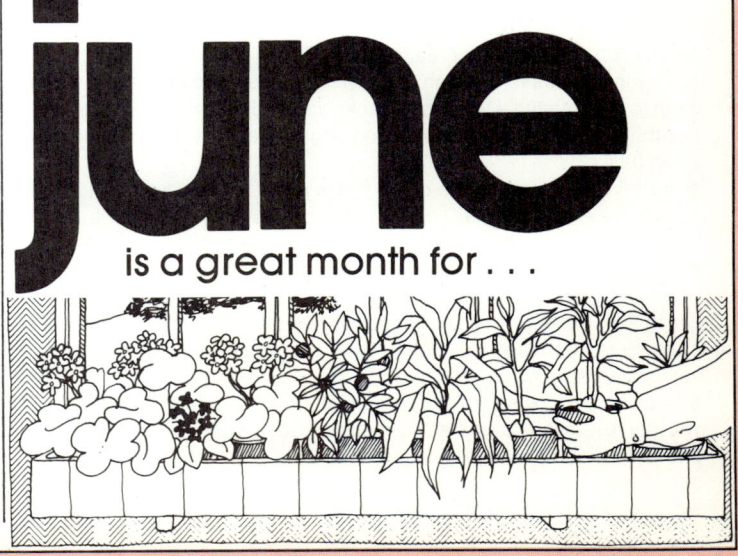

june
is a great month for...

months

july is a great month for...

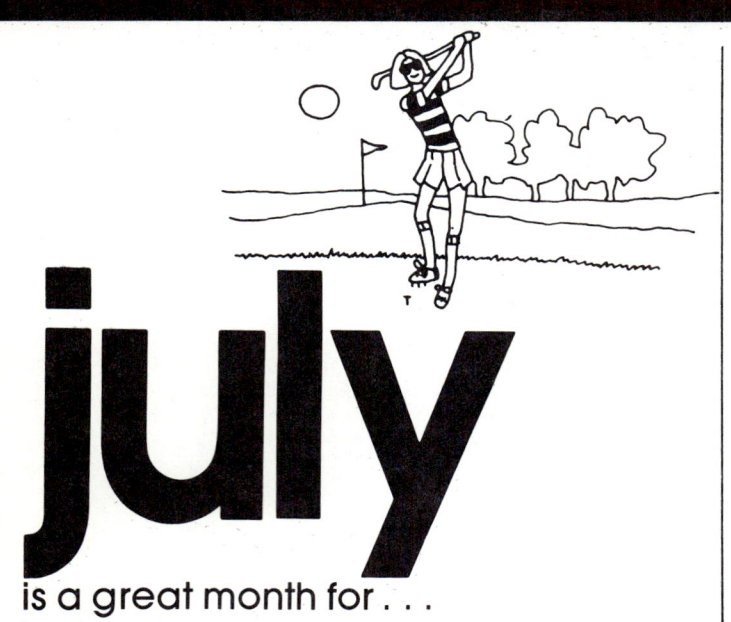

- Improving your tennis game fast with a concentrated dose of lessons and practice at one of the many tennis camps springing up all over the country. The sessions last anywhere from one to eight weeks, are open to advanced players or beginners, and can cost you anywhere from about $150 to a hefty $350 a week for room, board, and lessons. For a list of camps nationwide, send $1 to the U.S. Tennis Association, Education & Research Center, 71 University Place, Princeton, NJ 08540.
- Organizing a block bazaar to raise money for outdoor gardening or tighter security in your area. Be sure to contact the police a few weeks in advance to see if licenses are required to close off the street or set up sale booths. Also check with your department of parks and recreation; many will provide free puppet shows, game mobiles, and other entertainment.
- Dressing up your bed with new sheets and pillowcases in bright summer colors bought at July white sales. As an alternative to more expensive designer prints, why not try mixing and matching solids—maybe pillowcases in lemon yellow plus sky blue sheets.
- Taking stem cuttings from your favorite house plants, now that they're going through a summer spurt and will benefit from some cutting back. Just remember that not all plants propagate by stem cuttings. Wandering Jew, philodendron, Swedish ivy, and coleus do and are some of the easiest plants to work with. Check with your plant store if in doubt about others.
- Giving Irish coffee a summer twist by serving it iced. You'll need: 1 tray coffee ice cubes (crushed), ½ c. Irish whiskey, 2 c. strong coffee sweetened with 3 T. sugar, and chilled whipped cream. Fill 4 glasses with crushed ice. To each one add 2 T. whiskey, chilled coffee, and stir gently. Top with whipped cream.
- Turning the beach into an exercise mat—you don't have to just lie there to get your tan. Do jumping jacks, leg and arm stretches, upside-down "bicycling," or try organizing a game of beach badminton or volleyball.
- Sending for college catalogs if you're out of school but plan to take a course or two next fall. You'll probably have to register in early September, so decide now what you want—or can afford—to take.
- Taking advantage of blueberry season by whipping up this fresh blueberry sauce to serve over peach or another favorite ice cream. Crush 2 c. fresh berries in saucepan. Mix in ⅓ c. sugar, 1 T. lemon juice, ½ tsp. salt, and boil one minute, stirring constantly. Add ½ tsp. vanilla and chill. Makes 1½ c.
- Picking your own berries for the sauce above. Many farms will let you harvest bushels of fresh produce—berries, corn, green beans, whatever is in season—for lots less than retail price. And as a side benefit you'll soak up the sun and breathe clean country air. (Check with the local chamber of commerce for farms that welcome outsiders.)

- Planting a last-minute summer vegetable garden. Early in August, you can still sow seeds for carrots, spinach, kale, and radishes (check a garden-supply store for other possibilities), and you'll have fresh food to harvest right up to the first frost, usually in November.
- Doing as many of your regular exercises as you can in the water instead of out of it. If you're an exercise slouch, you might try this underwater hip and thigh shape-up for starters: Stand in chest-high water, right side to the dock or swimming pool edge. Hold on for balance and swing your left leg in wide circles—5 forward, 5 back. Then turn so your left side is to the dock and repeat circles with right leg.
- Checking out summer clothing sales for pieces that can carry you all through fall and winter. It's easy now that khaki and denim have become seasonless. Look for sundresses and pinafores that you can layer over long-sleeved T-shirts or sweaters as the weather becomes cooler. Look, too, for heavier cottons and synthetics in tartan plaids, muted or dark colors; they'll run you the year long and save money in the process.
- Buying camping equipment, which often starts going on sale during August—take advantage of the good buys.
- Getting the sneakers you spent a mint for back into shape if they've had a rough workout during the summer. For $13.95, Tred 2 will resole almost any pair of athletic shoes, patch up tears in the body of the shoes, and add new insoles and laces. Put check or money order inside shoes and mail to: Tred 2, 2510 Channing Ave., San Jose, CA 95131 (allow about two weeks for delivery); or see if a sporting goods store near you has a "Resole Bag" in which you can mail in your shoes.
- Keeping your beach towel or blanket neatly earthbound without piling up lots of loose clutter around the edges. Sew small ribbon or cord loops to each corner, then anchor loops to the sand with plastic tent pegs (6" pegs cost about 25¢ each at any sporting goods store).
- Brushing up your tennis vocabulary. Here's a quick guide: lob—a high, soft shot; volley—a ball hit before it bounces; overhead smash—hitting down hard on a ball; ground strokes—the most common tennis strokes, hit on the bounce in a straight line over the net; service ace—a serve hit so hard or placed so well that it can't be returned; fault—an unsuccessful serve; double fault—losing a point on two improper serves.
- Making a mini-plan for medical emergencies. If your doctor is on vacation (lots are in August, including psychiatrists), check who's covering and jot down the number. If you're deep in the country, call the nearest hospital or medical college for recommendations; note the number of the State Highway Patrol. If you're overseas, call the American embassy for its approved list of doctors.
- Buying that new car you've been eyeing for months in the showroom window. New models appear in the fall, so many dealers start to cut prices on this year's models during August.
- Cutting calories by thinking fish or seafood. For example, cod, flounder, and sea trout (East Coast), abalone and Alaskan crab (West Coast), or whitefish and carp (Midwest) are more abundant in summer and prices should be lower.

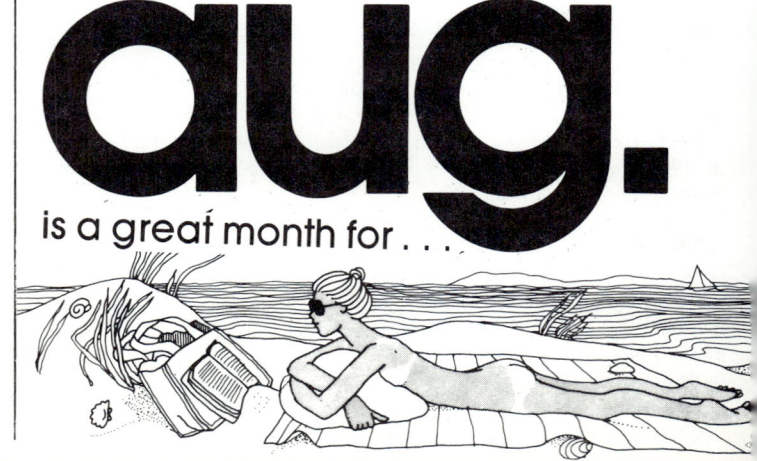

aug. is a great month for....

months m

sept.
is a great month for...

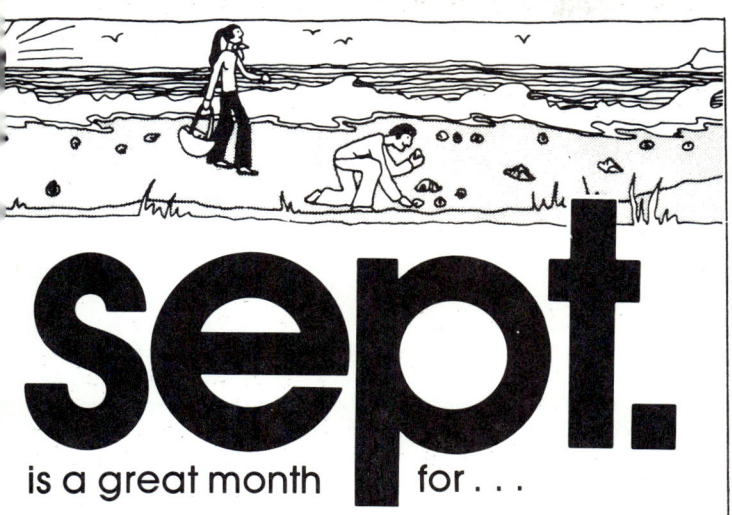

- Taking advantage of the "walking weather"—and whether you're interested in a nature walk or a mountain climb, you can write for coast-to-coast information on walking clubs to The Sierra Club, 530 Bush St., San Francisco, CA 94108. If you want more specifics about your state's club, write to its recreation department for names and addresses.
- Not being astounded if your nails grow more slowly or chip and break more easily now. That's normal in cooler weather. Give them extra care—perhaps nail hardener over a base coat.
- Brushing up on your "landlord-ese." The following are terms any apartment-dweller or renter should know, especially during September, which is a peak moving month. *Property manager/agent*—person or group running an owner's property for him, in charge of everything from negotiating leases to hiring the superintendent; *escalator clause* (in a lease)—lets the landlord charge you a percentage of his rising costs, (for example, the cost of fuel); *guarantor*—someone who either endorses the lease or signs a separate agreement to pay your rent if you don't (if you're a student, your parent may have to be one); *rider*—a clause added to a standard lease, (for instance a special ban on pets or waterbeds); *waiver*—lease clause that says you give up a right you're entitled to, such as a periodic paint job. If a waiver appears in your lease and you're not sure of its implications, consult a lawyer before signing the lease.
- Planting your favorite flower bulbs so you'll have blooming gifts for friends by Christmas or thereabouts. Crocus or miniature narcissus are good choices, and your local florist can suggest others (just make sure he knows you want them ready for the holidays). The Brooklyn Botanic Garden staff suggests this easy procedure for planting your bulbs: Fill a 3" to 4" pot with sandy soil and pot your bulb so that it is barely covered. Water well, then place plant (pot and all) in an airtight plastic bag to seal in moisture. Cover with a brown paper bag to keep out light and refrigerate for 6–8 weeks. (You're "forcing" the winter hibernation the plant would go through outdoors.) After that, remove your bulb from cold storage and gradually shift it from semishade to full sunlight on a cool windowsill (without a radiator underneath). It should bloom in a few weeks.
- Boning up on football terms in case you're not dedicated to what's going on out there during an average 150-minute game—and your husband or friends are. Surprise them by knowing such catchy terms as: *red dog*—when a swarm of linebackers tries to cross the scrimmage line (where each play starts) to stop the opposing team's quarterback from getting the ball into action after he receives it from the center lineman; *bootleg*—a sneaky maneuver by the quarterback as he fakes handing the ball to another runner and instead hides it against his hip and runs with it himself; *button hook*—pass pattern in which the receiver runs straight down the field, then turns and runs back a few yards to face the passer and catch the ball; *offside*—when either team crosses the scrimmage line before the ball has been put into action; *clipping*—contacting any player except the ball carrier from behind could cause serious injuries, so there's a 15-yard penalty for it.

- Trying Gourmet Popping Corn developed by Orville Redenbacher. Here are some of his tips: Use 3 parts corn to 1 part oil. If you use a pan instead of a regular popcorn popper, be sure the bottom is good and heavy—an iron pan, for example—and that there is a lid to allow the steam to escape. When the corn has popped, add butter, ½ tsp. each garlic and onion salt, grated Cheddar cheese and toss together. Place in a 325° F. oven for 5–10 minutes, stir gently, and serve.
- Putting your houseplants on a diet by suspending monthly feedings. Most plants have a dormancy period that lasts from roughly mid-October through February, and during this time they should not get their usual doses of plant food.
- Boning up on pumpkin consumerism. You're likely to get bargain prices at a farmer's market or rural roadside stand. A round shape is a plus for jack-o'-lanterns and there are prime varieties for carving (with names like Spooky and Funny Face). You can cook and eat them, too. But Cheese pumpkins or small Sugar pumpkins—both rare finds—have better texture, if cooking is your prime concern. Ask a grower if he has them. And watch for soft spots or punctures, which signal mold.
- Getting Halloween thrills with records such as "Tales of Witches, Ghosts and Goblins" read by Vincent Price, or stories of Hawthorne or Poe read by Basil Rathbone (all three on Caedmon Records).
- Cultivating the tradition of afternoon tea. Agree upon a time and place to meet with friends; it's a lovely at-home or going-out idea. Experiment by steeping some of the unusual teas—cinnamon, rose, or orange and spice. Or be more adventurous and try a jasmine with real blossoms floating in the cup. If you're going to be very traditional about it, try crumpets (little muffins) or take turns bringing cheese, crackers, and fruit to go with your tea. A plate of homemade cookies or sliced sweetbread would be a great idea, too.
- Getting a head start on some unique Christmas cards. Instead of the usual run-of-the-mill sort, use the beautiful art reproduction cards put out by famous museums. To get a catalog to order cards from, send 50¢ to: Boston Museum of Fine Arts Catalog, Museum Shop, P.O. Box 3, Boston, MA 02112. Or send $1 to: Metropolitan Museum of Art Catalog, 255 Gracie Station, New York, NY 10028. Allow three to four weeks for delivery. For the Los Angeles County Museum of Art catalog, send $1 to its Museum Shop at 5905 Wilshire Blvd., Los Angeles, CA 90036.
- Shaping up your legs for skiing with this exercise used by the U.S. Women's Ski Team: Stand on toes and lean forward—arms over knees—alternating jumps in place with short-distance jumps.
- Giving your diet and budget a hand by stocking up on local fish bargains such as East Coast mackerel, bluefish, and porgies, or West Coast halibut and king salmon. And for an exotic change of pace, why not try oysters, too?
- Getting some bright ideas on room-planning from home-furnishings promotions at local department stores.

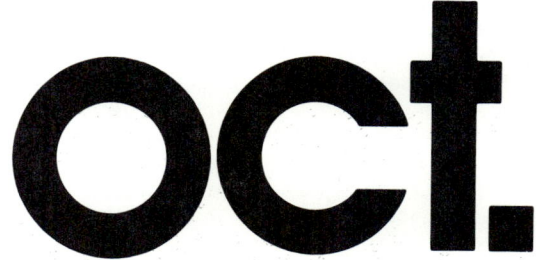

oct.
is a great month for...

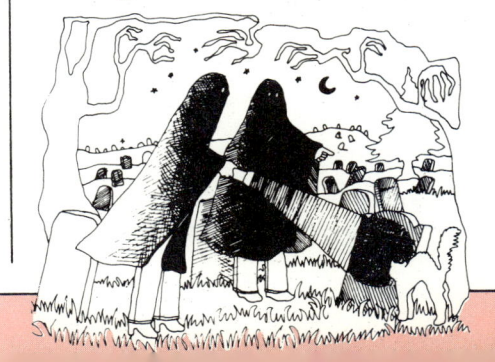

125

m months

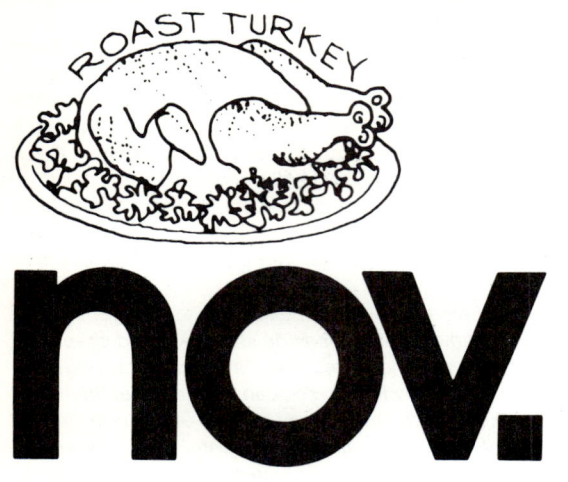

nov. is a great month for...

- Mailing Christmas packages to Asia by the first week of November, to ensure that they reach their destinations on time.
- Sharing your Thanksgiving dinner with a foreign student. For a student who'd like to be adopted for the day, call the International House of a nearby college and ask the head resident for help.
- Tuning up winter sports gear. A ski shop will adjust and release-check your bindings to see that they release properly, as well as clean and silicone them. Ski edges should be sharpened and the bottoms flat-filled and waxed. Ice skates should also be sharpened by a reputable shop—a bad job can make you veer to one side or stick to the ice. Rub boots with a penetrating leather conditioner (avoid heel area, or "counter," which must stay hard for good support). Also, protect soles with waterproofing enamel or spray.
- Giving your hands some cold-weather first aid. Be sure that the rubber gloves you use for household chores are cotton-lined; otherwise perspiration will add to dry skin irritation.
- Making last-minute holiday reservations by calling the Independent Reservations System—a computerized clearinghouse for over 1,400 hotels and motels in the continental U.S., Canada and seven European countries. Their toll-free number operates 24 hours a day (800-323-1776 all over the U.S. except Illinois, where it's 800-942-8888). You just phone in where you're going, when, and how much you can spend. The computer does the rest.
- Buying at least one glittery something to wear for the holiday parties. A sleek sweater with gold or silver threads knotted in would be a pretty touch for a long or short skirt or pants. If your budget is stretched about as far as it will go, buy a new golden, pewter, or bronzy eye shadow to glow on holiday eyes.
- Giving autumn salads extra flavor by starting your own mint, tarragon, chive, and other herb vinegars to use in the dressing. Steep 2 T. dried herbs (or ½ c. fresh) in a mixture of ½ pt. white vinegar and ½ pt. dry white wine for 2-3 weeks. Strain and bottle.
- Heading off the possibility of hitting rock bottom in your checking account two weeks before Christmas. It's easy if you apply now for credit cards that can give your checkbook a reprieve during those hard-pressed weeks. Some department stores even have special holiday plans under which you won't be billed for December purchases until January or February.
- Giving your pet a bath before cold weather makes it an impossibility. Six months is a long time to go with an unbathed dog leaping in and out of your lap.
- Taking advantage of Indian summer weather with a day trip to an Indian reservation. Tribes from Alaska to Florida plan special dinners on Thanksgiving and have craft exhibits, rodeos, and powwows other times during the year.
- Heading south to resort islands if you're a sea, not ski, girl. Most prices are still on summer's lower rates during November, and you have till December 15 to take advantage of them.

- Dazzling them. When you're off on the party circuit dressed in glittery evening wear, why not top off the look with some sparkle in your hair? Buy plastic containers of glitter in the notions department of the dime store—sparkling flecks of gold or silver or red—and brush the glitter into your hair. A little hair spray will help hold them in place.
- Jogging, jogging out into the cold, brisk air. According to Pete Schuder, track coach at Columbia University, it's a good idea to do a little stretching or jogging in place before you leave the house, to get your heart pumping faster; and bundle up a bit—a track suit would be good. Fingers and ears are the areas most sensitive to cold, so wear gloves and a hat or earmuffs.
- Giving yourself a beauty present for Christmas. Pick one thing you've never had done professionally (a facial, eyebrow tweezing, or deep-conditioning for hair), then duck into a good salon to have it done. Call first to check prices; they may be more (or less) than you expected. For example, a top-flight New York salon might charge $3.50 for an eyebrow tweezing, $15 for a facial, $10 for a conditioning.
- Stocking the trunk of your car with the essentials of winter driving. Include shovel, salt and sand, traction mats, a can of window spray de-icer, ice scraper, antifreeze, rags, booster cables, flashlight, emergency blinker, and first-aid kit.
- Knowing what items cannot be sent legally through the U.S. mail—especially when you're mailing Christmas packages. Among other things, the list of nonmailable materials includes intoxicating liquors (beverages of .5 percent or more alcoholic content—this does not include items such as rum-filled candies); perishable food if it cannot reach its destination in good condition within the normal transit time between the mailing and address points; narcotics; parcels containing furs, hides, skins, or pelts of wild animals that are not properly dried or cured, have an offensive odor, or are not plainly labeled; flammable material (this includes strike-anywhere matches; safety matches may be mailed if they are tightly packed to prevent movement and ignition); lottery tickets (this includes chain letters). If you have any questions, check the Postal Service Manual at your local post office.
- Treating the poinsettias you're given as houseplants rather than as holiday decorations. With proper care, they'll bloom for over a month. Place the plants near a sunny window and water them as soon as the soil feels dry. If you're not too impatient, you can have color again next Christmas. Trim off red as well as green wilted leaves and keep the soil moist through winter. When spring arrives, cut the stems back to about 6" and start watering more liberally. Cuttings can be rooted in vermiculite or damp sand. From October through November, the plants must have a completely natural light cycle—so put them in a dark closet when you turn the lights on in the evening and take them out in the morning. Then wait for the blooming.

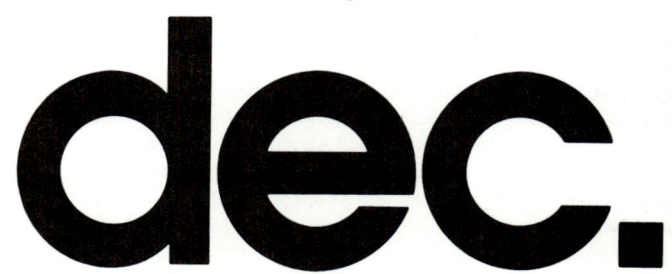

dec. is a great month for...

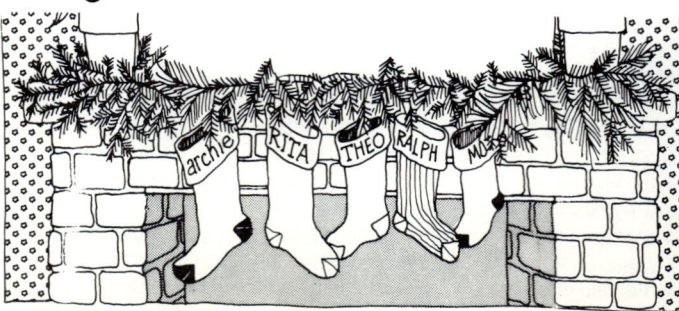

movies

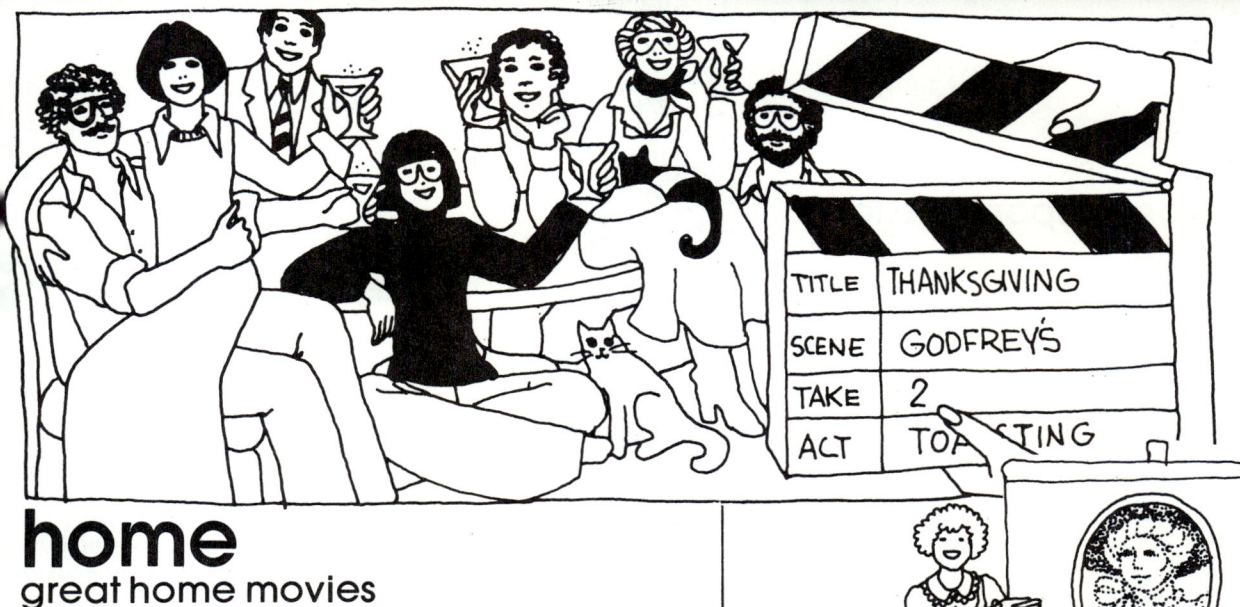

home
great home movies that let you keep your friends

Most people traveling in strange places become so overwhelmed by the subject they are filming that they pan for a moment, then realize that they have just passed something interesting, go back to shoot it, continue panning, and go through the same process at the next point of interest. The finished film looks as though the camera had been operated by an electric typewriter that automatically returned to the left when the bell rang.

Look carefully at the whole scene before you film—foreground, background, sky, details. Be sure you have a picture within the frame that interests you and shoot only that.

Collecting shots: What do you dig? Taxi drivers? Stray dogs? Buildings? Doors were the subject of one recently seen home movie. The traveler shot Georgian doors in Dublin and empty, forlorn-looking doorways in Paris.

Editing: Throw out your mistakes. Don't expose your friends to them. Or if you must save them, cut them out of your film and put them on another reel for your personal viewing.

Don't be afraid to change chronology. If the first few days of travel shots seem less exciting than others, edit the sequences by splicing in a few of your grander moments.

Sun and shadow: Don't leave your camera at the hotel on a cloudy day. A heavily overcast sky will give you some of the most brilliant color you ever shot. If you're shooting people on a very sunny day, try to shoot them in open shade; the dark shadows cast by features in the sun make people look like Frankenstein's monster.

The nature of movies: Don't photograph groups of people standing still. Have them walking or moving in some way; move the camera slowly over the subjects. Shoot from moving vehicles—trains, buses, cars. The results will be real motion pictures, not just very expensive stills.

Titles: Filming titles after the fact can be expensive and time-consuming. Look around for a title that already exists—the name of the city on a sign at the airport or on the road.

Showing your films: Call your friends, tell them you're having a screening, and let them decide if they want to come. Most of them will. After all, how many of them were in Greece, Turkey, or even Ohio last year?

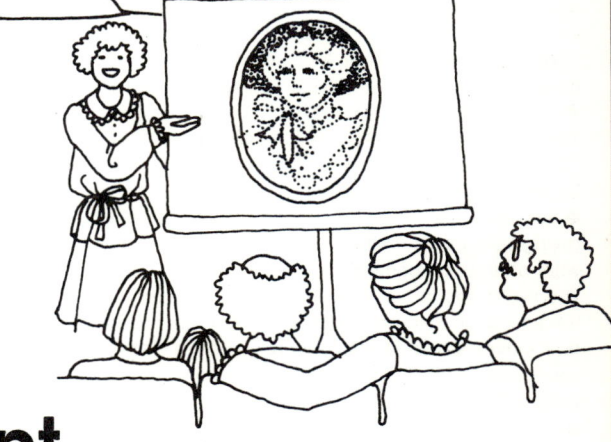

rent a movie
for a party or just for fun

Renting a movie isn't as expensive and complicated as you might have thought. For one showing on one day, rental rates range from $40 to $250 per film, depending, of course, on the prestige and glitter linked to the film and its stars. Usually, two of the conditions on renting are that no admission fee be charged and that the showings will not be open to the public.

Film libraries stock 16 mm sound, full-length motion pictures in color and in black and white. You can get anything from movies as well-known as *True Grit* and *Rosemary's Baby* to some that never quite made it at the box office.

Films Incorporated is one of the more extensive film libraries, with branches across the country in Atlanta, Dallas, Hayward (the San Francisco Bay area), Hollywood, New York City, Salt Lake City, and Skokie (Chicago). Write for their free 370-page, illustrated catalog, which includes short synopses of the films, rental rates, and conditions and order forms. (Send $1 for postage and handling to Films Incorporated, 440 Park Ave. South, New York, NY 10016.) If you rent films by mail, you must pay postage and handling both ways. You should place your order at least one month in advance of the date you want to show the film. Look under "Motion Picture Film Libraries" and "Motion Picture Equipment & Supplies Renting" (16 mm sound projectors can be rented for about $20 to $25 a day) in your Yellow Pages for more information.

m moving

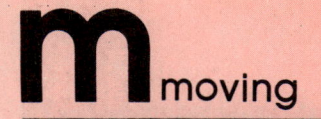

moving

rights
your moving rights:
what you're responsible for,
what movers are responsible for

One woman who moved from Massachusetts to Virginia found that her mover had lost or damaged 87 items en route. In Laguna Beach, California, another woman lost possessions and a chunk of her new house after a moving van rolled down a hill and crashed into it. Such rare catastrophes or other, minor problems inevitably cause headaches. To avoid them, know the responsibilities you and your mover have.

● **on local and intrastate moves**
Your rights depend on the state you live in because intrastate moves are regulated by state rather than Federal agencies. If you have questions, call the agency or department that regulates the moving industry in your state; in New York, for example, it's the Department of Transportation. This agency may have a booklet outlining your moving rights.

● **on interstate moves**
Your key rights are listed below; others are included in the booklet, "Summary of Information for Shippers of Household Goods," provided by your mover.

● An interstate mover is required by law to see your goods before giving you an estimate of how much it will cost to move them, so be wary of any company that gives you a final estimate over the phone. The exact cost of your move cannot be determined until your household goods are weighed after being loaded into the van.

● A mover is permitted to charge you extra for packing and unpacking your goods and for the cartons or containers the mover provides. But, if you prefer to pack or unpack yourself, a mover must allow you to do so.

● Plan to be at your new residence before the movers arrive. Most movers specify that they will wait only three hours for you to show up; after that, the mover can place your goods in storage at your expense. If your mover is a no-show without notifying you in advance, you may be entitled to the cost of motel rooms, furniture rental, or other expenses. (See below for how to file a claim.)

● At the time of delivery, a mover has a right to ask you to pay no more than 10 percent above the estimate you were quoted. (Payment must be made in cash, money order, or cashier's check unless other arrangements have been made.) If the actual cost turns out to be more than 10 percent above the estimate, the mover must give you fifteen business days to pay the rest.

● You should understand the mover's liability to you in case of damage or loss; this is by far the biggest bone of contention in moving. An explanation of the methods for declaring value on goods may be obtained from your mover or the "Summary." Whichever you choose, the most important thing is to ask your mover what any policy will mean in concrete terms. For example, if a mover assures you that your "entire shipment" is covered for $5,000, ask how much you can expect to be reimbursed if one glass-top coffee table is broken. Will you be repaid its full value or only a certain number of dollars per pound of its weight? Remember, too, that the mover's liability is usually not for what the goods cost new but for their depreciated value at the time of shipment. If you have valuable antiques, heirlooms, or anything that you want to be fully covered under all circumstances, then you will need a special "all risks" policy. Ask an insurance agent about a "trip transit" policy, which covers goods being moved from point of pick-up to point of delivery.

● You should file a loss or damage claim as soon as possible, but you have up to nine months after you move. Your mover must respond in writing to such a claim within thirty days and propose a settlement within 120 days. If the company seems to be dragging its feet, a call to your nearest Interstate Commerce Commission office may speed things up—and if you continue to get unsatisfactory response from the mover, you can sue.

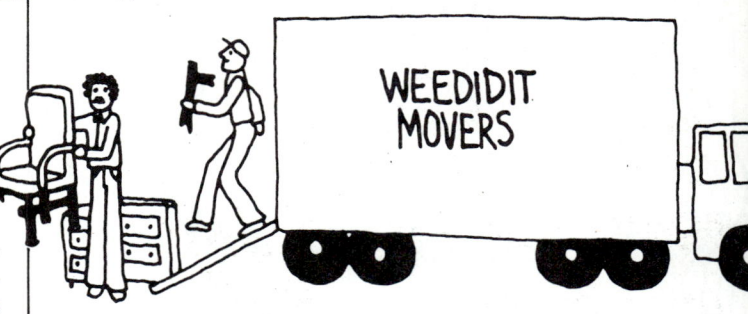

survival kits
for a new dorm, house, or apartment

Before moving day arrives, set aside two boxes, preferably marked or decorated to stand out clearly from the others you've packed. Label the first, "Indispensables—Me"; the second, "Indispensables—House (Dorm or Apartment)."

Into the first, put a handful of items you can't live without or that make you feel so much better you'd prefer not to. These might include a cup, pot, and small jar of coffee; a favorite book or magazine; stationery, pen, and stamps; aspirin; a pretty plant; cigarettes and ashtray if you smoke; and a small transistor radio. Try not to let this box be put into a car, truck, or moving van where it may become lost or buried. Kept handy, it can tide you over while you wait for your roommate to arrive, the movers to unload the furniture, or the telephone installer to show up. Without the box, you may face a few hours of thumb-twiddling in a barren room—especially if you move on a weekend, when stores are closed or less accessible.

In the second box, place the household items you'll need immediately—towels, washcloths and soap; light bulbs; toilet paper; a few cleaning supplies; one or two dishes, eating utensils; bed makings (sheets and pillowcases) for as many of you as are moving; and perhaps shelf paper and a pair of scissors. That way, if you have a long wait for the furniture to arrive, you'll be equipped to use the time constructively.

Remember your husband and child, too. Forgetting a child's favorite doll can trigger trouble if she can't understand it's not lost permanently. A husband may be delighted to find you've included his favorite pipe.

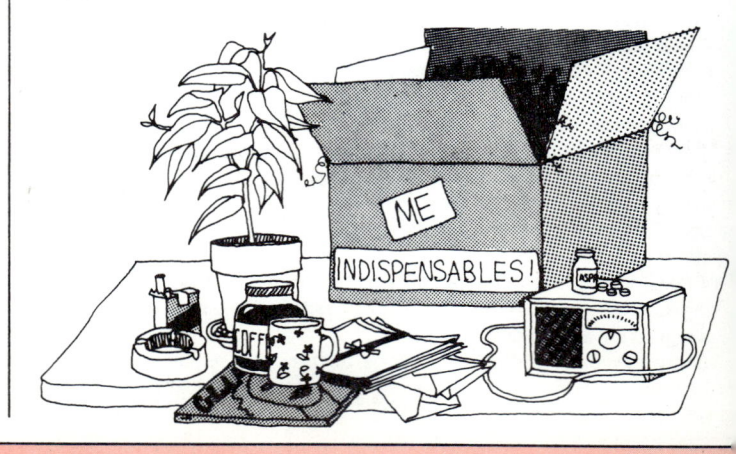

names

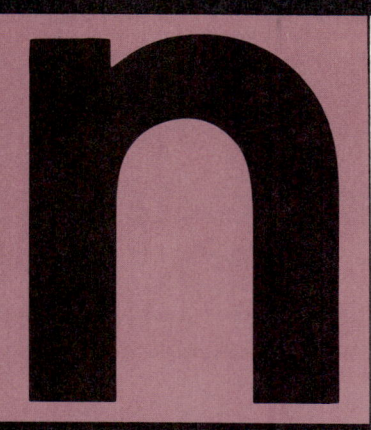

names nature

names

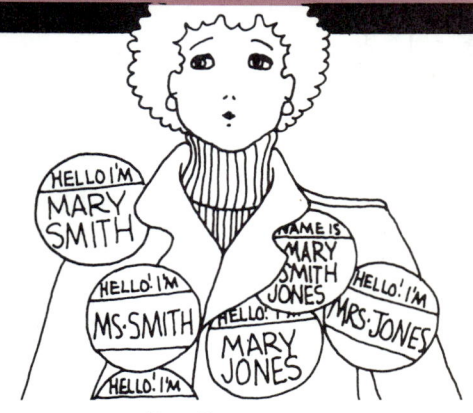

maiden info on keeping your own name after you get married

No state has a statute that specifically requires a woman to take her husband's name after she is married. However, many women who try to keep their own name after marriage, even when it is legal, run into bureaucratic and other snags. Banks, for example, sometimes insist that women use their husband's surname on their joint banking account.

To resolve such problems, the Center for a Woman's Own Name (CWON), which is a nonprofit organization, was formed. It has received thousands of letters and calls from women trying to retain their own name after marriage—or to revert to it after divorce. You may want to write for a guidebook listing the procedures for keeping or reverting to your own name in all fifty states. It also offers suggestions on such finer points as: What do you do about the names of children, if or when you have children? The 55-page booklet costs $2, plus 50¢ postage. To get a copy, write to The Center for a Woman's Own Name, 261 Kimberly, Barrington, IL 60010, requesting a copy of the "Booklet for Women Who Wish to Determine Their Own Names After Marriage." If you have a question that the booklet cannot answer, CWON will try to help, or put you in touch with someone who can.

nicknames
how to get rid of a nickname that's not really you

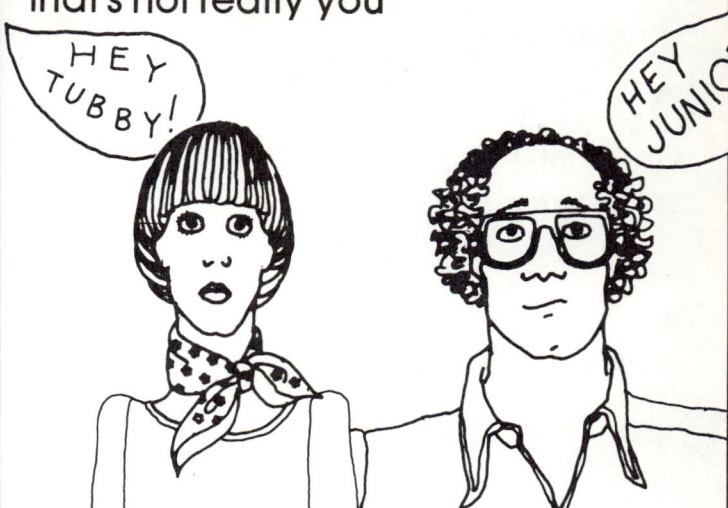

Are you stuck with a nickname that you'd rather live without? Perhaps you're a Vanessa who hates being shortened to Van, a Katherine called Kathy who'd prefer to be Kate. Or maybe you're still answering to the name you earned one Friday night in the dorm.

Here are some tips on how to trade in your old name and get people to call you by the name that's really you.

● As soon as you get the notion to change your name, wait a few weeks before doing anything about it to be sure you really want it and that you aren't just acting on a whim.

● The best time to start using your new name is when you enter another environment—school, a new job, a new neighborhood. Most people that you introduce yourself to won't know you ever had another name. And hearing your new acquaintances call you by this name without awkwardness will encourage you to try it on your old friends.

● Tell your friends and family about the change—you can't expect them to pick it up on their own. Try to explain your decision in positive terms so that you won't hurt the feelings of whoever gave you your old name. For example, if what you're relinquishing was the result of your younger brother's first attempt to say your name, tell him and your parents that you always loved it, but that you feel too old for it now.

● Make a point of using the name yourself. Even if people recognize your voice on the telephone, begin conversations with "Hi, this is —." When sending notes to your friends, be sure to sign your new name.

● The trick to getting people you know into the habit of calling you by a different name is to correct them gently each time they address you incorrectly. If friends don't seem to get the message and act amused, you could sit down with them and explain how important the change is to you and that it's more than a passing fancy. You may choose to let your very closest friends and family call you what they always have, but this will make it harder for new acquaintances to catch on.

● Use visual aids to help you and your friends get accustomed to the transition. Make new signs with your name in big, bright letters for your mailbox, your door, and your desk. You might also have stationery with your new name printed.

● Remember that if the new name you choose isn't the name on your birth certificate or a derivation of that name, and you intend to use it for business or legal reasons (such as your driver's license), you'll need a court order to change it.

● Finally, don't get discouraged. It will take plenty of time, even years, for everyone to pick up on the change. But as your circle of acquaintances expands, the number of people who persist in calling you by your old name will diminish. And then maybe the only time you'll have to answer to "Egghead" will be at your high school reunion.

129

nature

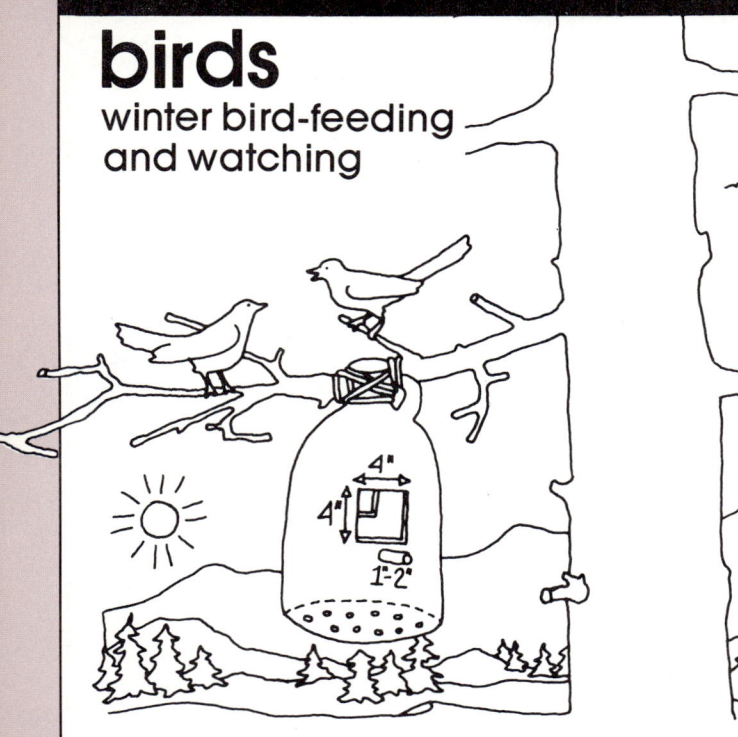

birds
winter bird-feeding and watching

A great way to stay in touch with nature is to "recycle" an empty plastic bleach bottle by making the bird feeder we've described below. And the cold months are a great time to make one because freezing, heavy snow, or anything that diminishes the birds' natural food supply will cause birds that might not ordinarily come to a feeder to do so.

Before you make a feeder, though, here are some dos and don'ts for bird-watching in general:

DON'T start feeding birds unless you can keep the feeder stocked at all times during the colder months. Birds can become dependent on your handout and starve without it. If you must be away, a friend should fill the feeder in your absence. How much bird seed you'll need depends on the number of birds you attract; a 5-pound bag of commercially mixed wild bird seed lasts an average of two weeks in a feeder like the one sketched above.

DO scatter some seed on the ground, too; some birds eat from the ground.

DO try to put water out daily in a shallow dish, particularly when other water sources are frozen.

DON'T place the feeder where cats can get at it—hang it from a tree limb, for instance. Or, if you can't make it inaccessible, make sure that your cats are collared and belled.

DO realize that you can suspend feeding during the summer when birds' natural food supply is more abundant.

DO buy a guidebook to help you identify the birds you attract. Roger Tory Peterson's *A Field Guide to the Birds* is the bird-watchers' bible.

To make the feeder: Scour a one-half-gallon plastic bleach bottle well, removing any remaining bleach and labels. Cut roughly 4" x 4" holes on two sides. Make holes in the bottom with an ice pick for drainage. About an inch below each big hole, punch another hole large enough for a ¼" thick perch (such as a dowel or tree branch). Then insert the perch so that it extends 1"–2" out from each hole. Attach the feeder to a tree branch or fence with heavy twine or wire wrapped around the neck of the jug, or to an exterior window frame with a long hook or nail through the neck.

woods
nature walker's guide to the woods— and its folklore

The woods are at their very best on a crisp autumn day—but before you go off exploring, you might want to know the truth about some of that old folklore surrounding things like wild mushrooms. We got the answers from Kaye Anderson, associate naturalist with the Teatown Lake Reservation Nature Center in Ossining, New York.

● *Eating wild mushroom will make you go mad.* Possibly. While some wild mushrooms are perfectly edible and delicious, others have been reported to be hallucinogens—and a good many are poisonous. There is a variety of tests for determining which ones can be eaten, but no one test is conclusive for all mushrooms, so unless you're a mycologist (mushroom expert), don't do any nibbling. Bring them home, leave them out on newspaper for a few days, and then put them in a wooden bowl with other dried things for a pretty table centerpiece.

● *The leaves change colors and drop from the trees in autumn because of the sudden frost.* False. The color changing and dropping of leaves in autumn is part of the natural life cycle of a tree. It's the shortening of days, not a sudden frost, that triggers the tree's preparations for winter. As days shorten, the tree has less and less sunlight to produce chlorophyll, and finally, the chlorophyll breaks down and disappears, exposing other color pigments that have always been there. Trees lose their leaves as a result of the tree closing some of its ducts in an effort to preserve existing moisture through the winter. In the Northeast, however, temperature changes *are* responsible for the brilliant hues. The sudden drop in temperature that occurs at night after a sunny day creates sugar formations in leaves that bring out the fiery red and orange pigments.

● *You can tell direction by noting how the sun travels.* True. Although the sun sets in the exact west only twice a year—on the first day of spring and the first day of autumn—you can get a general idea of west by noting the sun's movement. Press a stake into the ground and mark the tip of the shadow. Ten minutes later, mark the tip of the new shadow. A line drawn from the second mark to the first will point west.

● *You can tell if someone's approaching from a distance in the woods by listening with your ear to the ground.* True. The old cowboys and Indians really knew what they were doing. Sound vibrations are carried through the ground; that's how snakes, who have no ears, can detect the movement of other creatures.

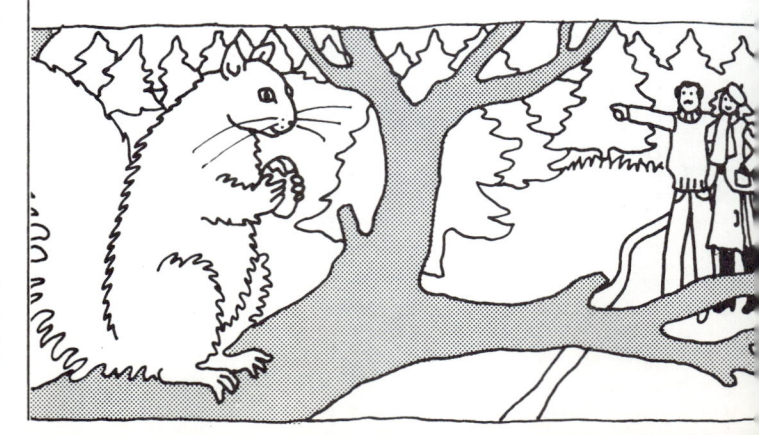

outdoors

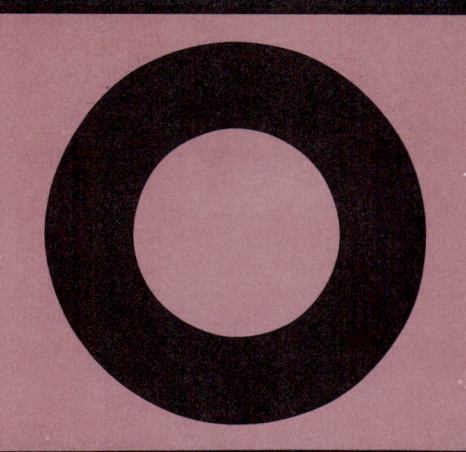

Oktoberfest outdoors

Oktoberfest

great ideas for your own Oktoberfest

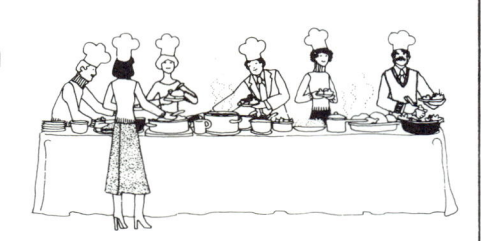

The first weekend in October is a good time to host an Oktoberfest to out-revel Munich's. The first Oktoberfest was a two-day celebration of a royal marriage; now it is a two-week period of extravagant eating, drinking, and wild fun. At your own, you might have recorded German beer songs, polka music, or selections from Romberg's light opera, *The Student Prince,* to set the mood. Then serve hot German potato salad (recipe below) with an assortment of zesty wursts, such as knockwurst, bratwurst, bauernwurst, frankfurters and, if you can find it, the traditional veal weisswurst. Don't forget sauerkraut and sweet mustard to go with the wurst, fresh loaves of pumpernickel or rye bread, and generous mugs of beer—served plain or as the traditional German drink, *Radler Mass:* beer mixed fifty-fifty with lemon soda. Serve apple strudel or German chocolate cake for dessert.

● **hot German potato salad (warmer Kartoffelsalat)**

6 med. white potatoes (about 2 lbs.)
½ c.—4 or 5 strips—diced bacon
⅓ c. minced onion
¼ c. vinegar
¼ c. water
½ tsp. sugar
salt and pepper to taste
2 T. chopped parsley

In a large covered pot, boil potatoes in their jackets in 2" of water until tender (about 30 min.). While warm, peel and slice into ¼" slices. In skillet, fry bacon until lightly browned, add onion, and sauté until tender, not brown. Add vinegar, water, sugar. Heat mixture to boiling and pour over potatoes. Season with salt and pepper and toss lightly with chopped parsley. (Serves 4–6).

outdoors

activity
great warm things to do outdoors in the chill winds of early spring

If you've been hibernating all winter, there's nothing like moving outdoors to clear your head, sharpen your vision, and send your spirits soaring. Why not try these ideas when winter makes way for spring?

● Hike into the woods. When it's still chilly out, hiking can be invigorating—just be sure to dress warmly. Bob Marcinczyk of Kreeger & Sons, a camping and backpacking equipment store, recommends wearing three layers of clothing; it's not the thickness of your clothes that keeps you warm, but the air trapped between the layers of material. Your layers should include insulated underwear, bulk insulation (a heavy sweater or down parka, depending on the temperature), and an element layer, such as a wind shell (keep the windchill factor in mind when dressing). Zippers or buttons in your clothes allow you to adjust the insulation according to your physical activity. Protect your feet with layers, too—try a single-walled padded boot with a pair of water-repellent liner socks and two pairs of water-absorbent wool socks over them to keep your feet warm, dry, and blister-free.

● Ride horses. People tend to think of horseback riding as a spring/summer/fall activity, but according to Laddie Andahazy, director of the Equestrian Center at Lake Erie College in Ohio, March is a great time because horses love the nippy weather. They'll be especially high-spirited and playful (they drag in summer heat just as humans do). Also, many stables keep their trails in good condition all year.

● Start work on your vegetable garden. Planting shouldn't be done till at least April, but Charles Mazza of the Brooklyn Botanic Garden recommends March as the time to fertilize the soil with organic material (because it ought to be present in the soil for at least a month before planting). Spread any compost material, rotten leaves from your yard, or peat moss over your garden area. Then work it into the soil with a rake. If the ground is exceptionally muddy from rain, just spread the material around and wait till things dry up a bit before working it in.

● Fly kites in the bold March sky. Follow these pointers from Mark Skwarek of the Go Fly a Kite Shop in New York City: The best way to launch a kite is to stand with your back to the wind, holding onto the string and unwinding it as a friend takes the kite about 100 yards downwind and then launches it. Once the kite is in the air, the flyer takes control. If a kite starts to nosedive, don't jerk in the string suddenly (the natural inclination), but instead release additional string and work the kite back into the air.

● Take rubbings of any interesting raised surface, from a manhole cover to a historical wall carving. Rubbing is easy with the right materials. Cecily Firestein, who has taught classes on rubbing and written a book about it—*Rubbing Craft*—suggests you use Aqaba paper (about 40 cents a sheet at an art supply store) and a rubbing wax such as Old Stone (about $2.50 for eight different colors). Cut the paper into a rectangle that fits over the area to be rubbed, secure it in place with masking tape, then simply rub with wax until enough of the design is lifted. Rubbings look great in inexpensive chrome frames.

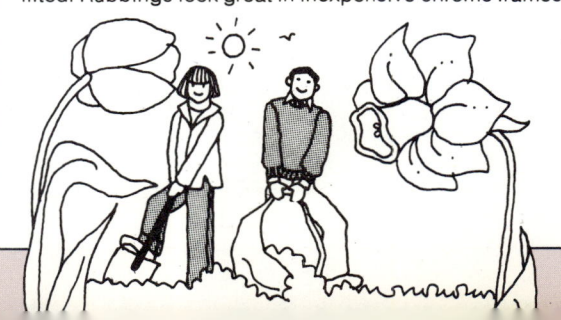

outdoors

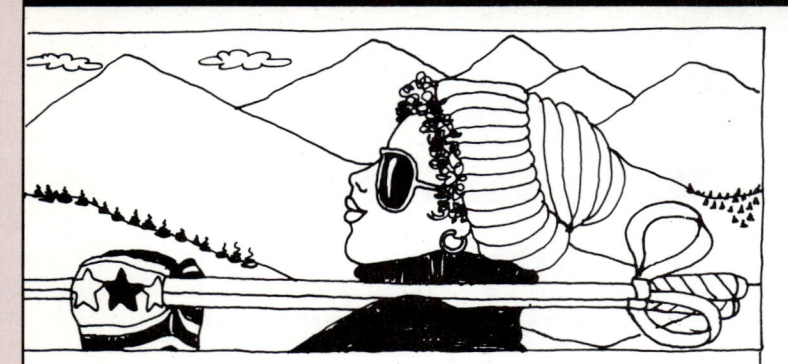

beauty
5 quick mid-winter beauty tips

● Turn down the heat in your home to 72° F. or less. Any central heating system is drying, but temperatures over 72° F. are especially drying to skin and can contribute to puffy eyes in the morning. You'll save on heat, too.
● Don't discount winter sun, especially if snow is involved. You might not get a real burn, but winter sun exposure contributes to the overall damage sun does to skin. Always wear a sunscreen on your face if you're going to be outside a lot. Dermatologists say it's best to pick a moisturizer that contains a sunscreen.
● Avoid soaking in hot tubs or taking long hot showers. Hot water is more drying to skin than tepid or warm water—it opens pores and lets natural moisture evaporate. Try a warm bath or shower instead. When you dry off, apply moisturizer, using body moisture as an added plus. Dust with powder if you like.
● Buy a loofah or slightly abrasive sponge and use it in your bath or shower a couple of times a week. It will help keep dry, flaky skin under control.
● Have a professional pedicure to get rid of the corns and calluses that usually come with wearing heavier shoes.

skin
the outdoor woman's guide to beautiful skin

Cold weather can stir you to a faster pace, a bloomier skin, and fresh pleasure at being out, but if you don't take a few precautions, being outside can turn that bloom to a chapped red. Here are a few easy ideas to keep you one up on winter.
Eyes: Wear sunglasses all year. They will help protect against the cold and wind that make eyes water. The eye area is the driest part of your face, so treat it with a rich moisturizer worn under makeup and while you sleep.
Cheeks: Cheeks are prime targets for chapping and windburn. Give them the protection of a good moisturizer or a moisturizing foundation during the day. Petroleum jelly applied to chapped areas at bedtime is very soothing. Use a cream, rather than a powder, blush if cheeks are chapped.
Lips: Always wear a protective lip pomade over, under, or in place of lipstick. If you don't, the moisture from licking them will cause chapping. If lips do get chapped, wear a clear or colored gloss, not a lipstick, which will only emphasize cracks.
Ears: If a hat or earmuffs won't work for you, try a ski band—the kind that goes around your head and covers your ears. They're good-looking and deliciously warm.
Hair: Don't forget that cold wind and weather make hair dry and brittle. Treat yours gently and deep-condition it once a month. Try using your dryer on the "warm" instead of "hot" setting to cut down on the effects of too much heat. Limit use of electric rollers and curling irons to three times a week.

work
beauty tips for women who work outdoors

Many young women have written to us asking for advice about looking their best and protecting hair and skin when they work outdoors. Here's what our beauty editors recommend:
● Put your emphasis—and your money—on skin care. It's very important for any woman who's outdoors a lot, especially if she works in a city or polluted environment.
● Buy a good quality, mild soap and use it twice a day. If you have oily skin, you might find a mild abrasive cleanser like Komex (available in drugstores) useful on oily spots like chin, nose, or forehead. Use this several times a week depending on how oily your skin is.
● Use a mild skin toner or astringent daily after cleansing.
● Use a light moisturizer, concentrating on dry areas, especially around eyes.
● *Always* protect your skin with a sunscreen. The paler your complexion, the stronger the screen should be. You'd do well to get the advice of a dermatologist on your skin's requirements and the best screen or block for you.
● If your job necessitates long-term exposure of arms and legs to the sun, be sure you also protect those areas with the sunscreen, too. If you plan on tanning, get a very slow, gradual tan and use protection even when you're actually tan.
● Cover your hair with some sort of hat or scarf. Sun exposure is very harsh on hair, especially if you color or permanent or chemically straighten it.
● Use a protein shampoo. It's especially necessary for anyone who's outdoors a lot, because sun and weather exposure can damage hair. Protein shampoos help replace some of the protein loss caused by exposure.
● Since air pollution makes hair dirty, anyone who is outdoors a lot will have to wash her hair more frequently than someone who isn't. An easy, wash-and-wear style will save you a lot of time and trouble. Put your money in the best haircut you can get. Ask for advice on upkeep of the style and follow it. Be sure your hair is trimmed as often as the style requires. Hair can become hard to manage when it's in need of a trim.
● As for makeup itself, use a minimum—too much build-up outdoors looks and feels overdone. A moisturizer, very light foundation if you want, some mascara, blush, and lip gloss—or at least a lip pomade for protection—should do it.

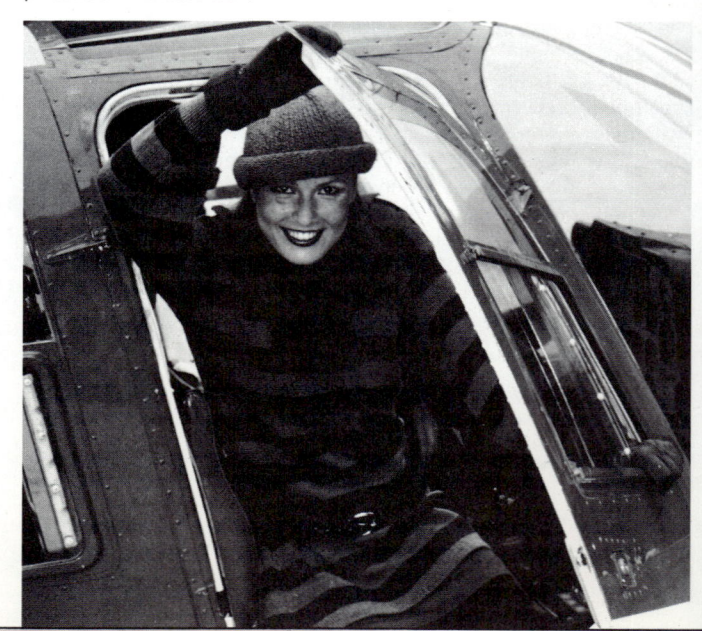

parties

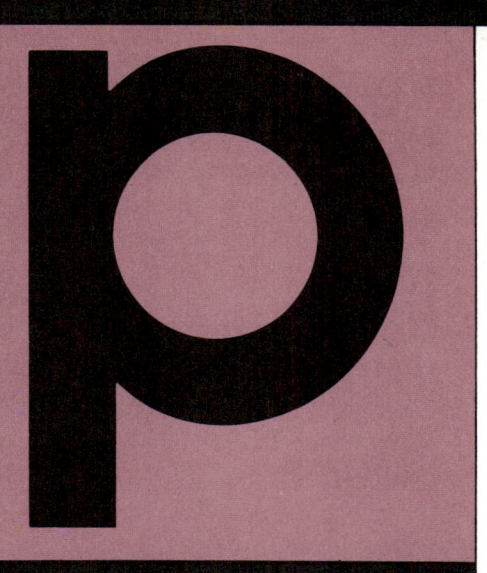

**parties
pets
plants
pregnancy**

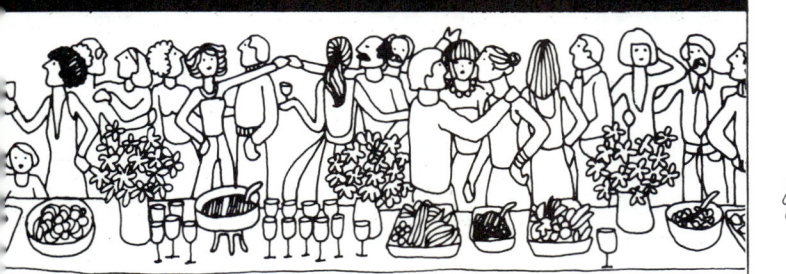

parties

food & drinks
how to program your party thinking if you've invited 20 or 40

Here are the basics you'll need in party snacks: roasted nuts; assorted cheeses and water biscuits or assorted thinly sliced meats—ham, turkey, salami—and crisp breads; ripe and green olives, raw cauliflorets, zucchini strips, scallions placed around a sour cream and dill dip, or cherry tomatoes and sour cream mixed with minced clams as a dip; dried fruits—raisins, dates, figs.

Bar build-up: This chart is based on average preferences—consider your guests' tastes when you buy.

- **20 guests**
  2 qts. bourbon
  2 qts. blended whiskey
  2 qts. vodka
  1 qt. Scotch
  1 qt. gin
  1 fifth rum
  1 qt. dry vermouth
  1 qt. aperitif, such as sherry
  1 gallon dry white wine
  1 gallon red wine
  8 qts. club soda
  1 six-pack ginger ale
  1 six-pack tonic water
  1 six-pack bitter lemon
  1 six-pack cola
  1 qt. each orange and tomato juice
  20 lbs. ice cubes

- **40 guests**
  4 qts. bourbon
  4 qts. blended whiskey
  4 qts. vodka
  3 qts. Scotch
  2 qts. gin
  1 qt. rum
  1 qt. dry vermouth
  1 qt. aperitif
  1–2 gallons dry white wine
  1–2 gallons red wine
  14 qts. club soda
  2 six-packs ginger ale
  2 six-packs tonic water
  2 six-packs bitter lemon
  2 six-packs cola
  1–2 qts. each orange and tomato juice
  40 lbs. ice cubes

nerves
how to psych yourself out of party nerves when you're giving a party

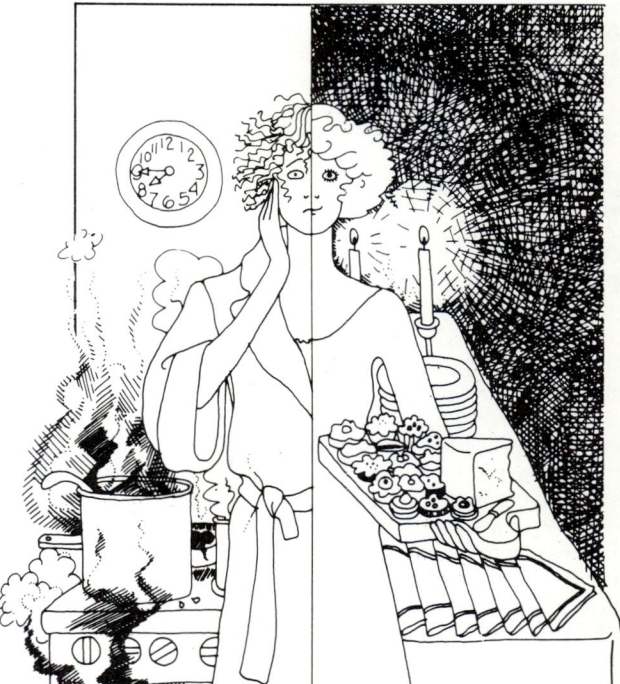

Giving a party is a little like swimming in chilly water. It takes some urging to get you in the water, but once you're in, the water seems just great. If you don't believe it, give a party and see for yourself!

- Don't feel you're the only one anxious about giving parties. *Everyone* is a little apprehensive. The trick is to calm down enough to have control but not to lose that little nervous edge that keeps you alert to the specialness of the occasion.
- Confront the fears behind your party nerves. One New York psychotherapist says worrying that guests won't like each other can tie in with fears about how much they like you. Recognizing this, plus realizing that many seasoned party-givers also worry, helps relieve the pressure.
- If this is a first party or you're terribly uptight, keep the party simple, say cake and coffee after a sports event or the theater. You might also

133

p parties

have a friend cohost a party with you to take some of the pressure off you.
- If you want to try a big party, pick a theme to give you something to plan around and to spark the fun. Themes could be anything from Valentine's Day to Halloween.
- If the party list is small, invite people by phone, starting with close friends first. This way, you aren't tense about RSVPs, and you'll get warm encouragement with every acceptance.
- Plan the party in writing. It helps keep you organized, and checking off things as you do them gives you the psychological satisfaction of getting on with the job.
- Don't knock yourself out cleaning just before the party. It tires you physically and emotionally. Clean the place a few days before the party, then relax. At zero hour, tidy the bathroom only; there will be too many people standing around everywhere else to notice a little dust.
- Serve something you feel at home with, not something brand-new. Try to make it ahead so all you will have to do is heat it and serve it. You can do this whether you're serving hors d'oeuvres or a meal.
- Be good to yourself. If you can afford it, buy a new dress so you'll feel really special and pretty, or if you can't swing that, wear something that makes you feel sensational.
- Don't panic if guests arrive late—they always do.
- Introduce guests as they arrive and try to give them something to start talking about. "Meet John, he has a Siamese cat, too," will give two strangers a point of contact.
- Keep people circulating. One way to do it is to encourage them to move from one food table to another so they can sample everything.
- Build up to a special surprise—have someone read palms, do handwriting analysis, or whatever. You don't have to hire a professional; just ask someone you know with a hobby to be part of the show.
- Try serving mugs of steaming coffee when you've had it for the evening and you want to send everyone home.

rentals
what you can rent for your next party

What can you do if you'd like to serve beef stroganoff but don't own a chafing dish that would keep it warm? Or what if you have a great milk punch recipe but no punch bowl to ladle it out of? One solution is to rent either item from a party rental store.

"Anything you've seen in a restaurant or at a party hall, you can rent," says Marty Gold of Party Time, a New York rental service that once rented 7,000 chairs, 2,000 champagne glasses, and 2 truckloads of dishes, silver, glassware, and garbage pails to the City of New York for the opening of the World Trade Center.

You can rent anything from a 48-cup percolator for a shower to torch lamps for a barbecue—but ask these questions before you do:
- *Is there a minimum order you have to place?* There may be no charge or a charge of as much as $20 to $25.
- *Does the charge include pick-up and/or delivery?* If so, you may be able to save by doing one or both yourself.
- *What happens if you break or damage an item?* Typically, a small portion of the fee is designated a breakage charge, and if your damages are under this amount, you pay nothing for them. Find out how much your breakage charge will cover, or, if there is no breakage charge, ask how breakage is dealt with. You should also know whether or not any part of the breakage fee will be returned to you if you return everything in good order.
- *What is the time limit on the items—and what will happen if you can't return them within it?* You'll probably be charged a late fee.
- *What else does the shop rent that might be used at your party?* Below are a few examples—some just for fun—of what Party Time has for rent and the rates for one day. Rental services in large cities should have similar items, sometimes at lower prices.

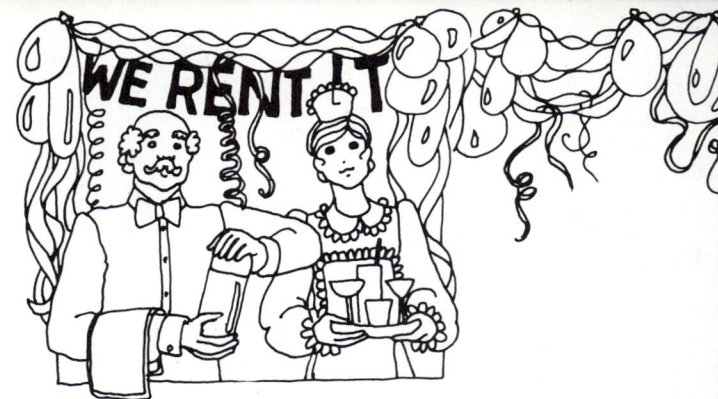

40-hanger coat rack	$9.00
silver chafing dish	$10.00
card table	$2.25
folding chair	$.55
45" x 45" cloth for card table	$1.50
glass punch bowl and 12 cups	$6.50
champagne or wine glass	$.20
dinner plate	$.16
knife, fork, or spoon	$.18
48-cup coffee percolator	$7.50
kerosene torch lamp	$1.50
record player	$35.00
25-cup samovar	$10.00
one hot-dog stand, with umbrella	$50.00
one 15 mph Tin Lizzie, with go-cart motor (for the guest of honor or birthday child to ride in)	$150.00

Finally, remember that if you'd also like a bartender to mix the drinks or someone to come in and clean up afterwards, you can get either of them, too. Look in the Yellow Pages under "Maid Service" for both; rates range from $4 to $6 per hour.

pets

aquarium
how to set up your first aquarium

Collecting tropical fish can be a great hobby—and as "pets" go, they aren't much trouble. Here are some tips for setting up a first aquarium.
- **buying fish**

Buy just a few at first to be sure your aquarium set-up is safe and works well. Try including egg-layers such as zebras or neons (30 cents to 40 cents each), and live-bearers, such as guppies or platys (30 cents), which are fun because they give birth to fully developed babies. Keep your tank clean by including two catfish for every five gallons of water (catfish cost about 70 cents each). They scavenge food from the bottom of the tank, keeping it from fouling up the water. Buy a few algae eaters, such as mollys or suckermouth cats (30 cents to 40 cents each), to keep algae from overrunning the tank.
- **setting up the tank**

You can buy a complete five-gallon tank setup for about $25. This size tank is pretty small, however, and limits the number of fish you can have. If you think you'll be an enthusiastic collector, you'll save money by buying a bigger tank to start. A 20–29 gallon set-up costs $50 and this is a roomy, fun-to-watch tank. The set-up includes tank, hinged lighted hood to keep fish from jumping out, filter, air pump, thermostatically controlled heater, and some gravel to line tank bottom.

pets

Rocks and live plants are good additions to your aquarium. Both provide hiding places for fish. If you have many plants, plan on buying an inexpensive strip reflector to give them adequate light.

A good aquarium shop—we checked with Aquarium Stock Company, Inc. in New York—can give you more advice. Or you can check the book *Tropical Fish* by Lucile Quarry Mann.

cats
what you can and can't expect from a cat... plus tips on how to pick one

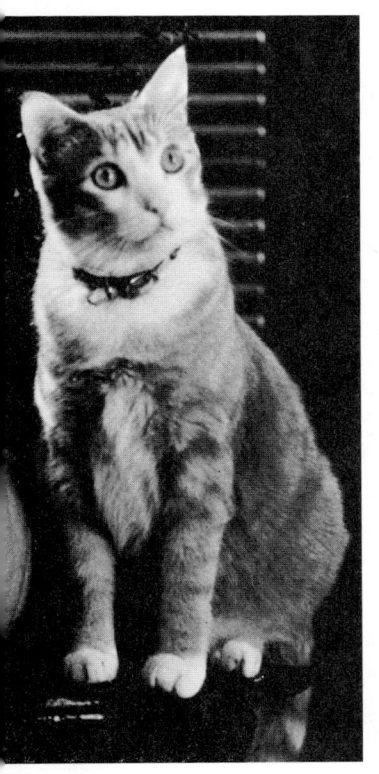

Few people can resist the lure of a tiny, big-eyed ball of fluff that seems to be looking just at you from the pet shop window. And any number of cat owners will confirm that giving in to the urge for a cat has been one of the happiest decisions they've ever made. But owning a cat can bring some surprises, too, unless you know these facts before you pick one out.

- *You can expect your cat to be pretty liberated whether it's male or female, to be able to stay alone without much fuss during the day and even for a weekend. For long periods, leave your cat with friends, hire a drop-in cat-sitter, or board it. Don't worry about psychological after-effects when you return—cats are usually easy-going enough to survive short separations with ease. But do be sure and point out your cat's special likes and dislikes—that Samantha can't stand catnip but loves to play a particular game—to a sitter.*

- Observe cats you encounter in friends' homes, or borrow one for a while. They love to climb, claw things, smell and rub up against fresh-cut flowers, get up on the table, and sometimes even join in the family dinner. Some people see these antics as adorable and cuddly—as aspects that make a cat even more fun to have around. Others find such activities inconvenient or annoying.

- If you want to start your pet life with a kitten, try to find one that will come over to you easily. It should have a good coat, no discharges from eyes or nose, and ears free of waxy brown materials.

- Wait until a kitten is seven weeks old before you take it home. In that time, its mother will take care of housebreaking it.

- A kitten should get one or two distemper shots when it's about six to eight weeks old. Cost is around $10 in big cities and includes a physical exam. Then, a final or permanent shot is given after the kitten is three months old.

- Spaying or castrating a cat is easiest when the cat is young. For a male, the simple operation should be arranged when he's seven months old or older, costs about $15 to $30, and there is usually no hospital stay. For a female, it's best to operate after her first period of heat—usually around seven months. Cost will run at least $35, higher with any complications or extra medication, plus the average hospital stay of two days at a typical $3 a day fee.

- One thing to watch out for—both male and female cats can have bouts of urinary tract infections, but males are more prone to them. If you notice your cat goes to its box frequently but cannot perform, take it to a veterinarian fast, before the blockage becomes critical—sometimes it's only a matter of forty-eight hours.

- Expect to spend about a couple of dollars a week for cat food. Packaged, prepared, semimoist foods provide a good diet, and you can add canned selections for variety if your cat seems bored by a steady menu of one thing. Avoid raw meats because they are the source of infection for the disease toxoplasmosis.

- The only equipment investment you have to make is a box for the cat to use, plus kitty-litter refills (under $1 a bag, which lasts about three weeks).

- You might also consider taking in an older, more grateful cat—say two, three, or more years old—instead of a tiny kitten. Older cats have more serenity and mysterious charm, which make up for all a kitten's seductions, and at the same time they are less wild with their claws and less given to the battle charges over sofas, chairs, and tables covered with valuable baubles. Their personalities are also more formed and consistent.

dogs
pick the right dog for you

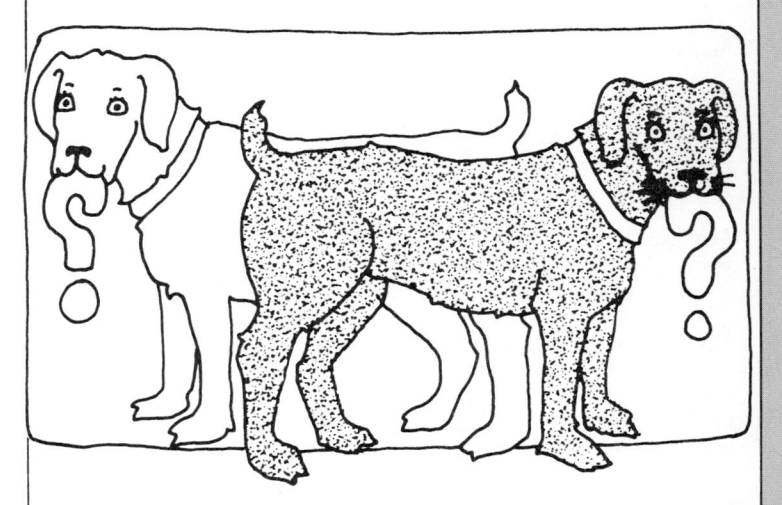

There they are in their cages at the local humane society or ASPCA, tails wagging, noses poking through the bars, all looking cute and lovable and promising enduring love. How do you choose the dog that will be a good companion and not take a bite out of the first male who enters your apartment?

According to the Bide-A-Wee society, a New York animal adoption agency, all dogs are born with good dispositions. Their personalities may vary from bold to placid, but only mistreatment by humans creates problem dogs. Here are some general rules to guide you in choosing a dog that has already had a master.

Don't let maternal feelings lead you into choosing the shyest and most frightened animal. It may need more attention and patience to overcome its fears than you have to give. The same is true for any dog that cowers or growls or seems totally indifferent to what's going on around it. You may be able to eventually coax it out of antisocial behavior, but it's not likely. Spend a half hour with the dog at the pound; walk it around the block a few times, ask to have it run free, out of its cage, and watch how it behaves with other people and animals. You should then have a pretty good idea of its disposition.

One New York psychologist believes that dogs, like people, will do what's expected of them. So once you've got your dog home, be firm about the behavior you want: walk it, feed it, play with it, and that free dog from the pound will be all you hoped for.

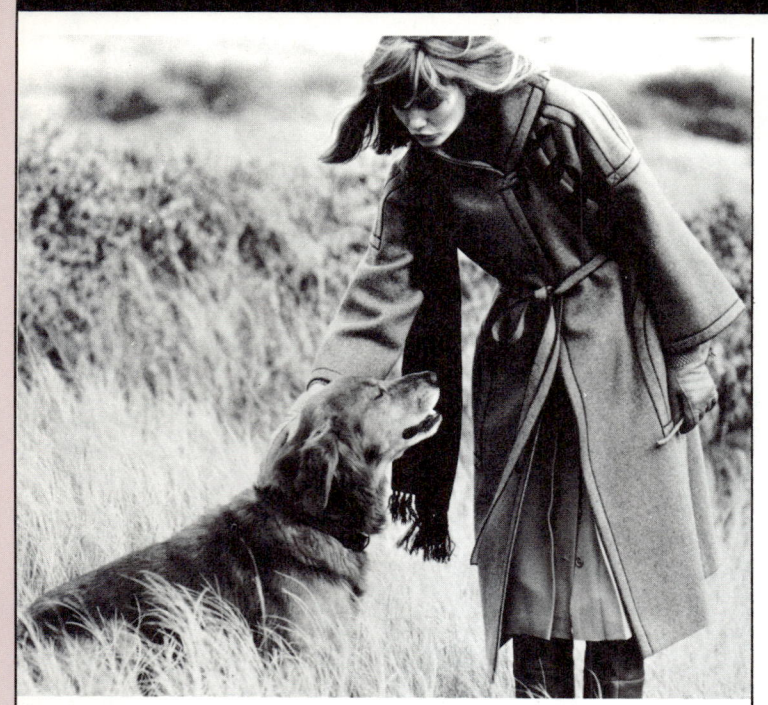

pets

sick
when to call the vet if your pet is sick

It's one thing when *you* feel achy and listless—you take an aspirin and fall into bed. It's quite another thing when your dog or cat is out of sorts. Pets react differently from humans to sickness, and even the most loving owner might read her pet's distress signals the wrong way. To find out when to act—and when to wait—we talked to veterinarians to get some guidelines.

● **guidelines for dogs and cats**
In general, any persistent vomiting or extreme changes in bowel movements that go on for more than eighteen hours are signs to call the vet. As for the old adage about a dog's (or cat's) nose being the barometer of its well-being, forget it. A dry nose is no reason to get into a tizzy. But not urinating for more than eighteen hours is. There may be blockage of some sort that, if left untreated, could lead to uremic poisoning. See the vet or go to a clinic immediately. Constipation for more than two days is another indication that something's wrong. And if your pet's been nosing into the garbage or eating plants, be sure to watch it closely for the next twenty-four to thirty-six hours for vomiting, diarrhea, changes in stools. If you remember that bones were in the garbage, call the vet right away.

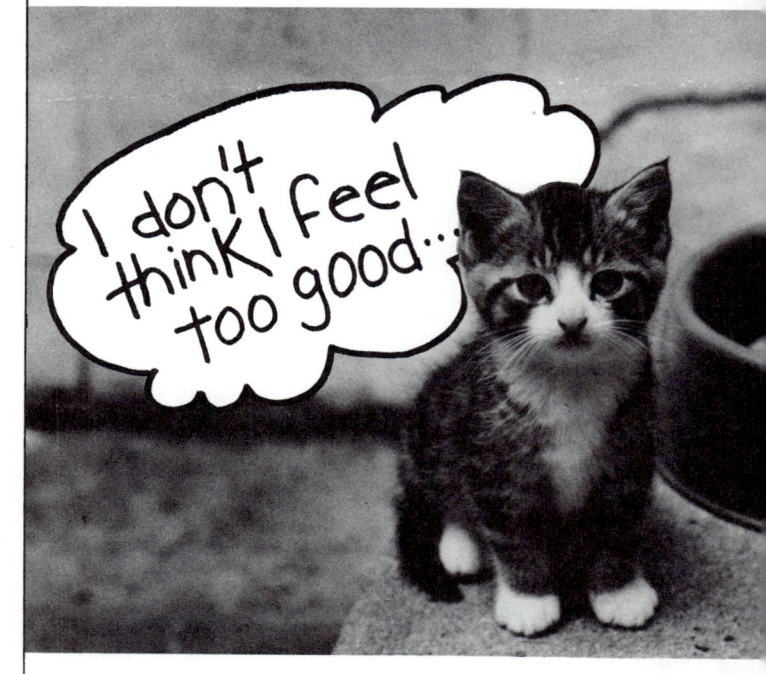

dogs
feed your dog well nutritionally — but inexpensively

Your dog may be a prince to you, but there's no need to spend a king's ransom to feed him. Here are some tips for sorting through the biscuits, burgers, special cuts, and meaty chunks.

● Don't pick a dog food because it sounds yummy to you or the price is so high you think it must be good. Nutritional content should be your main concern. Dr. Francis Kallfelz, Mark L. Morris Professor of Clinical Nutrition, New York State College of Veterinary Medicine at Cornell University, suggests you buy a product that meets the recommendations of the National Research Council. The NRC publishes a table of nutrient requirements that experts have established as necessary in a maintenance and growth diet. There are a number of dog food manufacturers that follow these recommendations and say so on their packaging. (You can find them at almost any supermarket.) This doesn't mean that companies that don't say their product has NRC approval produce inferior food—but when the statement does appear, it's a good guideline.

● Some dog food advertisements do a lot of barking about "extra meat," "extra protein," and "less cereal." But as long as a food is well-balanced according to NRC recommendations, you don't have to be concerned about cereal extras.

● When it comes to choosing between a well-balanced dry food and a well-balanced canned food, it's basically a matter of how much you want to spend. Canned food is more expensive than dry, but it hasn't been proved to be any better for your pet. Do take your dog's preferences into consideration—a small dog may want canned food because it's easier to chew. Some experimenting with your dog will help you come up with a reasonably priced, well-balanced product that he finds tasty.

● Table scraps aren't bad for your dog—in fact, try adding them to commercial dry food to increase the palatability and to add variety. But according to Dr. Kallfelz, they shouldn't constitute more than 10–15 percent of your dog's diet.

● Don't waste money on vitamin and mineral supplements. Your dog should get everything he needs from a well-balanced commercial dog food, and some research has indicated that overfeeding your dog with such things may be harmful.

● **guidelines for cats**
Because cats are pretty stoic creatures, it can be much harder to tell when a cat is sick than a dog. Their symptoms often come on rather suddenly; once the symptoms do appear be sure to keep a close eye on your pet. If the symptoms don't clear up within a day or so, call the vet. Any personality changes, loss of weight, general listlessness, or not eating for more than a few days are other indications all is not as it should be. If your cat seems to have a cold—sneezing, wheezing, coughing—don't panic, but do be observant. Cats are quite prone to upper respiratory viruses and many are not serious. If it gets worse or other symptoms appear, phone the doctor. And isolate the sneezing cat from other pets, especially other cats. While there's nothing you can do to absolutely prevent another cat from catching the virus, isolation may help. Another cause for worry, especially with young castrated male cats, is any irregularity in defecating or urinating. If the cat cries or if it defecates outside the litterbox, something is usually wrong.

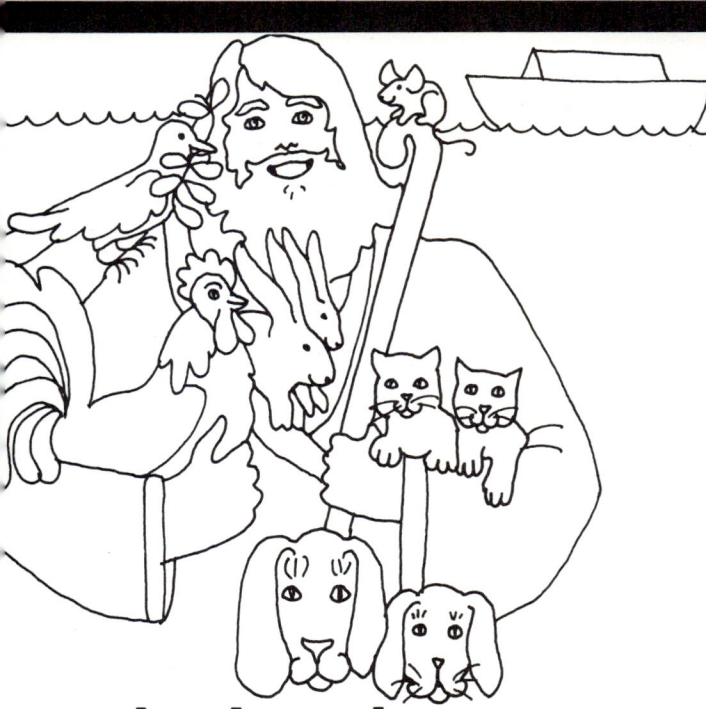

plants

veterinarian
how to find a reliable veterinarian

We've heard enough horror stories about nonsterile spayings and infected cat-fight wounds to know that pets can get poor or insensitive veterinary treatment. Here's how to get your pets the best of care.

The best sources for names of good veterinarians are other pet owners, so ask neighbors and friends. If you're still not satisfied, try the Yellow Page listings, which are complete if not too full of advice. If all else fails, write to the American Animal Hospital Association, P.O. Box 6429, South Bend, IN 46660 for members' names in your locality. Its standards are high, and only 10 percent of the nation's small animal hospitals and clinics and 35 percent of individual practitioners belong.

Before you visit a veterinarian, call for some typical costs. Says one highly respected veterinarian, "You usually get what you pay for," so beware of rates that are too low. An average female cat spaying runs $35 to $45; an average male, $15 to $30. Female dog spayings can run anywhere between $45 and $80 (about $10 to $15 cheaper for the males), depending on size, age, and general health of the animal.

Ask if a veterinarian is available for emergencies. If not, is a nearby clinic or hospital open at night? Emergency care is one of the top priorities, as most animals are fairly stoic, don't show early signs of disease, and are prone to accidents.

On your first visit to a veterinarian, look for these qualities:
● He is busy but takes time and shows real, sympathetic concern for your pet.
● He uses a minimum of physical restraint on a nervous animal and plays with it until he gains its confidence.
● He explains his diagnosis and treatment, confirms it with lab work, and tells you what steps he'll take if this initial treatment doesn't solve the problem.
● His staff is properly uniformed, friendly, and courteous.
● He has someone on night duty to care for pets that must stay over.
● His office is clean and neat, with a separate and closed operating room.

Recently, a number of veterinarians have begun combining their hospital practices in a central building. They handle out-patients in their own offices, but treat hospital cases that need specialized care or procedures in the combined facility. Pooled finances make a high-quality staff and equipment possible. If your veterinarian is into this kind of project, he's probably up on the latest in veterinary medicine.

accessories
ways to save on plant accessories

We're not going to tell you where to buy your plants—if you're a plant lover you've already discovered the local places to find healthy specimens. But a clay pot is a clay pot—so why not save money by shopping around for the lowest prices in plant care supplies?

● **the plant supermarket**
The huge plant stores and sheds that are sprouting up all over usually offer the best prices on supplies, like pots and soil. If you have a lot of plants under your care, these places are worth making a trip to. Many have their own greenhouses so you can pick up good-size quantities of soil at extra-good prices because it's bagged by the store. And when it comes to plant care, what could be better than roaming around a greenhouse to discover the ambience particular plants really love—see how the jade plants reach to the sun, the way Boston ferns nestle together in shadier spots.

● **the dime store**
Many dime stores—and even regular food supermarkets and novelty shops—now have whole sections devoted to plant supplies. You won't find a resident botanist to help you decide whether you need peat moss or humus for your philodendron cuttings, but you will find many things you need to make your garden grow—hoses, tools, plant lights, garden gloves—and a good selection of reasonably priced plant decorating items—everything from macramé hangers to pink terrarium gravel. The clay pots are likely to be higher in price than at a regular plant store, but bags of soil like those distributed by Swiss Farms are priced the same as anyplace else.

● **the little neighborhood plant store**
Most small plant stores concentrate on selling plants, not lots of plant accessories, but you'll usually find a small selection of pots, soil, and plant food. Service is good and what's nice here is that there's generally someone to advise you in buying your supplies.

To give you an idea of the variance in prices of plant supplies, here's what three New York City stores had to offer.

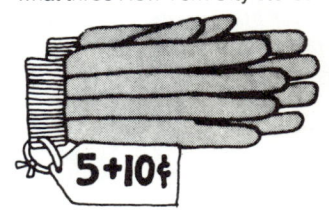

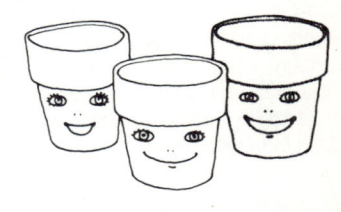

	dime store	neighborhood plant store	plant supermarket
Clay pots:			
8"	$3.79	$2.99	$1.75
7"	$2.79	$1.99	$.95
5"	$.99	$.59	$.40
4"	$.69	$.29	$.30
3"	$.49	$.19	$.25
Clay Saucers:			
6"	$1.39	$.69	$.60
4"	$.79	$.39	$.30
Peat Moss:			
(medium-size bag)	$2.99	$2.99	$1.50 (prepared by store)
Water mister:			
(plastic 32 oz.)	$1.98	$1.98	$1.99
Plant food:			
(8 oz.)	$1.59	$1.99	$1.50 (prepared by store)

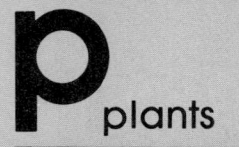

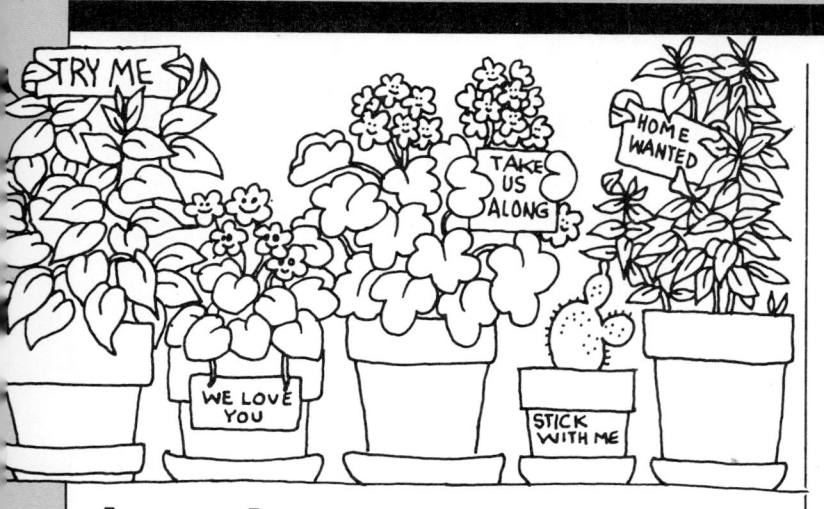

plants

buying
how to choose a healthy plant

How do you know that healthy-looking plant won't drop dead the minute it comes to live with you? There's no guarantee, of course, but these tips from Connie Athas of Tuilleries plant consulting service in New York will help.

1. Look for a perky plant with new growth and fairly thick foliage. Check leaves for healthy color. Pale new growth, yellow or cracked leaves, brown or trimmed-off edges (the store has cut off blemishes) are all danger signs.
2. Inspect leaves, stem joints, and soil for insects. And breathe deeply; soil should smell earthy-fresh, not sour (the soil may be badly aerated or be a poor mix).
3. Don't be fooled by a plant that's all foliage, few roots; this can happen if it's grown from a cutting or pruned-off branch. Check drainage holes for roots and tug gently at the stalk to see if it's secure—some movement is okay. The plant needs a good root structure to survive.
4. Try to shop mostly at a reputable country nursery or a plant shop. Dime-store or supermarket finds can sometimes be risky.
5. Ask the nursery if a plant you want has been acclimatized at least one to two months. Many houseplants are grown in Florida or southern California, then shipped to other areas. They need time to adjust to the move and the nursery should take charge during this period.
6. To ensure continued health, ask for care tips plus the popular and technical name so you can do homework. Bundle it up against winter chill by wrapping in a shopping bag and newspaper if the store doesn't provide paper sleeves.
7. At home, wash the plant leaves with mild soapy water to kill insects. Don't fertilize or transplant it for at least two months. And don't panic if your plant loses leaves the first three or four weeks; it's adjusting to a new home.

cures
do your plants have the droops? here's how to cure them

Anything from bugs to dry winter air or overcompensating for winter growing conditions could be getting your plants down. We drew up these rescue guidelines with the help of Dr. S. S. Hagar of Brooklyn Botanic Gardens, and *Flowering House Plants*, a Time-Life book.

If your plants are bugged, pick off the insects. Dab the leaves with a cotton swab dipped in alcohol. Wash the leaves gently with lukewarm suds or dip the entire plant upside down in warm soapy water; rinse with tepid water. Washing doesn't always get rid of the eggs, so Dr. Hagar suggests spraying them every seven to ten days for three to four weeks, or until the insects disappear.

● **caused by environment**
Symptom: Leaf edges are crinkly and brown.
Cause: Lack of humidity
Cure: Increase humidity by misting leaves and placing pots on bed of moist pebbles or by grouping plants in a planter with peat moss around them.
Symptom: Plant bears few or no flowers and an excess of foliage. Stems may be elongated. Green scum may be on sides of pot.
Cause: Too much fertilizer
Cure: Fertilize less often or at half the suggested rate.
Symptom: Stems become mushy, dark and rotten; lower leaves curl and wilt; soil at top of pot is wet.
Cause: Too much water
Cure: Do not water so much or so frequently. Water when soil is dry to the touch. Unclog drainage hole.
Symptom: Tips of leaves become brown and wilt; lower leaves turn yellow and fall off.
Cause: Not enough water
Cure: Water until water runs off the pot and do not water again until soil is dry to the touch.
Symptom: Leaves turn yellow or curl and wilt.
Cause: Too much heat
Cure: Move to cooler spot; be sure plant is not close to a radiator or hot-air outlet.
Symptom: Stems grow abnormally long, leaves become long and pale, and new leaves are undersized.
Cause: Not enough light; too much nitrogen
Cure: Move plant close to plant-growing light or to sunlight; reduce strength and frequency of fertilizer.
Symptom: Leaves curl under; new leaves are undersized.
Cause: Too much light
Cure: Give plant more shade or move away from plant light.

● **caused by bugs**
Symptom: Tiny insects take flight when you move the plant; leaves become pale, turn yellow and drop; leaf surfaces are sticky.
Cause: White flies, usually on leaf underside
Cure: Spray with malathion (8 oz. cost about $2.50), rotenone (8 oz. cost about $3) or isotox (8 oz. cost about $2.50).
Symptom: White, wooly spots appear on plant, leaves develop sticky patches, and entire plant looks stunted.
Cause: Mealy bugs—oval, covered with white powdery wax
Cure: Spray with malathion or isotox.
Symptom: Leaves and stem become shiny and sticky; leaves curl and buds may be malformed; insects are visible on undersides of leaves.
Cause: Aphids—pear-shaped, green, brown, yellow, black, or red
Cure: Spray with malathion (do not use on ferns or jade plants), isotox, or rotenone.
Symptom: White or brown dots appear on stems; plants become stunted and leaves sticky.
Cause: Scales—oval, hardshelled
Cure: Spray with malathion or isotox.
Symptom: Leaves show snow white speckles, then slowly turn yellow; tiny spider webs appear.
Cause: Spider mites—brown, red, or green
Cure: Spray with malathion.

decorating
tips on decorating with plants

When you're decorating with plants, a lot depends on your apartment, furniture, and the look you prefer. Here are some ideas to get your imagination started.

● For decorating clues, take a long, hard look at any plant—the way it grows, the shape, texture, and density of its leaves, even the curve of a

plants

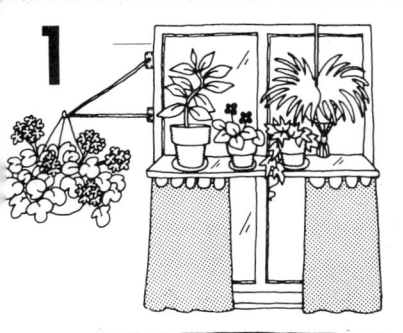

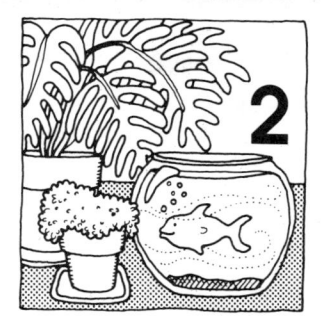

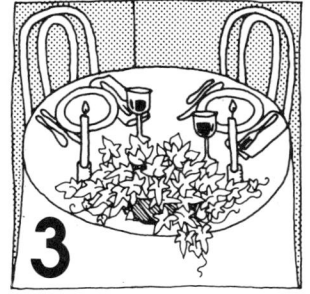

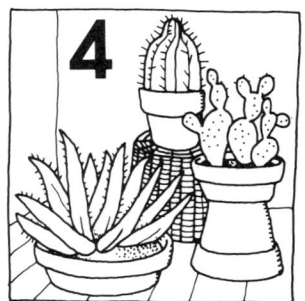

stem. For example, a rubber tree is clean-lined and contemporary; feathery palms and ferns look great with wicker and bamboo; stark succulents might enhance your American Indian rugs or pottery.
- Not all plants look best in groups. Your large cactus or delicate bonsai deserves its own spot as living sculpture.
- Curtain a whole window with greenery—or just the top half, leaving the bottom for café curtains or shutters. You might sit plants on glass shelves built into the window recess or hang them at different levels from the ceiling. Also try mixing pottery or basket containers with clear ones for some play of light through glass; use a hanging terrarium or a bowl with a philodendron or other plant that can grow in water instead of soil (Sketch 1).
- Use plants in odd spaces where furniture can't fit: under a staircase or in front of an unused fireplace, for instance. You might remove a closet door, keep bottom shelves for bright storage boxes, and leave the top area for plants. (Install special lighting to keep the plants alive in such spots.)
- For a feeling of space, give your eye a new direction to travel—up. Trailing plants look great in metal windowboxes sprayed white and suspended high by chains—or set on a ceiling-hung slatted wood tray. Floor plants set all along the narrow side of a room can also make it seem wider.
- Match plants up with other natural companions—a bowl of goldfish, gourds, driftwood, coral, seashells, even a clear bowl filled with water and colored pebbles. Small framed photographs peeking from behind foliage add a personal touch, too (Sketch 2).
- Think color. Your rust begonia might pick up copper tones in an area rug; set off coral, amber, or cinnamon tones in your china pattern; or add its own color accent to a neutral room. And don't forget that foliage comes in many shades of green, some more compatible with your furnishings than others.
- Set plants next to other things with an outdoors look, such as paper or fabric in floral, fruit or animal patterns, landscape photos, a synthetic grass floor covering (like Astroturf), or a natural woven area rug like sisal.
- Instead of cut flowers for your table, try a low ivy or shallow basket filled with small cactus plants. Or group plants with fruit: 3" herb pots with small baskets of strawberries or a bowl of fragrant lemons surrounded by daffodil plants (Sketch 3).
- Pots and planters play a big decorative role. Don't be afraid to contrast containers of varied size and shape, while keeping the look consistent. Terra-cotta or cork-bark pots match well with other "naturals." For a modern look, try containers made of plexiglass, covered with mirror, or enameled a bright color (with the name of your plant stenciled in bold letters). Stay alert to all kinds of amusing objects to set your plants on or in—old birdcages or folding metal salad drainers.
- When you do group plants, arrange at least three together and have shorter plants "step up" to taller ones. Also think up and down—not just sideways. Stagger plants on high and low pedestals or set them on a step ladder for a cascade of foliage (Sketch 4).

feeding
when and how to fertilize house plants

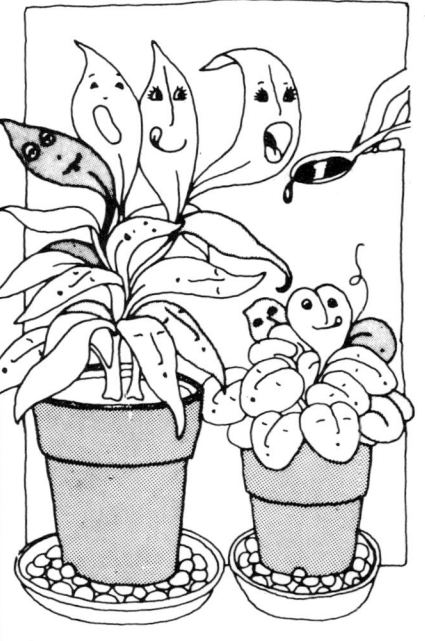

Fertilizing plants is necessary for optimum plant growth because it restores vital elements, particularly nitrogen, that are lost in watering and that *do* leave plants looking a little peaked if not replaced. However, most plants should be fertilized only from roughly March through September. From October through February, most plants have a dormant period, during which they should *not* be fertilized.

For common house plants, follow the directions of any commercial fertilizer; for more unusual or flowering plants, check with a plant shop or guide first. And in either case, remember that the cardinal rule of plant feeding is "better undernourished than overnourished"—so take it easy.

free
5 house plants that cost nothing

All you pay for is the soil and pots because all five of these house plants are grown from seeds or parts of fruit you eat all the time—grapes, oranges, grapefruit, lemons, kumquats.

For each plant, you'll need a terra-cotta pot, about 8" or 10" in diameter, and its saucer. A mixture of two parts potting soil, one part humus, and a handful of vermiculite are needed for each pot. Line the bottom of the pot with ½" of clean pebbles or stones for drainage. Add water to make the soil settle.

Grape vines frame windows with foliage that sometimes stays green all year around, sometimes turns a speckled red in autumn. Mix different kinds of grape seeds if you like. Dry the seeds, then plant about twelve in the pot you've prepared, ½" deep. (They probably won't all

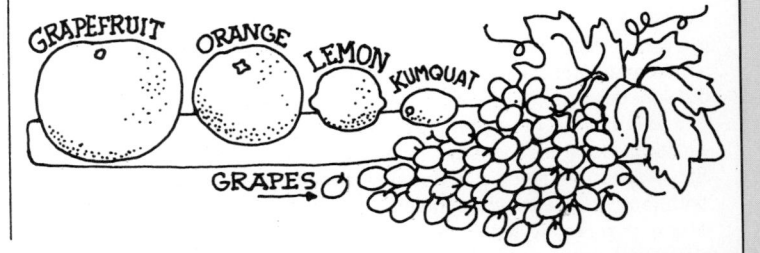

139

p plants

come up.) Keep soil moist. Put pots in a window where they will get no more than a few hours of direct sunlight a day until they have grown at least 6" or so tall. Only the older plants can take more sun. Give the little vines something to cling to as they come up—swab sticks or cocktail mixer sticks. Grape vines insist on growing upward.

Grapefruit, oranges, lemons, kumquats give any sunny or even slightly sunny window the feeling of a California or Florida fruit orchard. First add a handful of sand to your potting soil and mix it in. Rinse the seeds with warm water, plant them about ½" deep. Water well and sink the soil down close around the seeds. Water twice a week and spray the top soil with water every day.

lighting
a guide to plant lighting — and survival

The amount of light a plant gets is usually crucial to its survival, but it can be hard to know how much one should get—particularly when plant guides use terms like "direct" or "strong" sunlight. (You may think your apartment gets plenty of "strong sunlight," but will your *coleus blume*?)

To determine the amount of light any window gets, you need only to figure out whether it faces south, north, east, or west, and then find out how much sun it gets in the guide below. Each description is for a window not blocked by trees or apartment buildings.

- A north window never gets direct sun, but it does get good, bright light throughout the day. Almost any kind of plant will grow here, except those that require direct sun, such as cacti, jade plants, and geraniums.
- An east window receives direct sunlight a few hours in the morning and fairly low light for the rest of the day. A plant that needs direct light must have at least an east window.
- A west window provides good, bright light most of the day and direct sun in the afternoon. It gives better light than an east window because the light is brighter for a longer time.
- A south window gets the best (strongest) light: that is, direct sun almost all day. In a room with only a south window, many plants can be kept far away from it and still flourish. But fragile plants, such as African violets, may burn or wilt in direct sun and are best kept away from a south window.

repotting tips for repotting plants

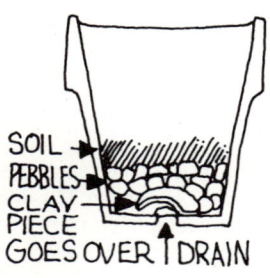

Houseplants have growing spurts during spring and summer. So if yours have been growing very slowly lately (or not at all) or if their roots are showing through topsoil or drain holes, they probably need to be moved to larger pots. There's no one method for repotting, but the tips below are simple enough for a beginner.

First, you'll need a clean pot a size or two larger than the pot your plant is already in—one with a top diameter 1" to 2" wider. Premixed soil from a plant shop is fine, although with experience, you may work out special soil formulas.

1. Place a piece of broken clay over drainage hole to keep soil from washing out later. Top with a layer of pebbles to ensure good drainage. Add a thin layer of soil and tap down gently. (Clay and plastic pots usually have drainage holes. If yours doesn't, add extra pebbles; or use a decorative container as a cachepot to cover a regular pot.)

2. If your plant hasn't been watered in a few days, it should pop out of its pot more easily. Tap all around sides of pot to loosen, then hold the plant gently—by the stem if possible—while you turn the pot upside down. Keep a hold on the plant so it doesn't crash out of the pot. Tap bottom of pot and lift the plant and soil out. (If it sticks, run a knife around pot edge and tap again.)

3. Center plant over the soil in the new pot; sprinkle more soil around sides and top to ½"–1" below rim. Tap down gently.

4. Water soil gently but thoroughly and let drain. This settles the new soil and removes air pockets. If your plant goes into shock, place in the shade and water normally. It should revive in a week.

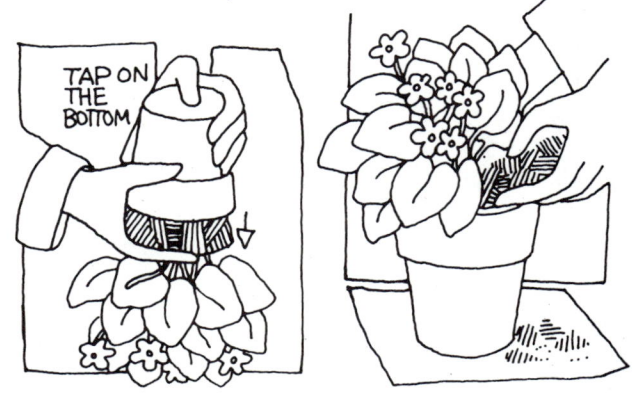

terrariums
how to make a bottle garden for under $5 in an hour or so

Beautiful as they are, bottle gardens, or terrariums, needn't take more time, money, and dexterity than you have to spare. Almost anyone can make the easy terrariums (see sketch) for under $5. With the directions below, it shouldn't take more than an hour to complete, and it will last for months with little or no attention.

- *Pick any wide-necked glass container, such as a fish bowl, brandy snifter, apothecary, home-canning, or candy jar. If it doesn't have a top, you'll need a piece of glass slightly larger than its opening. Any container must be clean, so wash it with soap and water, then let dry thoroughly before using.*

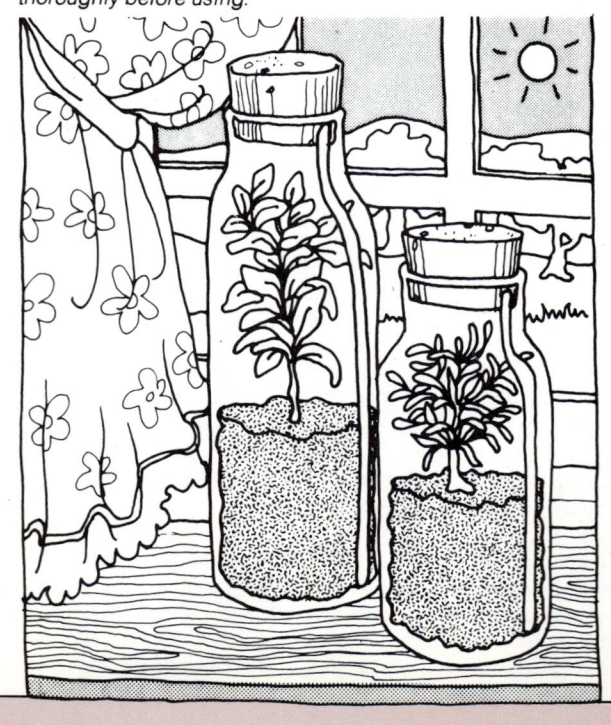

pregnancy

- Put a drainage layer of coarse sand or small pebbles such as bird or aquarium gravel about 1" deep on the bottom of the jar. On top of this, put an inch-deep layer of soil that is 1/3 crushed charcoal and 2/3 peat moss. You can buy both of these in dime or plant stores and mix them yourself.
- With a long-handled spoon (an iced-tea spoon or a regular spoon with a stick taped to it), poke a 1" deep hole in your soil. Then gently brush away as much dirt as possible from the roots of a small-size plant, such as a tiny fern, begonia, philodendron, peperomia, creeping fig, African violet, or dwarf gloxinia. Most plant stores have many terrarium plants for 50 cents to $2 each.
- Using your fingers, a pair of long tweezers (with tips taped if they're sharp), or wood or plastic tongs, place your plant in the hole and replace the dirt around it. Then surround your plant out to the edges of the terrarium with tiny "ground cover," such as moss or baby's tears and tamp it down slightly. Water just enough to dampen the soil without getting it soggy.
- Cork or cover your jar with its own top or lay a piece of glass across the opening. You must *cover the container's opening completely to create the controlled and uniformly moist environment the plants need to survive.*
- Keep your terrarium in a spot that gets good light, either on a bright windowsill or in the interior of a sunny room. Don't water it again until the soil dries out, which may not be for several months. If your plant grows too tall for its container, uncap it and let the plant grow out of its top—again, watering only when the soil feels dry.

pregnancy

back soothers
for pregnant women

More than any other group, pregnant women complain of backaches, according to Dr. Leon Root and Thomas Kiernan, authors of the book *Oh, My Aching Back.* But cheer up. An aching back doesn't have to be a part of pregnancy. Here are some tips to help avoid it.

Good posture is more important during pregnancy than at any other time. Stand with your pelvis tilted slightly forward (tightening your buttock muscles will help you do this). Pull up your upper torso and let your shoulders go down slightly and back. As you walk, you should almost have the feeling of gliding. To help you learn to tilt your pelvis forward, lie on the floor and slip your hand under the small of your back. You'll probably feel a space between the floor and your back. Now roll, or gently tilt, your pelvis forward until the space disappears or at least minimizes. If you start doing this early in your pregnancy, you'll be able to teach yourself to stand and walk with your pelvis tilted forward without having to think about it.

You can get a backache from *sitting* slumped over, too. Sit with the small of your back nestled comfortably against the chair and keep your upper torso straight.

If you have to stand for any period of time, shifting your weight from one foot to the other will help redistribute the stress placed on the muscles of the back and spine.

Toward the end of your pregnancy, you may sometimes feel as if your bones just won't support you. Hormonal changes cause you to lose fibrous tissue in the pelvis and ligaments loosen prior to delivery. You can compensate by being meticulous about how you stand and sit.

If your doctor approves, you might find this mini-exercise relaxing, too. Lie on your back, keeping your legs on the floor, and stretch first one leg and then the other out in front of you, trying to touch an imaginary object with your toe.

feelings
think you're the only parents-to-be with these feelings?

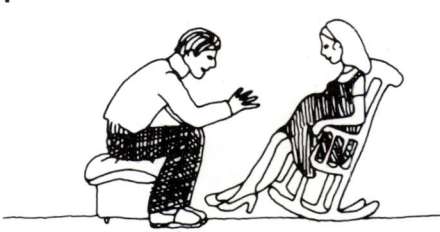

Psychiatrist Arthur D. Colman and his wife, Libby, have discovered that most couples can't quite sort out their thoughts during pregnancy. But in *Pregnancy: The Psychological Experience,* the Colmans describe pregnancy not as a time of simple waiting, but as a life crisis with great emotional impact on "the pregnant family," *father* as well as mother. By learning about them, the Colmans hope you will recognize yourselves and participate in your own experiences more fully.

Do you realize that many pregnant women:
 . . . develop "car phobia"?
 . . . are gripped by sudden, compulsive urges to clean house?
 . . . have a continual fascination with newspaper articles on death and dying?
 . . . dream about their own or the baby's death and worry about their "untested competence as a mother"?

Do you know that many expectant fathers:
 . . . do not imagine the newborn in their fantasies, "but see themselves walking with their two-year-old or playing ball with a teenager"?
 . . . feel a sense of deep frustration—even rage—when they are not permitted in the delivery room?
 . . . have minor psychosomatic symptoms that express the conflicts triggered by their wife's pregnancy?

These instances may occur during the three "phases" or "trimesters of pregnancy." The first trimester (first through third months) is often a time of great joy, coupled with an awareness of coming changes for both husband and wife. The second (fourth through sixth months) consists of "the quiet months," in which the most overwhelming experience is feeling the baby move. The third (seventh through ninth months) usually entails much anxiety about the imminent unknown and about sexual awkwardness.

Many prospective parents, the Colmans say, feel they are alone in heightened sensitivities or unexpected moods that occur during pregnancy. On the contrary, they assert, you may have more company than you ever expected.

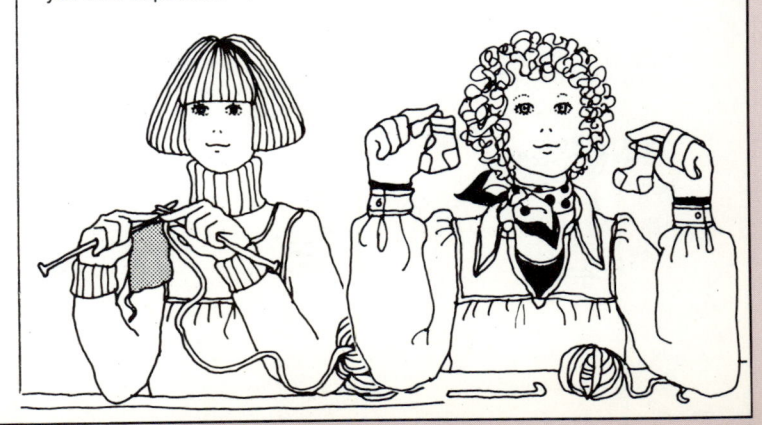

p pregnancy

wardrobe
the maternity wardrobe that pulls together like a dream

Trying to pull together a maternity wardrobe that's both comfortable and good-looking throws a lot of first-time pregnant women into a frenzy. One *GLAMOUR* reader made careful note of what worked well for her and decided to pass her tips along to us. We liked them so much we thought we'd share them with you—and added some of ours.

- Many smock dresses have pretty little yokes that extend just below the bosom and give a soft fullness over the stomach.
- A long cardigan sweater—one that reaches well past your hips—becomes a little body coat to be worn with any number of loose-fitting tops underneath.
- A favorite pair of jeans can be converted to maternity jeans by inserting a stretch panel in front. Many maternity shops or notions departments have the panels ready for inserting.
- Your husband's shirt over your jeans can be wonderfully comfortable to work in.
- If you like to sew, don't limit yourself to maternity patterns. Loose-fitting tunics or empire dresses work beautifully. Hem circumference should be at least 53" to allow enough fullness.
- All your regular shirts and blouses can be worn under maternity jumpers or tunics. Just leave the bottom button or two open.
- Try shopping in the loungewear departments for exciting-looking clothes that are cut loose and easy.
- Shirt jackets in regular sizes can look snappy worn open over a maternity shirt.
- A wrap dress or top bought or made a little on the big side is a super idea.
- A butcher's apron jumper in any bright solid or print fabric you like is handsome over any of your shirts, T-shirts, and sweaters.
- Kimono wrap tops can work for maternity wear if the wrap is full enough and you wrap and tie it just below the bosom.
- Shops that carry "folk" clothes can be great sources for unusual maternity clothes. All the embroidered peasant shirts and dresses around are usually full and pretty enough for dress-up.
- Many women find that buying a smashing maternity bathrobe for mornings and nights during the last six or eight weeks is worth the money.

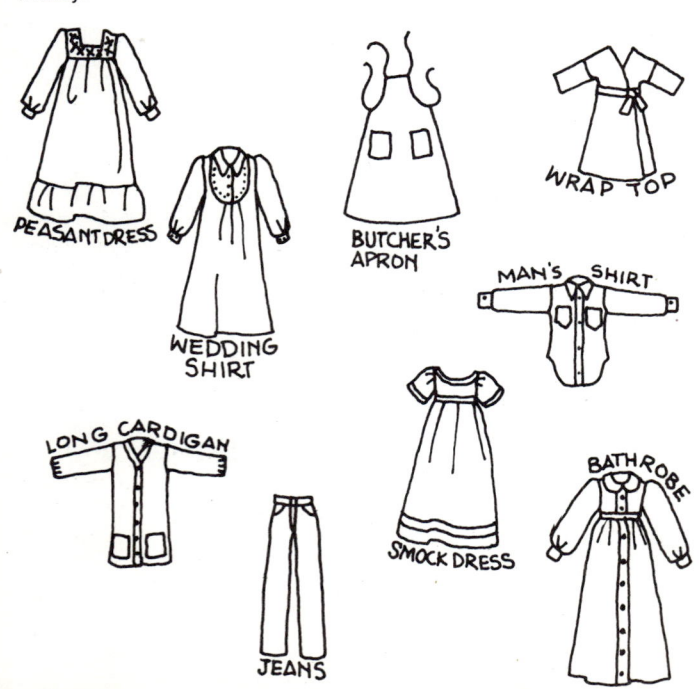

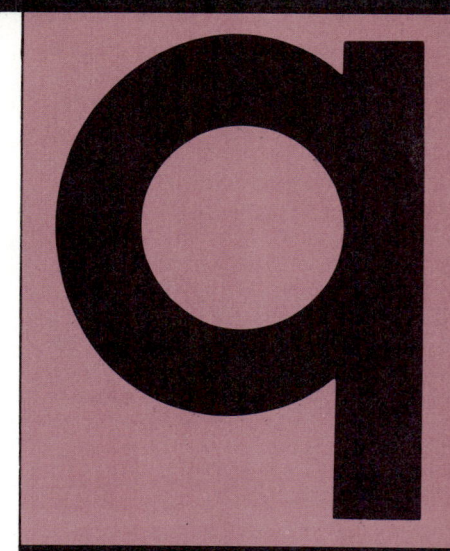

q quilts

tips on getting your old quilt through many more winters

Quilts have such charm that you're very likely to come across one that you can't resist. Antique ones are unusual, and old family quilts probably contain a bit of history that make them even more interesting. If you already have an old quilt or if you'd like to buy one, here's how to keep it in one piece for a longer time.

- Old patchwork often rips open at the seams. Topstitch grosgrain ribbon over the ripped seams, working the ribbon into an allover pattern. (It's important to reinforce the patches surrounding the ripped ones, too, as they will be the next to go.) Try ribbon in various widths, and choose colors to blend or try those in strong contrast, such as black on red or brown and orange.
- Sometimes whole patches must be replaced; use as similar a fabric as you can find. Then topstitch them on with your choice of a machine zigzag stitch. Many quilt experts recommend that you stitch around every patch in a particularly weak quilt—or one that is going to get a lot of wear and tear. If you use a thread that contrasts with the backing fabric, it will create an attractive "vermicelli" outline pattern on the reverse side.
- If you don't have a sewing machine or your quilt is too thick for your machine to sew, you can add patches and/or outline old ones with hand cross-stitching.
- Have your quilt dry cleaned by only the very best cleaner and ask him to take special care of it.

Finally, if you can't save the whole quilt, you might try any of the following:

- Sew it into a jacket, jazzed up with wooden toggles or satiny frogs.
- Hang it as a "painting" or as a dressing screen, and conjure up romantically cold mornings, flannel nightgowns, and china wash basins.
- Make sofa cushions with it.
- Make big, floppy-brimmed hats to give as presents.
- Or simply snuggle back down under it—being very careful not to put your foot through!

records

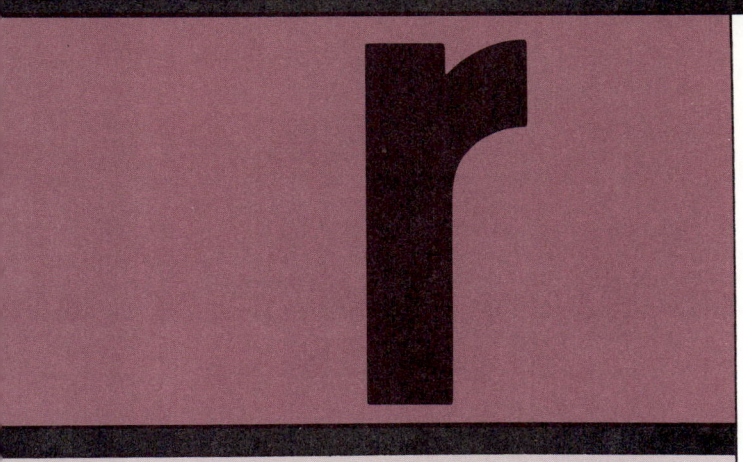

records romance

records

care
7 ways to make your record albums last longer

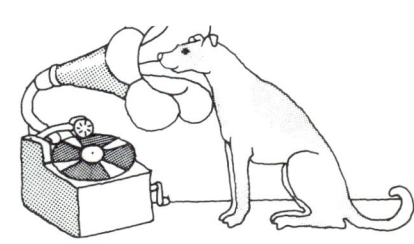

Whether your taste runs to Carly Simon or Stravinsky, there's no remedy for a damaged record. Prevention is the best medicine. You can avoid trouble by following these simple precautions:

• Remove the cellophane jacket-wrapping as soon as you buy a record. Cellophane tends to shrink, which can bend the jacket and warp the record.

• Protect records by keeping them in their cardboard jackets and paper undercovers when not in use. Jackets will last longer if you tape around their edges with a ½" strip of clear adhesive-backed paper or adhesive tape. If the originals should tear, you can buy replacement jackets for about 25 cents each. New soft-plastic undercovers are also a good investment; paper ones can cause minor scratches if they tear.

• Handle records only by their edges or centers. Oily fingerprints on the grooves attract dust and cause scratches. To remove surface dirt, don't wash the record but wipe it before and after use with a chemically treated, antistatic cleaning cloth. Cleaning kits with a bottled solution and an applicator are also available, but the solution must be used sparingly to avoid leaving a film on the record. Remember to wipe in a circular direction, not across the grooves.

• Always keep your needle in top shape. It should be replaced if it jumps over various parts of different records. If it skips consistently over a particular spot on a record, the record—not the needle—is probably worn or scratched. Remember, too, that the needle may be narrower but not wider than the record groove, so a needle geared for stereo records is fine for monaurals but not vice versa.

• Don't overstack records on the spindle. In fact, audio experts say a good rule is to stack only half the number considered acceptable by the company that makes your turntable.

• To avoid warping, always store your records vertically at moderate room temperature—not on a sunny windowsill, near a radiator, or in a hot car.

• Finally, if your favorite Beatles album is slightly the worse for years of wear, there's no need to throw it out; you won't damage your needle by running it over mild warps and scratches. Just make sure that you keep your turntable's tone arm weighted properly by following the instructions in your owner's manual.

clubs
a guide to record and tape clubs

If you'd like to build up your record or tape collection by mail *and* at a discount, check into the clubs listed below. We've also included mail-order companies that offer special albums not sold in stores.

Before you sign any agreement, read brochures and contracts carefully so that you know (1) how many records/tapes you're obligated to buy if you join a club, and (2) how the club operates. For example, under a "negative option" plan, you must return a card if you *don't* want the main club selections. With a "positive option" club, you initiate all orders; there is no minimum purchase. Under an "automatic ship" plan, you receive records/tapes for a ten-day trial. Here, too, returning a record can be inconvenient and may be at your own expense. Also keep in mind that records can take anywhere from two to six weeks to arrive and that postage/handling costs may be extra.

The key to abbreviations in this list follows.

COLUMBIA RECORD AND TAPE CLUB (1400 North Fruit Ridge, Terre Haute, IN 47811): All music categories, stereo, many labels. IO 11 rec/tapes $1.86, must buy 8 more in 3 years; D list price; SS 50%+; NO.

RCA MUSIC SERVICE (6550 East 30 St., Indianapolis, IN 46219): All music categories, stereo, many labels. IO 6 rec/tapes 5¢, must buy 4 more in 3 years; D list price; SS ⅓ to ½ off and more; NO.

INTERNATIONAL PREVIEW SOCIETY (175 Community Dr., Great Neck, NY 11025): Sets of 3- or 4-record albums—mostly Deutsche Grammophone, Phillips. Bonus certificate with every order entitles you to one record at half price. IO 4-record set $7.98 (value $31.92). After that, no minimum purchase required; D albums cost $15.99 each or ⅓ off; NO.

THE GREAT AWARDS COLLECTION (Same address as International Preview Society): Monthly series of classical LPs, all winners of top international music awards. Catalog every 4 wks. Bonus certificate. IO 4-record set $6.98; no minimum purchase; D—each LP ordered is $1 off list price of $6.98; NO.

TIME-LIFE RECORDS (Time & Life Bldg., Chicago, IL 60611): 6-record series—*Beethoven Bicentennial Collection, Wagner—The Ring of the Niebelung, Great Men of Music, The Story of Great Music, The Swing Era, As You Remember Them* (popular instrumentals). For each series ordered, you get multirecord album plus informative book/booklet every other month. With BBC, WRN, GMM, you get bonus book(s) with first purchase. No minimum purchase. Each volume ordered costs from $14 to $30, depending on series.

COMPANIES OFFERING "TOP HIT" ALBUMS NOT SOLD IN STORES: Categories range from classical to country to rock and jazz, from hits of one era or one artist to hits along a particular theme.
1) Tele House: 299 Park Ave., New York, NY 10017.
2) Sessions Records: 477 West Butterfield, Lombard, Ill 60148.
3) Brookville Marketing: 420 Lexington Ave., New York, NY 10017.

Key to abbreviations:
IO—introductory offer plus minimum purchase requirement
D—discount for monthly choice
SS—special higher discounts for other selections
NO—negative option plan
AS—automatic ship policy
PO—positive option plan

r romance

romance

flowers
put some romance in your life

Start spring, celebrate good news, or for no special reason at all, send him flowers for a change. It doesn't have to be a dozen "long stems"—one rose can be more dramatic, or send bachelor buttons or a bunch of daisies. Better yet, send him a plant for his bedroom or office to remind him of you all year round.

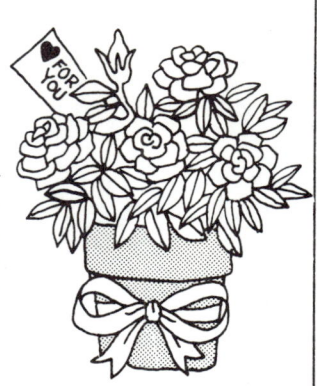

summer romance
what not to do about a summer romance, especially at the end of summer

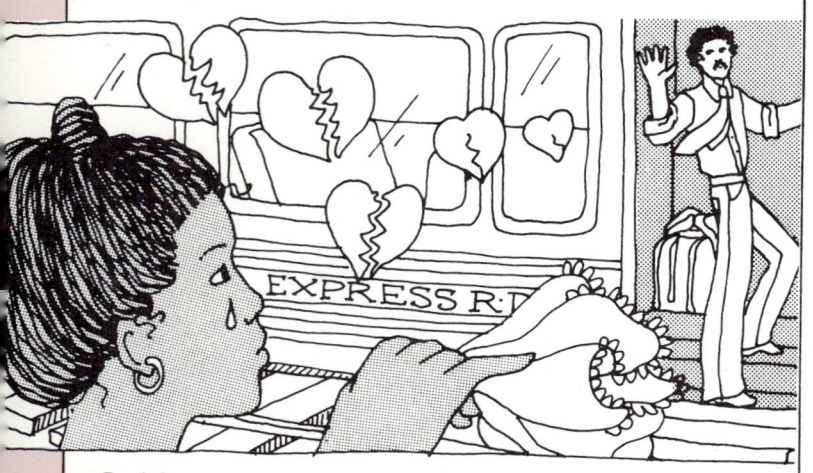

Don't forgo a summer romance just because you're afraid it won't last. But don't let summer's seductiveness blind your perspective. What worked under a full Spanish moon may not do as well back on home ground. By Cleveland moonlight, he may seem more ordinary.
- Don't blow the relationship out of proportion. If you've got a bad case of Roman fever for the man you lingered with at the Coliseum, maybe what you're really experiencing is the difficulty of reentering the nonvacation world and a normal routine. Get busy with new activity.
- Don't always consider the romance an all-or-nothing matter. Stay in touch with him periodically even if you aren't going to continue the romance. It's nice to have contacts in other cities, people who will give you an insider's view should you ever visit.
- Don't make the correspondence that immediately follows long or intense. You can never go wrong with the space allowed on a postcard—pick some up at a local museum; or send him a goofy souvenir from the town you live in—a tie or a coffee mug painted with one of its landmarks.
- Don't get into long, nothing-is-the-same-without-you letters or expensive phone conversations that are usually the product of a melancholy mood. They make you seem only one-dimensional—and get you nowhere.

telegram
send him one anytime

Who said it had to be opening night or a special occasion to send a telegram? Give someone the thrill of tearing one open—the message inside can be as simple as "You're the best." A Mailgram costs $2.75 (100 words or less) and will arrive in the next day's mail. A telegram—same-day delivery—starts at $4.75 (15 words or less), depending on where it's going; specify if you want the message hand-delivered rather than telephoned ($3 extra).

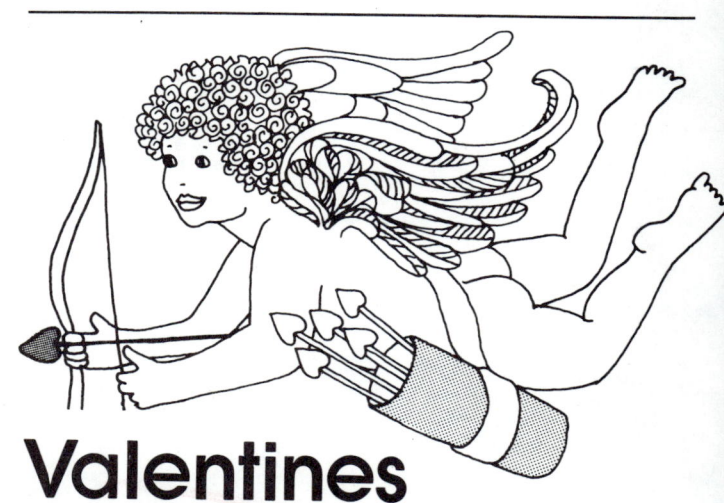

Valentines
12 mushy Valentines to make him fall in love with you all over again—or for the first time

Valentine's Day, the oldest holiday celebrated in the Western world, stems from an ancient fertility festival for lovers. You don't have to go as far as the Romans, but you can make it an excuse for being your most sentimental, romantic, and tender-hearted self. Here are some mushy Valentine gestures that are sure "to win his affection."
- Make him a real old-fashioned Valentine card—cut a big heart out of red construction paper, glue it to a paper doily, then fold it in half with an original or favorite poem of yours written inside.
- Give him a Valentine's Day wake-up call with Frank Sinatra's "My Funny Valentine" playing in the background.
- Serve him a luscious breakfast or brunch.
- Send his parents a thank-you letter for having him.
- In your sexiest, Lauren Bacall voice, tell him: "I'm hard to get. All you've got to do is ask."
- Surprise him with "penny" Valentines, secret love notes, and candy hearts (the kind that says "Be Mine" and "Kiss Me") that you've hidden in all the places that he'll reach into during the day—pockets, drawers, medicine chest, refrigerator (if he's very fastidious, put them in plastic bags).
- Give him a signed photograph of yourself in a lacy paper-doily frame.
- Send flowers.
- Bake him a loaf of bread in a heart-shaped cake pan. It's a real homemade Valentine, and if you paint it with clear polyurethane, it will last forever (even if your love affair doesn't).
- Treat him to a night on the town—you buy the dinner and tickets to a play, concert, or hockey game.
- Present him with the Valentine gift for the liberated man: a butcher's apron, a pot holder, and rubber kitchen gloves wrapped in tissue paper and tied with red ribbon.
- Muster up your courage and say what you really feel—"I'm crazy about you," "I think you're terrific," "I love you."

self-improvement

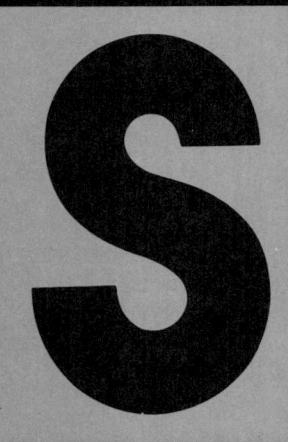

S

self-improvement
sewing
shoes
shopping smart
skiing
skin
sleep
smoking
sports
spring
sticky situations
summer
swimming

self-improvement

courses
find a course on almost anything

If you want to learn more about a particular subject or to develop a new job skill but don't know how, a center for life-long learning in your area may be able to help. These centers act as information clearinghouses for courses and programs available to adults at local colleges, vocational schools, museums, libraries, and community service organizations. Centers are now operating in most major cities, including Denver, Salt Lake City, Portland, St. Louis, and New York. The New York City Regional Center for Life-Long Learning (part of the City University of New York), for example, offers free information on over 20,000 courses at 550 institutions; it also offers telephone service, a printed directory, and workshops. Other centers also offer individual course and career planning. Some charge a fee, others don't. To find a center in your area, check the Yellow Pages of your phone book under School Advisory Services or call the office of the dean of continuing education at a local college or the adult education office of your local school board.

You might also try *The New York Times Guide to Continuing Education in America*. Or write for *On-Campus/Off-Campus Degree Programs for Part-Time Students;* send $4 to the National University Extension Association, One Dupont Circle, Suite 360, Washington, DC 20036.

family tree
how to trace your family tree

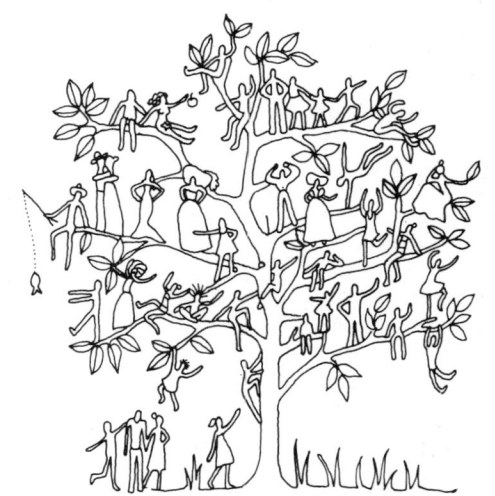

If you're curious about how and when your ancestors came to America or what they did before they got here, you may want to start a serious genealogical search back through your family tree. It can be a time-consuming but diverting process. If you get into the kind of snags that require professional help, a consultation fee could cost from $50 to $100. A warning: Don't fall for flat $200 promises to prove that you're directly descended from a duke—more than likely the fee will be real, the pedigree won't.

- *Begin by getting what information you can from parents, grandparents, aunts, and other relatives.*
- *Check birth certificates, naturalization papers, and wills via county and court records.*
- *Prepare a card index of family members starting with your generation. Use full names and list wives' maiden names.*
- *Talk to the librarian in your public library to find out where special genealogical collections are that might be helpful.*

S self-improvement

- Write to the Publications Sales Division of The National Archives, Washington, DC 20408 for their free genealogical information leaflets: "Genealogical Records in The National Archives" (GIL5) or "Genealogical Sources outside the National Archives" (GIL 6).
- Contact The Genealogical Society of The Church of Jesus Christ of Latter-Day Saints, 50 East North Temple St., Salt Lake City, UT 84150. It has launched a world-wide project of filming vital records, and its teams are working everywhere, even in previously inaccessible areas. Through their branch libraries—there are over 200 in the U.S.—you can order films on England's probate records, Sweden's birth list, etc. Write also for a list of private genealogical researchers who can provide professional assistance.

memory
remember names, faces, facts, and anything you don't want to forget

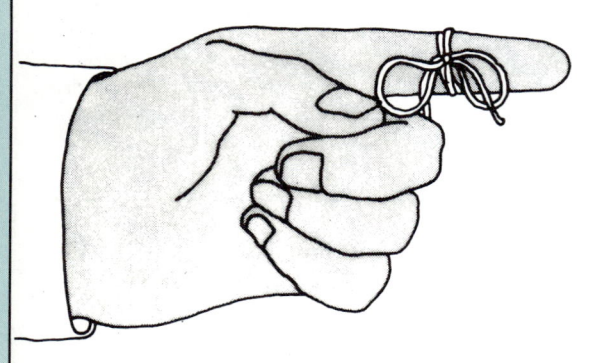

Have you ever remembered every comma of a "Dear John" letter you wrote six months ago but drawn a blank when you tried to recall the date of your mother's birthday? If so, you know that most of us have very selective memories and that no two are identical. You may be able to repeat verbatim passages from *Fear of Flying* or *The Prophet* but forget half the items on your weekly shopping list, while a friend does just the reverse. These differences, however, aren't simply a matter of one person's having a better memory than another. As Dr. Bruno Furst points out in his fascinating book *Stop Forgetting*, memories aren't so much "good" or "bad" as trained or untrained. Regular workouts will tighten slack memory muscles in much the same way as you'd tighten any other muscles. Try these tips for your problem areas:

● **names**
● To remember a name, make sure you hear it clearly and distinctly during an introduction. Then use the name as often as possible during the conversation immediately following. Next, try to make an association with the name. For example, a name may have a meaning of its own (such as Starr, Brown, Short, or Coffey) or it may recall a famous person (Whitney), product (Lipton), or place (Paris). Even if it doesn't, you may be able to make an association by breaking the name down into parts (Braverman) or translating it into English (Boucher into butcher). If you still can't make an association, you can always resort to a "sounds-like" ("devil" for Devlin, "dash in" and "skis" for Dashinsky). Then create a mental picture around the name and the image you have of it. For example, picture Ms. Carpenter dismembering your living room sofa with a hacksaw. The more colorful the picture, the more likely it is to jump to mind each time you see a person—and remind you instantly of a name.

● **faces**
● When it's important that you remember a face, pick two or three of the person's most salient facial features: maybe bat's-wing eyebrows, flaring nostrils, or pointy earlobes. Then mentally exaggerate these to make a caricature. Color your caricature with a characteristic facial expression (say, humility) that will be sure to leave a vivid imprint on your mind. Or try connecting a face to that of a famous person.

● **errands and calls**
● If you've written a letter you have to mail today, connect the letter with something you're certain to observe, say, a mailbox. You might visualize the recipient sitting on top of the box. If you habitually forget to mail letters, you can make a regular practice of asking yourself who is sitting on top of the mailbox today?
● Do you often forget to make an important phone call? Associate the person you have to call with your phone. Or, move the telephone to a spot you don't usually find it in—its new location will remind you.
● A good way not to leave behind a specific item, such as an umbrella, is to form a mental picture of the item when you put it down—your umbrella suspended from the center of your elevator, for example.

● **book or movie plots**
● After you've read a book or seen a movie, sit down as soon as possible and summarize it either in your head or for a friend. Wait even a day and your grasp of it will slip. You have to review a plot, theme, anecdote, or snappy punch line about four times to make it a permanent part of your repertoire.

shyness
5 steps to overcome shyness without going to a shrink

Being shy is like going through life with perpetually dirty hair and runs in your stockings. You feel miserably conspicuous, and no one else notices. Unless you are exceptionally shy—few people are—taking these five simple steps will help loosen you up.

1. Dr. Jerome L. Singer, author of *The Inner World of Daydreaming* and a professor of psychology at Yale, says that shy adults often were shy children who withdrew and consequently didn't acquire the social graces. They often can't dance, flirt, or make small talk and, thus, find social gatherings painfully unenjoyable. So learn to dance. It's the classic confidence boost.
2. As for learning to small-talk, it's basically a matter of opening your

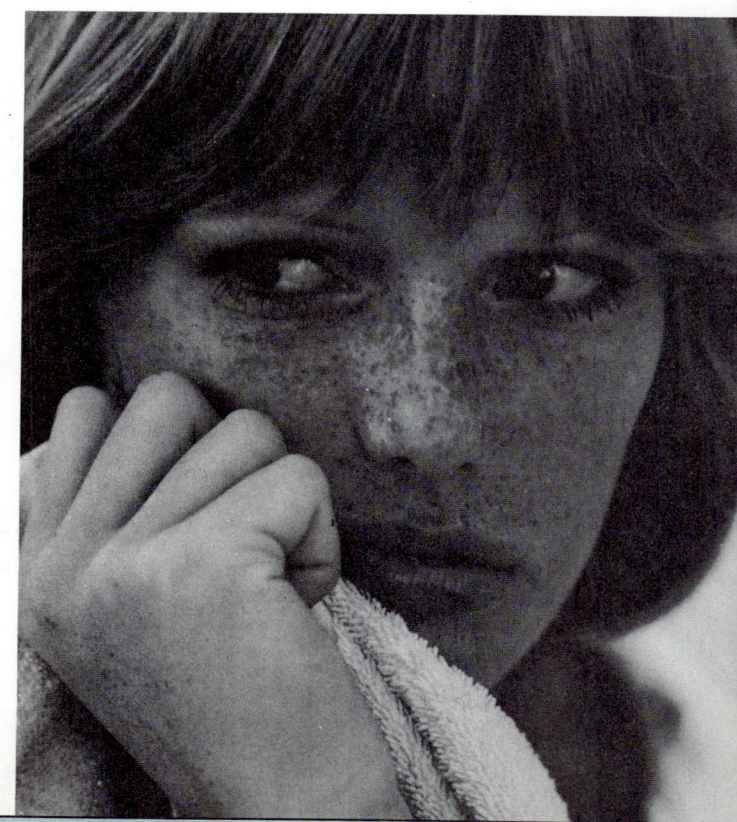

self-improvement

mouth and just saying it before the words get cold and the cat gets your tongue. According to Dr. Louis Hott, Medical Director of the Karen Horney Institute, shy people often place unreasonable importance on what they say and do. Probably the biggest hurdle to clear in overcoming shyness is taking yourself too seriously; no one else is expecting the ultimate profundity or witticism, so take the pressure off yourself.

3. Another good way to crack your shell is to enroll in an exercise, sport, or yoga class. A good workout is relaxing (just don't overdo it and get constrictive body muscles); afterwards, you'll be much less likely to tense up in difficult social situations. Make it a routine, and you'll begin feeling more confident of your body movements. Deep breathing exercises will also help calm you. Posture-improving exercise—ones that stretch the back muscles—will do wonders for your ego via your carriage. In no time at all, your arms will never again feel like lead pipes screwed, for some ridiculous reason, into your sides.

4. Emily Cho, a New York wardrobe consultant who owns and operates her own personal service, "New Image," says a shy woman can dress herself right out of her shell. Ms. Cho has found that the shy woman usually has a closet full of dark, drab dresses that hang loosely or are too big. She tries to hide in her clothes, but they offer her little real security. Ms. Cho recommends that a shy woman "compensate for initial shyness with clothes that express who she really is." To find out who you are and what image you want to project, go shopping. Try on anything that strikes your fancy and look at all the different you's. Ask a close friend to come along and react. Gradually, pick up several things and give yourself time to get used to them so that you won't feel in costume and on stage.

5. Often, shy people arm themselves at parties or other social gatherings with someone who is socially adept. But it rarely rubs off. The shy person merely ends up receding into someone else's shadow. Next time, try your own wings and go alone. You won't feel any pressure to live up to anyone else's poised behavior—and you just might surprise yourself.

singles
consciousness-raising groups: what do you find particularly difficult about being single?

"Like women, single people are, in some ways, second-class citizens," says Karen Terninko, leader of a singles consciousness-raising group sponsored by NTL Institute (National Training Laboratories), a consulting and training organization for sensitivity groups. "In singles consciousness-raising, you can find out that a lot of the things you thought were your own hang-ups or inadequacies are really the result of things society does to you through stereotyping." Some of the questions that come up in the sessions: What do you find particularly difficult about being single? How would you like your life to be diffferent?

As yet, singles groups are not available to most people. Ms. Terninko operates out of the central office of NTL Institute, Roslyn, Virginia. If you're interested in forming your own group, she suggests getting a qualified leader who has had experience running sensitivity or encounter groups, not just therapy groups. "A lot of therapists think that they can run any kind of group, but they can't because they don't understand small-group dynamics well enough to be able to turn it into anything but a therapy group," Ms. Terninko said. "Consciousness-raising has a therapeutic effect but it is not 'therapy.'" To find a qualified leader, you might check with the business schools or counseling departments of colleges in your area.

Or, as many women's consciousness-raising groups were started, you might just get together a group of singles yourself and discuss your own situations, as well as singles topics you've read about in books and magazines that focus in on the singles world.

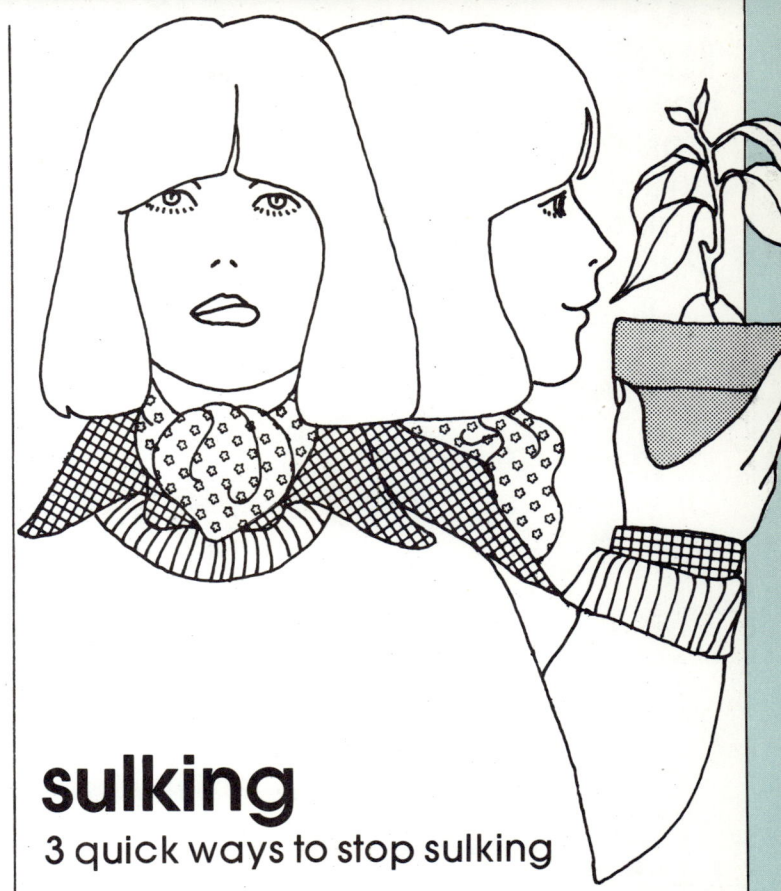

sulking
3 quick ways to stop sulking

We usually sulk when we want people to know that we are angry with them or hurt by them, according to psychologist Robert Tyson. But sulking around the house or office is the least effective form of communication because it puts the very person you want to notice you on the defensive—why should *he* have to do the guesswork about what's troubling you? What's in order is a straight statement from you, but often when you've gone into a sulk, you're too emotionally confused to be clear about your feelings. It's something akin to a mild depression. Here are Dr. Tyson's three easy, sensible steps to get you up and out of your sulk.

1. The worst thing that you can do when you're in such a low state of mind is *nothing*—lying on the sofa staring into space is no good because that cuts you off from exactly the stimulation you need in order to resurface. If you give in and withdraw, you will only prolong your misery. So go into action.

2. But no big-deal actions, nothing hard or important. The best first aid for a depressive sulk is called the "graded-test" method. This recent, effective therapy is based on the fact that the do-nothing mood deprives you of the main source of encouragement—the feeling of success. Try a new recipe, clean up those accumulated dribbles of office work or housework that you've been putting off, repot plants, weed and groom the garden. Do anything that's simple, that you can do well and easily, so that you get the positive feedback of success.

3. The chances are nine out of ten that you are being too hard on yourself. It is you, not the world, that is being so strict and expecting so much from you. It's you who is telling yourself that you should demand more cooperation from him, not him; it's you who wants to hate yourself because you fumbled the tennis game, not your partner. Be a bit more lenient on you. Have an ice-cream supper. Why not, for once? Or go buy the too-expensive T-shirt or strappy sandals you wanted. Then get yourself dressed up in them immediately—for the simple reason that we all tend to identify with how we look and act. If you identify happily with the new you, if you give another person even a half smile to show that you're rising out of your depths, he, or she, will respond to you positively instead of withdrawing to let you sulk it out.

S self-improvement

time
how to stop wasting time — and start making things happen

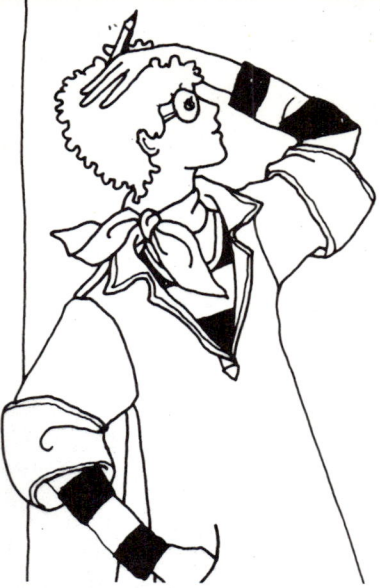

Wasting time—whether it means lounging around the pool or catching the breeze in a hammock—is one of the luxuries you're entitled to every so often. But there are also times when you need to get organized, to make things happen. We talked to Alan Lakein, a time-planning and life-goals consultant, who made some very good suggestions on how to get started.

- The most important thing, according to Mr. Lakein, is "not to feel guilty about any unfinished projects," for the times off and vacations that get in the way are good for you. Now's the time, however, to make fresh commitments to the goals you really want to achieve.
- Make a written list of everything you want to accomplish by a certain time. Label each item A, B, or C, according to priority. Your A's should be of high value, activities that will help you achieve important goals, such as taking on an extra project at work or getting your apartment painted at last. Your B's should be of medium value and your C's of low value, such as washing your car when you know it's going to rain. Always make A's your first consideration and C's your last—you may eventually find that many C's don't really need to be done at all and that by dropping them, you have more time for valuable A's.
- Now start planning your time. Write up a daily "to-do" list that contains the A's, B's, and C's you want to work on. Block out periods of the day for them, making sure that most of your time will be used for A's. (But be sure to keep your schedule loose, in order to allow for any changes.) Also, reflect for a moment to determine when during the day your "prime time" is. Since prime time is the part of the day when you feel most on top of things, that's when you should be working on your A's.
- Even though you've made a daily schedule, make it a habit to ask yourself several times a day, "What is the best use of my time right now?"
- Practice the "Swiss cheese" technique. It's Mr. Lakein's plan for using any short period of spare time to get started on A projects. For instance, when there are five minutes to kill before lunch, don't leaf through the same old magazines; instead start that book you have been wanting to read.
- Train yourself not to procrastinate. Whenever you get the slightest hint that you're wasting time on a C, say it. Say "I'm wasting time." The more you hear it, the more it will sink in and you'll finally go back to your A's.
- With a little planning, you'll soon be getting control of your time and be able to make the things you want to happen, happen. But don't make the mistake Mr. Lakein feels many people make—"trying to do too much too soon." The essential thing is to stay flexible. What good is your time if it isn't any fun?

Note: If you'd like to know more about Mr. Lakein's philosophy, you can find it in his book, How To Get Control of Your Time and Your Life.

volunteering
what to do if you'd like to volunteer— but don't know how to get started

If you've ever considered doing volunteer work but haven't known who needs your help, you may want to get in touch with the Voluntary Action Center nearest you. Nearly three hundred of these centers nationwide act as liaisons between people who want to help out and organizations —ranging from Planned Parenthood to recycling centers—that need them.

"Volunteering is a great way to refresh a tired psyche," says Felicia A. Fox, a coordinator of the Voluntary Action Center in Portsmouth, Virginia. A national staff member adds that many young women do it to make friends, to get paraprofessional experience for graduate school, or to "try on" careers they're thinking of switching to.

Check the White Pages of your phone book for the center in your area, or write to the National Center for Voluntary Action, 1214 16th Street N.W., Washington, DC 20036. Or call toll-free 800-424-8630.

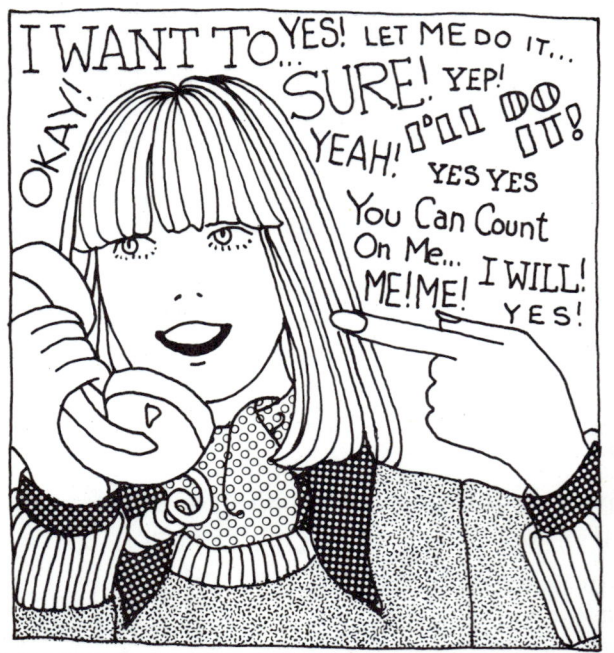

world records
10 world records waiting to be broken by you

If you have despaired of achieving immortality as an actress, best-selling novelist, or criminal defense lawyer, you may still be able to leave your mark on the world—or at least the record books—by setting a new record for donut-eating, Frisbee-throwing, or cucumber-slicing.

Records for all these and more appear in the 1975 edition of the Guinness Book of World Records, a classic 687-page collection of life's most fascinating superlatives. Among other things, the book tells the title of the best-selling novel of all times (Valley of the Dolls), the most common surname in the world (Chang, borne by roughly 10 percent of all Chinese), and the world's highest I.Q. (210, held by a 12-year-old South Korean prodigy).

Even more intriguing than such facts, however, are the following records, any of which might be broken but so far haven't been. Should you decide to try to topple one, the procedure for claiming your recognition is fairly simple; see the introduction to the Guinness Book of World Records for details.

148

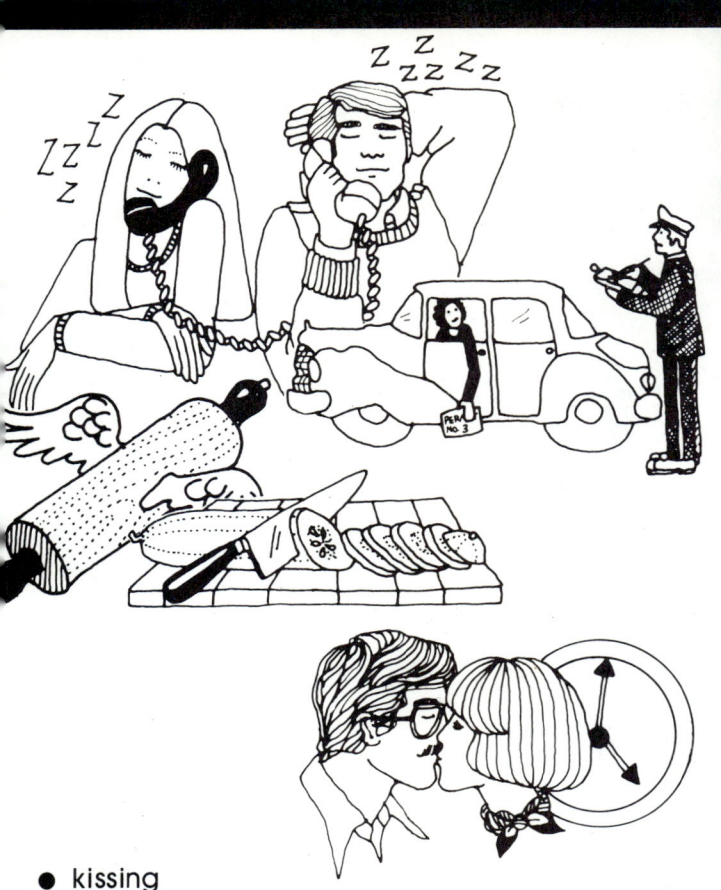

sewing S

sewing

dress
30-minute evening dress: make it today, wear it tonight!

The soft, bare dress below is such a snap to sew that even nonsewers can make it. It's also inexpensive—the cost of a couple of yards of fabric and trim for straps.

The secret to making this dress is to use the right kind of fabric—it must be soft and drape well. Lightweight jersey or any soft knit, not a double knit (most are too stiff) is a good choice. A soft challis would be pretty.

Using a tape measure, measure your body from underarm to the floor and add 5". Then buy that length of fabric, preferably 54" to 60" wide, or a tube fabric that's at least 50" in circumference to make a size 8 or 10 dress. The dress shown here is 52" around at the hem and will fit a size 8 or 10; for a size 12 or 14, add 1½" to 2" to the width.

Fold your fabric in half lengthwise and cut it, if necessary, to a width of 27" for sizes 8 to 10. Then seam the two raw edges together, leaving a 1" seam allowance—this will be the center back of the dress. Next, turn down 2½" at the top to form a casing for elastic. Stitch 1¼" down from top fold around, leaving a small opening for inserting the elastic.

To measure the elastic, hold a strip of 1" wide elastic firmly but comfortably around your chest, just above the bosom. To that length add 1" for a seam, and cut. Insert elastic in casing, seam elastic, and blindstitch the opening in casing. Slip on dress and arrange gathers so that you have a little burst of fullness in the center front and back, with the rest of the gathers evenly arranged around top of dress.

The prettiest straps can be made from rows of rhinestones or sequins, available by the yard in notions shops or department stores. A yard should be plenty for two straps. If you're using sequins, make double straps for strength. Pin straps in place, front and back, so they look right and feel comfortable, then tack them securely in place by hand. Hem dress. You can make a soft tie belt from the remainder of your fabric, or wear a suede or leather belt.

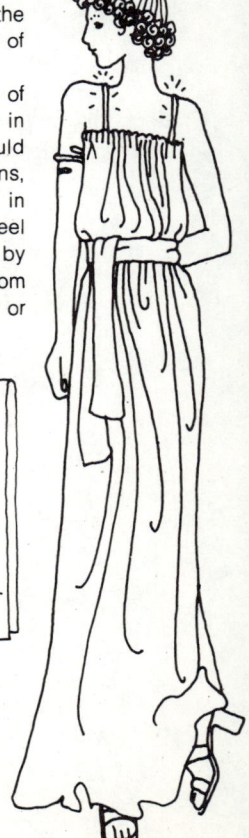

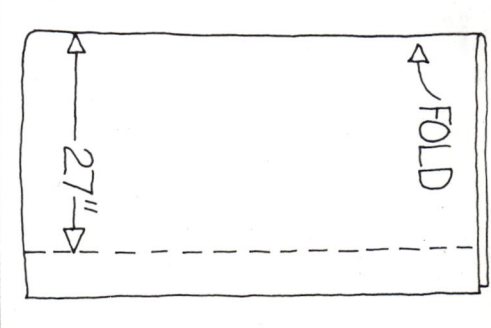

● **kissing**
You'll know it's "true love" if you can beat the world's record for kissing and come out of it still speaking to each other. All you have to do is top the one set at a "smoochathon" in Fort Lauderdale, Florida, on April 20 –24, 1974, when Vincent Torro and Louise Heath kissed for 96 hours, 32 minutes.

● **showering**
If you've ever been accused of monopolizing the shower, you may be able to scrub your way to a record. The current one was set in 1973 by David Foreman at Niagara University, who showered continuously for 175 hours and 7 minutes.

● **eating donuts, hamburgers, or potato chips**
Guinness lists 34 separate records for eating different foods in record times. For example, the one for donut-eating was set by Gary Edwards, a 27-year-old Californian who last year consumed 37 in 15 minutes. (Hint for prospective record-breakers: *Guinness* as yet lists none for eating McDonald's French fries.)

● **failing a driving test**
If you've flunked your test more than once, cheer up. Maybe you can unseat Miriam Hargrave, 62, of Yorkshire, England. She finally passed her driving test on her fortieth try, but by that point, she had spent $720 on driving lessons and could no longer afford a car.

● **telephoning**
To immortalize any club or organization, you might try to produce the world's longest busy signal. The longest telephone connection on record was 724 hours, between Sigma Nu fraternity and Kappa Delta sorority at Morehead State University in Kentucky.

● **throwing a rolling pin or Frisbee**
When it comes to unleashing frustrations, primal therapists might take a lesson from Oklahoman Sherri Salyer, who threw a 2-pound rolling pin 144 feet, 4 inches. The longest Frisbee throw on record is 285 feet by Robert F. May in San Francisco.

● **cucumber slicing**
Don't think of it as fixing a salad; think of it as training for the world's heavyweight title for cucumber-slicing. The incumbent? Norman Johnson, a British student, who sliced a 12-inch-long cucumber into 20 slices in 24.4 seconds, on the BBC-TV program, "Record Breakers."

149

S sewing

dress
make a sensational holiday dress — fast

The soft, bare dress below is easy to make and sensational to wear in three different ways. Here's how to sew it.

You'll need approximately 2½ yards (depending on your height) of 36" or 42" fabric. To determine the exact length you'll need, use a tape measure to measure from your underarm to the desired length of dress. A mid-calf hemline is the most versatile. Add 2" for hems. A soft, crapey fabric is best. A jersey, single-ply knit, or panné velvet would work well. First, cut two identical panels of fabric at your determined length down the width of your fabric. Next, make a casing across the top of both pieces by sewing on matching bias hem binding. Stitch binding to the top edge of dress fabric, right sides together, making a very narrow seam. Turn binding to inside of dress and stitch to dress, close to bottom edge of binding, to form a casing. Seam panels together down length, leaving 3" open at top and 12" open at bottom. Machine-stitch or handhem seam allowance of slit openings to the inside to finish. Insert a 40" length of ribbon or trim into the casing to tie over shoulders. You can also make a self-belt by stitching together two 40" long, 1" wide strips from additional fabric.

One way you can wear the dress is to tie straps over your shoulders and belt with matching sash or a purchased one, or you can wear the dress loose. Another way is to wear it as a strapless dress by tying the straps under your arms at the sides. Or you can wear it as a skirt by tying it at your waist.

If you want to make a self-belt, you'll need about ¼ yard more fabric.

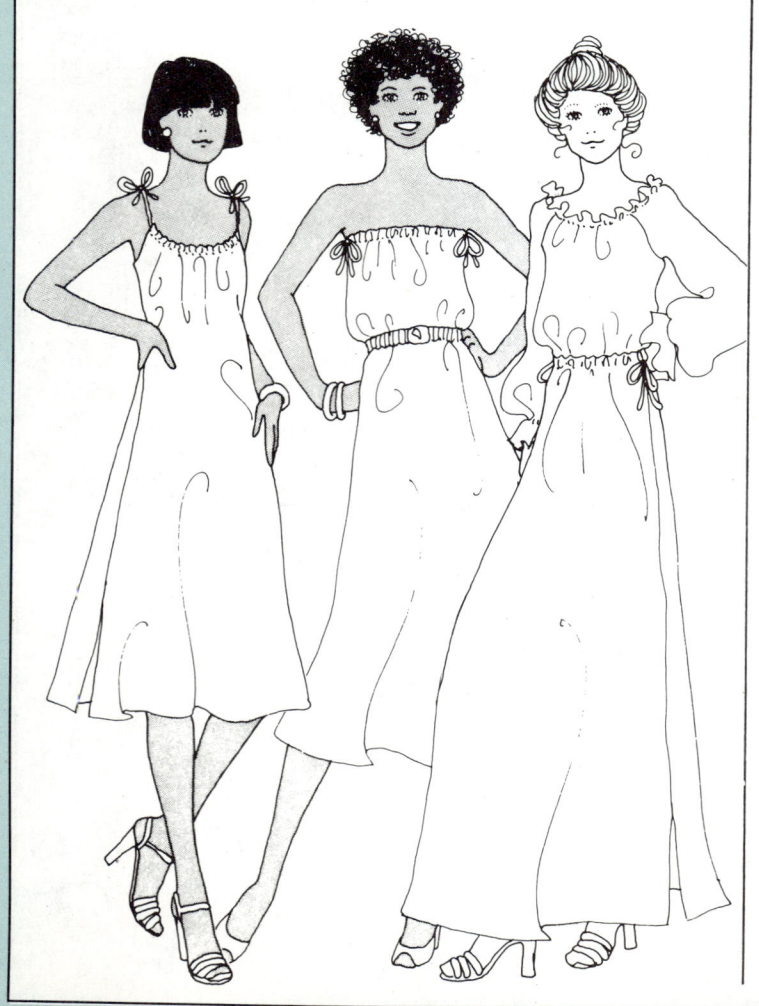

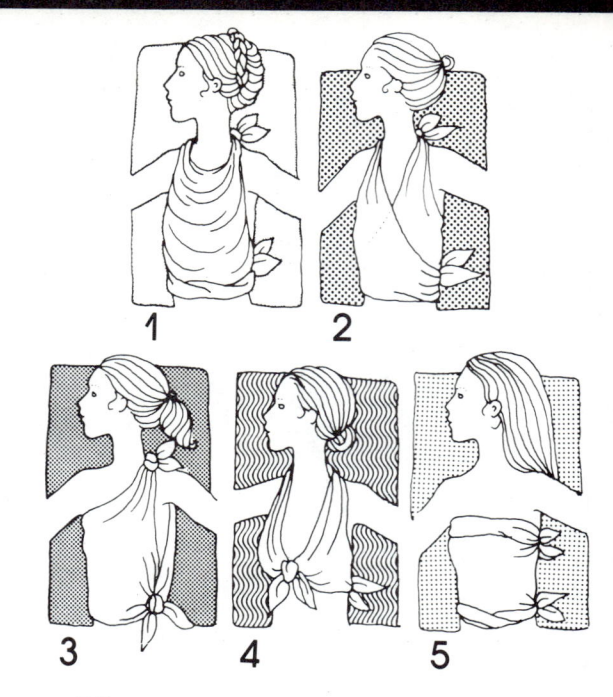

halter
a halter to make in 5 minutes to wear 5 different ways

This halter is probably the easiest thing you'll ever make. There isn't one single stitch to sew! Just cut, tie, and go. What is essential is that the fabric be a *single-knit nylon* that drapes very softly. (Don't buy a bonded knit.) It can be a print or solid color. Buy 1 yard of 45" or 1¼ yards of 42" fabric. Don't even hem edges, because hemming will limit the stretch and drape of fabric. The sketches above show five ways to tie the halter.

1. Hold fabric by corners in front of you, longer sides—if you're not using a square—hanging vertically. Tie top corners behind your neck and arrange neckline folds softly, forming a big, soft cowl neck. Gather fullness at waist, and tie remaining two corners in back at your waist.
2. Place fabric on any large, flat surface—a floor, a bed, or a table—with longer sides, if there are any, vertical. Bring one bottom corner up to the opposite top corner to make a triangle. Grasp the top ends, one in each hand, and tie behind your neck. Tie two bottom ends in back at your waist.
3. Hold fabric before you, with long sides vertical. Place top edge under one arm, bring up two top corners, and tie over opposite shoulder. Tie remaining two corners at waist, with knot off to one side. Arrange folds to cover underarm area.
4. Arrange fabric into a long, narrow strip and hang, scarflike, over your neck with loose ends toward waist. Tie two inner corners in front, under bosom, and remaining two in back at waist.
5. Place fabric over midriff of body with longer sides running horizontally. Tie top corners in back; tie remaining two in back at waist.

Another idea: Tie fabric around your waist, sarong-style, over a bikini.

hems
can you let that skirt down?

Some skirts made of certain fabrics are good candidates for lengthening, while others will give poor results. Know these tips before you let that old skirt down:

- Without undoing any stitches, roll the hem around to see if the

sewing

crease is very worn or soiled. If it is, you'll probably have a permanent mark. Light-colored skirts that have been dry cleaned often will also show a mark. Permanent-press fabrics are other poor bets to rework.
- Avoid most polyester fabrics, velvet, corduroy, or silk. The crease is there to stay.
- Creases can usually be steamed out of wool or a high wool-blend flannel, tweed, printed challis, or plaid, but not out of wool gabardine. One way to check when you don't know fiber content is to see if ordinary wrinkles press out easily from the skirt.
- Cotton skirts are usually easier to let down if they haven't faded or worn at the crease from too many cleanings. If you alter a cotton skirt that you usually dry clean, dampen the new hem with a sponge and press it, then send to the dry cleaner.
- Finally, ask your dry cleaner if he can steam out the crease from a particular skirt that you want to alter. If he says no, don't tackle the job.

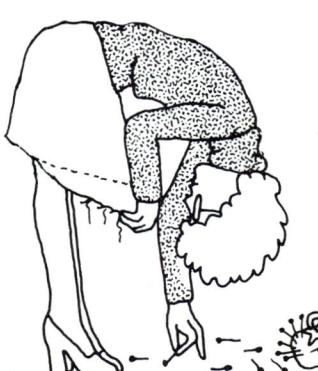

hems how to let down hems without leaving a mark

Your favorite coat is two inches shorter than your new skirts. Your old skirts look too short this year, and you can't afford to ditch them. Start on a skirt and see what kind of professional job you can do with this hint.

Take out the old hem and put in a new one as you normally do. Steam press the mark lightly, so that hem lies flat but mark is still quite visible. Machine-topstitch in matching or contrasting color thread right over the mark, using it as a stitching guide. Make another row of topstitching ¼" above or below the first. Press again to smooth stitching lines. What you have now is a smart-looking topstitched hem with no mark! If you want to lengthen a coat that's too thick for your machine to accommodate, take it to a good dry cleaner-tailor and clue him or her in to the trick. A professional machine will stitch through the thickness of your coat.

hems painless way to hem bias skirts

If your bias skirt needs to be shortened, you can be in for some tricky work, because any fabric cut on the bias has a tendency to stretch. So here are some tips:

The hem of a bias skirt should be as narrow as possible, which probably means you'll have to cut off the excess if the skirt is really long. After the hem is cut, run two rows of machine stitching parallel to raw edge to keep fabric from stretching. Then, before you hem, hang your skirt on a hanger overnight or longer to allow for any stretching. Unless the fabric is very sheer, don't use hemming tape; it can make the hem pucker. If you must use tape, use only narrow stretch lace tape. When you hem your skirt, keep stitches loose so they won't pull. When you press, don't press the very edge or fold of hem; stop just above it (see sketch). Pressing the fold will only make an unattractive edge.

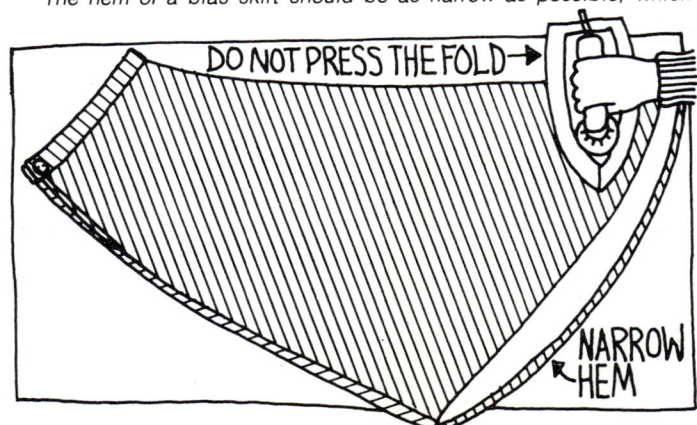

If your sewing machine has an adapter for a stretch or zigzag stitch, you can hem your skirt by machine, provided the style is sporty enough that you won't mind the stitches showing.

When your skirt is hemmed, fold it in half over a hanger to store instead of hanging in the conventional way. This method will help prevent further stretching.

jumper
make a super apron jumper in almost no time

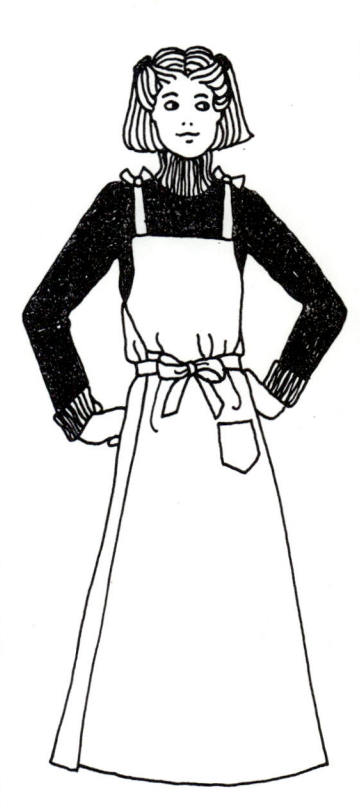

Butcher aprons are good for more than just cooking: two of them can turn into a super jumper with almost no sewing at all. Just buy two aprons in a fabric and color you like—you have a choice from printed cottons to sturdy denims. Cut the neck strap on each apron in half (the neck straps on some aprons are already in two pieces, so leave those as is). Then put on both aprons, one on your back, one on your front, and tie the front to the back neck straps so they become shoulder straps. Take the belt from the front apron and tie it around the back; bring the belt from the back apron around and tie it in a pretty bow in the front. If you want the sides closed, pin together the sides of both aprons, cutting off excess fabric if the skirts are very full, and stitch side seams together. Layer the jumper over a shirt or turtleneck and you've got a smashing look in almost no time, with almost no effort.

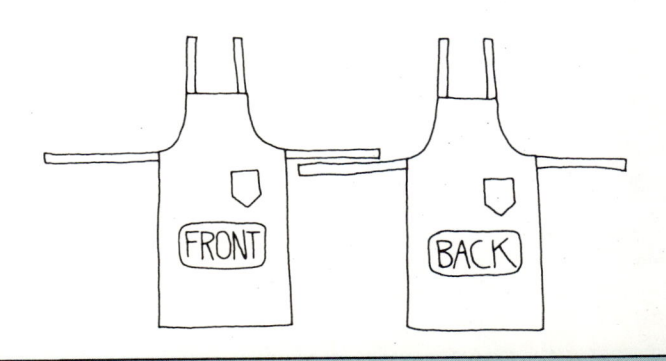

S sewing

leather & suede
tips for sewing leather and suede

Leather and suede, both the real thing and imitation, require special handling when you cut or sew. Here are some ideas to keep in mind:
- Don't pin your pattern down; instead, use mending or masking tape. You can use chalk or a tracing wheel to mark the pattern for cutting.
- Be sure you have good, sharp scissors for cutting the pattern accurately.
- Don't sew any seam until you're sure of it. If you rip out stitches, you'll find needle holes are permanent.
- A special foot for your sewing machine will help to feed the material more evenly. Singer's Even Feed Foot is good if your machine will adapt to it; otherwise, check with the manufacturer of your machine for a recommendation.
- Buy a special needle for leather to do any hand stitching, and use the recommended sewing-machine needle to machine-stitch.
- Rubber cement can be used to reinforce seams and to put up hems.
- Leather and suede skins usually have thin spots in them. Reinforce these areas with iron-on tape on the wrong side. Cut areas of your garment that get most stress from center of skin—it's the strongest part.

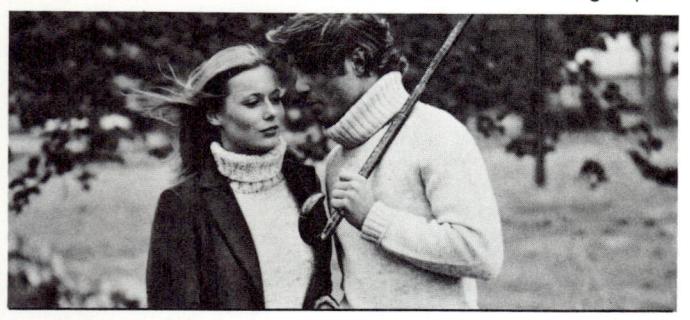

nightgown
make your own bow-tied nightgown in just half an hour

You can bow-tie yourself into this nifty gown, above right, about a half hour after you take the first stitch. It's so easy, you'll wonder how it can be so pretty.

You'll need 3 yards of 36" wide fabric. Drip-dry cottons like gingham and seersucker are good fabrics, or even nylon or other drip-dry synthetics. You'll also need 6 yards of grosgrain, velvet, or embroidered ribbon (8 yards if you want to edge the hem with ribbon). Be sure the ribbon you pick is washable too.

Start by cutting four pieces of fabric, each 17" long by 6" wide. Next, cut the remaining fabric into two rectangles, 42" long by 36" wide, to form the skirt. Sew two of the small pieces, right sides together, along one long and two short sides, taking a ½" seam. Leave one *long* side open. Turn to right side and press. Repeat with remaining two small pieces.

Next, sew the two rectangles together down the long sides to form skirt. Leave the top 6" open on each side. Press seams, and topstitch raw edges down on 6" you've left open.

Make a row of machine gathering along the top of each piece. Pull in gathers to fit the two top pieces you've just made. Sew tops to skirt. Cut four 1-yard lengths of ribbon. Machine-stitch ribbon to top edge of gown leaving equal ends free on each side to tie with. If you're using ½" or ¾" ribbon, you'll need two rows of stitching, one along top and one along bottom of the ribbon. Stitch another piece of ribbon over seam that joins skirt to top on both back and front of gown. Cut four ½-yard lengths of ribbon for straps. Machine-stitch one length about 3" in from corner on top of gown to form one shoulder strap. Stitch down securely, turning under raw edge of ribbon. Do the same with the other three pieces of ribbon.

Put on nightgown, tie sides and shoulders, and pin up length of hem. Cut off excess fabric so that your hem is 1" deep. Stitch hem by machine. If you want to edge the bottom with ribbon, measure, pin, and machine-stitch the ribbon in place.

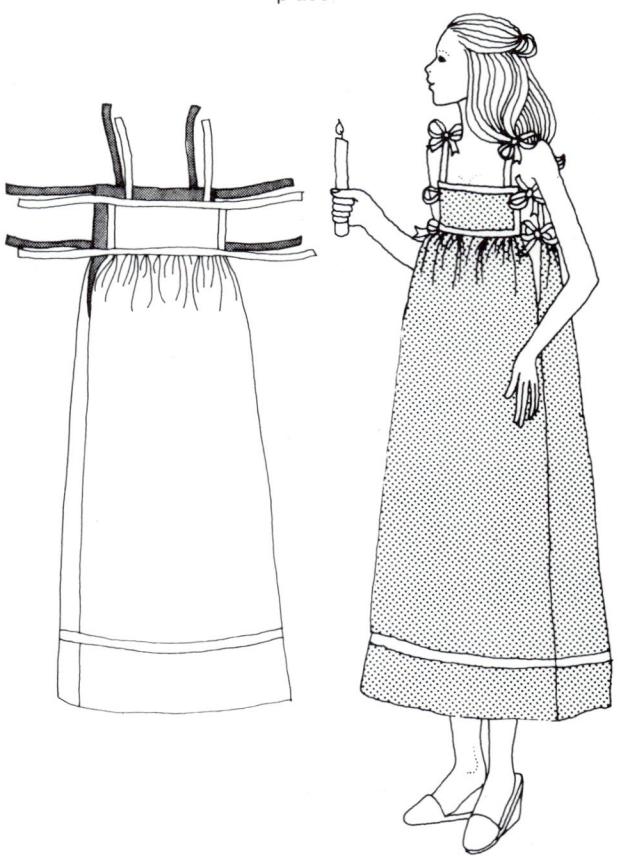

pants
quick way to shorten cuffed pants

You don't have to take the whole cuff apart to shorten cuffed pants. There's a much quicker, simpler way to do the job. Here's how:

Try on pants and decide how much shorter you want them to be. Then make a tuck *half* that deep on the inside of the leg, just below top of cuff so it won't show on the outside (see sketch). For example, if you want your pants 1" shorter, the tuck should be ½" deep, which will actually shorten the pants 1" because of its double thickness. Once

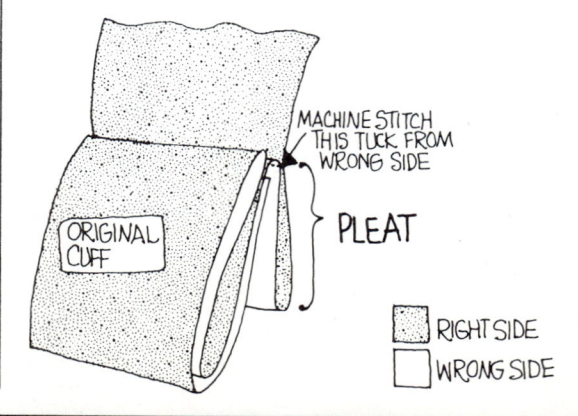

152

sewing

you've formed the tuck, pin in place and stitch by hand or machine.

If your pants have a wide cuff and are only a little too long, it's possible to hem the bottom of the cuff under and press flat. You will, of course, have less of a cuff with this method. If pants are of a very heavy fabric, however, make the tuck described above for the most professional-looking finish.

rain poncho
to cover you, books, packages

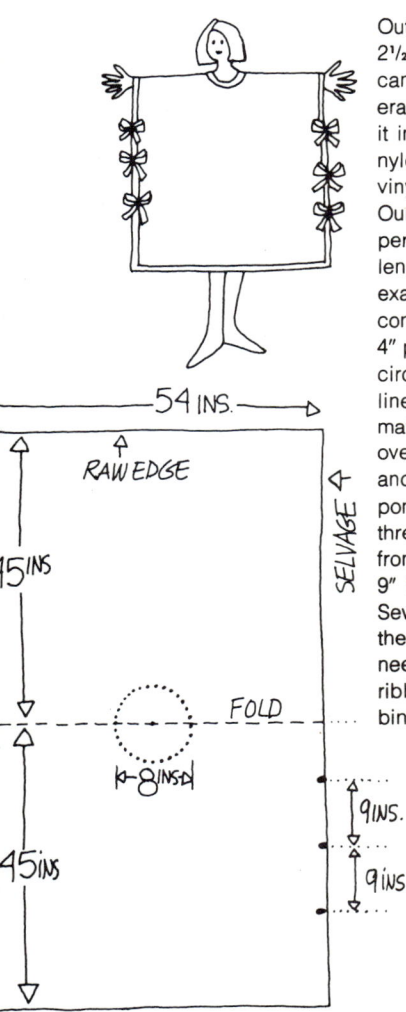

Out of this rectangle of material—2½ yards of 54" wide fabric—you can make your own portable coverage against rain or snow. Make it in ciré (light as wind-breaking nylon), plain or cotton-backed vinyl, or water-repellent canvas. Our dimensions will cover a 5'8" person down to about knee length. Fold the length of fabric exactly in half. With a marker or contrasting color pencil tied to a 4" piece of string, swing a semicircle from the center of the fold line. Cut out the circle with the material still folded. Slip poncho over head, adjust sides; remove and hem to desired length. Fold poncho lengthwise and mark off three points that are 9" apart on front and back sides, beginning 9" from fold and moving down. Sew on 6" pieces of ribbon at these points to tie poncho. You'll need ten 24-inch sections of wide ribbon to sew on for ties and binding around edges and neck.

shirts how to make an ordinary shirt into a great new jacket

Any shirt you've grown a bit tired of or feel is too "blousy" to layer under sweaters can be turned into a great new nonpro baseball jacket. You can make the transformation in just a couple of hours using any nonclingy shirt. Bodyshirts with darts will work if you open the darts first. The straighter and looser the shirt, the more fullness you'll get at the waist of your jacket.

To start, you need a shirt, plus about 1 yard of knitted ribbing, available in many notions sections of department stores and fabric shops. We used Lowenthal's Ribbed Banding, which comes in 2", 4", and 6" widths in fashion colors and stripes. Cut your shirt 2½" below your natural waistline. You can taper the length slightly longer toward the center back if you're longwaisted. Turn up a ¼" hem around the bottom, then run a row of long machine stitches around the bottom. Pull thread to gather. You'll be able to arrange the gathers better if you gather the two front parts and the back separately. Pull in the gathering threads until the jacket fits comfortably at your waist. Leave about 1½" ease.

Next, cut a length of ribbing to fit your waist comfortably, adding ½" turnback on each end. Pin ribbing to right side of gathered edge of shirt, leaving the ½" turnbacks loose. Stretch slightly if necessary to adjust fit. Be sure gathers look even all around. Machine stitch ribbing. Sew ends to inside; finish with snaps or hooks.

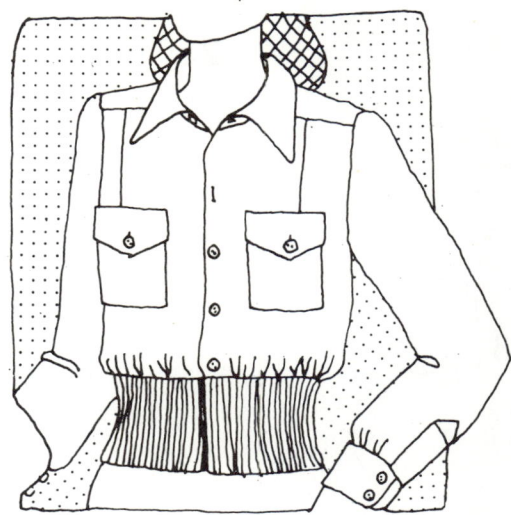

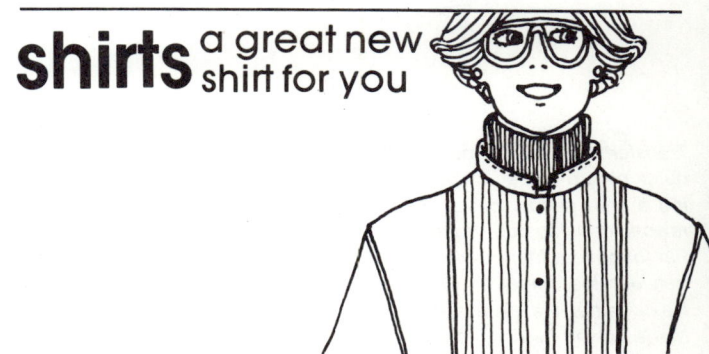

shirts a great new shirt for you

A man's tuxedo shirt with tucks or ruffles down the front has the makings of a sensational shirt for you—with just a little work. Pick one that's a bit blousy on you for a soft, easy look. If the collar and cuffs are frayed; it doesn't matter. Here's what to do with the shirt:

1. Carefully remove the collar from the collar band by slitting the stitches with scissors. Then, stitch the collar band together again (see sketch). This will give a sleek, band-collar look that's pretty.
2. If the sleeves are too long or the cuffs frayed, cut off the cuffs and stitch a small hem. Wear sleeves rolled up to just below the elbow.
3. Find tiny white pearl buttons to fit through the stud holes. For even less sewing, use studs.
4. You can leave the shirt as is—soft and white—or you can dye it.
5. Layer it over a T-shirt in warm weather, a turtleneck in cold. You can wear the blouse belted, tucked in, or left loose.

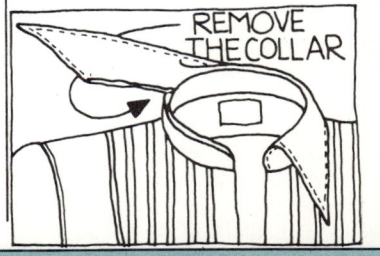

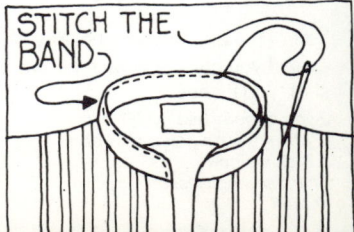

153

S sewing

shirts — taper his (or your) shirts

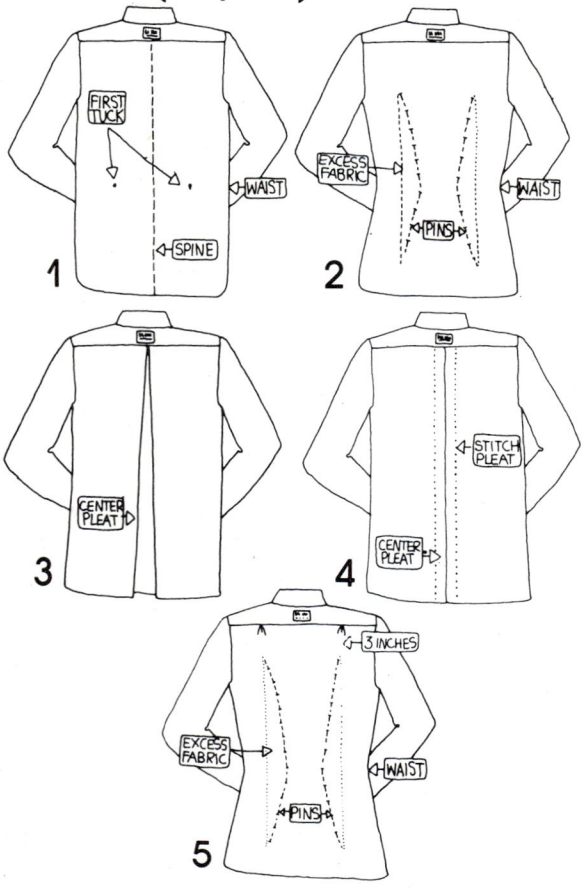

Transforming box-shaped shirts into tapered-body ones can be a quick pin-up-and-stitch procedure. To determine the amount of tapering a shirt needs, put it on inside out (the sketches show the shirt reworked inside out). Button it up, but leave the shirttail hanging free. Pin (or have a friend help you pin) a tuck at the waist at the midpoint between the center and either side. See Sketch 1; note "first tuck." Next, gather the excess material and pin to the bottom of shoulder blade, taking in less fabric as you go till the top tuck is just 1/8". Then pin down from the waist to 2" from hem. Repeat on the other side, taking in an equal amount of fabric, as in Sketch 2. Take a sit-down test: If the shirt feels tight or uncomfortable, release an even amount of fabric on each side and repin. The last step is a snap of a sewing job. Place each dart flat on the machine and stitch up, taking out the pins as you go. Should your shirt have a center pleat, as shown in Sketch 3, sew it down the back with two parallel rows of top stitching as in Sketch 4, before sewing in darts. Some men's shirts also have two small gathers on either side at the shoulder blade. To taper this style, stitch up the two tapering darts, stopping about 3" below each gather, as in Sketch 5. The dart should point to the center of the gather.

skirt — make this holiday skirt in 30 minutes

You can make the gala holiday skirt, above right, in thirty minutes, and even if you can't sew buttons, we guarantee you'll be able to make this skirt. You'll need:

2 yds. of good quality 72" wide felt.
1 yd. inch-wide grosgrain ribbon
1 7" skirt zipper
Sharp sewing scissors
Thread

The felt comes with a lengthwise fold in it; *don't* open it. Fold the entire two-yard length in half widthwise so that you have a 36" square. Find the corner that has *all* double folds with no raw edges. Measure down 3" from this corner. Make a light pencil mark. Make several more marks 3" down to form a cutting line, (see sketch). Cut on the line through all thicknesses. Then, place zipper on one of the folds so that the top of the pull is even with the edge you've just cut. Make a pencil mark at the end of the metal teeth. Slash the fold to your pencil mark to make an opening for the zipper.

Next, measure down 33" from the top of the skirt (where you've just cut). Measure down to different points several more times, until you have a cutting line. Cut through all thicknesses.

Try on skirt, and with your fingers, gently stretch felt at waist to fit comfortably. Take off the skirt and pin the grosgrain ribbon around the inside of the opening to prevent it from stretching further. Pin zipper into the opening you've cut, folding narrow seam allowances of felt to the inside of skirt before pinning. Layer the skirt, zipper, and ribbon with the zipper in the middle. Turn under raw edges of grosgrain to make a neat finish at ends. Trim off the tape "ears" at top of zipper. Sew ribbon and zipper, using a backstitch if you don't have a machine.

Try on the skirt for length. It can be cut as short as you like. You may want to trim it with glitter. A decorative belt will give the waist a smooth finish.

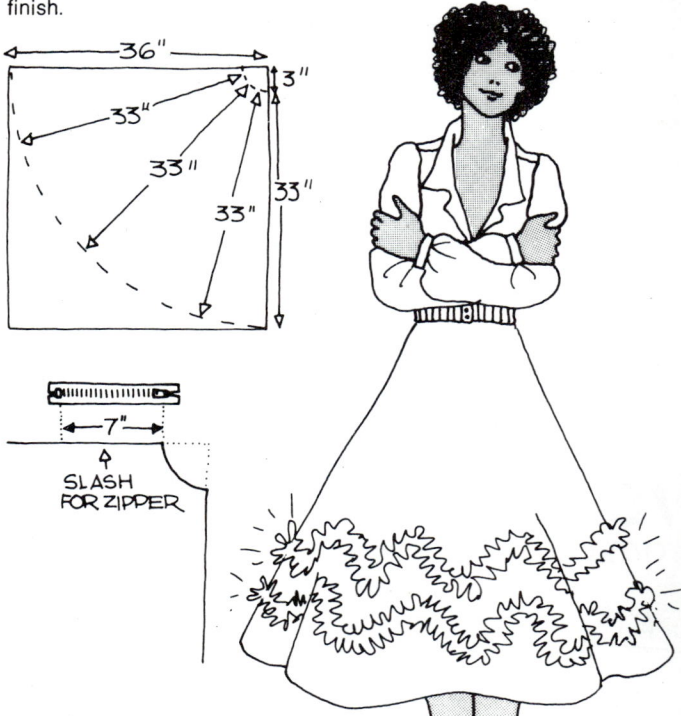

tops — a pretty peasant top to make in less than an hour

Come spring and summer, anyone can use a soft, pretty peasant top like the one sketched here. It's fabulous with long skirts or pants, and you can stitch it up in about an hour. You'll need:

1¾ yds. 45" fabric
½ yd. ¼" elastic for wrists
2 yds. narrow ribbon for neckline
Stretch lace seam tape

Fold fabric into quarters and lightly chalk in measurements (see sketch). Cut out "body" and two "sleeve extension" pieces. With right sides together, attach sleeve extension pieces to sleeves of the body along the 20" lengths. Topstitch with two rows in same or contrasting color thread. Then pin and stitch arm and side seams from wrist to hem

shoes S

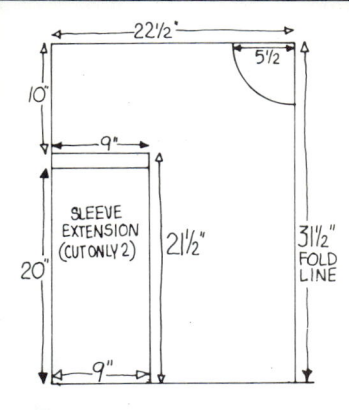

in one continuous seam, clipping corners at underarm. Turn fabric under ½" at wrist and stitch to make casing, leaving 1" open. Insert elastic through opening, gathering to size you want. Stitch the ends of elastic together, and hand-stitch casing closed. At center front of neckline, ¾" from top edge, sew a buttonhole. Stitch stretch lace tape to right side at neckline. Turn to inside, press, and stitch. Tunnel ribbon through buttonhole and around neckline, leaving enough ribbon to pull to size, and tie in a bow. Fold up bottom edge ¼", press, then hem to desired length.

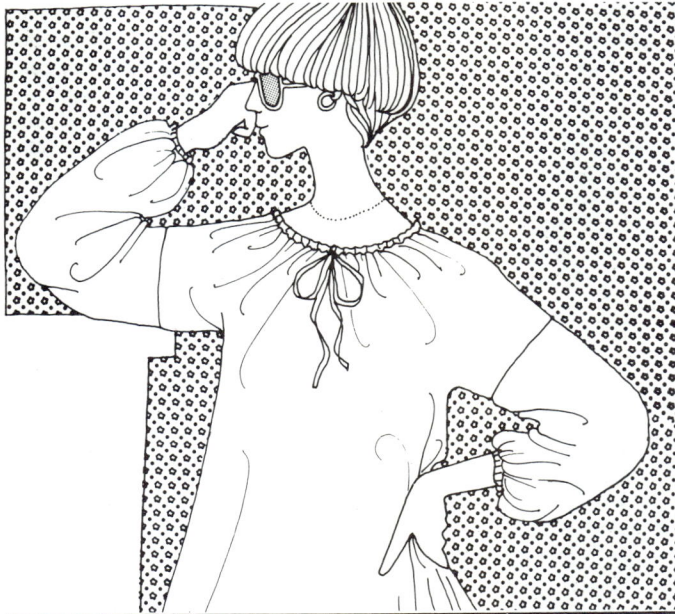

vest make a great new vest from what's already in your closet

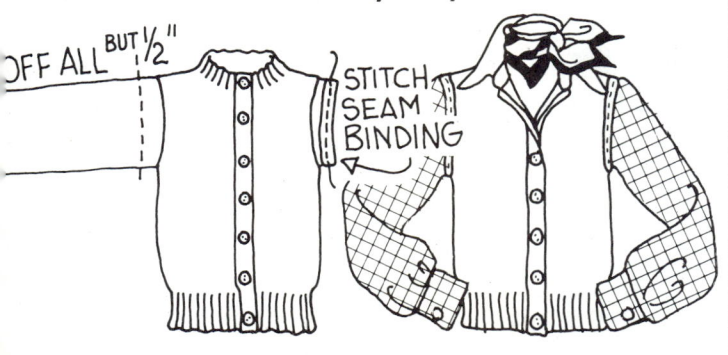

Vests are important fashion year round. You can have a vest without buying one new by looking through your closet for any good but not too-often worn cardigan sweater with a regular set-in (not raglan) sleeve, or a denim or other lightweight jacket. Here's how to turn the sweater or jacket into a super vest.

Cut the sleeves off your sweater or jacket, leaving a ½" extension beyond the shoulder seam (see sketch). Machine-stitch seam binding to the extension. Use stretch binding on knits, regular binding on woven fabrics. Next, turn back the binding and extension at the shoulder seam (see sketch), and hand hem in place on wrong side. That's *it*. You've got a great new vest to layer over shirts or turtlenecks!

shoes

boots
summer care and feeding for boots

Here are tips for cleaning your boots before storing them for summer:
● *Leather* is animal skin, and like your own skin, it needs cleaning and moisturizing. For delicate leathers like kidskin, a neutral cream is a good cleansing and moisturizing agent. Saddle soap works best on heavy leathers like cowhide. It's too harsh for fine leather and can dull the finish or crack the leather.
● *Suede* boots need brushing with very fine sandpaper or a dry sponge.
● *Vinyl and cloth*—Wipe with a sponge dampened in nondetergent soap. To repel stains, spray with Scotchgard®. To prevent tarnish and chips on metal ornaments, paint them with clear nail polish.
● *Summer storing and protecting*—Don't let your boots crumple up in the back of a closet; stuff them with inflated oblong balloons, crumpled newspaper, or dress cardboard, or clip them onto a skirt hanger. Cover boots during summer months. You can buy a vinyl boot-storage bag with openings on top that allow air to circulate. A cheaper covering method is two paper shopping bags, one inverted over the other.

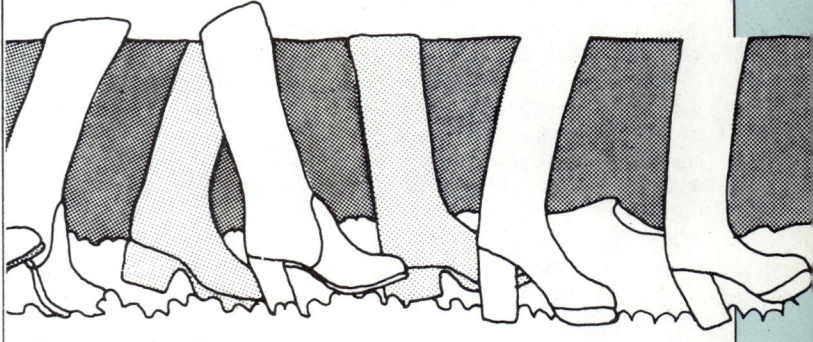

boots easy ways to help your boots take winter in stride

New leather boots should be treated with one of the many good *waterproofing sprays* on the market. If your old boots are not too far gone, waterproofing can give them added life. Follow the directions on the product you buy to the letter. Sloppy application might make the spray ineffective. Some of these products can be used on suede boots as well, but never put any product on suede boots or shoes unless directions specifically state that the product is safe for suede.

Saddle soap new leather riding or sturdy outdoor boots to nourish and protect the leather. The same goes for your old faithfuls. Many manufacturers of leather boots recommend a weekly saddle soaping to keep them in first-rate shape. However, for dressier kidskin boots, use a protective neutral cream.

If your boots do get waterlogged or stained, let them *dry out naturally* (never near a radiator) before treating them. Wash off salt stains with clear water before letting boots dry. If you have a good pair of boot trees, put them in your boots while they dry to help them keep their shape. If you don't have trees, gently stuff boots with newspaper until the shape looks as close to new as you can get it, and let the boots dry with the newspaper inside.

There are a few commercial products on the market that will help

155

S shoes

remove salt stains, but nothing does a perfect job. Waterproofing the boots before they get stained will keep the salt from penetrating too deeply and help to make the salt-removing sprays more effective. You may have to look in several shoe shops before you find one of these products, but they are made, and with persistence you'll find one. If your boots are suede, check product label to be sure it's okay to use.

To *remove matted spots* on suede boots, brush with the fine side of an emery board or very fine sandpaper, then apply one of the many suede-renewing products on the market. A mild solution of vinegar and water applied to the suede, followed by a brushing with a good suede brush after it dries, will also help restore matted areas to original finish.

And last but not least, remember that real blizzards or heavy rain storms call for waterproof boots, such as rubber or vinyl ones. Suede or smooth leather boots were never meant to stand up to this kind of weather.

buying how to buy shoes that really fit

Probably the biggest mistake most people make when they buy shoes is buying shoes that hurt in the store, then expecting the hurt to go away after the shoes are worn a while. It usually doesn't happen. Shoes you have to "break in" will, more than likely, break you, leaving blisters, corns, and whatever as memories. Here are tips to help you keep the "ouch" out of the shoes you buy from here on in:

- *DON'T buy shoes after you have walked all day long. Your feet are swollen after a whole day of walking and you'll never get a perfect fit.*
- *DON'T count on shoes stretching much after you buy them. Sometimes they will, but most times, the amount of stretch won't compensate for shoes that are plain tight.*
- *In general, suede or a soft kidskin "gives" somewhat more than calfskin, but don't buy even suede shoes that are really too tight.*
- *Always wear the kind of stockings or socks you plan to wear with new shoes when you buy them. If you're buying clogs to wear with thick, bulky socks, for instance, that's what you should wear in the store; sheer stockings will give you an entirely different fit.*
- *Check fit carefully when you buy high, chunky heels. They tend to push your feet forward and you may need a half size larger. Try your regular size and a half size larger and compare which feels better.*
- *Remember that size varies. You may not always be a size 6B, so don't buy it just because it's "your size." Try another size if a shoe is uncomfortable. Judge the shoe by how it feels, not by what size it is.*
- *Always ask the shoe clerk to measure both feet. As you get older, your feet tend to lengthen. Also, most people have unequal size feet; the larger of the two feet should be your shoe size.*
- *Don't hesitate to ask for a spot stretch. Clogs may need some stretching across the instep, while other shoes may pinch only in the toe, and so on. An innersole is a possible solution if a shoe is slightly loose. Since the trend is to consolidate sizes, you'll be seeing less of AA, A, B, or C, and more narrow, medium, or wide, so adjustments may be in order. Be sure to find out if you'll have to buy the shoes after they're worked on. Adding an innersole usually is reversible, but stretching is not—and you may be obliged to buy. Don't even suggest changes if the shoes aren't basically comfortable.*

comfort wear your shoes and boots happily

Shoes and boots that hurt end up in the back of the closet; no one can afford that kind of waste these days. Unless you have a special foot problem that should be taken to a physician or podiatrist, here are some happy ways to avoid the usual foot aches and complaints. They were suggested by Dr. Edward Stamm, past-president of the Podiatry Society of the State of New York.

- **the higher heels**

By pushing down your toes and tilting up your heels, *high-heeled shoes* shorten hamstring and calf muscles at the back of your legs. Stepping down to low heels or bare feet stretches them again. You can minimize strain by easing out of (or into) high heels gradually. For example, if you wear flats to work and plan on high heels for evening, wear medium-heeled shoes for a half hour or so in between, maybe while dressing for your date.

You can also keep muscles and tendons limber by trying the following stretching exercise half a dozen times (about two minutes) daily. Stand barefoot and erect with palms against the wall (an arm's length away and at shoulder height). With a slow, continuous motion, bend elbows, and come as close to the wall as you can without bending your body or lifting your heels. Count five, then push back slowly and repeat (see sketch).

- **tips on boots**

Cossack or cowboy boots are great outdoors, but if they're heavy (not all are) you may be in for some foot fatigue unless you limit wearing time. Switch to lighter shoes or slippers at home, or at the office.

Leather boots are porous; *synthetics* aren't. Perspiration can evaporate through a leather boot but may become trapped inside a synthetic. The solution: wear only thin cotton socks or "footies" under your stockings to absorb moisture and provide insulation.

Loose-fitting boots are great looking with big skirts and full-sweater and dress styles. But if you have *close-fitting boots*, be sure to put them on the right way. (Support stockings, incidentally, should be put on the same way.) Make sure your feet are drained of excess fluids—that is, elevate them for about two minutes. Keep your foot raised when you zip or pull on a boot. This way the snug fit will support your leg.

- **everyday shoes**

A good rule of thumb is to fit shoes to function. More flexible sandals or flat espadrilles are fine for walking on softer country roads or indoors. But for hard, city pavements, you need better arch support. Sturdy walking shoes are a good choice for a lot of city-street walking.

- **general tips**

Remember that skin care can help eliminate odor. First, lightly rub away dead skin with a turkish towel or loofa sponge while you bathe. Then use a good moisturizer (if you have dry skin) or witch hazel (if your skin is too moist).

Alternate wearing different shoes every day, to prevent foot odor and to get more wear out of all your shoes.

espadrilles
wrap up a new look for espadrilles

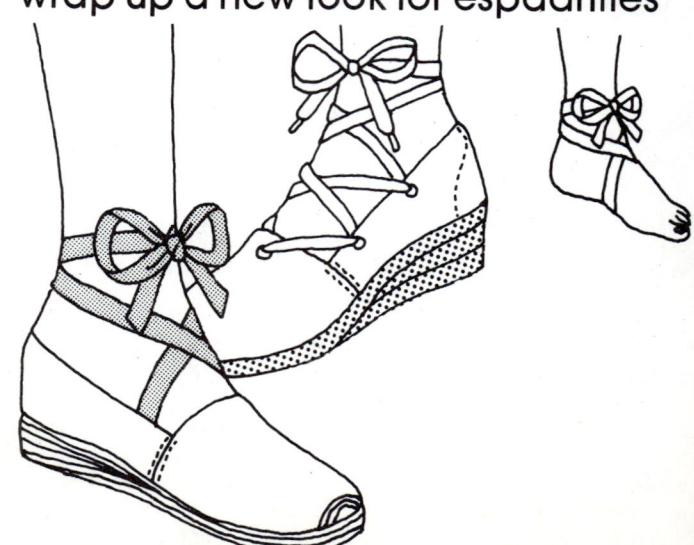

shoes S

A super look for espadrilles is this one—ankle-wrapped with grosgrain ribbon. These shoes look great with bare tanned legs and a soft, flower-print skirt. Just crisscross your ankles once with ribbon, and tie a bow in front, as in the sketch. For variety, try doing the same thing with long shoelaces or contrasting ribbon. Then put on your espadrilles—and voilà!

You might also turn an old pair of plain espadrilles into permanent lace-ups by attaching eyelets along the border, as in sketch. You can find an inexpensive kit with eyelets and attaching tools at any notions store. Just thread ribbon through eyelets and wrap it around your leg.

espadrilles
get your money's worth from your next pair of espadrilles

While some espadrilles are great buys, others are rip-offs. To get what you paid for, check these points:
- *The sole*—For longer wear, pick a pair with a crepe sole glued on the rope. Check to see that it's glued on securely. Another good feature is a rubber-reinforced heel; it will last longer and can be replaced. Crepe-soled varieties can usually be reheeled, too.
- *The size*—Espadrilles stretch with wear, so don't buy a pair that tends to be loose. Your big toe should fit comfortably. If it's too tight here, your toe may come through, but a little tightness over the instep or at the heel will work out quickly. If you have a narrow foot and the espadrilles seem wide, insert innersoles to take up the extra width.
- *The wedge*—Make sure the roping is "clean" (unfrayed) and securely glued down. If it isn't, this is a sign that the rest of the shoe is poorly made. If the roping does come loose after some wear, glue it with rubber cement.
- *The seams*—The edges should be double-stitched or reinforced. Seams at the back and sides should be secure.
- *The laces*—Espadrilles with laces should have reinforced holes (either topstitched or eyelets) or loops that are securely sewn on. Unfinished holes will tear after one or two wearings.

repair
8 things we bet you didn't know you could do with old shoes

A good shoe repair shop can do almost anything with old shoes—from widening, to tightening, even to changing heel heights on some shoes. If the shoes in question are top quality, it's worth the effort and money to save them. Here's a rundown on the more unusual changes you can make:

1. Heels can be lowered or built up a bit by the addition or subtraction of a lift for about $10. Or you can have an entirely new heel in a completely different shape put on; prices start at about $13.
2. If you've had your new shoes "stretched" and they still hurt, a shoemaker can open up the shoe where the leather meets the sole and add an extra piece all around.
3. If your shoes are tight across the instep, a gusset under the vamp will give you more ease.
4. Loose shoes can be altered to fit more snugly for $6 and up, depending on what's involved.
5. Boots that are tight in the calf can have leather or elastic gussets added.
6. If you have a pair of boots or shoes with salt stains around the toes, they can be covered up with a piece of matching leather or suede, giving the shoe a "wing tip" or "spectator" look.
7. If the rope or straw parts on your wedged shoes get destroyed, you might have them replaced or covered in leather if you think your shoes are worth saving. Prices begin at about $12.
8. If you've got a great pair of good-looking, comfortable shoes that shout old age, think of having the toes cut out or the backs cut off for a slingback look.

sneakers
how to sneak up on a great pair of sneakers

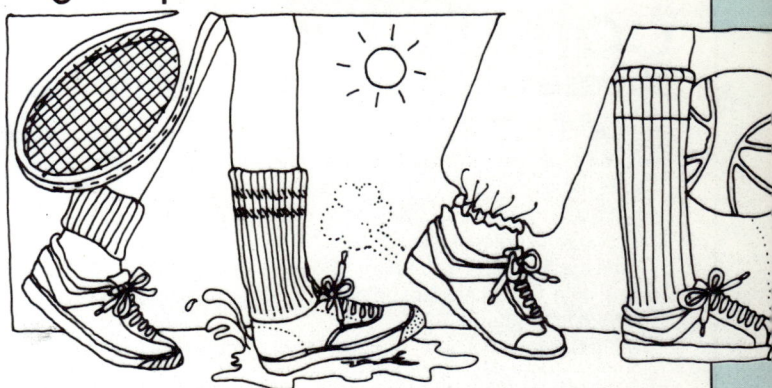

Remember when sneakers were plain canvas shoes with rubber soles and laces? Now there are literally hundreds of varieties—for everything from jogging to sky diving. How do you find the sneakers that are best for your needs? John Weiss of Runner's World is our sneaker expert.

- **good basics to look for**
- Sneakers should fit as well as regular shoes. Try on sneakers with the socks you'll be wearing since they can change the size you need by as much as one size. Don't buy sneakers just because you like the electric-green color or the bargain price.
- Look for a heel that's slightly raised to lessen strain on your Achilles tendon. A padded ankle band, innersole, and padded tongue add snugness and help prevent foot and leg fatigue.
- Expect to pay about $12 for inexpensive sneakers, $20 to $30 for top makes like Adidas, Puma, Tiger, and Tretorn. Remember that good sneakers last much longer than inexpensive ones and can be repaired and resoled much more successfully.

- **special sports requirements**
- Joggers should pick a nylon sneaker—good because they're light and don't usually cause break-in blisters as leather or heavy canvas models do.
- Tennis fans like nylon or canvas sneakers. Leather ones are fine if they're supple and lightweight. If you play a lot on clay courts, be sure the soles aren't deeply grooved; grooves will damage courts. A tennis-shop sales clerk can advise you further.
- Boating sneakers *must* have slip-proof soles to keep you from sliding on wet decks. Some soles have hundreds of tiny slits on the bottom for traction.
- Basketball sneakers should give good ankle support because of the side-to-side motions players make. Try a leather model with a rigid strip ("foxing") around the sole.

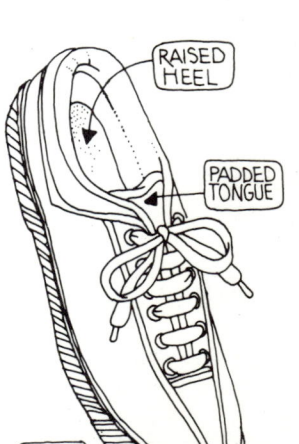

157

shopping smart

shopping smart

calculator
choose a calculator for your needs

The bank claims you have overdrawn your account by $6.37. You think you are $87.50 in the clear. Who made the mistake—you or the bank?

If one roommate made six $3.47 calls to Albuquerque, another made one $15 call to Rome, and you made a $2.10 call to Detroit, who owes what, and what percentage of the tax?

There are 557 calories in a Big Mac and 317 in a chocolate shake. If you are on a 1,500-calories-a-day diet and have already had 452, can you afford to eat them?

With a pocket calculator, these kinds of calculations are as easy as pushing a button. The question is, which calculator?

Those on the market range in price from $10 to $300 and in dimension from roughly the size of a cigarette pack to a standard telephone. But the choice isn't as complicated as it might seem. If you are not a scientist, engineer, or mathematician (or studying to be one), it's unlikely that you will ever need or want a calculator that costs more than $50 to $60. The main advantages of those that cost more are that they perform complicated trigonometric or other functions and have "memories" that let you store answers and retrieve them later on. If you could use either of these features, you probably know it, but if not, don't even consider them.

On the low- to medium-priced models, or those that cost between $20 and $100, look for an established brand name and at least a one-year warranty on all parts and labor. Texas Instruments, Bowmar, North American Rockwell, and Hewlett-Packard are generally considered to be among the most reputable.

It's also a good idea to buy a calculator with what's known as a "floating decimal point." This means that the decimal point will place itself in the right spot in your answer. On machines that do not have one, you must first do your calculation, then figure out for yourself where the decimal point should go. (Remember that all computations involving fractions, whether in recipes, measurements, or anything else, must be converted to their decimal equivalents before the calculator can work with them.) Check also for a readable digit display and buttons large enough to be easily depressed. One disadvantage of some of the least expensive models is that it's hard to depress one button without accidentally hitting another.

You might also consider how you're going to use your calculator. For example, if you're planning to travel with it, using your calculator for foreign currency conversions, a shirt-pocket-sized one would be most convenient. Don't forget that you might also be using the calculator to compare supermarket prices-per-pound, to tally up card or other game scores, and in restaurants to check out the casualties—either caloric or financial.

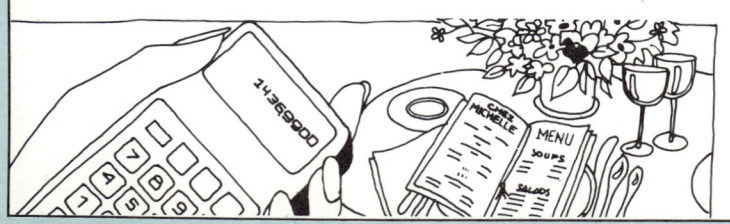

clothes 9 ways to spot quality in clothes you buy

To learn how to spot quality when you buy, take these tips from two experts GLAMOUR talked to—Victor Joris, designer for Cuddlecoat in New York, and George Kiss, a New York tailor and owner of Elegant Fashions. You'll save yourself a lot of disappointments if you follow their tips.

Size is the first clue to quality. If you're usually a size 8 and the size 8 pants you're trying on seem snug and skimpy, the manufacturer probably skimped on more than the fabric—unless you have gained weight!

Look at how the seams on a garment are finished. If they're overcast at the edges with machine stitching or bound with seam binding, that's quality, and you won't have a problem with ravels or rips.

If the garment is a knit or a stretch fabric, give the seams a gentle pull to see if they give, too. If they don't and feel stiff and taut, they're going to split open when any strain is put on them.

With the garment you'd like to buy hanging on a hanger, check if the back and side seams fall straight. If you see any puckers or "bellies," watch out. Don't let a salesperson talk you into thinking the seam will iron out flat: it won't. If it would flatten out, the manufacturer would have pressed it out in the first place.

If you're buying a bias-cut skirt, pick one that's lined at least to the hip. It will hang much better than one that's not lined at all.

Check buttonholes. Most are machine made, but they can be as good as the bound type. Be sure there are no loose threads and that the hole is reinforced by enough stitching to withstand the strain of a lot of opening and closing.

If fabric is plaid, striped, or a large print, it should match up at all seams. Sleeves should match with plaid or print across jacket front, for example. Pants should match at all seams, too; however, it's impossible to match the inside leg seam much above the knee.

If garment is lined—like a coat or jacket—the lining shouldn't be too stiff. Stiff linings tend to "crack" and pull apart at the seams. If jacket or coat is unlined, it should look as clean and neat on the inside as it is on the outside with no loose threads or unfinished seams.

Be aware that hard-finish fabrics like twills, gabardines, and most synthetics give better wear than softer ones like loose tweeds, soft cottons, and so forth. To check wrinkle resistance, crumple a small area in your hand and release it. Fabric should bounce back into shape if it's fairly wrinkle-free.

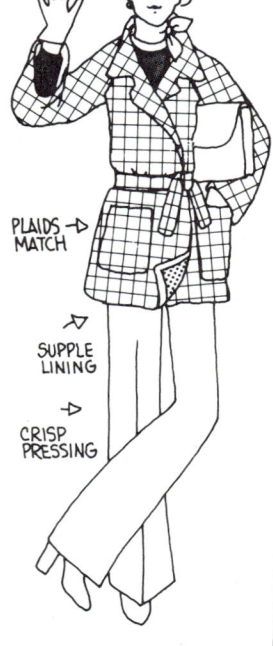

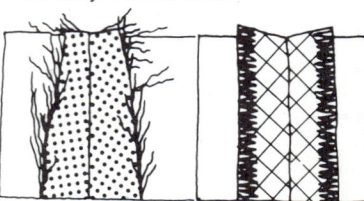

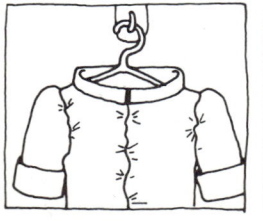

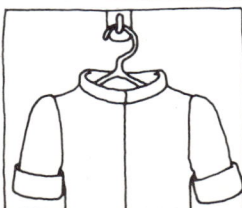

shopping smart S

drugs save on prescription drugs

With most things you buy, you feel free to shop around and get the best price, but there's something serious about prescription drugs that makes the idea of price shopping difficult, especially when you're sick. However, if you acquaint yourself in advance with some of the more common prescription drugs listed here, plus the tips on effective ways to cut drug expenses, you won't feel so helpless when the time comes to buy.

● Ask your doctor if what he's prescribing can be prescribed by its generic name (the common name for the drug) rather than by a specific brand name which often, though not always, costs more than the generic equivalent. For example, penicillin V is the generic name for a drug supplied by a variety of drug companies, but doctors might write a prescription for it as "V-cillin K®," the brand name used by only one of these companies. "V-cillin K®" is not only one of the most commonly prescribed drugs, but it is also one of the more expensive brands of this drug. The chart below gives examples of the money saved by using generic drugs.

● Tell the pharmacist you want the best price. In many cases, even if the doctor writes the prescription "generically," the pharmacist will still fill it with one of the more expensive brand names. In some states, if the doctor writes a brand name, the pharmacist can make a generic substitution. If the pharmacist can't and there is a less expensive option, have him call your doctor for permission to make the substitution.

● Call a few drugstores to get the best price. In all states, it's permitted to quote prices over the phone; in some, a pharmacist is required by law to do so if asked. The prices below are from a chain discount drugstore in New York City.

drug	brand name	generic
	(cost per capsule)	
ampicillin 250 mg *antibiotic*	29¢	8¢
tetracycline hydrochloride 250 mg *antibiotic*	29¢	6¢
penicillin G 250 mg *antibiotic*	16¢	6¢
propoxyphene (Darvon® Compound-65 mg) *analgesic*	10¢	6¢
Librium® *tranquilizer*	8¢	no generic available
Valium® *tranquilizer*	10¢	no generic available

drugstore
how to get the most for your money

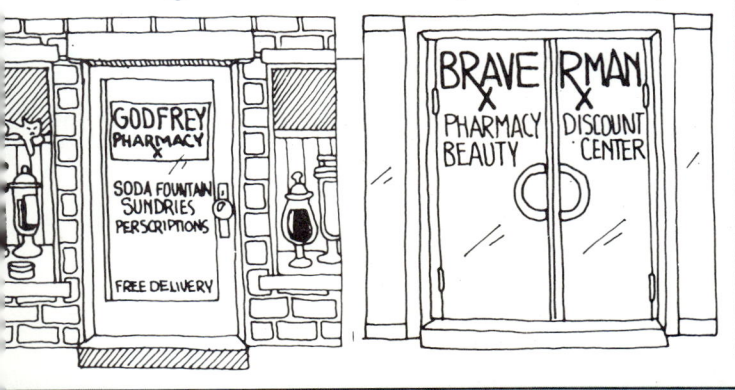

With the variety of drugstores and all the signs shouting "discount," "cut-rate," and "special," it's hard to know where to find the best prices *and* the best service. These profiles may help you:

● **neighborhood pharmacy**
It's probably right on your corner. The service is usually excellent and the pharmacist will take the time to answer questions and offer advice. Other attractions may include ice cream floats, charge accounts, and free delivery—which certainly matters when you have the flu. But all that attention does cost more.

Some of the health and beauty items are likely to be priced high. They might also be unmarked or stored on hard-to-reach shelves and behind glass cases, making shopping difficult. One pharmacist admitted the store didn't display toothpaste because "it's just too expensive here." Which means the customer has to ask for it and then, once it's on the counter, is too embarrassed to say "never mind."

● **pharmacy/"discount center"**
The terrific feature here is bargain prices on a variety of items; the not-so-terrific feature may be a long line at the cash register. As one manager of a chain discount store put it, "The service just isn't the same as a small pharmacy's."

The very low-priced items here are what are known as "leaders." Things like shampoo, tampons, and birth control pills are often sold at a loss and are designed to woo you into the store, where you'll buy other undiscounted items on which they make up that loss. All prices are not equally low.

Leaders vary from one discount store to the next, and the way to really save money is to shop around and note who offers the lowest price on *each* particular product and size you need.

It's also important to remember that other less popular items, as well as many prescription drugs, may cost the same as in the neighborhood pharmacy.

● **health and beauty aid discount**
No prescription drugs are sold here, but it's a great place to pick up drugstore basics, as long as you're not too fussy about decor. This store may be farther than the corner, but the savings you get could be worth more than whatever trip you have to make. (Discount department stores and dime stores sometimes have health and beauty aid sections that advertise "low, low prices." Again, shop carefully—some items are bargains; others are not.)

Here's a sample of what three such stores in New York City had to offer in price on the same brand-name products.

	neighborhood pharmacy	pharmacy/ discount center	health and beauty aid discount store
shampoo *(11 oz.)*	2.29	1.69	1.49
toothpaste *(5 oz.)*	1.00	.83	.69
deodorant *(14 oz.)*	2.89	2.35	1.99
face and body cream *(6 oz.)*	1.59	1.59	1.19
tampons *(40 reg.)*	1.98	1.59	1.39
aspirin *(200 tabs.)*	2.29	1.79	1.49
contraceptive jelly *(4.44 oz.)*	3.50	3.19	2.79
birth control pills *(21 pack)*	2.95	2.25	*
tetracycline *(250 mg. caps.)*	.10/@	.06/@	*

*Not available

shopping smart

factory outlets
what you should know about shopping in factory outlets

If department-store shopping can be compared to a smoothly guided tour, then factory-outlet shopping is more like a safari through often uncharted aisles. Outlet stores don't offer all the comforts of more traditional ones—for instance, they rarely accept credit cards—but shoppers in these stores often turn up real finds on anything from leather skirts to light fixtures.

There are just a few things to keep in mind if you venture in a factory outlet. First, factory outlets are simply stores where you buy directly from a manufacturer, usually in a factory or warehouse. Second, the quality of the merchandise you find in them varies widely but consists mostly of surplus material that a manufacturer could not sell. For example, if a department store refuses to accept a late shipment or certain items do not meet specifications, a manufacturer will often try to sell this merchandise through an outlet. Third, when you are shopping in one, it helps to brush up on unfamiliar terms. Jean Bird, author of several Factory Outlet Shopping Guides to areas from Maine to Virginia, lists the following basic terms any shopper should know:

- Samples—These range from mannequins' garments to samples a salesperson might show to a prospective store buyer. (Occasionally, a style does not suit enough buyers and is never sold to stores. Samples of it are labeled in outlets as "one of a kind.")
- Overcuts, overstocks, overruns—These terms refer to surplus merchandise made up after an original order is filled (in anticipation of reorders), but never sold.
- Mill ends and remnants—These are ends of rolls and surplus fabric, carpet, etc., not used up in the manufacture of an item.
- Seconds, irregulars, flaws—These can include holes, pulled threads, or other defects that may or may not alter the appearance of an item.
- Cancellations, discontinued floor samples—Styles not being produced at the time.
- First quality—Merchandise that has no defects.

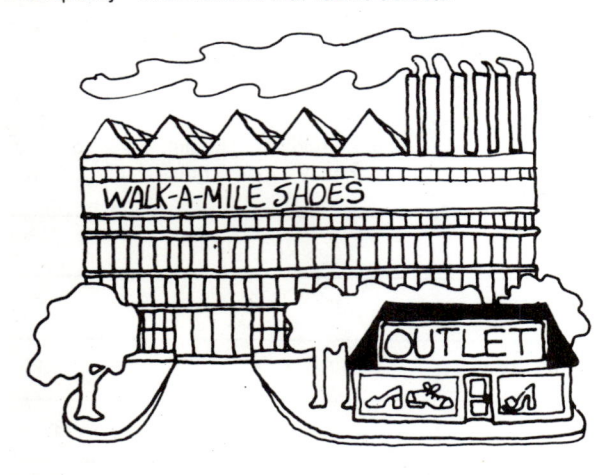

fur
tips on buying used furs

Fur coats are big fashion with big prices to match, so you might consider buying your fur secondhand. Flea markets, thrift shops, used-clothing stores, and furriers sell them quite inexpensively, but to get a real bargain you've got to know which fur has only one short season left, which is repairable, and how much repairs cost.

- Keep in mind that black-dyed Australian rabbit, raccoon, and skunk are most durable. However, raccoon—like mink—costs more to have repaired because of its striped pattern. Muskrat and fox are popular but weaker furs and often need repair. Natural rabbit sheds heavily.
- Check seams and hard-wearing spots on any fur (underneath the collar, the back seat) for brittle hide. This must be replaced to make your coat durable, which would be an added cost to the coat. Check with your local furrier for an estimate on the price.
- Also check the hide of vertically striped fur to see if the coat has been "let out" or vertically seamed. A many-pieced coat gets structurally weak with age and cannot be patched. A protective coating can be put onto the back of the fur to strengthen it, but this is a fairly expensive process which must be done by a furrier since the coat is completely disassembled. If you're considering remodeling (cost runs $100 up), however, it would be wise to have any aging fur coated.
- Make sure the hide of Persian lamb is bluish; white hide indicates age, and if the fur has not already begun to rub off, it soon will.
- If fox has begun to shred (and fox has this tendency), nothing can be done but extensive patching, possibly a whole sleeve or two. This can become expensive, but many companies are using leather trim to patch at reduced prices.
- If you're going all out on a used mink, concentrate on color. A ranch mink, for instance, is naturally black-brown. As it ages, it lightens; so a reddish brown fur coat is probably between 15 and 20 years old and would run around $200 to $400. Since most minks begin to break down around this time, plan on putting even more money into it. Pastel mink browns with age, so when the pinkish tone goes, the fur is on the downhill side.
- The experts don't recommend that you cut your own full-length fur into a jacket yourself, but if you've had sewing experience (and didn't pay dearly for the fur), you might want to try. Use a razor-blade cutter, and cut only through the hide on the wrong side. This way the fur can lie smoothly instead of being blunted. The hem can be finished with seam tape.

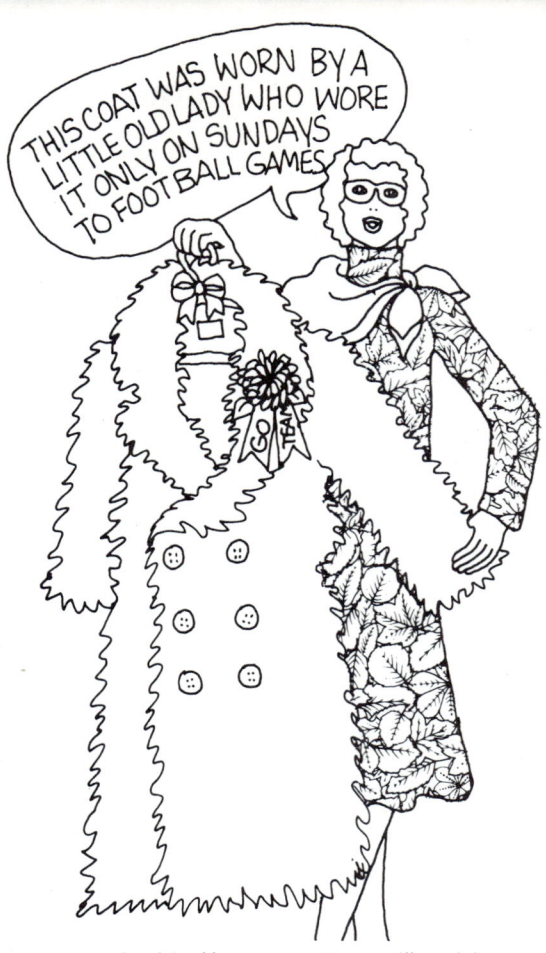

shopping smart

guitar
fast shopping tips for guitar buyers

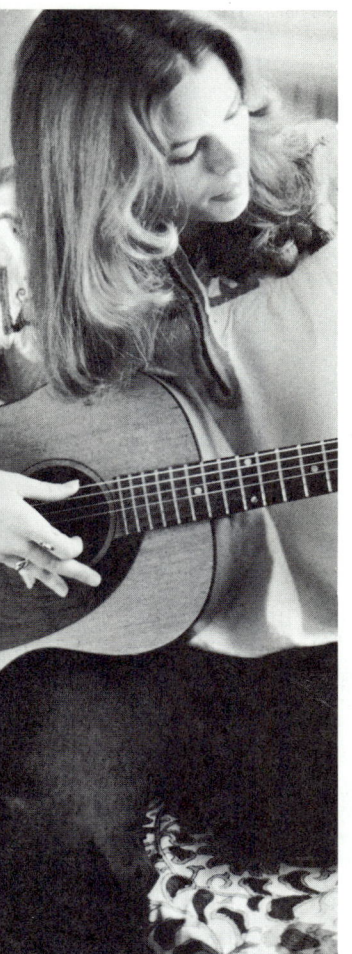

Top guitars like a Martin, Gibson, or Guild cost $200 on up, but you can find good guitars for $90 to $150.
• Nylon-string guitars are best for classical music. Steel-string ones ring sharper and are better for any other music but classical.
• Try playing difficult chords on guitars you're considering. If you have trouble, find out if the "action" —the distance between the strings and fingerboard—can or should be lowered.
• Check for a warped neck; this can cause a buzzing sound or make the guitar hard to play. Look down from the neck to the body. If straightening is necessary, find out whether it's a simple or complicated adjustment.
• Listen to guitars in your price range. Trust your ear. Don't overlook lesser-known brands—they often give you the most for your money. For example, Angelica, Carlo Robelli, and Ibañez are three Japanese imports worth looking into, according to Arnie Rosstad of Sam Ash Music, Inc., in New York City.
• Hunt for bargains, but beware of a store that won't allow returns. Try to buy from a store with its own repair shop since it's difficult to send back guitars to the manufacturer.

mail
dos and don'ts for shopping by mail

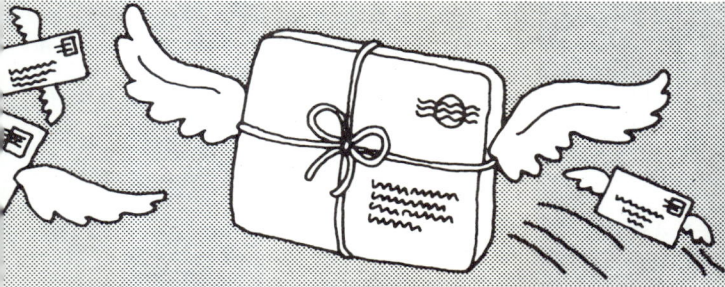

• DON'T be less cautious than if you were shopping in person. Compare prices, beware of utopian claims, and study written descriptions, not just slick photographs. Find out company policy on returns or exchanges. Also check company reputation with the local Better Business Bureau if you have any doubts.
• DO be precise about color, size, quantity, etc., and specifiy what you will or won't accept as a substitute. Say, a blue hat if they're out of red ones.
• DO check catalog for shipping and handling charges to include with your order. If you're doing mail order from abroad, have items sent by air mail, especially around Christmas; surface-mail delivery may take months after reaching the U.S.
• DO avoid the holiday rush by placing Christmas orders early or in mid-November. If you won't accept a package after a certain date, say so in your order.
• DON'T, under any circumstances, send cash. Pay by check or money order from your local post office, or if you place a mail order abroad, by an international certified check at your bank. You can also have the bank send a speedier cable or mail transfer of funds to the shop's bank or one nearby for a charge of about $2.
• DON'T forget that most imported items are taxed from 1 percent to over 50 percent of their value at customs, depending on what they are and where they're from. (For example, the rate for Communist countries is the highest.) Since you can't pay duty in advance, have any gift sent to you if you don't want a friend stuck with the bill; mail again after paying the duty.
• DO keep complete records of all domestic and international orders. Ideally, you should have a duplicate copy of the filled-in order blank, including any extra directions about substitutes, delivery date, etc., but if that isn't possible, keep a complete description of all items, including catalog number and date ordered.
• DON'T put off opening a package and returning damaged or mistaken items. Some companies will take back merchandise late, but most set a deadline of 10 to 30 days for returns. It's also a good idea to send gift cards in advance, asking friends to let you know if something doesn't arrive or if it comes in poor condition. (Since you have receipts, you can clear up the problem faster.)

motorcycle
tips on buying your first motorcycle

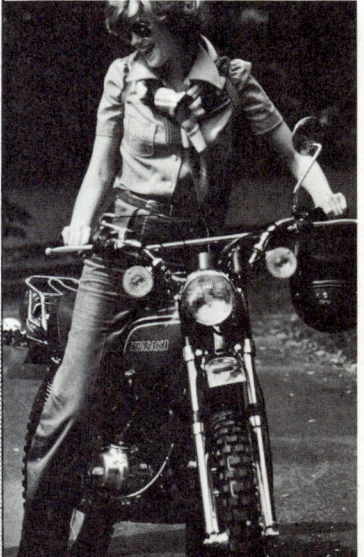

If you're a backseat motorcyclist who would like to move up to the driver's seat, here are tips on buying your first motorcycle:
1. Before buying, test your enthusiasm and get basic skills by taking a motorcycle safety course that requires at least 20 to 40 hours of instruction, some of them on a motorcycle. For a course near you, contact the police, a local school board, or a reputable motorcycle dealer. Or write to the Motorcycle Safety Foundation, 6755 Elkridge Landing Rd., Linthicum, MD 21090.
2. When you're ready to buy, remember that motorcycle engines are measured in cc's: small motorcycles run from 70cc to 250cc; medium commuters from 250cc to 500cc; large touring motorcycles up to 1200cc. Your best bet as a beginner is a motorcycle in the smaller range. It's not for superhighways, but is fine for zipping around city or suburban streets. The cost: $700 to $900 new, about half that used.
3. You'll have three basic models to choose from. On-street motorcycles are your most likely choice, since they're designed for normal pavement riding. Combinations, or dual-purpose, have the advantage of being legal in the streets as well as designed for off-road, country riding. Off-street motorcycles, designed strictly for riding on dirt or sand, are illegal on public streets.
4. Plan on buying these safety accessories. A helmet that comes be-

S shopping smart

low your chin costs at least $30 for a good one. You should also have *eye protection*—either goggles or a chin-length plastic face shield attached to your helmet. Goggles cost $8 to $15, the shield, $2 to $4. (Eyeglasses are not a safe substitute.) *A luggage rack* to leave your hands free of packages runs about $25 to $40.

5. Your motorcycling outfit is an extra expense and should include leather gloves; over-the-ankle boots with heels and slip-proof soles; long, narrow pants, plus a long-sleeved jacket or shirt made of durable fabric like corduroy, denim, or leather. (Increase your visibility by wearing bright colors and adding reflective tape to clothes and cycle.)

6. Before buying any motorcycle, keep in mind that it will need the same regular maintenance as a car, plus daily checks of brakes, cables, headlights, and gas or oil leaks.

7. Also check state insurance laws since motorcycle insurance costs range widely, depending on area, driver, and motorcycle. (You may or may not be able to include motorcycle coverage on your car policy.)

8. Finally, check with your state department of motor vehicles for motorcycle regulations. Rules of the road that apply to cars also apply to motorcycles, but you may have extra requirements, too, such as driving with headlights on even during the day. Also, not all states require a written or driving test and only 38 states have special licensing procedures for driving a motorcycle.

rights
your rights as a shopper— and how to cash in on them

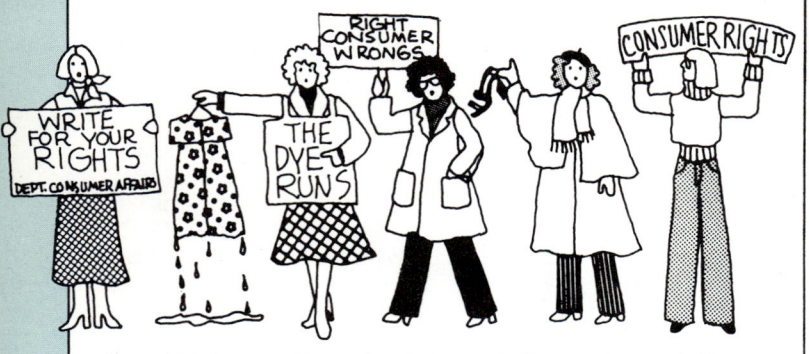

It would take more than a legal degree to figure out your rights as a shopper in every situation. Many "rights" aren't strictly legal, but have to do with accepted store policy regarding complaints, returns, credit, and so on. Here are some situations you might encounter if you're dealing with a large, reputable store:

● There are no hard-and-fast rules about what's considered a legitimate complaint. So if you're dissatisfied with the quality, wear, or fit of an article, speak up. For example, if an expensive skirt looks shabby after a month of normal wear or a dress shrinks when you've washed it according to directions on the label, ask for a free repair, a replacement, or a partial or full credit. If a defective item spoils something else, you might be entitled to extra compensation. For instance, one store we spoke to reupholstered a chair soiled by dye from one of their dresses—and credited the dress, too.

● Don't be afraid to complain about reduced merchandise. It might be tired looking but it's supposed to wear well and not be damaged (unless it's tagged "damaged," "as is," etc., or it's from a bargain area where prices are slashed and customers are warned to beware).

● Some stores will pay the difference if you buy something from them, then find a competitor charges less—or if you paid the regular price and the item is put on sale within ten days or so.

● If your local chain store has run out of what you want, they'll usually track it down at another branch, even if it means ordering from Chicago when you live in New York. Or if your heart is set on a slightly soiled garment, ask for a spot cleaning; there's no charge and no obligation to buy. You might even ask the manager for a price reduction.

● Doing your own alterations? The store seamstress may save you time by pinning things up free or for just a few dollars.

● Check store policy on returns before you buy. Is there a ten- to fifteen-day time limit? Are some items not returnable (like bathing suits, intimate apparel, hats, expensive evening dresses, handbags, or altered garments) or not returnable unless a special tag is kept on (like jewelry)?

● For returns, you will receive cash if you paid cash and have the receipt, credit if you lost the receipt or charged the purchase. Credit should last indefinitely. But the Federal Trade Commission found that some large stores were notifying customers of their credit balances for just a month or two, then dropping the credit. So protect yourself from this abuse by keeping all credit slips, canceled checks, or early statements that reflect a credit balance. If after three months you haven't used the balance, write the store and ask them to send you a check for the amount.

● Most stores try to discourage shoplifters with store detectives, two-way mirrors in dressing rooms, and electronic garment tags that trigger an alarm system unless properly removed by the salesperson. They're all legal but not infallible. So if a bell goes off by mistake or a detective stops you because you took a scarf from one part of the floor to match it with a blouse in another, remember: Don't be intimidated into signing anything. Aryeh Neier, executive director of the American Civil Liberties Union, points out that many innocent people have been embarrassed and frightened into signing an agreement not to sue the store for false arrest if the store agrees not to prosecute for shoplifting. What you're not told is that your name is sent to a credit agency, which for years can affect your ability to get a job or an apartment, or be accepted to a school.

● As to advertisements: if a garment is mistakenly advertised at the wrong price, and it's not a gross misprint (like $1.98 for a $198 coat), you might be able to get that price if you refer to the ad. If you think advertising has been purposely misleading, check the law with your state or local Department of Consumer Affairs or District Attorney's office.

sales a guide to shopping at the annual January sales

January is big-sale time and, faced with racks and racks of "bargains," you can hardly expect to know what's a good buy and what isn't. Here are some ideas to help, plus a few tips on the kind of sales you'll be seeing advertised in the local papers.

● *An ad for a "special purchase" sale means the items are not the store's regular merchandise marked down, but merchandise bought from one or two manufacturers—perhaps an overstock of clothes already too late for the regular selling season—at a low price. You'll find good bargains, but don't expect to find that sweater you saw in the fall but couldn't afford.*

● *When the store marks down its regular merchandise, the ad will usually say "mark down"; this is when you can expect to find that sweater.*

● *A sale that advertises "seconds" or "irregulars" means there's some irregularity in the merchandise. It can be a slight or a real flaw. Just be certain you know what's wrong with anything you buy.*

● *Here are some good buys to watch for in winter. A winter coat—a good special purchase and mark-down item—can be a real bargain. Pick a classic style like a trench, duffle, wrap, or a short jacket coat that looks terrific with pants. These styles are never out of fashion.*

● *A fur jacket, if you've been wanting one but couldn't afford it, is a good buy, too. A bulky wrap sweater would be another "look for." A classic V-necked cardigan sweater to wear over shirts and turtlenecks is always great to have.*

● *A sweater or shirt in a great off-beat color may have seemed risky at full price, but on sale it could be just the brightener you need.*

shopping smart

- A silky shirtdress, if you can pick one up, would be a real find.
- A pair of classic pumps or high-heeled moccasin shoes will always work, as well as simple sling-back pumps or pretty, dressy sandals.
- Check out the lingerie sales at the same time. You might find your favorite bra on sale, a supply of bikini panties, or some beautiful sleepwear.

sales
there are sales, and there are sales — do you know one from another?

Special, clearance, close-out. It all sounds very tempting—and very confusing. What are you really getting when you respond to all those sale ads? Here are a few helpful translations to give you an idea of what you're buying. Our list of sale terms comes from the New York/New Jersey Better Business Bureau, but similar terminology is commonly used across the country.

Sale means exactly what you'd expect, a reduction from the advertiser's own previous price. A clearance sale is a reduction in price on merchandise previously offered at a higher price. Merchandise sold in clearance sales is clearly not new stock and any ad that implies it is, is misleading—perhaps deliberately so—and should be regarded with some degree of suspicion.

Merchandise sold at a clearance center should be composed of items previously offered at the retailer's store. The Better Business Bureau recommends that you buy at such centers with caution because, all too often, the merchandise has not been offered for sale before and is not of the best quality.

A liquidation sale is one where the retailer intends to go out of business and wants to convert his assets into cash. You can get a good buy provided it really is a liquidation sale. Frequently, however, this is just an advertising ploy to get customers into a store.

A comparable value indicates that the advertised item is similar but not identical to merchandise selling at the "comparable value" price. The ad usually reads something like this: "Curling irons, $9.95, comparable value, $15." This can be a good buy, but you should check out the differences between the sale item and the regularly priced ones to be sure you are getting all you think you are.

sales calendar
calendar of annual bargains to help you keep inflation in tow

Probably the best time to buy almost anything from a hair dryer to a car would have been last year. But second best is the traditional sale periods listed below:

- **general-merchandise sales**

Many stores have across-the-board reductions keyed to special holidays. Practically every month has one, so if you can hold off the urge for instant gratification, you might keep the following in mind: December, January (after Christmas); February (Lincoln's and Washington's Birthday); April (after Easter); May (Memorial Day); July (Independence Day); September (Labor Day); October (Columbus Day); November (Thanksgiving, Election Day).

- **special-item sales**

In general, prices are reduced on items just before or after their peak selling season. For instance, coffee-table books have a special rate just before and after Christmas. New models of cars, TVs, stoves, etc., also mean a price cut on old ones.

- **clothing**

Furs (January, August); summer fashions (June, July); winter fashions, underwear (January); coats (January, Columbus Day).

- **crafts**

Fabrics (January, February, June, July); notions (any time, but be on the alert before Mother's Day and Christmas); sewing machines (anytime, but one giant company usually has special promotions in September and March).

- **home appliances**

Air conditioners (February); small ones from irons and blenders to hair dryers and makeup mirrors (January, February, March, July, August).

- **home furnishings**

Dinnerware (September, October); furniture (January, February, July, August); rugs/carpets (May, October); white-sale items—towels, sheets, pillows, blankets, etc. (January, August).

- **home entertainment**

Audio equipment—stereos, radios, tape recorders (February, March, April); TVs (April, May); toys (January).

- **sports**

Camping (August); fishing, golf (April, May, September); skiing/skating (September, February, March); tennis (late August); underwater (April, May, September).

- **travel**

Bicycles (January, February); cars (new—August, September; used—November, December); motorcycles/motorbikes (October, November); luggage (January, February); tires (March, April, September).

sewing machine
how to save time and money when you're out to buy a sewing machine

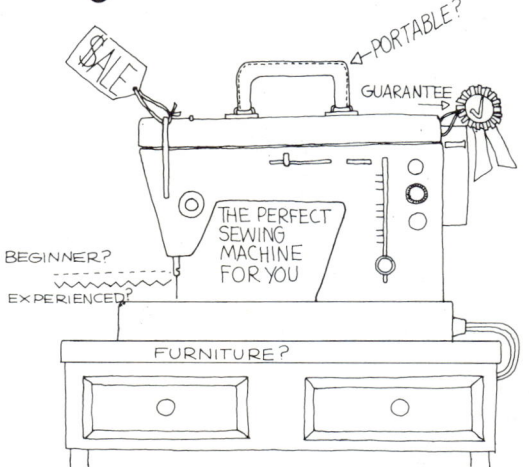

With so many models to choose from, and prices ranging anywhere from $50 to $500, the first thing to decide is just how much sewing you expect to do.

If you're a beginner, look into simple zigzag or straight-stitch models (or anything you can use on stretch fabrics, if you expect to be working with them). You can learn how to use a simple machine quite rapidly. Some models offer a number of special attachments for feather and satin stitching, embroidery, and so forth.

If you're more experienced, you might want one with disks for automatic chain or decorative stitching. The higher price tag will be worth it if you plan to do a lot of fancy embroidery or appliqué work on fabrics, leather, etc. The weight of your machine is important too, so check it by carrying it around in the store before buying. (A cast-iron portable, for instance, can be a burden.)

Some experts think that portables give you the most for your money unless you're in the market for cabinet furniture. Once you've narrowed

S shopping smart

down the models that interest you to a few, give your selections a good try. The right one is the one that feels right, seems comfortable to operate, and handles easily and smoothly for you. Also check out the guarantees for all parts of the machine. Buying from an authorized dealership protects you no matter where you move if you have any difficulties later on.

Inquire about any free training lessons. Some models are offered with just one lesson, others with two or more. You could possibly sign up for a course at a discount at the time you buy the machine.

You might also keep an eye out for slightly used machines or floor samples and demonstration models that have been reduced in price.

size charts
to help each other with your shopping

What men and women give each other as presents has changed so much that the usual etiquette-book rules about what you can and can't give now provide more laughs than help. Anything seems to go—from a ski parka to a loaf of banana bread still warm from your oven.

With so much freedom, giving presents is apt to seem a lot more complicated than when your biggest decision was the color of the stripes on his tie. Take the problem of sizes: even if a man wants to buy you a silky shirt or a pair of velvet jeans, how will he react to a saleswoman who impatiently wants to know whether you're a 7/8, 9/10, or 11/12—and is that a junior or misses size? Do you take a petite, small, medium, tall, or extra-tall length? You, too, might have similar problems the first time you walk into a menswear shop or department store, intent on buying something bigger than a cuff link. Even buying a belt requires knowing his waist size and the width of his belt loops.

To help both female and male shoppers, we've compiled two charts you can copy and carry. One has spaces for you to fill in the key sizes for three men—say, a father, brother, and friend. The other has spaces for a man to fill in the key sizes for three women—say, his mother, sister, and you. After picking your three, you can simply tell each man, "I'm updating my files and need a complete list of sizes for the important men in my life—you included." Even if you're only planning to buy each a belt, the chart will spare your having to ask pointedly for their waist size. Of course, by giving the other chart to a man, you spare his having to ask the same kind of embarrassing questions.

Here are some other ways you can help each other with your gift shopping.

Remember that many gifts miss their mark because they reflect the image the giver has of you rather than the image you have of yourself. So why not find out the other person's self-image before you do your shopping? Flip through men's and women's fashion magazines together, with each of you trying to pick out the clothes you feel the other would like. For example, as you're going through the men's fashions together, you can say, "I think you'd look great in this," and if you get a resounding "yecch," you'll know you're off target. You can ask him and hope he'll take the cue, "What on this page do you really like? What don't you like, and why?" To polish his image of you, leaf through copies of fashion magazines together, asking him what he'd most and least like to see you in, making sure you point out how his choices compare to what you're most and least likely to wear. Or tell him about the funniest present you ever received, one that was totally, hopelessly not you. Has a well-meaning relative given you an oversized cape that makes you feel like Florence Nightingale? A sweater scattered with red-nosed reindeer? A set of crocheted egg warmers?

If he asks what you'd like for a present, try not to give him the usual, "Oh, anything," answer. It's more honest and easier on him to give him a half-dozen choices in several different price ranges, from a Flair pen to a Mercedes-Benz. You can also lightly point out a few of the things you want to avoid—the color that makes your skin look a warmed-over gray or chocolate, which gives you hives.

● for him to take shopping			
Dress or skirt *junior or misses*			
Blouse			
Sweater			
Pants *size and length*			
Coat or jacket			
Gown or robe			
Belt			
Slippers			
Gloves			
Stockings			
favorite Perfume			
"Don't likes"			
Favorite colors			

● for you to take shopping			
Shirt *neck sleeves collar cuff links?*			
Sweater			
Slacks *waist length*			
Coat or jacket			
Pajamas or robe			
Belt			
Slippers			
Gloves			
Socks			
After-shave			
"Don't likes"			
Favorite colors			

shopping smart

sports gear co-ops
how to join one

If you're gearing up for anything from backpacking to tennis, you might check into a profit-sharing group called the Recreational Equipment Co-op. It operates through mail order as well as in their four stores in Seattle, Berkeley, Los Angeles, and Portland, Oregon. Here's how the co-op works:

You become a member by paying $2 the first year, then buying at least $5 in merchandise every year after that. Even nonmembers can order from the catalog; however, members get a yearly dividend based on the group's profits. For the past two years, the refund was about 10 percent of the cost of items the member bought during the year.

It takes three to four weeks to receive an order. You can call for a catalog by dialing 800-426-4840 (this call is toll free) anywhere in the U.S. except Hawaii and Alaska. Washington residents can call toll free 800-562-4894.

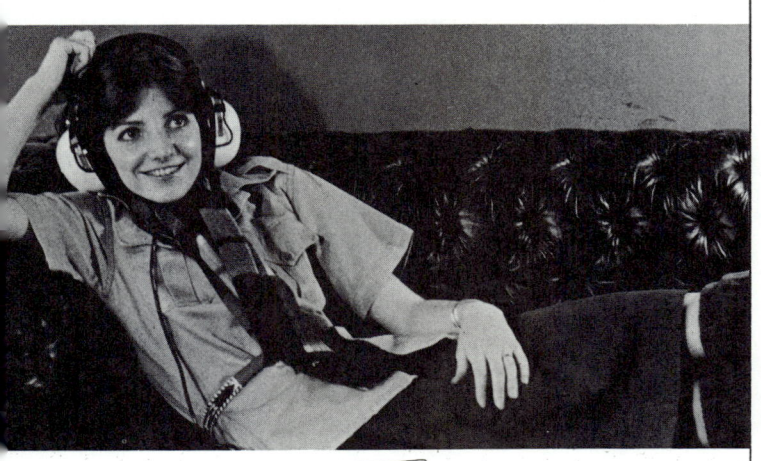

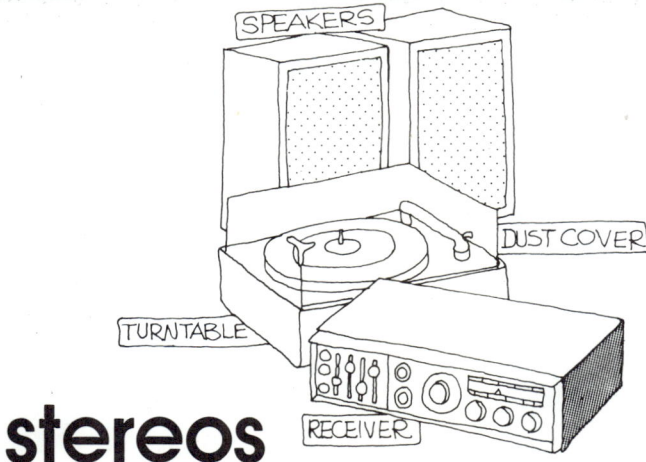

stereos
tips for the stereo equipment buyer

No matter how large or small your stereo-equipment budget, these tips will help you make the best selection for your budget and needs:
- **buying guidelines**
- Buy a name brand. Lesser-known brands might not be easily serviceable.
- Make sure each component (or unit) has a warranty. The three basic components you will need are a receiver—made up of an amplifier, a pre-amplifier, and a tuner; a record changer or manual turntable— preferably one with a dust cover for protection; and two speakers.
- "Compact" sets with fixed or noninterchangeable components are great for small apartments and for college students pressed for space. The sound is adequate, but it can't be upgraded by trading in one part for a better unit.
- If a stereo is on sale, ask why. If a store is merely cleaning out last year's discontinued model, you're safe. Some models, like cars, can be lemons and have acquired substandard reputations. Ask friends for opinions and be as friendly with the salespeople as possible to get straight answers. Beware of models with a "90-day guarantee"; good models carry one- to five-year guarantees.
- **your purchase strategy at the store**
- Make sure the salesperson has left all tone controls at the flat or mid-range position and the "loudness" control is not turned all the way up.
- **for receivers**
- Make sure the salesperson hooks up the speakers and receiver so you can see how far the volume has to be turned up for suitable volume. If dials must be at a 3 o'clock position in order for you to hear the music at standard volume, the receiver is not strong enough for the speakers.
- **for speakers**
- Because there are sales on speakers all the time, the list price can usually be ignored. Unless the speakers are "fair-traded" or sold at a fixed price, there is usually a discount of about 20 percent.
- Remember that different ears hear in different ways and people favor different types of sound. Some speakers give a "warm" or "colored" sound—one in which the mid-frequency range is emphasized—and although coloration is frowned upon by hi-fi buffs, your choice should depend on what *you* prefer. Don't be influenced by what you've been told is "the best."
- **in general**
- Take your favorite, familiar, and undamaged record and play it on each system you're considering.
- Installation of stereo sets—that is, hooking up speakers, turntable and receiver—is complicated. Ask if installation comes along with the price of the set; it often does. If it does not, make sure the turntable, tone arm, and cartridge are assembled at the store (some come already assembled, some don't). Once you're home with your new system, have an experienced friend help you hook it up.

study light
how to choose a good study light

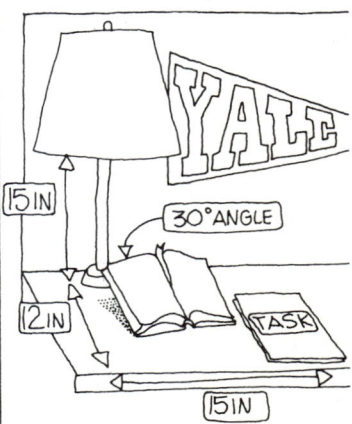

It's best *always* to use a 200-watt incandescent bulb with any study lamp. The bulb should reach just above the bottom edge of your shade to give a wide spread of light. The lamp you're using, whether it's a table or hanging model or is attached to the wall by a swivel arm, needs to be placed so that the bottom edge of the shade is 15" from the surface of a desk or table. The best shade should be translucent so that light can come through (but not so sheer you can see the fixture) and should open at the top to minimize glare.

Put the light about 12" to one side of your reading or writing project. The Better Light, Better Sight Bureau, after testing study lamps and making sure that they meet the requirements developed by the Illuminating Engineering Society, has tagged with a BLBS tag the ones that meet its specifications for eye comfort at a reasonable cost. That means better light, better sight. These lamps usually cost about $20.

165

shopping smart

typewriter
buy a typewriter that's right for you

Whether you zip along at 70 words per minute or can barely hunt-and-peck your way on the keys, these questions can help you pick the best typewriter for you:

● **how much can you afford to spend?**
Manual typewriters range in price from about $35 to $150; electrics, from under $100 (for a lightweight portable without extras) to $700 (for the fanciest office models). So first comparison shop to see what's available in your price range. If you're on the tightest possible budget, don't forget to check your Yellow Pages under "Typewriters" for stores that sell reconditioned, secondhand typewriters at bargain prices. Regardless of the type of machine you're considering, type on several before you decide. *Always* type on the machine you're planning to buy.

● **do you want a stationary or portable machine?**
Unless your house or apartment is literally your office—or you nourish a secret dream of one day turning out a Greater American Novel than Philip Roth's on your typewriter—a portable is best. Obviously, a portable is a must for a college student or anyone else who has to type in a spot other than her room. Within the portable category, there exist both lightweight (7 to 12 pounds) and average (17 pounds or more) typewriters. The lightest typewriters are usually cheapest and may be great for anyone who plans to do a lot of traveling with it, but they can also be harder to type on or may have fewer special keys than others. In any case, a good, well-balanced portable should not "walk" across a table or move in any other way while you're typing on it.

● **do you need a manual or an electric?**
Electric typewriters tend to be less tiring to type on for long periods, such as when you're doing term papers or reports. These machines may also give neater results, particularly if you're only a fair typist. (Even if you slam down on one key and barely touch the next, you'll get a uniform printout.) However, some people find the constant hum of an electric typewriter distracting. If you're used to a manual machine, the quick action of an electric might take getting used to—you might even *prefer* the heavy feel of a manual. Because electric typewriters are more delicate than manuals, they might pose problems (such as keys sticking more frequently) for anyone who tends to pound them furiously. Although your electric might remain trouble-free for years, if something does go wrong, repairs can be more complicated and costly. If ribbon changing has always seemed like a drag to you, you might also want to consider buying a typewriter that has a cartridge instead of a ribbon; you just push a button to eject the old ribbon cartridge, then insert a new one.

● **do you need any special features, such as a carriage or unusual keys?**
The usual carriage is 9" to 10" long, but on some models a 12" to 13" carriage is available for people who use longer paper or envelopes. If you'll be typing in a foreign language, you might want a typewriter with special accent-mark keys. In some cases, these can be added to a machine that doesn't have them. For people who'll be doing lots of charts or statistical reports, special tabulator keys are available that move the carriage to preset positions quickly and accurately. Vertical half spacing is another handy extra if you'll need lots of subscripts for biology reports or superscripts for math formulas or footnotes.

● **what kind of typeface do you want?**
Most models are available with either pica typeface (10 characters per inch) or elite (12 characters per inch). The choice is largely a matter of personal preference. More unusual typefaces—such as those with script or squared-off letters—are considered too difficult to read or too unusual to use on business letters, reports and résumés. However, people who use their typewriters mainly for personal correspondence often prefer this more stylized look.

warranties
from hairdryers to transistors— what you should know about warranties

Don't wait for your new hair dryer to break down to find out what kind of warranty it has—or worse, that it has no warranty at all. The following tips should help you know what to look for in warranties (often called guaranties).

Manufacturers are not required to provide written warranties, but when they do, they must follow the guidelines in the Magnuson-Moss Warranty—Federal Trade Commission Improvement Act. The Act helps tighten up warranty requirements and makes the language in warranties easier to understand. Warranties on products manufactured after July 4, 1975, and over $10 in value must be conspicuously marked *full* or *limited*. A *full* warranty provides that defective goods will be replaced or repaired free of charge within a reasonable period of time. A full warranty may be valid for a finite period of time, but this must be clearly indicated on the warranty (as in "full 90-day warranty"). If after a number of repairs the product fails, you can request a refund of money or replacement of the product or the part of the product in question.

A *limited* warranty is a warning signal to buy with caution, although it doesn't mean that you should automatically avoid the item. It may take care of only certain parts of the item, require that you pay for labor costs yourself, or carry other restrictions. Make sure you know what parts are warranted and whether or not they are important parts. Find out how long the warranty will be in effect and if different parts are warranted for different lengths of time. Be sure you know what the warranty covers—leakage, breakage, malfunctions—and who pays for labor and shipping fees. If labor or shipping costs are high, the warranty is worth considerably less to you.

Be sure to send in any required warranty forms immediately after the purchase. If you don't, the warranty may not be valid. Find out from the seller or the warranty document itself whom you should contact if something goes wrong and exactly who will replace or repair the item: the manufacturer or seller. Also, keep a copy of any warranty material.

Remember that a warranty that you don't fully understand can often be as ineffective as no warranty at all. Questions about specific products should be directed to the seller or manufacturer.

watches
digital watches— is one a good choice for you?

Digital watches used to be associated with big price tags, but not anymore. You can buy a digital watch for under $20—or if money is no object, you can spend several thousand dollars for a gold and diamond one. Most digitals run in the $30-to-$40 range.

● In general, digitals are more accurate than regular watches, so if *precise* accuracy is important to you, this could be a big plus.
● Digitals generally need very little adjustment to keep them accurate.
● Routine cleaning and oiling is unnecessary, so there is practically no maintenance expense. You do have to change batteries every year or so, but you can do it yourself on many models. Cost is usually minimal—$5 or less.
● You can choose between a constant display digital (where numerals showing the time are always visible) or models where you must press a button to display the time. Many models also display the date when the button is pressed a second time. People who don't like wearing a watch because it's a constant reminder of the time may

skiing

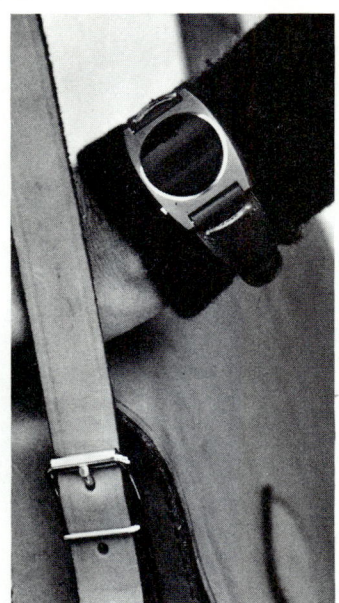

find a push-button digital a good choice.
- On the negative side, digitals need to be somewhat larger than regular watches to allow for batteries and a readable number display. If you want a really small watch, you won't find one among the digitals. The smaller the digital, the smaller the batteries, so you may have to change them more often on the smaller sizes.
- Repair, if it's necessary, can be more of a problem with a digital. Many jewelers just don't have the know-how because these watches are so new, but this situation is improving rapidly as digitals are becoming more popular.
- Digitals that require a push button to display the time are sometimes hard to read in bright sunlight but are being improved.

skiing

after-ski
parties to give without spending a lot of time in the kitchen and money

If you want to feed dinner to lots of ravenous sportsmen or women, try this super dinner for skiers:

- **hamburger stroganoff**

3 lbs. ground beef
2 onions, finely chopped
2 T. butter
2 4-oz. cans mushrooms, drained
2 tsp. tomato paste
2 T. sherry or white wine
3 c. sour cream

Shape beef into meatballs and cook in heavy frying pan until brown. In clean pan, sauté onions in butter until golden. Add mushrooms, tomato paste, sherry; cook 2 minutes. Add meat and cook a few minutes until hot. Add sour cream, stirring until smooth and warm. Serve immediately. Preparation should take 45 minutes. Serves 8. Salad, French bread, and brandy-topped coffee ice cream complete the meal.

If you prefer to gather ten or more friends around a blazing fire as the lifts begin to close, set up a rustic spread of wine, bread, and cheese. (If you are commuting to a weekend ski house, you might transport a few specialties from your city bakery, especially if they have ethnic loaves—maybe Syrian bread, Russian pumpernickel, Irish soda bread, Vienna twists, Norwegian raisin fruit bread—as well as standbys like bagels, brioches, whole-wheat rolls.) On a wooden cutting board, set out soft (Gourmandise, Camembert), semisoft (wine Cheddar) and hard (Gruyère) cheeses. Or, serve just butter: salted, sweet, herbed, or whipped. Winter fruits—apples, oranges, and pears—will add color to your feast. Ask friends to bring their own wine, or try serving this *vin chaud*:

- **hot wine**

3 qts. Burgundy wine
1 ½ c. white sugar
½ c. light brown sugar
Peels of 2 lemons
3 sticks cinnamon
36 cloves
1 c. brandy
3 oranges, sliced

Combine Burgundy, white sugar, light brown sugar, lemon peel, cinnamon, cloves. Bring mixture *to a boil* over medium heat. Turn heat to low; simmer for 15 minutes. Add brandy and serve with slice of orange in each glass. Serves 10.

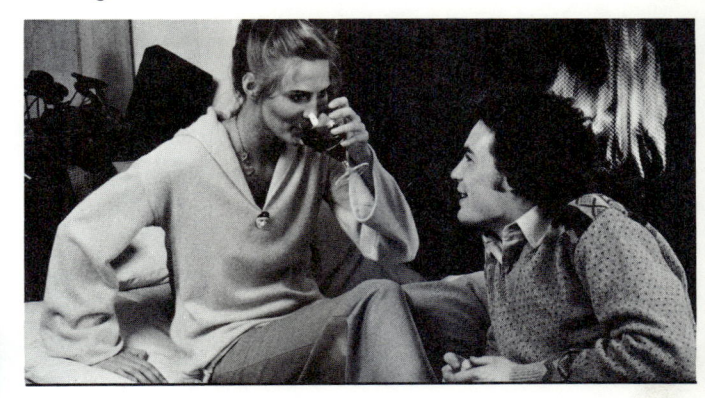

cast how to shower or bathe when you're wearing a cast

During the ski injury season, some arms and legs invariably end up in casts, and coping with the problem of how to shower or bathe without wetting the cast doesn't come naturally. We asked some successful cast-wearers and the Rehabilitation Department of Lenox Hill Hospital in New York for ideas. Check them out with your doctor first.

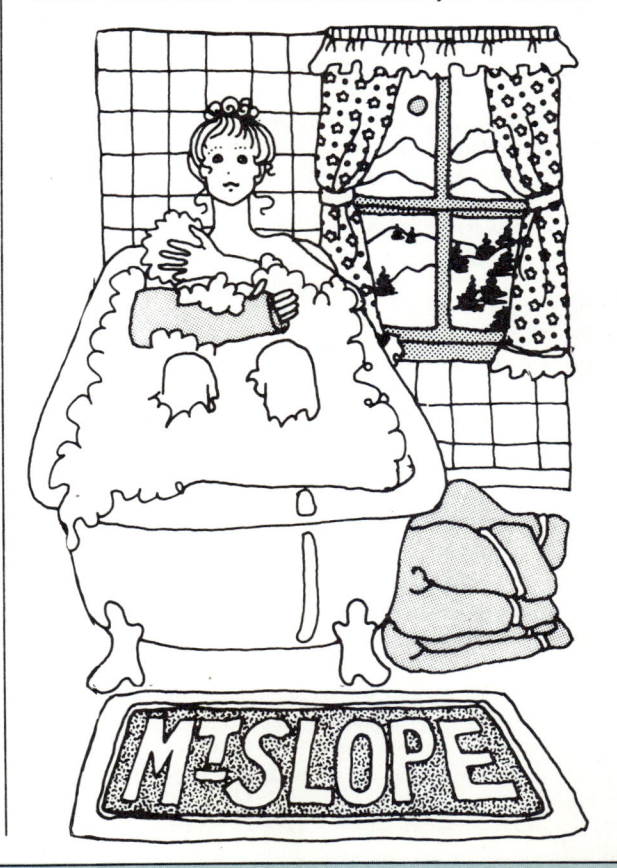

167

S skiing

If you have a leg cast, buy giant-size plastic garbage bags and a roll of masking tape. Slip the bag over your cast, and seal it with tape. Even with this protection, don't take chances getting the cast wet. If your cast doesn't cover your knee and you can bend your leg, you might try sitting on a low stool in the tub with your leg in front of you, resting on the tub's rim. This way you can take a sponge bath and let the water run into the tub.

If you have an arm cast, use a smaller-size plastic garbage bag and masking tape when washing. Again, don't count on the bag being a total seal.

Most doctors stress caution in the bathroom. A cast will make you somewhat clumsy, and wet surfaces are normally slippery, dangerous places. It's a good idea, especially at first, to have a friend there to help you maneuver in and out of the tub or to respond if you need aid.

Also, be careful to wash the skin between fingers and toes because it tends to dry and crack. Exercise fingers and toes by wiggling them a bit, and keep them well moisturized with a body lotion or cream.

cast
what skiers should know about the light cast

Here are some facts about the light cast that may make recovery from an injury easier than a traditional plaster cast does. The light cast, introduced by Merck, Sharp & Dohme, is made of plastic material topped with fiberglass mesh tape, which hardens in minutes under ultraviolet light. It's called Lightcast II and is an improved version of an original light cast developed during the late 1960s. Stronger than a plaster cast but half as heavy and bulky, it can be fitted under loose clothing, and you can move around better. A light cast is immersible (unlike plaster, which falls apart when wet), so you can bathe or get hydrotherapy to heal a skin wound or keep your muscles in shape, which means you're stronger and will recover faster once the cast is off. A light cast is also porous, so skin stays cooler and itches less.

What are the drawbacks? Not all physicians are equipped to put on a light cast. In a ski emergency, you would probably get a plaster cast first; then, if your doctor is in favor of it, you can switch to a light cast. (This isn't necessarily an extra step, since physicians often remove a plaster cast to check healing, then put another one on.) A light cast also works best on "undisplaced" fractures, where the bone is broken but not knocked out of place, says Dr. James Parkes II, attending orthopedic surgeon at Columbia Presbyterian Medical Center and Roosevelt Hospital in New York City, and team physician for the New York Mets. A light cast can cost twice as much as plaster, say, $50 versus $25 for an average-size one. Autograph hounds, beware—the surface of a light cast doesn't take to signatures and art work.

cross-country
a beginner's guide to cross-country skiing

If you spend the winters envying friends who ski but haven't had cash or courage to attempt downhill skiing yourself, why not give cross-country skiing (or ski touring) a try? Though you can tour almost anywhere—from snow-covered golf courses and bike paths to abandoned fields—you might start at a ski touring center near one of the major ski areas. They have marked trails, instructors, and rental equipment, plus après-ski events to share with the downhill skiers.

Good cross-country boots, skis, bindings, and poles cost about $75 to $100, but rentals run about $10 a day and are a better bet your first few times skiing. You can test your enthusiasm before investing much, and the rental shop will wax your skis. (Most cross-country skis must be waxed to suit snow conditions, or they won't slide when you want them to or grip well when you're skiing up mild slopes. Waxing is tricky for a beginner.)

Compared to downhill equipment, touring skis are lighter. Poles are usually longer and have curved tips and larger baskets (disks near tips) to help you push ahead. Boots are comfortable and light, like track shoes. They attach to the ski only at the toes so your heels can move up and down. Sliding on snow is like sliding in backless slippers.

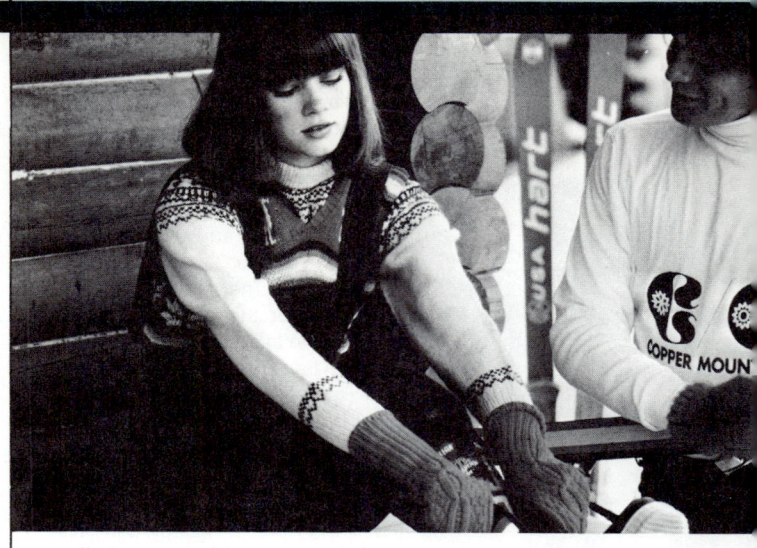

Any light, loose clothing is fine, though knickers and knee socks are the classic look. Dress in layers: thermal underwear, knickers/jeans/slacks, turtleneck, a sweater if it's cold, and a lightweight jacket. Try wool socks with thin cotton or silk socks underneath, light gloves, and a cap. You need less coverup when you ski, more when you rest or stop for a snow picnic. Sunglasses are also advisable, and a small, cross-country fanny-knapsack is handy for toting food and extras.

If you've kept in shape with indoor tennis, winter hikes, or calisthenics (like leg and thigh exercises, sit-ups, and push-ups), you may be up for longer tours. Otherwise, a two-hour trip is a good beginner's limit. Ski, then rest; stick to flat land and gentle slopes if you can't tackle steeper ones.

cross-country
everything to pack for a cross-country ski weekend

A weekend of cross-country skiing is an easy ski trip to pack for: You need water-repellent clothes that cut wind and don't burden you with too much weight or bulk.

Pack one basic outfit with a change of socks and shirt for each outing. The classic suit for cross-country skiing is a nylon windshirt or jacket (Sketch 1) and water-repellent knickers (2). Underneath, a double-knit cotton turtleneck (3), and, if it's very cold, a heavy wool sweater (4). For a weekend, take at least two cotton turtlenecks. Two layers of socks are important unless it's late in the season or fairly warm. The bottom layer (5) should be lightweight and allow for movement—tights are fine if they don't squeeze your toes—and over that, heavy knee socks (6).

For a weekend that includes two separate ski tours, you'll need to pack four pairs of socks and bring along an extra pair of outer socks to carry in your ski pack. Your legs will get splashed, so don't try to make it with one set of socks for two jaunts, and do add a pair of waterproof ciré bands that fit over ankles and boot tops to keep snow from getting into your shoes.

Sturdy leather gloves (7) with silk or synthetic liners give you more flexibility for poling, but if it's really cold, mittens are a better choice. Add goggles or wrap-around sunglasses (8) to cut glare, and a stocking cap to cover ears and head (9).

Half the fun of skiing cross-country is picnicking in the snow, so take along a knapsack (10). Pick a small one that doesn't take up much room

skiing

in a suitcase but will hold a picnic lunch with a vacuum bottle of hot wine.

Try to keep after-ski packing simple, too. The best strategy for any resort is three smashing pieces in coordinated colors. Try a lush winter-bright sweater or leotard with velveteen pants and, for a second night, the same top with your favorite wool skirt.

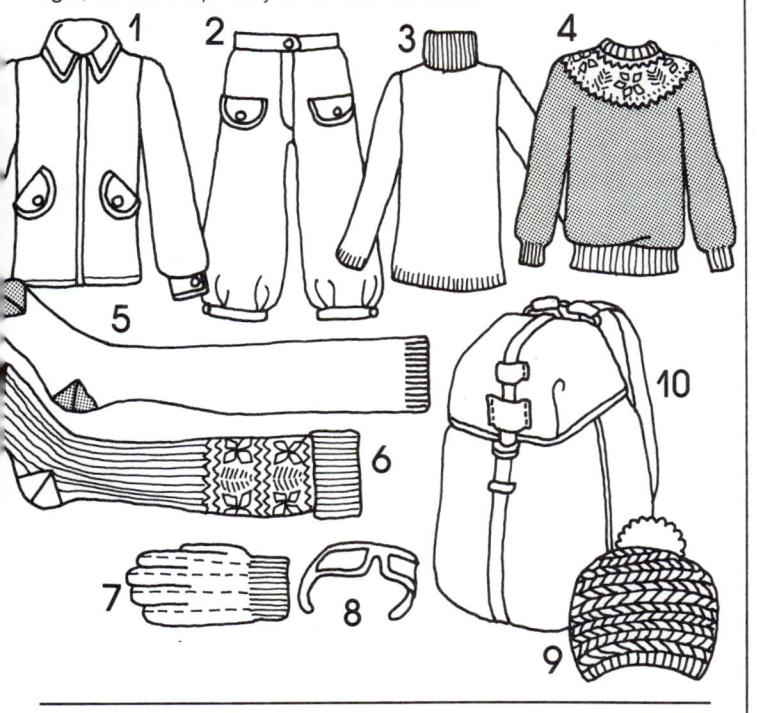

gear
how to buy your first ski gear

If the closest you've come to skiing to date is watching Rosie Mittermaier on TV and now you want to move onto the slopes, then rent equipment for your first few attempts to see if you like it. If you plan to learn by the graduated length method (GLM), popular at many resorts, you'll start on extra-short skis and need a few days to ease into the longer ones that are worth keeping.

When you're ready to buy, head for a shop specializing in ski gear; it's your best bet for expert buying advice and proper binding adjustment. Good starter skis, bindings, boots, and poles cost about $200 to $300. You can cut costs with "package" deals, good secondhand equipment, or a simpler outfit—e.g., wear warm-ups over pants, not ski pants. Remember these tips, too:

- BOOTS—Plastic buckled boots have replaced leather laced boots, and a low model is usually best for a novice because they give more control. Proper fit means your toes can wriggle but ankle and heel are secure (so your foot won't lift when you press forward to ski). Wear heavy socks when you try on boots. If boots are uncomfortable after a few days of skiing, go back to the store to have pressure spots eased or other adjustments made. You can expect to pay $50 to $100 for a good beginner-intermediate pair.
- BINDINGS—They hold boots to skis and are your main protection against possible injury. If spring tension is properly set for your weight, age, skiing ability, and strength, they'll release when you fall—not before. Avoid older "cable" (or "bear trap") bindings that don't release as easily as "toe-and-heel" or "plate" models. Good bindings cost about $30 to $100. (Note: You should check your bindings at the beginning of the ski season and periodically thereafter to see if the setting needs adjustment. The local ski shop or ski patrol will check them.)
- Inexpensive ANTIFRICTION DEVICES—Teflon plates or mechanical devices put on skis below the ball of your foot and SILICONE SPRAYS (for bindings and boot soles) also help ease boots from bindings if you fall.
- SKIS—Good fiberglass skis are rugged and durable. Shorter skis are a plus, too, because they're lighter and easier to turn. Your skis should reach from the floor to somewhere between your chin and just over your head. Expect to pay about $75 to $125 for a pair.
- POLES—Most new ones are made of aluminum, not bamboo. To check for the right size, turn the pole upside down. With your arm straight down at your side, bend elbow, forearm parallel to the ground. Your hand should fit under the circular "basket" near the pole tip.
- WHAT TO WEAR—Basics are a parka, ski pants and/or warm-ups, sweater, thermal underwear, a cap, and two pairs of socks (silk liners plus one thermal pair). Mittens are warmer than gloves but both protect you from cold and from rope-tow burns. Try a layered look with sweaters so you can take off your parka and maybe one sweater to keep from getting overheated. As for goggles with interchangeable lenses, yellow lenses help you see on dark days, and dark lenses prevent glare and help you make out snow contours on bright days.

knickers make your jeans into ski knickers

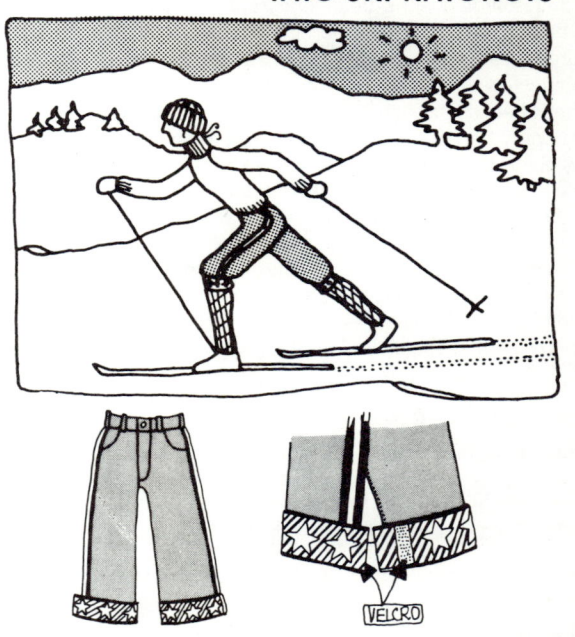

The knickers illustrated here make great-looking, comfortable ski garb or just fun pants. Here's what you'll need and how to make them.

1 pair of jeans
¼ yd. VELCRO® fastener, ¾" or 1" wide
1¼ yds. decorative ribbon for knee bands, 2" wide
2 yds. decorative ribbon for side seams, ½" wide

With jeans on, squat down and mark one leg with a straight pin 1" below your kneecap. Remove jeans and mark the same length on back of leg. Cut off jean leg straight across at pins. Cut other leg to match. Measure 3½" up from raw cut edges, marking around with pins. Cut off these 3½" strips and save to use for knee bands. Open outside leg seams about 3" up from cut edge. Reinforce at top. Machine-gather both legs ¼" from cut end and draw threads slightly. With right sides together, sew the 3½" bands to bottom of jean legs, allowing about 1½" overlap on bands for closure (see sketch). Make a ¼" machine hem in raw edge of knee bands. Cut pieces of VELCRO® fastener to fit inside bands and handstitch them on. Try the jeans on before doing this to be sure you place fastener so that bands will be comfortable when closed over heavy socks. Handstitch 2" ribbon over the bands, turning under raw edges at closure. Handstitch ½" ribbon down the outside seams of jeans.

S skin

skin

acne treatment
you may not have heard of

Cryosurgery or freezing with liquid nitrogen is not new—it's been used successfully to treat many kinds of skin lesions, including skin cancers. Increasingly, it's being recognized as a very successful treatment for acne, both active cases and resulting scars.

Dr. Douglas Torre, a dermatologist and a leading expert in cryosurgery, has treated many acne cases with cryosurgery and says it's most effective with cystic acne, a severe form marked by large, deep-seated lesions and scarring. While the acne is active, the patient is given liquid nitrogen treatments at two- to four-week intervals; then as it is controlled, treatments are less frequent. These cryosurgery treatments are not usually expensive, and Dr. Torre says they're best combined with other standard acne treatments, such as the antibiotic tetracycline, drying lotions, and so forth. Once the acne has cleared up, cryosurgery can help diminish scars.

The affected area is sprayed with the liquid nitrogen, which is so cold that it freezes the skin on contact. The dermatologist, by choosing various spray heads, can control the area he or she treats. The treatment is quick and not painful. With active acne, you can expect treated areas to look red and scaly for a few days. Treatment for scars requires two or three treatments. The skin blisters and swells a bit at first, then forms crusts and finally peels in a week or so. This peeling reduces scars. Although less effective on scars than dermabrasion (mechanical peeling of the skin), cryosurgery is less expensive and less risky.

If interested, call the nearest teaching medical center and ask for a referral to a dermatologist equipped to give cryosurgery treatments.

facials
what are they and who really needs them?

If the word facial *conjures up visions of your great-aunt Sophie with gobs of cream smeared on her face, we're not surprised.* Facial *is an old-fashioned word; "skin treatment" or "professional cleansing" are more to the point.*

Autumn is an especially good time to have one. After summer sun exposure, the outer layer of skin is hardened, making it more prone to clogged pores and breakouts. A professional cleansing is the best way to get rid of this dry, dead layer. Here's what the average treatment in a salon includes.

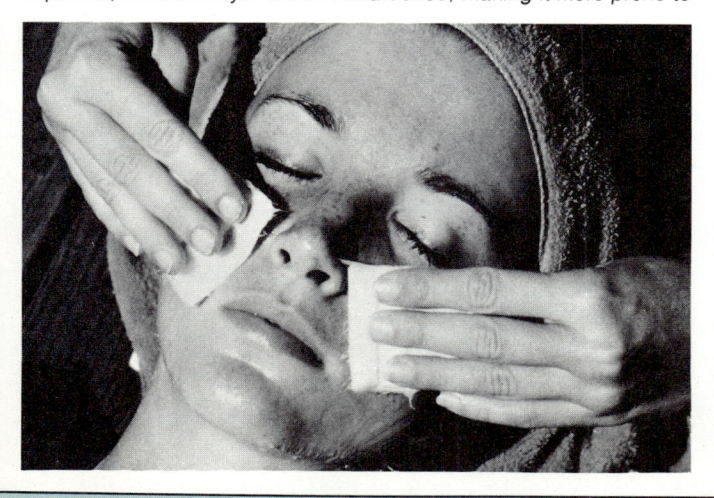

Cleansing is first, usually with a standard lotion or cream cleanser, and sometimes with the help of steam or a sloughing lotion that loosens the outer skin layer. The cleansing is generally followed by a mask —anything from a clay type that hardens on your skin and is rinsed off, to a peel-off mask, depending primarily on your skin type. Some salons follow the mask with a gentle facial massage. The final step is moisturizing. Sometimes heat is applied to help the moisturizer penetrate the skin.

Depending on where you go for your skin treatment, you may find everything done by hand or you may be confronted by an army of octopuslike machines. They are pleasant, soothing, and harmless—providing you go to a reputable salon. Don't expect even the best facial to cure an acne problem. Go to a good beauty salon or to the facial salon in a good department store. Expect to pay $10 to $15 and to stay at the salon for about an hour.

The ideal might be to have a facial once a month, but most people haven't either the time or the money for this. A good rule of thumb is to go when you feel you need it, whenever your skin begins to look dull and gray and doesn't seem to respond to your home ministrations.

problems
common skin problems— what you can do about them

Smooth, clear skin is something everybody wants—but, unfortunately, not everybody gets. Some of the most common annoyances—blackheads, whiteheads, tiny broken veins—can be coped with fairly easily if you know how. Others, like acne, acne scars, or stretch marks, are more troublesome but not impossible. Here are some tips that can help eliminate a few skin bugaboos from your life.

Many young women complain of small, spidery broken blood vessels, which are most commonly seen on the cheeks and on the sides of the nose. There are a variety of causes for these—heredity, extremes of temperature, and the sun. The sun is probably the most common cause. Using a high-quality sunscreen or sunblock is the most effective preventive measure. Once broken vessels appear, you can have them removed by electrodesiccation, a process done by a dermatologist using a very fine needle and an electric current. There is a slightly uncomfortable sensation for a fraction of a second while the vessel is being destroyed. If done properly, the vessels will disappear for good.

Almost everyone is occasionally troubled by blackheads and whiteheads. The terms are also frequently confused. Whiteheads form when an oil gland is covered by a thin layer of horny skin. An irritation develops, and a tiny drop of pus forms underneath, resulting in the white spot. Whiteheads respond well to gentle scrubbing with a good antiseptic soap. Scrubbing removes the thin, horny layer, so that the infection heals.

Blackheads are a mixture of natural oils, bacteria, and other substances in an oil gland opening. Exposure to air causes the material to dry out, harden, and oxidize to a dark color. This dark, hard matter that forms a blackhead has nothing to do with dirt, but careful cleansing can help dry up the excess oil that causes blackheads. Gently steaming the face or using a facial sauna to open the skin's pores makes blackheads easier to remove. If you're cautious, you can remove an occasional blackhead yourself. First, cleanse the face and follow with a mild steaming to open pores. Then, using a piece of sterile gauze, *gently* press on each side of blackhead to remove it. Don't apply strong pressure, and if the blackhead doesn't lift easily, don't persist. If you have numerous blackheads, it's best to have a dermatologist remove them.

Breakouts, or pimples, are probably the most frequent skin annoy-

skin

ance. Occasional pimples are no problem, but in large numbers—constituting severe acne—the situation can be difficult. Most small breakouts will respond to drying lotions or creams, combined with thorough cleansing twice a day. Any druggist can recommend a good drying lotion, and it should be used according to directions. Anyone with severe acne should consult a good dermatologist. Only a physician can determine and prescribe proper treatment for severe acne.

Acne scars can often be helped by a treatment called dermabrasion, which involves rubbing the skin, usually with a wire brush, to help level the scarred area. Not everyone is a good candidate for the process, the results of which depend on the extent and kind of scarring. If you have scars, it can be worthwhile to consult a dermatologist. Dermabrasion doesn't yield peaches-and-cream skin, but often there is noticeable improvement. The treatment does carry certain risks—the chance of increased scarring or a change in pigmentation—so it is important to find a dermatologist who has had considerable experience with the procedure.

Many young women complain of stretch marks after pregnancy or after losing a great deal of weight. There is no really successful treatment for them except to let nature take its course. The redness, quite visible in stretch marks after pregnancy, fades with time. And although the breakdown in the underlying tissues remains, the stretch marks do become less noticeable with time.

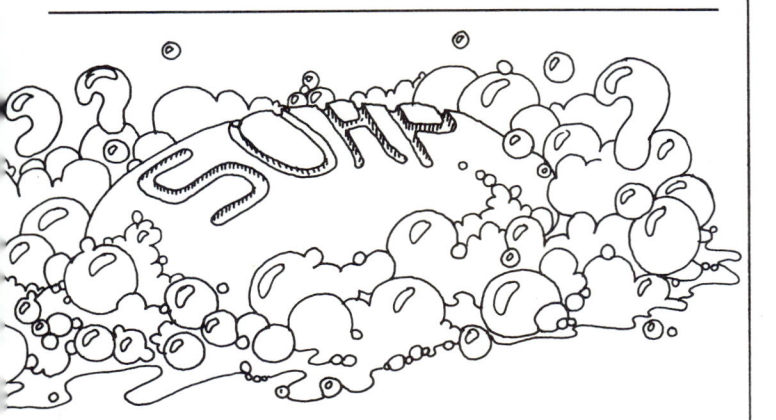

soap   pick the right soap for your skin

Choosing the appropriate soap for your skin can be confusing, so we put together the following guide with the help of Dr. Robert Auerbach, a well-known dermatologist.
MEDICATED SOAPS *usually have an ingredient to remove surface oil from the skin; they're good for oily skins prone to acne and blackheads.*
DEODORANT SOAPS *usually contain an antibacterial agent. Their odor-reducing properties are debatable, but they may make you feel fresher.*
SUPER-FATTED SOAPS *are rich in oils, such as coconut oil, lanolin, or olive oil (as in true Castile soap), etc.; they are also high-lathering. They remove a minimum amount of surface oil from the skin and are best for dry skin. They are also for people who find that regular soap irritates their skin, especially facial skin.*
ABRASIVE SOAPS *contain pumice or a similar ingredient with particles that help scrub off dead skin by friction. They're not for your face or other sensitive areas but are great for hard-to-remove dirt on your hands. (Do not confuse abrasive soaps with the grainy beauty scrubs, which are not soaps and don't cleanse; they only remove dead skin.)*
GLYCERIN SOAPS *are transparent and soft. They are good for dry skin because they remove a minimum amount of surface oil.*
SOAPLESS CLEANSERS *(liquid soaps) are made of synthetic detergents and emollients and lather well; they are good if you have hard water, but are not always milder than soap. Heavy-duty soapless cleansers for industrial use are also made, but don't use them on the face or sensitive skin.*
PERFUMED OR "SPECIAL INGREDIENT" SOAPS *are just that: soaps to which some other ingredient (oatmeal, honey, apricot, and so forth) or scent has been added.*
Note: *The terms* hard-milled *and* soft *refer to soap manufacturing processes. Soft soaps are oilier, wear more quickly, and tend to be more expensive.*

summer
a doctor tells you what to do about end-of-summer skin problems

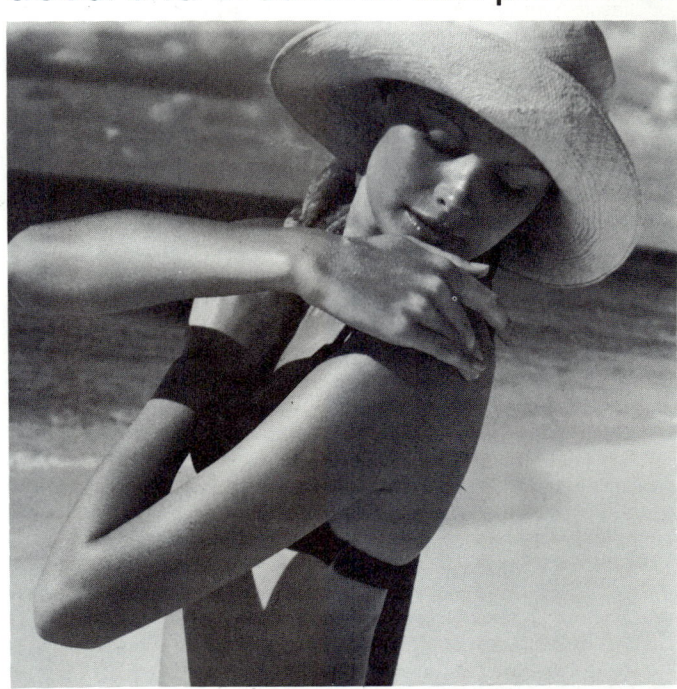

Dermatologist Dr. Robert Auerbach says that most skin specialists see many cases of breakouts, specifically acne, in September or early October. The cause, he says, can be one of two things. Mild sun exposure may have helped the skin, making it clear up and break out less during the summer. Once the "sun therapy" is gone, the skin responds by breaking out. The other cause also has to do with sun, but for a different reason. Sun exposure thickens the outer layer of the skin. This can block oil glands, so that they get dammed up and breakouts result.

No matter what the cause, it's not a welcome situation. Dr. Auerbach recommends keeping the skin scrupulously clean when breakouts occur. Wash it as often as necessary to keep the skin's surface free of oil. For mild cases, use an astringent or plain rubbing alcohol on a cotton pad to help dry up the excess oil. For more serious cases, a prescription astringent might be necessary. If you notice an increase in blackheads or stopped-up pores, it's usually worth the money to see a dermatologist and have them removed. Dr. Auerbach suggests that you ask your dermatologist to teach you the correct procedure. Then you can do it yourself or show someone how to do it for you when new blackheads appear.

You will probably find a cover-up lotion useful for a few weeks—either a commercially available cover lotion or stick, or one your doctor prescribes.

If you don't have oily skin, you may find that summer sunning dries out your skin. Your therapy is the opposite of oily skin types. Keep your skin clean using a mild cleanser made for dry skins, and apply a good moisturizer at midday. A tinted moisturizer can help keep your tan glowing and moisturize, too.

171

S skin

sunlamps
what you should know about sunlamps

- Sunlamps have the same potential for damaging skin as the sun does, including drying it out and aging it prematurely or even causing skin cancer. However, because the time most people spend under a sunlamp is considerably less than the time they spend under the sun, the lamps are responsible for less damage.
- *Under no circumstances should you use a sunlamp without wearing dark glasses or goggles.* If your sunlamp came complete with goggles or glasses, wear them. If not, drugstores sell eye protectors made especially for use with sunlamps. Don't rely on ordinary sunglasses, which allow ultraviolet rays to "leak" in at the sides and may not provide adequate protection.
- If you're wondering about sun lotions for sunlamp sessions, remember that it's best to cut down on exposure time and to apply a moisturizing lotion *afterward*. Instead of exposing your skin for four minutes and using a sunscreen, it's best to stay under the lamp for only two minutes and use a moisturizer afterward.
- Always follow the manufacturer's directions for the distance at which to use the lamp. Never stay under the lamp longer than recommended times or use it at less than the recommended distance. Always tan your skin without makeup.
- Use the lamp only to give your face a nice glow. You may also find using a sunlamp helpful in drying up occasional breakouts, but don't use a sunlamp as regular acne therapy unless your dermatologist has advised it.

frame of mind, rather than the actual lost sleep, is most likely to affect how you function the next day, so try not to worry about it.
- DON'T blame dark circles or puffy eyes necessarily on a lack of sleep. *Continuous* lack of sleep can indeed give you dark circles, but the common shadow below the eye is usually hereditary and has nothing to do with sleep. The same is true of puffy eyes with the exception of some morning puffiness which comes from the normal accumulation of fluid in sensitive undereye tissue. This type of puffiness usually disappears in an hour or so.

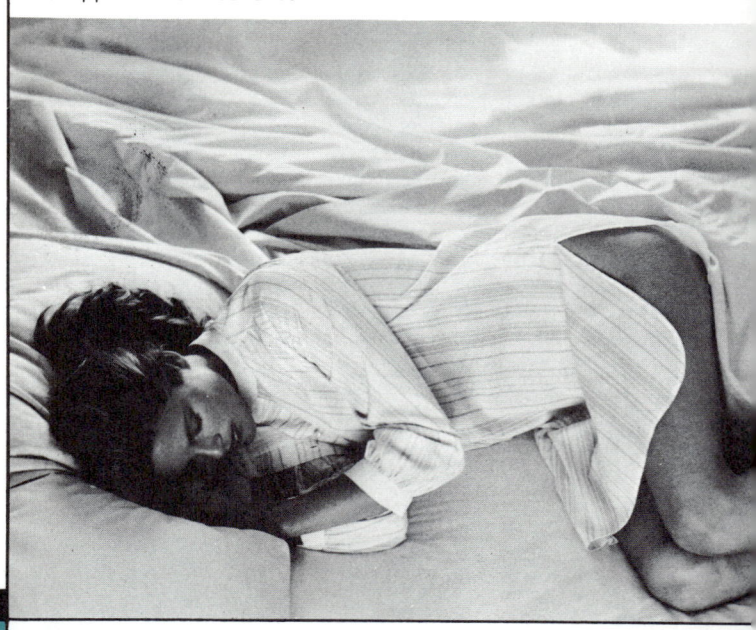

sleep

dos & don'ts for sleep

- DON'T frustrate yourself by vowing that eight out of every twenty-four hours must be spent in sleep. Statistics indicate that seven to eight hours of sleep are gotten by 62 percent of all people; another 15 percent sleep only five or six hours; 13 percent sleep nine or ten hours; and 8 percent sleep five or less hours; with 2 percent sleeping more than ten hours. As you can see, there's a wide range of "normal" sleep patterns.
- DO try to go to bed at about the same time every night. The regular bedtime will encourage your body clock to make you drowsy at this hour. Another tip for hard-to-fall-asleepers: Save your bed for sleep only; don't read or watch TV while in bed. Experts say building the mental association of "bed–sleep" helps you feel drowsy when you actually get into bed.
- DO elevate your head and chest while sleeping if you have a cold or any respiratory trouble. Try putting a couple of books under the two "head" legs of your bed. If you're going to do this on a more or less permanent basis, have a lumberyard cut you two 6" wood blocks to put under the bed legs.
- DO try to get used to sleeping on a firm bed. Some support for your back will help prevent your developing lower-back aches and pains. Sleeping on your stomach also stimulates lower backache by putting too much strain on the lower back.
- DON'T panic if you can't sleep the night before a big occasion. Your

dreams
catch a dream— and then interpret it

Dreams are more than just the idle chatter of a dozing mind. They are a way to explore your unconscious, to learn more about yourself. You may be surprised to learn that the average adult dreams three times every night and has a total of about one thousand dreams a year. The fact is that most dreams disappear without leaving a memory trace; even those that wake us tend to evaporate within minutes unless they are particularly vivid or unless we make a special effort to remember them.

Even if you are a nonrecaller, you can learn to catch dreams and to interpret those you catch. The trick is to sleep with pencil and paper or a tape recorder beside your bed, together with a dim light or flashlight. Then think about dreaming before you fall asleep; tell yourself you will awaken from a dream. When you do wake up, sit up very gently, switch on the dim light, and write down or record the dream; include what you think it might mean, what might have triggered it, and how you felt during and afterward. If you try for a night or two and don't succeed in catching any dreams, try again using an alarm clock; set it for about two hours after the time you expect to fall asleep (most people are into a dream period by then) and for 5 or 6 A.M., since dream periods become longer as morning approaches.

The next day, try to analyze your dream. Dr. Ann Faraday, a psychologist and author of *Dream Power*, suggests that you explore on three levels. First, check for objective facts that may have eluded your waking mind: If you dream you forgot a dentist's appointment, look at your calendar and see if you are actually forgetting one. Then, even if the dream does seem mainly a practical nudge from your unconscious, try the second level of analysis and treat the dream as a kind of mirror that reflects inner conflicts and feelings. If, for example, you dream of someone close to you—a sister, a husband—you can explore the plotline for what it reveals of your feelings toward that person. If you dream of someone once close to you whom you haven't seen in years, that person may simply embody qualities you once learned from him or her.

When you dream about a public figure, such as Queen Elizabeth, that is almost always symbolic, and you must ask yourself what people, situations, virtues, or vices you associate with the figure. Animals are also usually symbols unless you dream of a real animal that is very much part of your daily life. If you associate to the dream animal and its presumed personality, you may find that a lap dog stands for one particular friend, a snake for another. Vehicles often represent a lifestyle, so if you dream about a car, you might ask yourself what sort of car and whether you were the driver or just a passenger. Dreams of a car stalling often reflect sex problems. Not always, though: Dream symbols can be interpreted only through the very personal associations of the dreamer. A dream about standing on a mountaintop obviously means something quite different to a rock climber than it does to a person afraid of heights.

At the third level of analysis, you reenact the dream, taking on the roles of each major element in it, including objects and animals. You might find yourself playing the part of a tree, describing how you feel about having squirrels for tenants, and role-playing a squirrel. When an argument develops, usually between an underdog character and a scolding, bullying top dog, you know you've struck pay dirt: these are facets of yourself that are in conflict. It is here that dream analysis has so much to offer, for if you can get in touch with these secret parts of yourself and begin to accept them, you will be a happier and freer person.

less
how to sleep less and get more done

The standard eight hours of sleep nightly is probably more than many of us really need, according to Dr. Robert Van de Castle of the University of Virginia Sleep and Dream Laboratory. A twelfth-century scientist named Maimonides came up with the eight-hour figure when he wrote a miscellany of health rules, but recent studies have indicated that the amount of sleep necessary to function well is an individual matter.

You may need eight, you may need even more, but Dr. Van de Castle believes that many of us could function well on seven or even six—and that could mean at least an extra 365 hours of waking time each year! If you're interested in reducing sleep time, it's best to do so gradually, going to bed about the same time at night and rising earlier in the morning. Set your alarm for a half hour earlier and try getting up then for two or three weeks. Next, repeat this procedure taking off another half hour. If you feel good, try a little more. If you start to feel irritable and droop early, it may be necessary to add more sleep time, or take one or two catnaps daily (ten to fifteen minutes) to refresh yourself.

morning
ease yourself out of bed in the morning

Every morning when your alarm sounds, your impossible dream is to burrow back under warm covers. You're not alone. More than eighty percent of us have to drag ourselves out. Here's how to make rising a delicious, new-air experience.

● *Yoga does beautiful things for a morning-tight body,* says Michaeline Kiss of New York's Yoga for Health School. The slow stretches and muscle poses, which increase circulation, make you feel like you're waking to a massage. Here's a simple exercise to get you started:

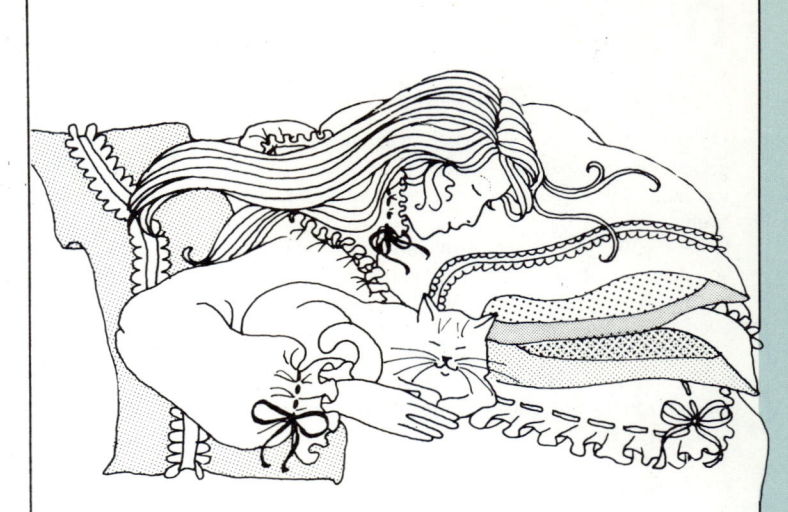

While still lying flat on your back in bed, stretch your arms straight back behind your head. Push your waist back against the bed. Keeping your limbs in contact with the bed, slowly stretch your left arm and leg about 15 seconds; release. Repeat on the right side. This movement stimulates circulation through your trunk and limbs and flexes your spine. Deep breathing exercises will make you alert earlier.

● *Ease yourself into the morning with music instead of a sleep-shattering alarm. On days you have an extra early appointment, switch to an unfamiliar radio station—a foreign language might jolt you to with a seductive accent.*

● *If you get "sleep hangover" (stumbling in and out of the bathroom and not functioning until 10 A.M.), get ready for morning the night before. Put out clothes, organize your bags, make children's lunches. Keep instant oatmeal, breakfast drinks, fresh fruit, frozen waffles on hand, and navigate half-awake the first half hour.*

● *Set a timer on an electric coffeepot so that it will begin perking a few minutes before your alarm. The aroma will entice you out of bed, the brew will warm and wake you. If you can preset your oven, tempt yourself up with a warmed coffee cake or baked apples you popped in the oven the night before.*

● *If you take prescription sleeping pills, you probably get up groggy —it takes at least ten hours before they lose their effect. Even some over-the-counter pills may deprive you of your deepest REM (rapid eye movement) dreams that are needed for satisfying sleep—especially if you're a naturally short sleeper or take the drug every night.*

To kick the habit (tranquilizers and barbiturates can be addictive), Dr. Richard Phillipson at the National Institute on Drug Abuse recommends switching pills and gradually reducing dosage under a doctor's care. Withdrawal can be physically and psychologically painful; even discontinuing over-the-counter type pills after six weeks can result in increased and/or disturbing dreams. But they're temporary, and the refreshed wake-up is worth it.

● *If you're on sleeping pills prescribed for pain or some other medical condition, ask your doctor for a short-acting pill and see if you can switch brands frequently.*

● *Depression or anxiety over an event of the coming day can make it even harder to get up. So think positively.* Shirley Linde, coauthor of The Sleep Book *with Louis M. Savary, suggests filling your mind the night before with thoughts of good things that will happen the next day. If there's not much to look forward to, plan to do something pleasant early in the morning. Invite a friend over or out for breakfast, take a scented bath, watch the kids gobble blueberry pancakes, or ride a bike through the morning air.*

● *Don't avoid your problems. Decide how to face them so they won't pull you back under the covers.*

S sleep

night
how to go to bed beautiful

Many women feel that going to bed looking beautiful means sacrificing good looks the next day—unset hair, dry skin, and smudged mascara. Instead, think of your looks in terms of twenty-four hours instead of twelve.

HAIR: If you choose a simple style with its beauty in the line of the cut, you don't have to wrap and twist it up in rollers at night. There are many such cuts for straight or curly hair—shaggy ones, graduated lengths, even all around—all uncontrived. If your hair is straight or limp and you like a little wave, put in a few rollers in the morning, leave them in while you're showering or bathing. Once or twice a week, give it a lift with electric rollers. Set-while-you-wear hairstyles are another way to avoid rollers at night. Try these:

1. For long hair, pull hair into a ponytail, turn the ends under, fasten with bobby pins.
2. For medium-length hair, fold a pretty square silk scarf into a narrow strip and tie it around your head like a headband. Roll the ends of your hair under the scarf, slide bobby pins under to fasten.
3. Long hair can be parted in the center from forehead to neck nape, each half caught in a coated elastic band. Pull one section to each side and roll into a plump coil.
4. For crinkly waves around your face, make several small braids around the hairline and tie with ribbons.

SKIN: Whatever your skin needs—moisturizer or something creamier—look for an effective, quick-absorbing one. Apply it liberally a few minutes before you go to bed. Allow the lotion or cream to soak into your skin, then blot off any excess. Try a scented body moisturizer all over your body.

EYES: Clear lip gloss slicked on brows will give them a sexy shine and lubricate them. If your lashes and brows are extremely fair, consider having them dyed professionally for a soft, natural effect.

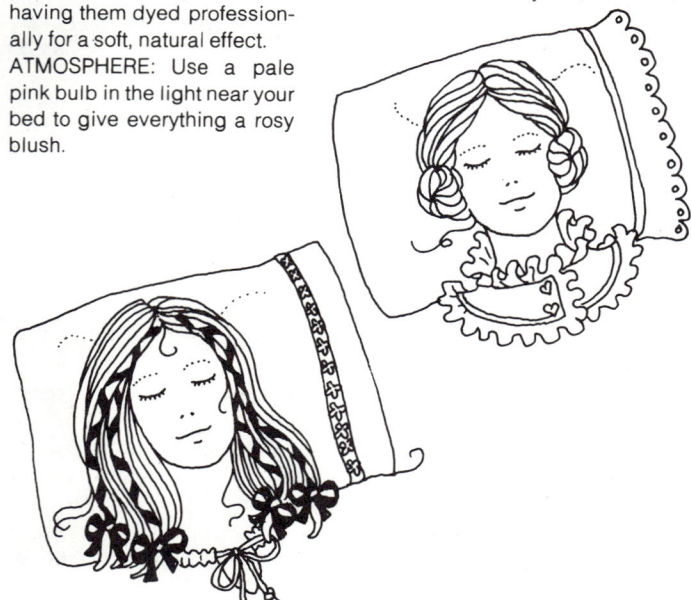

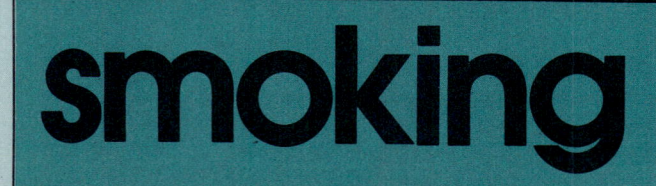

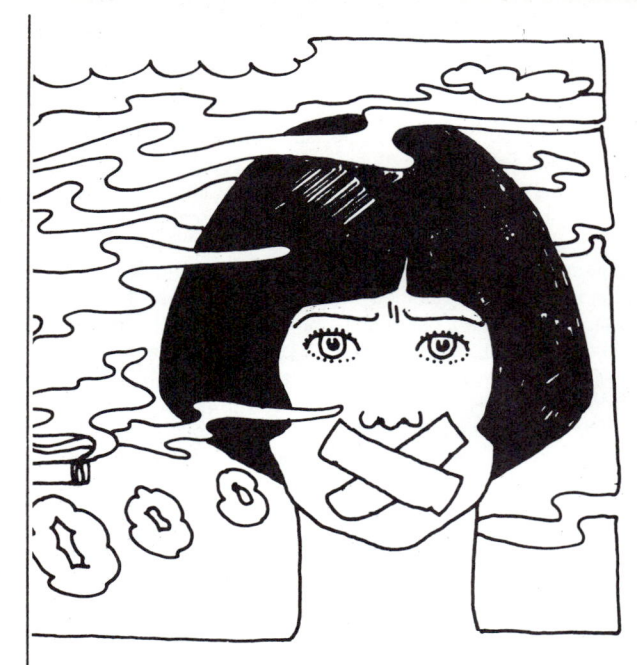

ATMOSPHERE: Use a pale pink bulb in the light near your bed to give everything a rosy blush.

smoking

heart disease
one more reason to quit?

If you're one of millions of smokers who've switched from plain to filter-tipped cigarettes for health reasons, you may want to think about quitting altogether when you consider the findings of an Oxford University study.

The study shows that, although smoking filter-tipped cigarettes reduces the risk of lung cancer, you're trading tar for increased carbon monoxide in the filtered smoke, and carbon monoxide has been linked with heart disease. The British physicians thus concluded that smoking filter-tipped cigarettes increases your risk of coronary heart disease. They compared the changes in type and quantity of cigarettes smoked from 1953 to 1973 and found that, as the use of filter tips increased, the number of lung cancer deaths decreased, but the incidence of coronary heart disease rose.

nonsmokers
do they have rights, too?

This group says yes . . . if you are a nonsmoker who has suffered in silence while breathing secondhand tobacco smoke in public places, you can find a friend in GASP. GASP (Group Against Smokers' Pollution) seeks to ban smoking in public places, such as doctor's offices, hospitals, grocery stores, theaters, and restaurants, and urges people to help prevent indoor air pollution.

Literature available from GASP includes excerpts from the 1972 report on the "Health Consequences of Smoking" by the U.S. Surgeon General. According to the Surgeon General, the hazards tobacco smoke pose to nonsmokers include, among others: "complex pharmacologic, irritative and allergic effects" and a possible "adverse effect on the protective mechanisms of the immune system."

The group publishes a periodic newsletter, The Ventilator, and distributes buttons, bumper stickers (GASP—Nonsmokers have rights, too), and posters (Please don't smoke—people are breathing). Its poster for smoke-filled rooms reads: Please don't breathe—people are smoking.

For more information on joining the group or forming a new chapter, write to GASP, Box 632G, College Park, MD 20740, enclosing a stamped, self-addressed, business-size envelope.

sports

quitting
why women may find smoking harder to kick than men – plus some aids to breaking the habit

Why do women—more than men—find smoking such a difficult habit to kick? Researchers learned that of the 10.2 million who quit smoking during a four-year period, only 3.8 million were women. It seems, too, that women have a 25 percent higher return rate and are the first to popularize new brands. In addition, the number of women smokers is steadily increasing.

Psychologists have various explanations for the reasons why so many women seem to be hooked: Cigarettes signify women's desire to break with old social restrictions; smoking helps women handle role confusion; the housewife's environment is more conducive to smoking, especially if she is alone much; in the business world, smoking creates a sense of equality with men; women, biologically, tend to be more masochistic; women are more fearful of weight gain.

Since we live in a society that tends to avoid emotion, cigarettes for many people tend to serve as three-cent tranquilizers that soothe unruly feelings. With each puff, rage, fear, tension, anxiety, or stress is being pushed down rather than resolved. Also, the movements tied up in the smoking ritual—striking matches, flicking ashes, inhaling—distract you from dealing with conflicting emotions.

"Probably the biggest problem for most smokers who want to quit is getting started. So begin by cutting down in some way . . . the number of cigarettes isn't important," says Dr. Donald Frederickson, Project Director for the Inter-Society Commission for Heart Diseases Research. June Walzer, director of the Stop Smoking Clinic for the American Cancer Society's New York City Division, emphasizes persistence. "Even after you've built up momentum, you have to keep pushing," she says.

The important thing to remember is that if you really *want* to quit, you can. The tips that follow are mostly from Ms. Walzer and from a book that you might want to read: *You Can Quit Smoking in 14 Days*, by Walter S. Ross.

● Wrap your cigarettes in a sheet of paper and whenever you light up, jot down the time, situation, and how badly you want the cigarette on a 1–3 scale. You'll learn to spot situations that trigger smoking and you may be able to avoid them. You'll also become aware of every light-up and this alone can help you cut down dramatically.
● Cut down by eliminating low-priority cigarettes (check your notations and try to eliminate all those you have wanted least).
● Try to get oral gratification—without calories—in other ways. Sip diet drinks through a straw. Or for the nip tobacco gives your tongue, munch ginger root, cinnamon sticks, or cloves.
● Brush your teeth and use mouthwash immediately after meals. It gets you away from the table—and those after-meal cigarettes—and cleans out traces of food which often trigger a craving to smoke.
● Keep your hands occupied with anything but a cigarette—try worry beads, a pencil, knitting, needlepoint.
● Make cigarettes hard to get. If you carry them in a handbag, switch to your coat pocket or hand your pack over to a friend at work. Never buy cartons.
● Relax . . . not by smoking but with exercise, yoga, deep breathing (you might inhale broadly as if taking a slow drag on a cigarette). Try closing your eyes and taking a "mind vacation."
● Don't use cigarettes as a reward. Pamper yourself with a bubble bath, professional massage, or small luxuries bought with money saved from not smoking.
● If smoking is your way of coping with boredom or loneliness, don't get homebound now. Go places, especially those where smoking isn't allowed—museums, libraries, movies, department stores. Try to go with nonsmoking friends.
● Talk to yourself. Repeat over and over that you will not smoke. And, probably most important of all, change your self-image—think of yourself as a nonsmoker.
● If you're a person who responds well in group activity, you might consider any of the following:

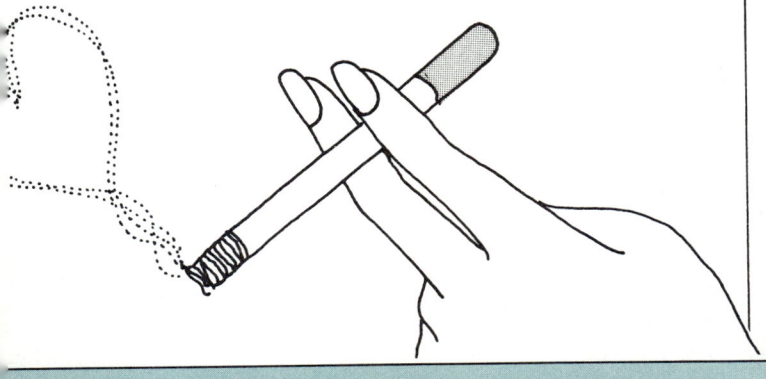

The American Cancer Society sponsors clinics across the country. They cost $5 to $25 and run four to five weeks with two group meetings a week. Similar clinics are run by the American Health Foundation.

SmokEnders, Inc.—a commercial group with chapters nationwide—runs nine-week seminars with once-a-week meetings for $100 to $175 (worth it if you need a stiff economic investment to keep you interested).

Also, the Seventh Day Adventist Church runs nonsectarian, five-day crash programs worth looking into.

sports

good sports, good fun, good for you

beach volleyball

Volleyball can be a fast, fun, and sometimes furious summer game for you and your friends. There are official rules for playing that are used by college teams, but if you're just out for a good time, you can stick to what Karl Skoog, director of men's intramurals at the University of Miami, refers to as "jungle rules."

Here's basically how the game is played. Each team has six players, who divide up equally in a front and back row on one side of the net. If you're playing jungle rules, any number of people you can round up on the beach can play. The right-hand back player of one team serves the ball over the net, and then players use any part of their body above the waist to keep the ball volleying back and forth across the net, attempting to hit a shot the opponents can't return and to keep the ball from hitting the ground in their area. If the team that serves misses a play—for example, the ball touches ground on their side, is hit more than three times consecutively by the team's players, is hit illegally, lands out of bounds, or is hit twice in succession by the same player—the

175

sports

serve goes to their opponents. If the opponents commit any faults, the team that served receives a point and continues to serve. A team must be serving to score. A team wins when it scores 15 points by a 2-point margin. (When playing by jungle rules on the beach or in the park, the main concern is just to get the ball over the net—even if it means doing a few dives in the sand.)

Equipment needed: a ball and a net (sets available for about $11 to $15) and sneakers if playing indoors or on dirt or grass.

Health and beauty advantages: Volleyball is a great general conditioner—you'll be running, jumping, improving coordination. And if you do your volleying on the beach, you can tan and keep busy, too. Be sure to wear some sun protection.

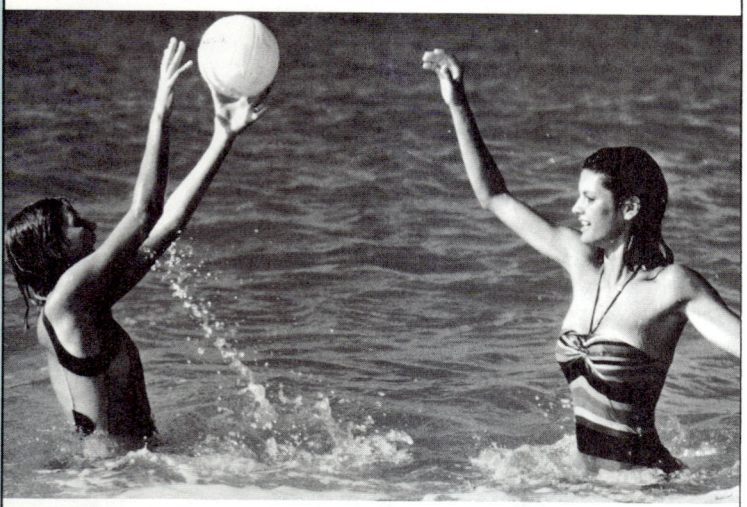

canoeing

Canoeing is a great way to get in touch with nature. If you've never held a paddle before, the first step is to check into beginning canoeing courses and guided trips offered by many local YWCAs, Red Cross chapters, and canoe clubs. Half the trick of learning to canoe is watching others who know how. Another trick is perfecting the basic "propelling" stroke—the bottom arm pulls directly backward as the top arm drives forward from the shoulder in one continuous motion. It's also safest to travel in a group. (For a free list of U.S. canoe clubs, write to the American Canoe Association, 4260 East Evans Avenue, Denver, CO 80222.)

Though you'll probably begin with rented equipment—canoe, paddle, and life preserver rent for about $10 to $15 a day—these buying tips may come in handy later on. They're from Ralph Frese, owner of Chicagoland Canoe Base.

CANOE: Your best bet is slightly round-bottomed, 16–18 feet long, and at least 75 pounds. Good canoes start at about $275.

PADDLE: Measure it from the floor to your nose. Top grades cost $15 to $20.

PERSONAL FLOTATION DEVICE ("life preserver"): A Coast Guard approved P.F.D. is legally required in the canoe at all times. Simple horse collar models cost under $10 but aren't as comfortable for long trips as jackets that run $20 to $30.

CANOE CARRIERS: For toting your canoe from home to water, the safest ones attach to your car roof with gutter clamps, not suction cups. Cost—about $25.

Whether you rent or buy basic gear, it's a good idea to take along these safety extras on any trip: a first-aid kit, waterproof patching tape in case your canoe springs a leak, a big sponge for bailing, and a spare paddle. Keep your clothes comfortable and light—because anything bulky can weigh you down if the canoe capsizes. A bathing suit plus sneakers are fine in warm weather, but keep a broad-brimmed hat, light slacks, and a shirt or windbreaker handy for too much sun and wind.

croquet

If you've never or only rarely played croquet, make it a summer habit for fun, coordination, and mind relaxation. Larry White, head of the Harvard Croquet Club, says, "The game takes a great deal of strategy and coordination—a fine touch." It's usually played on a lawn, using wooden balls and mallets. The object is to use the mallet to hit the ball through a figure-eight pattern of nine wickets (small frames stuck in the ground for the ball to pass through). Four to six players take turns hitting the ball. Free shots are gained by hitting your ball through the right wicket or by hitting an opponent's ball and sending it away from the wicket he's trying to get through.

Health and beauty advantages: Playing keeps you out in the fresh air and sunshine and the leisurely pace gives you plenty of time to think happy summer thoughts. Croquet is very good for improving your hand-to-eye coordination and consequently can help improve your tennis, golf, or basketball game. If you practice swings while you wait your turn, your waist will get some slimming exercise.

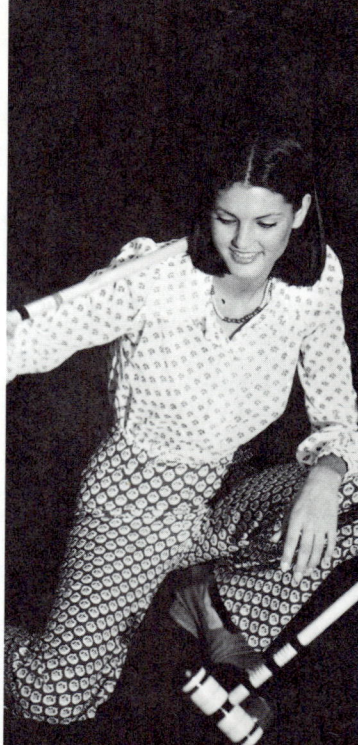

Equipment: Wooden croquet sets range from $14 to $60 for groups of four to six players.

Where to play: Take a set to the park, to a packed-sand, low-tide beach, a village green, or your own backyard.

Croquet has a tradition of confused and changing rules, so you may want to write for the booklet, "Know The Game: Croquet" ($2) from General Sportcraft Co., Ltd., 140 Woodbine St., Bergenfield, NJ 07621.

fencing

"Most people are attracted to fencing by romantic sword fights in the movies. But it's really a nonviolent sport that takes lots of discipline, stamina, and concentration," says Denise O'Connor, an Olympic fencer and assistant professor of physical education at Brooklyn College in New York.

Instead of swords, fencers use foils—thin, flexible blades with dull points and hand guards. The fencing game is played on a narrow strip 6' wide by 41' long. A bout ends when one fencer touches the other with the point of her foil five times.

Health and beauty advantages: Fencing shapes up your figure—particularly legs and thighs. The quick thrusts of your sword arm and the overhead position of the other arm for poise tone up arms and stomach. Good posture and a graceful walk are side benefits, because top fencers learn to stand tall and move with light, crisp, precise steps.

Clothing and equipment: You'll need loose-fitting pants and sneakers, plus a protective mask, padded jacket, glove, and foil. Classes often supply students with equipment; buying your own costs $50 to $70.

Where to study fencing: You might check out classes at local YWCA, adult education center, college, or actor's studio. Or ask the Amateur Fencer's League of America for the name of a fencing administrator in your area. Write to the Secretary of the A.F.L.A. at 601 Curtis Street, Albany, CA 94706. Group lessons cost about $4, private lessons about $8. Two lessons a week are recommended.

sports

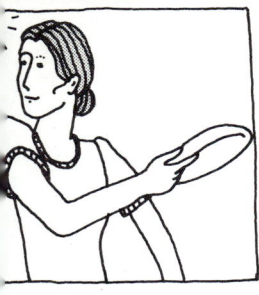

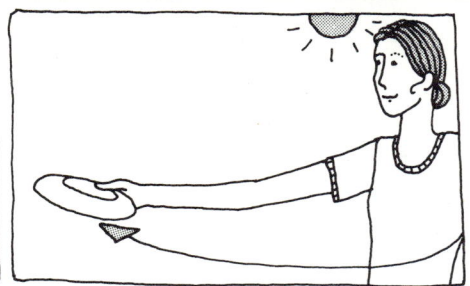

Frisbee

If cut-offs are the first sign of summer in many places, Frisbees are the second. Frisbees, in fact, have become so popular that there are Frisbee throwing contests; there's an *Official Frisbee Handbook,* and you can even buy a Frisbee that glows in the dark for nighttime play.

What if you haven't even mastered throwing the good old 9" Frisbee that started the whole thing, and your Frisbee throws fizzle in midair? Here's where you may be going wrong. Just remember that, according to Goldy Norton, author of the "Official Handbook," there are some twenty-seven possible throws. Here are two of the easiest:
1. For the backhand throw, hold the Frisbee with your thumb on its domed top, index finger along rim and other fingers underneath, as in the sketch above left. Face target (or opponent) or stand at an angle to it, whichever is comfortable. Then bring the Frisbee across your chest, cocking elbow and wrist. Extend arm fully, snap wrist, and step forward with your right foot (if you're right-handed; reverse if left-handed) as you release the Frisbee, as in the sketch top right. (If your aim is to throw *straight,* keep the Frisbee flat and parallel to the ground. To make a Frisbee curve, dip its right side for a curve to the right, and its left for a curve to the left.)
2. For the sidearm throw, hold the Frisbee with your thumb on top, index and middle fingers together along the inside rim, and other fingers curled underneath, as in sketch top right. With your throwing arm extended, not cocked, to your side, and with hand and wrist parallel to the ground, cock wrist back; then snap it forward and release Frisbee.

Catch a soaring Frisbee in the space between thumb and forefinger. You catch one more easily above the waist with palm down; below the waist with palm up.

gymnastics

"More than any other sport, gymnastics develops total coordination... which is one reason why many top athletes study gymnastics to improve performance in other sports from skiing to tennis," says Scott Crouse, head coach for the women's Southern California Acro-Team, Inc. You start doing tumbling and balancing exercises on the floor, then adapt these basics to stunts on balance beams, uneven bars, and trampoline. It's not just *what* you do but *how* you do it.
Health and beauty advantages: Gymnastics are great for overall body conditioning and problem areas that you can shape up with special exercises for legs, back, stomach, and so on. Good circulation, improved posture, and a graceful walk are natural spinoffs . . . so is a mental pickup, because it takes concentration—not just physical skill —to perform even a simple somersault well.
Equipment and clothing needed: *All you buy is a leotard. Gymnastic schools provide mats and other equipment.*
Where to study gymnastics: *Most "Ys" have classes in gymnastics, or your college may offer them. You can also find a local gymnastics institute by writing to: U.S. Gymnastics Federation, P.O. Box 4699, Tucson, AZ 85707.*

For a more concentrated program, you might ask the U.S.G.F. about gymnastics camps (they don't run any but can supply names); like tennis camps, gymnastics camps are run by top professionals, usually last a week, and are open to all levels from beginner to advanced.
Cost: *For group lessons it's about $3.50 to $10, depending on your level and the school; one week at a camp can cost $85 to $125 including lessons, room, and board.*

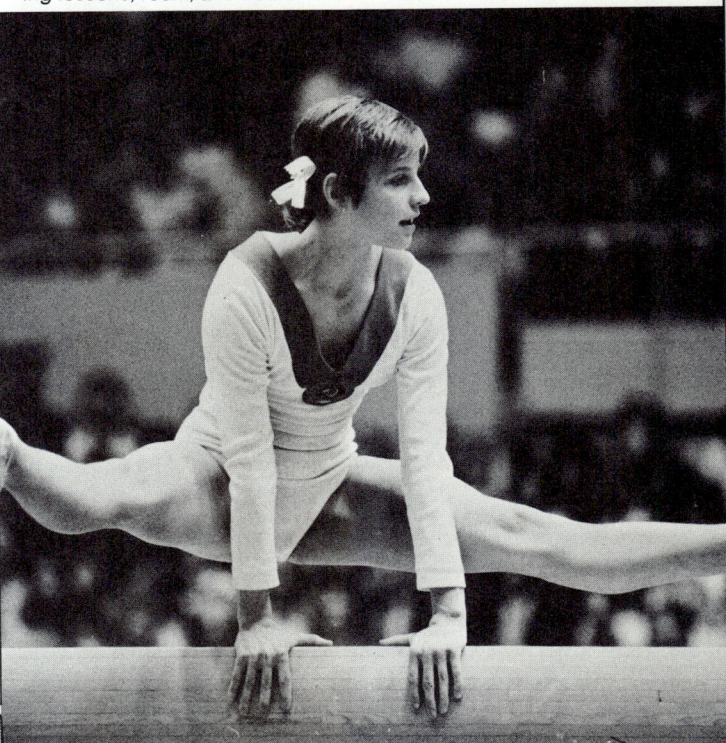

hiking

Hiking is an activity that people with any level of strength and endurance can enjoy. Beginners can start in their local parks, hills, or woods and work up to Mount McKinley. Any season is the perfect time to start: flowers are blooming in spring and summer, squirrels are scurrying in fall and winter.
Health and beauty advantages: Hiking is great for firming up leg muscles, toning up your body, revving up circulation. All that fresh air gives your skin a glow no makeup can match.
Equipment needed: For short, day-long rambles—leather hiking boots with 5" to 8" tops (for ankle support) are a must. Look for lightweight ones with padding (for comfort and to keep pebbles and twigs out) and lug soles. These cost anywhere from $25 to $40. If you plan extensive hiking, look for heavier boots. A canvas and leather knapsack or "day pack" ($5 to $20) is good for carrying your gear. This includes some simple first-aid items, canteen, knife, matches, candle, pencil, paper, map, compass, sunburn lotion, moisturizer, and some snacking food.
Where to go: Any biking or backpacking book will list places to contact for trail information, maps, facilities; a good one is *The Hiker's Bible.* You can also contact your state park or forest service, American Youth Hostels, and the Sierra Club.

177

sports

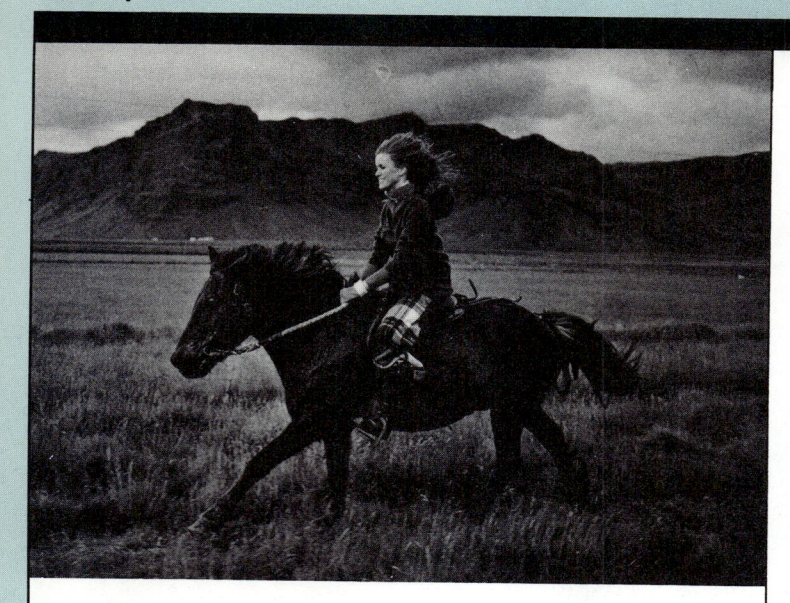

horseback riding

If you love horses and the challenge of physical and mental discipline, horseback riding could be the sport for you. You'll need lessons, so contact a stable in your area.

There are two basic styles of riding: the formal English style and the more relaxed, yet equally controlled, Western one. Riding schools often specialize in one or the other, so you'll have to select a school accordingly. Beginning lessons should cover the basics of the care and preparation of the horse for riding; teach correct procedures for mounting and dismounting; introduce you to the principles of the walk and trot, among other things. With more experience, you'll build up to the canter and jumping, if desired. Lessons can vary considerably in price, depending on the stable and region you live in. A half-hour private lesson can range from $5 to $15; a group lesson from $4 to $13 an hour.

Health and beauty advantages: Riding provides general body toning and muscle strengthening, with particular benefits for the calves and thighs. It requires endurance, coordination, and concentration, but you'll be rewarded by a great sense of accomplishment and a wonderful feeling of harmony with your horse.

Riding gear: This can be very expensive, so it's best not to spend a fortune before you're certain you want to take up the sport in earnest. For starters, wear your most comfortable jeans, and shoes or hiking boots with hard soles and low heels (sneakers and other soft-soled shoes are not appropriate). Later on, boots that cover your ankle may eliminate possible rubbing and irritations, and reasonably priced high rubber boots that can double as rainboots are available in many riding shops (starting at about $14). A hard hat or hunt cap is highly recommended (and often required) for protection when riding English (starting at about $14).

Where to ride: Check your phone book for the names of local schools, and ask other riders you know for information. Then visit the stable to make a general investigation. Check to see if the horses look well cared for and if the facilities are reasonably clean. Then, relax and enjoy yourself and your new equine friends.

ice skating

During and after the 1976 Winter Olympics—which featured Dorothy Hamill's dazzling performance on ice—many ice skating rinks around the country saw a 10 to 35 percent boom in attendance, according to the Ice Skating Institute. There are an estimated 25 million recreational skaters in America—and the number increases every year.

With so many artificially frozen rinks these days (about 1400), ice skating is a sport for all seasons. If you haven't touched ice since you were a kid, don't be intimidated. Nina Marfulius, a skating instructor with Sky Rink in New York City, says most adults have little trouble learning to skate or picking it up again, especially if they've been active in other sports. As for the old myth about "weak ankles," Ms. Marfulius claims, "That's a lot of baloney." When new skaters move along the side of their skates rather than the blades, it's usually because the boot doesn't fit or isn't laced properly.

Fabulous exercise: Skating is great exercise for your whole body—and your head. Try a few solo sweeps around the ice. "It's such freedom, such a creative way to express yourself," says Susan Berens, one of the stars of the Ice Follies.

Equipment: Instructor Marfulius recommends that you rent skates at a skating rink until you feel comfortable on the ice. A new skater with stiff, new boots has a double handicap. But once you're into it, invest in a good pair of skates from a skate shop or department whose staff will take the time to fit you properly—the boots should be fitted separately and then the blade attached afterward in accordance with your body balance. Quality skates start at about $35 to $40. Happy skating!

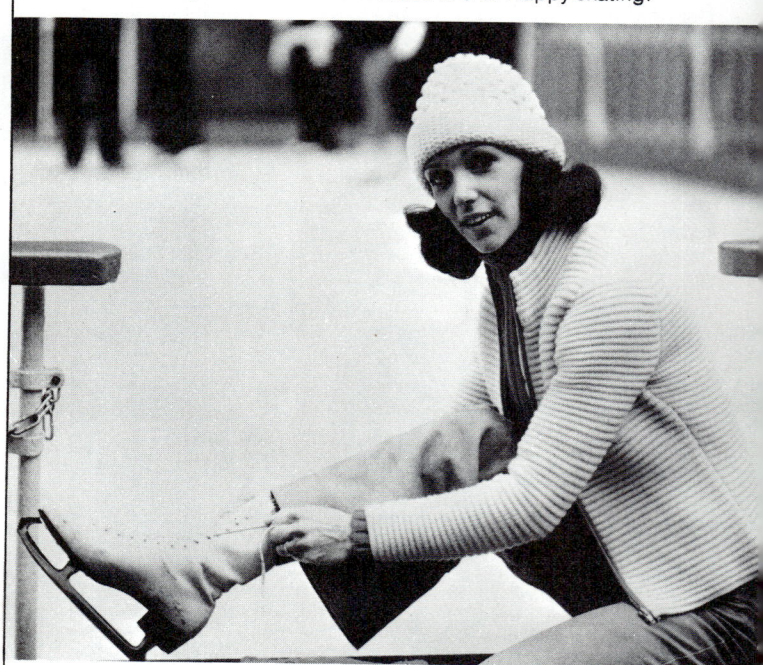

jogging

Don't let the usual image of a jogger, huffing and puffing for long stretches in baggy sweatpants, mislead you about the sport. Jogging actually requires no special shoes, clothes, or track—and can recondition anyone from an Olympic hopeful to an exam-weary student.

But the main goal of any jogger should be to make haste slowly; beginning joggers inevitably jog too fast, with sore muscles a frequent result. A comfortable schedule for beginners is jogging one to one-and-a-half miles three times a week (alternating jogging with walking when needed), with stretching exercises and walking on "off" days.

"If jogging 55 yards leaves you gasping and too breathless to talk with your companions, you're going too fast," say William J. Bowerman, a nationally known track coach, and Dr. W. E. Harris, a cardiologist, in their book Jogging. Other dos and don'ts for jogging include:
- DO wear clothes you find comfortable, and sturdy shoes. Rubber, crepe, and ripple soles ("track shoes") are all good choices. If you prefer sneakers, heavyweight ones are best.
- DON'T lean forward or backward when you jog; keep your body straight.

sports

- *DO breathe with your mouth slightly open when you jog; you'll get winded quickly if you use only your nose.*
- *DO find your best "footstrike." Some joggers run "flat-footed," while others land on the balls of their feet and then settle back onto their heels. In general, however, the heel-to-toe footstrike is the least tiring.*
- *DO try to jog on a surface that has some "give," such as grass. But any surface can work; just remember that on harder ground, you need shoes with good cushions inside.*
- *DO remember, finally, that if you can walk/jog ¼ mile in 3 minutes, you'll burn up 50 calories; 1 mile in 12 minutes, 100–149 calories; 2 miles in 24 minutes, 200–249 calories.*

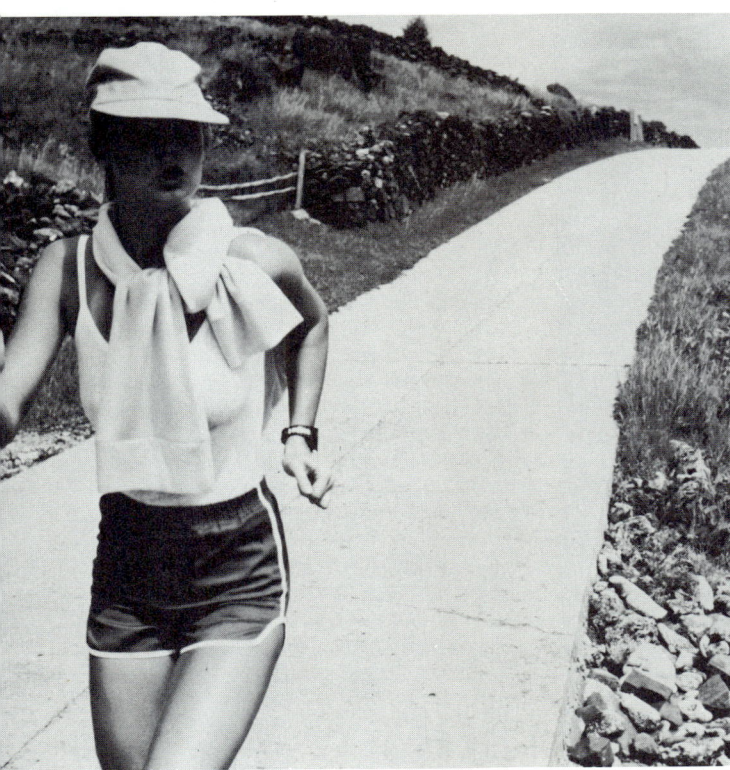

paddleball

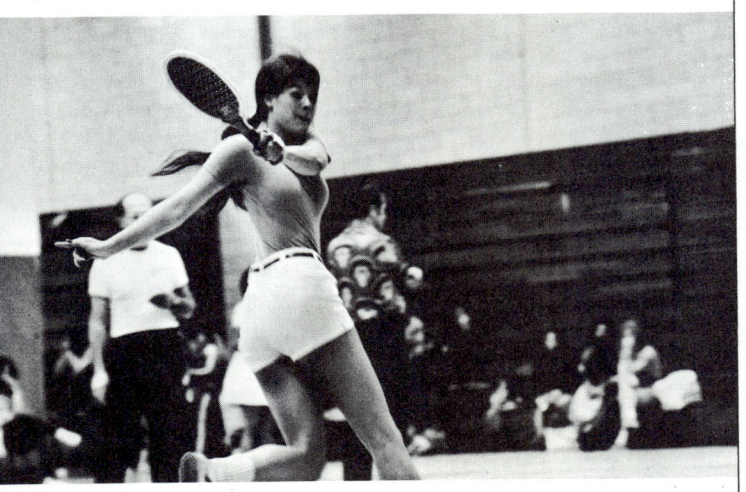

Paddleball is where the action is if you like to think fast, move fast, play hard—though even a nonathlete can have a lot of fun playing at a slower pace. It grew out of handball, with lots more volleying and wrist action than tennis.

You use a wooden paddle to hit a small black ball against a 16' high by 20' wide wall. (Four-wall versions are also played.) One bounce on the floor is allowed. Twenty-one points win the official game; only the server or serving team can score. A big plus is that you can learn the basics quickly.

Health and beauty advantages: You use practically every muscle in your body and vitalize your whole cardiovascular system. Athletic coaches recommend paddleball to build stamina and agility for other sports.

Clothing and equipment: You'll need sneakers, shorts, and a shirt; a small black handball (you can substitute with other balls); plus a paddle. The paddle is shorter—about 17" long—than a tennis racket and has a solid wooden face. It costs $4 to $20.

Where to play the game: Anywhere you can find a wall 16' high by 20' wide with 37' of playing space in front. Handball courts in parks and gymnasiums are perfect, but spunky players might get permission to use the side of a supermarket building or garage during off-hours.

With whom: You can practice alone or play with one to three other people.

For more information: Check *Paddleball: How to Play the Game* by Howard Hammer.

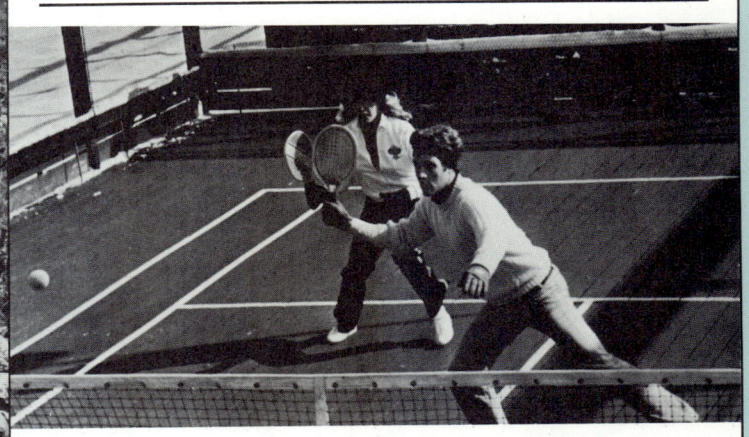

platform tennis

Platform tennis was "invented" by two frustrated tennis players on a dismal November afternoon in the winter of 1928. By 1973, over 55,000 people had discovered this great year-round sport. Last year, more than 400,000 people played, and over half of them were women.

Why? Platform tennis combines the best aspects of a sport: you can learn to play well in a month (this month!); it's competitive, social, mentally challenging, and invigorating. Plus, you can play all year round, outside, and at night!

"A tennis background helps but certainly isn't necessary. The basic strategy is like tennis, but it's more of a giggle game," says Gloria Dillenbeck of the American Platform Tennis Association.

The traditional court looks like a tennis court but is one-fourth the size. It's a "platform" made of wooden slats. Many are heated from beneath.

Platform tennis equipment is nominal. If you have access to a court, all you need is a 17" perforated paddle (they can be made of a combination of hard woods, aluminum, and laminated woods, or made of all aluminum or plastics and range from $10 to $35), a hard sponge-rubber ball (75¢), and a good pair of sneakers. Dress can be anything from a kilt to a warm-up suit—anything that lets you move freely and stay warm. The "pros" wear lots of layers and peel off when the game gets hot.

There are now more than 7000 courts in the U.S. and more are being built at a growth rate of 25 percent a year. The APTA reports that parks, YWCAs, and colleges are catching wind of the sport's popularity and are building courts.

If you want more information about the sport, write to the American Platform Tennis Association, 52 Upper Montclair Plaza, Upper Montclair, NJ 07043.

sports

pool

Pool enthusiasts credit Paul Newman with more than a box office hit in "The Hustler"; they claim he hustled the game of pool back into America's recreation spots and into women's lives, too.

A half million pool tables have been sold since 1974; over 30,000 tables are sold a year, and over 45 million people are playing the game. Most of the tables bought are for the home. Many pubs have even started their own pool leagues. Within the past few years, women are becoming prominent participants.

Why play? It's a great way to meet men and carry on a legitimately prolonged conversation (most coin-operated pool tables cost 25¢ – 35¢ per game).

How much skill... Conrad Burkman, chief referee at the 1976 eleventh U.S. Open Billiards Tournament, says anyone ought to be able to play the game after a month of practice.

And exercise? "You use as many muscles as you do in any other sport except swimming," says Mr. Burkman. "You bend, squat, stretch, sit ... you may walk two miles in a game."

Equipment? Regulation pool tables for a home are 4′ × 8′. They come in all sizes, range from approximately $99 to $2,000. A professional-quality table with a slate surface costs about $800. For "The Official Rule and Record Book" ($1.95), write to Billiard Congress of America, 717 N. Michigan Ave., Chicago, IL 60611.

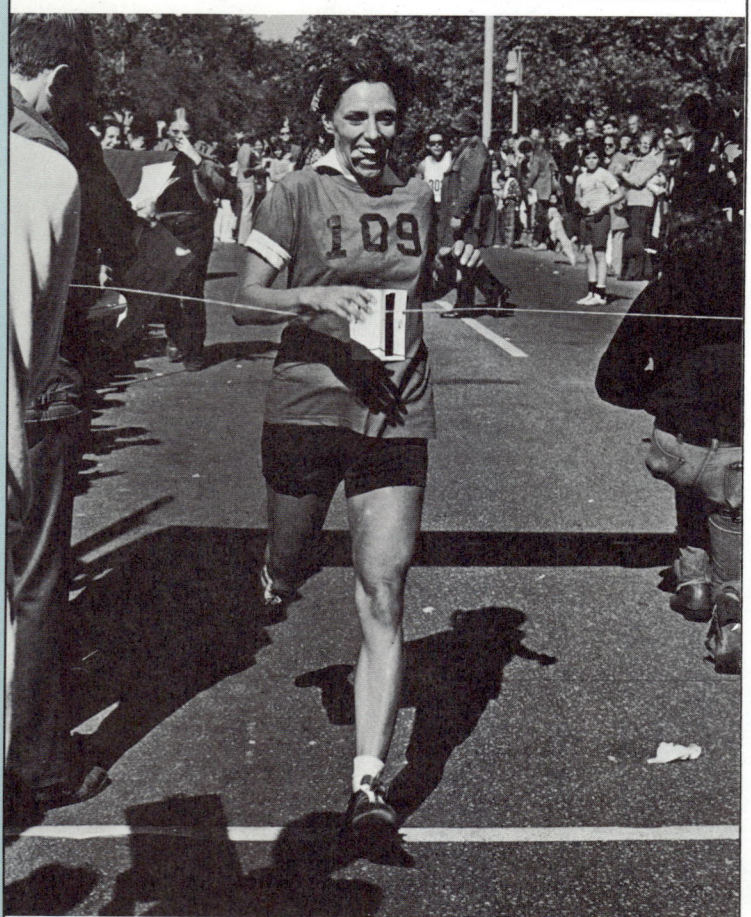

running

Running is almost certainly the world's oldest "sport." Yet even today, few others can match its physical and psychological benefits. It's free; it's good for your entire cardiovascular system; you can do it virtually anytime or anywhere; and you don't need to be well-coordinated or have a partner. Perhaps most important, it's fun.

Many female runners enjoy competing in the regular local events sponsored by the Road Runners Club of America. (By popular definition, a "runner" competes in organized races, a "jogger" does not.) Road Runners sponsors two kinds of running events open to anyone who pays a small membership fee: noncompetitive "run for fun" events and competitive distance, or "road," races from one to twenty-six or more miles. (Good news: In some events, you get a trophy, certificate, or ribbon just for finishing!)

Health and beauty advantages: *Besides promoting overall physical fitness, running can result in loss of weight or inches. Exercise doesn't, as many people believe, increase your appetite. If anything, after a good run, you'll probably only want a cool drink. Running also improves your breathing capacity and makes you very aware of all the vital functions of your body.*

Other advantages: *Competitive distance running has only recently been open to women, and male runners still outnumber female runners by about ten to one—which makes road races a great place to meet men.*

Clothing and equipment needed: *Good running shoes are strongly advised—a must if you'll be running on city pavement or other unyielding surfaces. In the winter or if it's chilly where you live, you'll need several layers of thin clothing, including a warm-up suit for serious runners; for warmer weather, just a shirt and shorts.*

Where to get more information on running: *For the address of the Road Runners Club of America near you, send a stamped, self-addressed envelope to Jeff Darman, 2737 Devonshire Pl. N.W., Washington, DC 20008. Information is also available from the National Jogging Association, 1910 K St. N.W., Room 202, Washington, DC 20006.*

Caution: *If you're running on your own, take it easy. According to Jeff Darman, president of the Road Runners Club of America, you should start by walking briskly for a week or more. Walk about a mile, less if you feel tired. Let your body gradually get accustomed to the new activity. Then speed up to a slow run, letting your body guide you. If you can't carry on a conversation while running, slow down.*

sledding

Whether you're tobogganing with the gang on a sunny, sharp winter afternoon or gliding with him and snowflakes on a night ride, sledding is fun at its best. If you can't do it right in your own backyard, maybe there's a hill close by.

Olympic sledder Katy Homstad found a big one when she was fifteen and slid down the "Luge" track at roughly 70 m.p.h. in the 1968 Winter Olympics in Grenoble, France. Now, at twenty-four, she anticipates competing again in the 1980 Olympic Luge competitions to be held at Lake Placid, New York.

The "luge" is an extremely flexible competition sled from Europe—the driver lies on her back and steers by changing body positions and with her feet. Lake Placid, home of the Olympic Bobrun and Luge teams, has the only professional track in America. Over 3,000 people visit there on winter weekends to watch the competitions.

Great exercise: Successful sledding, at any level, depends on how much you let go of your cares—and body. Noncompetitive sledding offers old-fashioned thrills plus a thorough workout. The cold air, the slightly out-of-control feeling going down the hill, and the many times you hike back up, all give an invigorating tone-up.

Simple equipment: a snowy slope, warm woolens, and something to slide on. The cheapest sleds (besides cafeteria trays) are Slide-A-Boggans and Flying Saucers: plastic roll-up sheets or concave disks with handles. Others include the Banana-Ski, a short, fat ski with a rope on the tip, which you ride as a surfboard, and the Skipper, a regular ski with a seat on it. Prices range from $2 to $15. Traditional sleds and toboggans range from $6 to $45. Discount toy stores and chain stores are your best bets for the cheapest prices and greatest variety.

snorkeling

The next time you go off for a sun-and-surf vacation, why not plan on getting more than a good tan? Take along a mask, fins, and snorkel and explore the underworld of the sea.

Snorkeling is a fabulous sport that just about anyone can learn quickly. You don't even have to be an exceptionally good swimmer—the mask provides great underwater vision, the snorkel allows you to breathe normally through your mouth, and the fins make you feel like you're part porpoise. Pete Philip, a certified scuba instructor with World Wide Diver, Inc., recommends that everyone have at least an hour lesson to learn to adjust the mask properly, clear the snorkel of water, and dive in water as deep as 15 to 20 feet. (A dive shop will probably offer lessons.)

Health and beauty advantages: When you snorkel, you swim, of course, an activity that many experts consider the best overall exercise for both health and figure benefits. You'll be diving, too, which helps develop good breath control and coordination. Probably most important, snorkeling opens up a rare world of quiet and privacy.

Equipment needed: You need a mask ($8 to $30, and for about $26 more you can get your eye prescription ground into it), fins ($10 to $25), snorkel ($2 to $9), and possibly a safety vest if you don't feel totally at home in the water. Most resorts have a dive shop, where snorkel equipment can be rented for a nominal fee if you want to give it a try before investing.

Where to snorkel: The best places to see marine life are in warm water oceans near coral reef formations—off the Hawaiian Islands, the Florida Keys, the Caribbean islands, and in the Mediterranean. But you can enjoy it almost anywhere.

Whom to snorkel with: For safety's sake, always snorkel with a buddy.

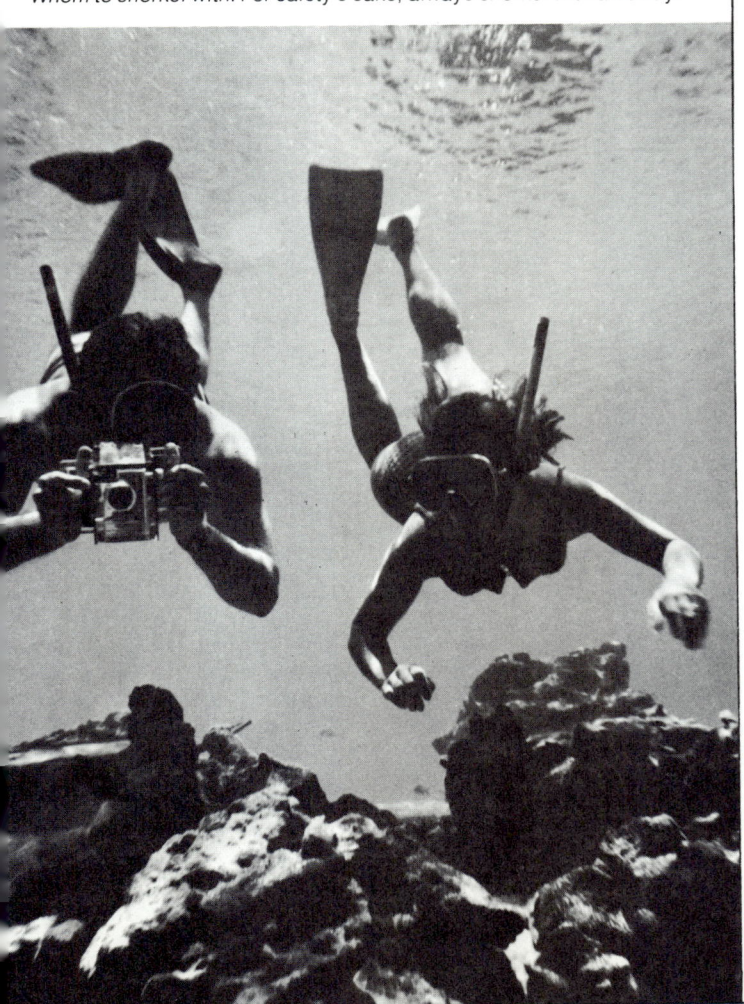

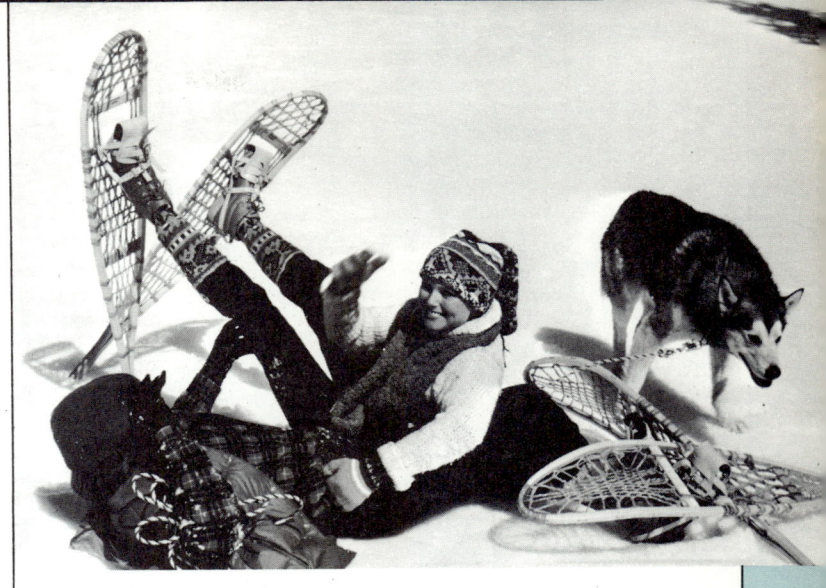

snowshoeing

If you can walk, you can snowshoe—it's that simple and takes minutes to learn. Experts climb mountains on snowshoes and even compete in speed and hurdle races. Whatever your level, you can explore quiet winter landscapes, stop to picnic, sketch, photograph scenery, and spot animal tracks.

Health and beauty advantages: *It's great for firming up muscles—particularly leg muscles—without strain. You might want to ease into more strenuous winter sports by building up your hiking endurance slowly. You breathe outdoor air and provide a ruddy glow for your complexion.*

Equipment needed: *Snowshoes plus bindings cost about $45 to buy—$2 a day to rent. You should start with a "Michigan model," which has a short tail in back that helps lift the front of your shoe over the snow as you walk. Later, you might try oval-shaped "bearpaw" snowshoes without tails (see sketches).*

Where to snowshoe: *Anywhere there's snow, from your backyard to marked hiking trails in state parks.*

With whom: *You can snowshoe alone, with friends, or with a snowshoeing group. Find one through your college outing society or your local chapter of groups like the Sierra Club, Appalachian Mountain Club, or Adirondack Mountain Club. Or write to the American Snowshoe Union for the name of a snowshoe club near you. The Union will also provide information about large snowshoe races—like the national competition in Maine at the end of January or the international races at the end of February. Their address: 138 Barlett St., Lewiston, ME 04240.*

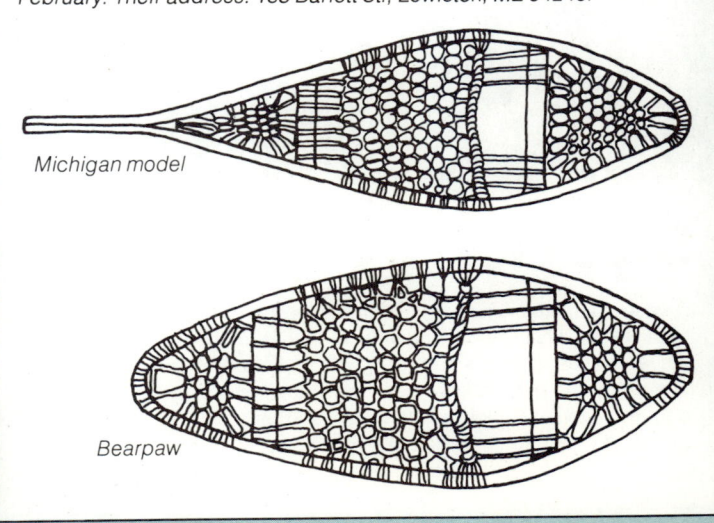

Michigan model

Bearpaw

S sports

softball

Organizing a softball team is a great way to get some neighborhood, campus, or office camaraderie—or competition—going.
How to play: *Softball is a two-team sport played with nine players per team. Each team tries to score the most runs by hitting the ball and touching four bases without being put "out." Games run for seven innings; three "outs" per team end an inning. Balls are pitched underhand to a batter who stands about 40 feet from the pitcher.*
Health and beauty advantages: *The running you do to touch bases, catch fly balls, and so forth is good for your respiratory and circulatory systems—and it burns off calories like mad. While waiting your turn at bat, exercise a little more by practicing your swing with an imaginary bat. It's good for waist and arms. Because softball is such an active sport, you get the benefit of an outdoor sport well into autumn without minding the cold.*
Clothing and equipment: *You'll need a hardwood or metal bat and four base markers, plus a regulation softball. Each player can have a glove, but only the catcher and first-base player may wear mitts. The catcher should wear a mask. Shoes can have spikes, but a good pair of sneakers and any clothing that lets you move and run freely is fine. Add a shirt with your team's name on it for spirit.*
Where to play: *Any field large enough for four bases, an outfield, players, and a peanut gallery of fans.*
With whom: *Anyone and everyone who likes the sport. Join the 26 million people playing softball and get the "ASA Official Guide and Rule Book" by sending $1.50 to: Amateur Softball Association, 2801 N.E. 50 St., P.O. Box 11437, Oklahoma City, OK 73111.*

squash

Squash is an indoor sport that resembles tennis. Walking into a squash court is somewhat like walking into the set of a futuristic science-fiction movie; the "court" is a small room with four stark white walls. Players hit a rubber ball off the front, back, and side walls of the room using a racquet slightly smaller than the one used for tennis. Squash strokes are slightly different from tennis strokes. Because of this, some disagreement exists as to whether playing squash will hamper your tennis game and vice versa, but many people can and do play both squash and tennis well. Here are the basics of the game:
Advantages: It can be learned quickly; after three or four lessons from a squash pro, you and a friend can play an energetic and enjoyable game. Because it's played indoors, squash can also be played year-round and regardless of weather condition. It burns up more calories than an energetic game of tennis, and it's great exercise for arms and legs as well as your entire cardiovascular system.
Number of players required: Usually two, but doubles can also be played.
Equipment needed: Tennis shoes are a must. White tennis clothes are preferred but are not mandatory. Squash racquets cost roughly $12 to $30 new; balls, $1 to $3 apiece. Both can be rented.
Where to play: On private or public courts. Many Y's, indoor tennis clubs, and colleges have squash courts, as do public squash clubs. For the name of the squash facility nearest you or any other information concerning women's squash, send a stamped, self-addressed, legal-size envelope to Ann Githler, United States Women's Squash Racquets Association, 59 Walden Rd., Rochester, NY 14610.
Cost of playing: None if you belong to a university, up to several hundred dollars for joining a private club. Depending on the facility, there may be a per-hour court fee of $3 to $16 for the court—not per person.

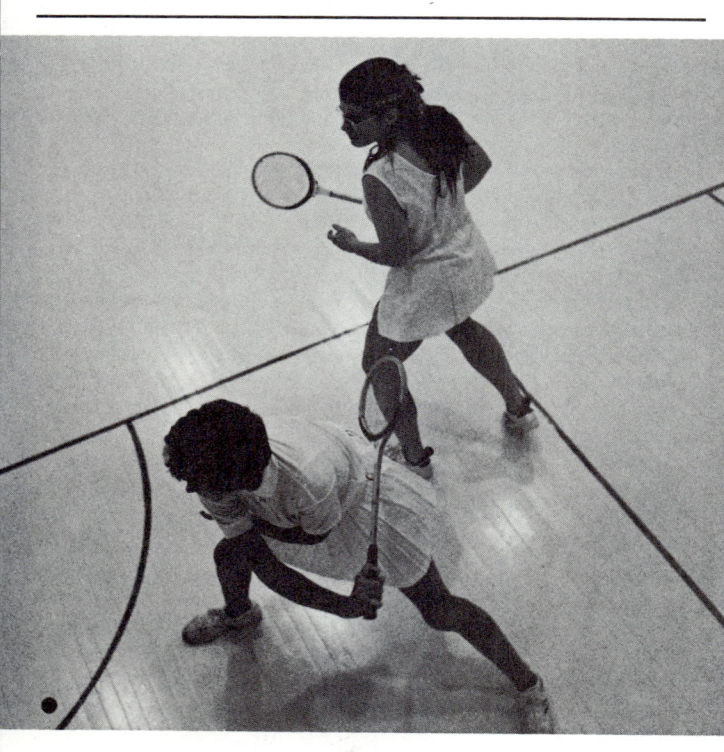

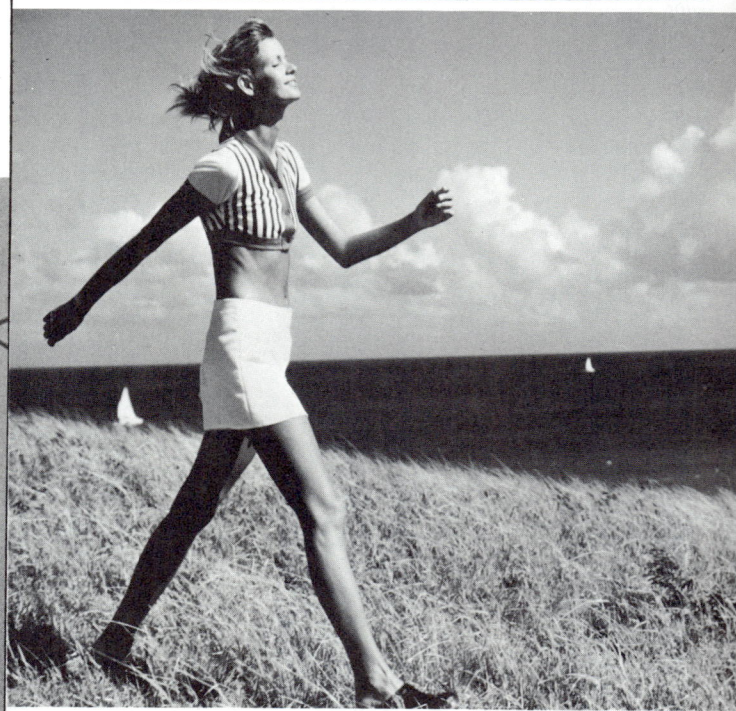

walking

You may have noticed that some people swing their arms at odd angles, others lean their head or torso to a side or point toes in or out instead of straight ahead, so their feet move in a weaving pattern instead of following a straight line. These are examples of "poor alignment"; they may *feel* natural, but they're actually only a few ways you may be using body energy inefficiently while walking, so you become tired and achy even after a nonstrenuous day. Both walking and running start with good alignment, or with each body segment centered over the one below—your head evenly held over your shoulders, shoulders evenly set over hips, and so on. "Many people walk properly if they're walking at a normal pace," one physical education teacher says, "but when they walk faster, they lean forward from the waist, which not only *won't* help you go faster, but puts an extra strain on your

spring

back muscles. If you need to go faster—say, because you're late for work—the efficient way is to lengthen your stride and lean slightly forward from your ankles, still keeping head, shoulders, and hips in line." Here are more ways to make walking benefit you the most.
- *DO* ask a friend to watch you from the side and then from the back to check your posture. You may be lifting your chest up like a general—but holding your head at an angle.
- *DON'T* let your feet cross over each other; keep them both moving along an imaginary straight line.
- *DO* place heels down first, then roll to the balls of your feet even when you want to speed up. Coming up on your toes places extra strain on calf muscles.
- *DON'T* stretch to an unnatural stride; if it's too long for your height and leg length, you won't shift weight over your feet soon enough—and won't move gracefully or faster. Too-short strides waste energy with extra leg swings. Let comfort be your guide.
- *DO* distribute package weight evenly. Have groceries put in two bags instead of one. Alternate the side on which you carry a heavy shoulder bag.
- *DO* carry packages close to your body; the farther out you hold a package, the more you throw off your alignment.
- *DO* walk for enjoyment and health, as well as necessity, since walking has physiological, as well as psychological, benefits like strengthening your cardiovascular and circulatory systems. Blood is constantly being pumped to all parts of your body and returned to heart, and the steady contracting of muscles in the calves and thighs when walking helps to squeeze blood back to your heart. When you don't work these muscles hard enough, they become slack and make the heart work harder to distribute blood (and the oxygen it carries).
- *DON'T* feel you need special shoes for most walks; unless you're planning on real hiking over rugged ground, almost any round-toed shoe with a low, wide heel is fine.
- *DO* alternate walking and jogging, if walking alone seems too tame, but try to follow the same straight-backed, heel-first form when jogging —and wear sturdy sneakers or tennis shoes.

spring

silk tree
the first sign of spring

The delicate branches, sketched left, have an Oriental quality about them. But they don't take Oriental know-how to make—this "silk" tree is incredibly easy.

Find a few bare branches with graceful shapes. Then buy ½ yard stiff silk or silklike fabric in a soft pastel or white. Cut pieces shaped as in the sketch. Each piece should be about 2½" long from leaf to end of stem, with leaf about 2" wide. Experiment before you cut all the pieces. Tape your leaves tightly on the branch in groups of two or three. (Brown florist's tape is ideal for attaching them.) Attach petals one by one. Put your branches in a vase, and enjoy them until the first real flowers of spring are ready.

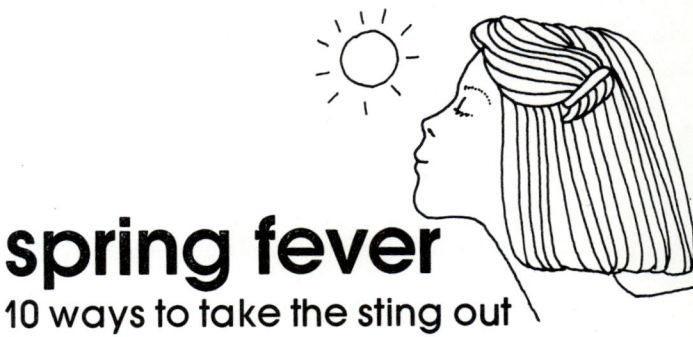

spring fever
10 ways to take the sting out

Spring is the prime time for depression, according to Dr. Ronald Fieve, author of *Moodswing: The Third Revolution in Psychiatry*. The blues you're feeling may be left over from winter, and are intensified now when spring begins making lots of promises but none in particular to you. You're like the ground hog who lies low through the cold months and then pops up only to be taken aback by the shadow it sees over spring. Here are remedies to get you in harmony with the season:

1. Take care of your body. As you come out of "hibernation," your metabolism changes and you may feel sluggish. Dr. Mark Imberman of Mount Sinai Hospital recommends that you get some extra rest and eat sensibly—instead of popping vitamin pills, enjoy fresh vegetables and fruit. It's also the time to start warming up for summer sports like tennis.
2. Get out of winter clothes. Lighter fabrics and colors will feel nice against your skin and give you the psychological lift you need. If it's still a little cool out, wear a sweater.
3. Play hooky—and do something you don't ordinarily have time for. A "mental health day" may sound unprofessional, but it could be just what you need to kick you out of the unproductive doldrums. Instead of saving your vacation days for summer, use some now.
4. Throw your hair back away from your face so you can really feel the warmth of the sun. Barrettes, combs, or a ribbon will hold it back with style.
5. Alter an old routine. Discover a different route to work, a new place to have lunch, or brown-bag it and take a long walk. Have your own private picnic. Pick up the telephone and call the man whose ring you're usually waiting for.
6. Have you been staring off into space lately, wishing you could splash naked in a pond of water lilies? Well, ask yourself if it really isn't something else you're longing for. A new job? A new lover? Make a list of things that have been bugging you and then act on at least one.
7. If classes or work keep you from making the most of spring days, there are still the spring nights to look forward to. Go to an outdoor café or sit on your stoop, watch the dusk change to darkness, and count the stars.
8. Consider how you can see the world—or your apartment—and brighten up the scenery. Wash your windows, take up winter rugs and enjoy the coolness of bare floors. Try to add just one new springy item.
9. Find any excuse for getting out-of-doors. If your schedule's too tight for escaping to become "one with nature," make time to walk home from the office, to carry your plants to the backyard or fire escape.
10. Fall in love, maybe with a homeless cat or dog, have a love affair with your city, cultivate a friendship with a woman. And if you're lucky enough to have a new man in the wings, spring belongs to you.

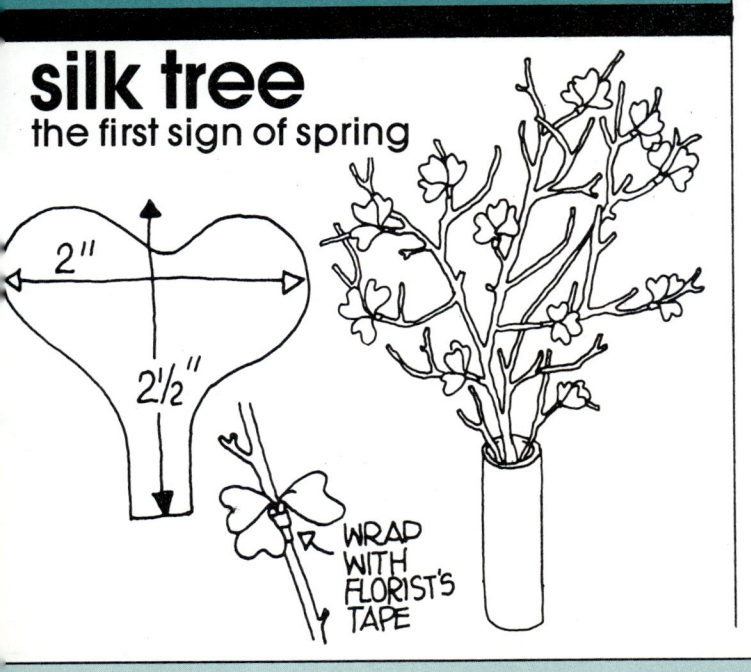

S sticky situations

sticky situations

bad breath
your friend's dinner menu is still on his or her breath . . .

SITUATION
A friend whom you're on the way to the movies with has apparently just finished a dinner of sardines, garlic, and onions—all of which are now working their effects on his or her breath. You don't really know this new friend well enough to joke about it, and—television commercials to the contrary—you just can't pull out a bottle of mouthwash and say, "Listen, Ed (or Jane) . . ."
SOLUTION
Tell your friend you'd like to stop off and get some mints before you settle in to the movie because you ate onions (or garlic or sardines) at dinner, and are afraid that your entire menu is now on your breath. Then offer him or her a mint, too.

borrower
your friend is always borrowing petty cash

SITUATION
You have a coworker, roommate, or other friend who's always borrowing small amounts of money and "forgetting" to pay it back. You're embarrassed to remind him or her about it, but the tab is adding up. You're also tired of being a petty cash machine. What can you do?
SOLUTION
Next time you're asked for money, why not say that the smallest thing you have is a $5 bill—and offer that. Five dollars is too much for your friend to forget about easily. But if he or she still does, you can ask for it back without feeling nickel-and-dime stingy.

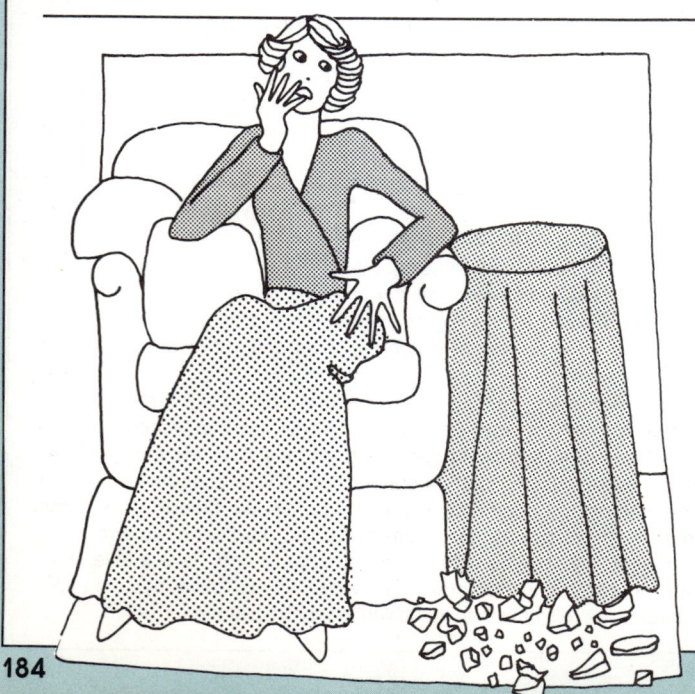

broken ashtray
you're at a party and break a friend's beautiful crystal ashtray

SITUATION
Your regret isn't relieved by any number of apologies for having knocked an obviously valuable ashtray or bibelot off a friend's coffee table and shattering it.
SOLUTION
First of all, don't offer to pay for it, even if you can afford to. And don't try to replace the broken object, unless you can get an exact duplicate. Instead, try to find something else you know your friend will love—and send it to her as soon as possible with a note that says something like, "Thanks for being so understanding about the ashtray . . . I know this can't begin to replace it, but I hope it will add in its own way to your apartment."

dating is he treating
or are you going Dutch?

SITUATION
A guy you've been going out with casually invites you for an impromptu dinner and a movie. You can't tell whether the night's on him or you're going Dutch. How do you avoid embarrassment when the waiter brings the dinner check?
SOLUTION
You can probably assume he's paying tonight if he's always paid before. If you think his budget is as tight as yours and you'd like to continue the relationship, this could be a good time for you to offer to pay your half.

In the case of previous dates when you've sometimes been treated *and* sometimes gone Dutch, you should ask what the situation is tonight. Ask directly, or if you find this hard to do, try something like, "I'd love to see you, but I'm really broke." If you are actually too broke to go Dutch, invite him for a "cook what's in the fridge" dinner at your place. He can then decide whether he wants to treat or accept your invitation.

diet you're on a diet and the
hostess's food is a caloric nightmare

SITUATION
You're invited to a friend's house for dinner with two other couples. You're on a diet and determined to stick to it, even on special occasions. How can you keep your diet and your friend?
SOLUTION
If it's an old, comfortable friend, tell her ahead of time that you're on a diet. Maybe she'll opt for a light dessert instead of chocolate mousse. Even if she doesn't, she's been warned and her feelings won't be hurt if you don't clean your plate.

If you don't know your hostess well, push the high-calorie foods around on your plate while you actually eat the low-calorie ones. Eat very slowly, spearing tiny bits with your fork. If you just can't resist the temptation of a rich dessert once it's in front of you, tell the hostess you're on a diet and pass it up.

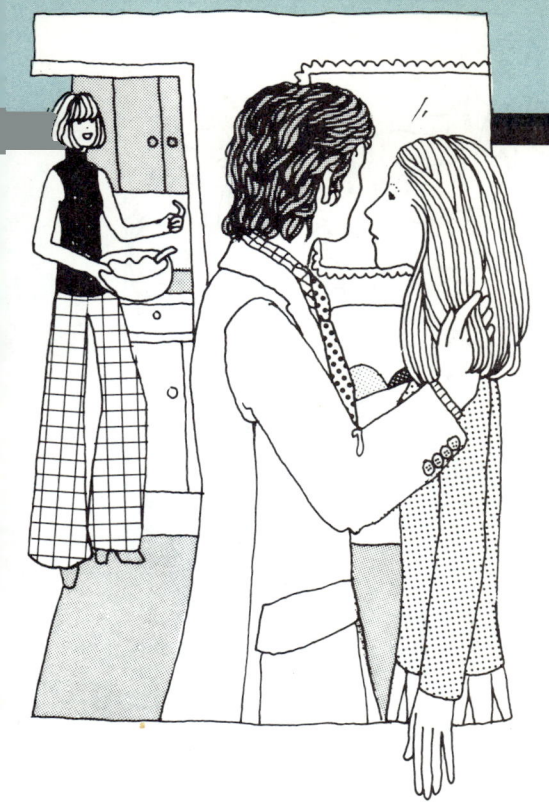

sticky situations S

drunk guest
a guest at your party is insulting another guest

SITUATION
After a few drinks, a guest at one of your parties has turned into its resident aggressor. Most of the others have either ignored or laughed off his or her insults, propositions, or verbal assaults, but he or she has now cornered a shy guest—who seems to be uncomfortable. As the hostess, should you intervene?
SOLUTION
Yes—to say that you need some help in the kitchen and wondered if the shy guest could give you a hand. If the insults (or badgering or pawing) were making her or him uncomfortable, you're providing an out—and if they weren't, he or she can go right back. If it seems that the aggressor is becoming a real problem, enlist his or her aid in the kitchen. If the aggressor provokes you, you have a perfect right to ask him or her to leave.

embarrassment
his public display of affection embarrasses you

SITUATION
You and your friend are invited to a dinner party where there are lots of people you really don't know well. His constant display of affection—kissing your cheek, standing with his arm around you—embarrasses you. What do you do?
SOLUTION
If you've been embarrassed by his caresses before, the best approach is to tell him nicely *before* you go to the party that you'd like to save the affectionate behavior for later when the two of you are alone—that is, if you do like him and mean it. Otherwise, why bother to go out with him? If you're unprepared for his behavior, you can subtly try to discourage him. Move away from his encompassing arm to talk to someone; stop his cheek-pecking in midair, etc. If this doesn't work or if it seems to be calling even more attention to the situation, take him aside and tell him that you're embarrassed and you'd appreciate his stopping.

favor
how to make it clear that tickets you picked up for a friend aren't a gift

SITUATION
An out-of-town friend who's planning to visit you writes and asks you to pick up some concert tickets for her in advance. You purchase them with your own money and want to make it clear you aren't making a gift of them. How do you do it tactfully?
SOLUTION
Actually, the situation could include anything a friend asked you to buy—from theater tickets to a Fair Isle sweater while you were touring Scotland. Here's one way to clarify things without having to come right out and ask for the money. When you hand over the purchase, simply tell her, "Don't worry about giving me the $20 right now. Pay me when it's convenient." Then she will know it's not a gift and if she forgets to reimburse you later, just politely remind her.

gossip
someone is gossiping about someone who's hearing it all—how do you warn him/her?

SITUATION
You are at a restaurant or in an office when one friend starts sounding off about how she can't stand so-and-so—not knowing that "so-and-so" is within earshot. How do you tell her?
SOLUTION
Don't compound the problem by announcing loudly that the person is nearby; he or she can hear you, too. Instead, try as unobtrusively as possible to pass your friend a note telling her who is listening. Or you might consider this: One way to get almost anyone to lower her voice is to drop yours almost to a whisper. Unless she's unusually thick, she'll probably notice the contrast quickly.

late date
what to do about someone who always keeps you waiting

SITUATION
You've got a good friend who's late every time you meet. Usually you grin and bear it, but one night those fifteen minutes throw the whole schedule off and ruin the entire evening. How do you keep it from happening again?
SOLUTION
Explain your angry feelings. Most people who have a tardy friend are usually so relieved to see the person that they squash whatever anger they felt while waiting—and this only reinforces the friend's behavior. If it happens again, give him or her five minutes—and then leave. When your friend checks in with you later, explain without sounding angry that you really had to get going and couldn't wait any longer.

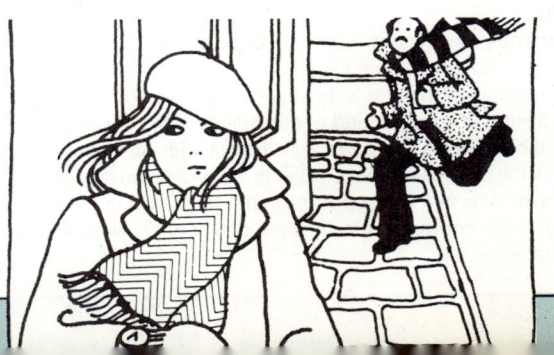

185

S sticky situations

late guest
your other guests have arrived, your roast is ready— and one guest is 45 minutes late

SITUATION
You have invited a man and another couple to dinner. The couple arrive on time—6 P.M.—but it is now 6:45 P.M. and your date is nowhere to be seen. You're impatient (and hungry) but can't decide what to do. Calling to ask if he's forgotten the date could embarrass him; if it has slipped his mind, you're not giving him a way to save face. Besides, now you're worried that you gave him the wrong date. What do you do?
SOLUTION
Presuming you want to see him again (and he isn't always late), call and say, "Jim, I forgot to tell you to come really informal tonight— jeans, in fact." That way, you give him a way out. He can say, "Thanks, I'm on my way over," or admit he forgot or has gotten delayed.

marriage
your friends keep asking when you're getting married

SITUATION
You've been dating a man for six years and couldn't be happier with the status quo. Neither could he. However, your friends are constantly asking you, "When are you two getting married?"
SOLUTION
The best response depends not so much on what you say, but on how you say it. Pick any one that suits you:
 "When we get old enough."
 "When would you suggest?"
 "When I'm pregnant with child."
 "When the world crisis is over."
It doesn't really matter which one you choose, but rehearse it before your mirror. Deliver your line like the blithe assured spirit you wish you were. No hesitancy, no stumbling. It isn't anyone's business but yours and his.

office Romeo
the office Romeo sees you as his Juliet

SITUATION
The office Romeo keeps flirting with you and goes out of his way to walk by your desk or be wherever you are. Now he's just come up to you at the "water cooler" while several other people are standing there, slipped his arm around your shoulder, and said, "So when are we two going out?" What do you say?
SOLUTION
That depends on whether you want to go out with him or not and on what type of Romeo role he fits. There are two. One is the "all talk, no action" man, and the other is so shy, he can only flirt publicly with the idea of asking you out instead of actually doing it. If you don't want to go out, the same delaying tactic will work with both. Say something like, "Ask me again next year around this time." If you do want the date, you'll have to assert yourself with both types and set the day by answering, "Why not make it for lunch today?" or "How about having a drink after work?"

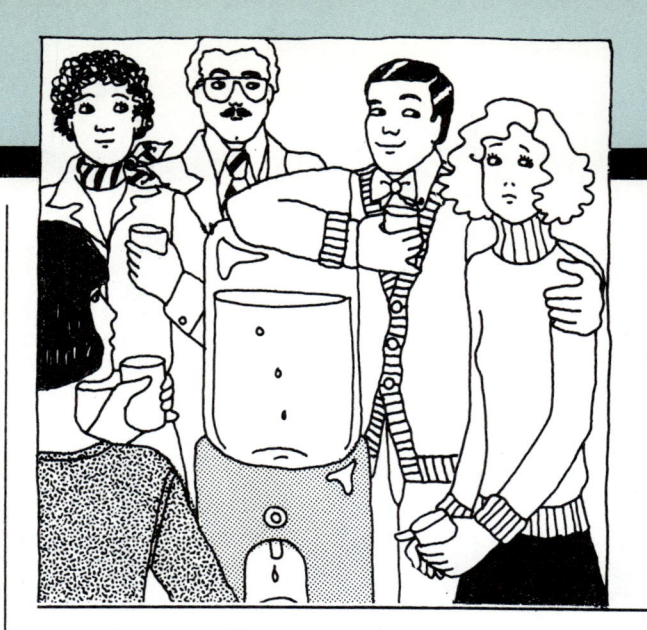

overslept
you've overslept for an important exam or job interview

SITUATION
You wake up two hours after you were supposed to have taken an exam or had a job interview. What can you do to remedy the damage that's already been done—and to make sure it won't happen again?
SOLUTION
Once you actually *have* overslept, it's best simply to admit the truth and hope the person in charge will agree to reschedule. But why let it happen in the first place? On days when you just can't afford to oversleep, you can back up your alarm clock with a professional wake-up service. (Check the Yellow Pages under Wake-Up Call Service.) For roughly $5 to $10 a month, a wake-up service will call you every morning at an agreed-upon time. So it's a good idea for someone who is chronically late to work. If you need only a one-shot boost, many will call you on only one day for $2 to $3. Granted, it's not a cheap phone call, but what's more expensive—that or sleeping through your Law Boards?

parents
your parents pretend to others that you aren't divorced

SITUATION
A few months after your divorce you go home to visit your parents. They're warm and welcoming. One night your aunt and a couple who are old friends of the family drop by. You tell your aunt that you plan to spend the next six months on a special work-study program at Columbia University. She says, "You're lucky to have such an understanding husband; not many men would let their wives leave home for six months." How do you reply?
SOLUTION
That depends on how sensitive you are to your parents' feelings. If they haven't told those closest to them, you can assume their value system has been deeply shaken. If you can, it would be best to save them the discomfort of an immediate disclosure. Later, when you're alone with them, point out that their pretense is disturbing to you and that you do not intend to keep it up in the future. If they don't inform the family and friends, you will.
 If, on the other hand, you feel their values needn't rule your own about honesty, you might say simply, "I'm sorry, I thought Mom and Dad would have told you, but George and I have been divorced several months." Don't get yourself involved in a rehash or justification of the divorce. Change the subject— you owe no one an explanation.

sticky situations

reunion
you can't remember the names of old chums at your reunion

SITUATION
You're back on campus, celebrating your fifth or whatever reunion. You see several familiar faces, really familiar, but you just can't remember the names that go with them. How do you handle the situation without offending anyone?
SOLUTION
What you want to do is let people know that you remember them even though their name escapes you. You might try starting the conversation by saying that you remember *he* was the football team's best tackle, or that you remember *she* was down on Freud long before the feminists got into the act. Go on to say that you're terrible at names and worse than ever with the excitement of the reunion. Another trick that will help if done in advance is to take along your old yearbook and study it for a half hour to try to connect names and faces again.

salary
friends want to know your salary and you want to turn off their curiosity

SITUATION
You and some friends are discussing jobs and you're asked how much you make. You feel it's no one's business, but you don't want to offend anyone by saying so directly. What do you do?
SOLUTION
You can usually make it clear that you don't want to quote figures by giving a funny answer. You might try something like, "Well, I make *above* five thousand and *under* fifty." Or laugh and say, "Not enough," when asked, "How much do you make?" If the friends persist in pressuring you for an answer, simply say you've found it best not to discuss your salary with anyone.

unexpected guests
two extra dinner guests show up without notice

SITUATION
After you've planned on having dinner for four, five or six guests show up. It's too late to go out and buy more food—what can you do now?
SOLUTION
First off, there's no need either to apologize or clutch. With a few minor alterations, you can stretch almost any meal to accommodate a few more guests. The solution depends on what you're serving: If you're having a steak, for example, it will go farther if you don't try to serve it whole. Turn it into shish kebab by cubing the meat and threading it on skewers with whatever vegetables you have on hand—tomatoes, onions, peppers, mushrooms, or zucchini. Then broil. For steak or other single-portion items—such as pork or lamb chops or chicken breasts—you can also cook the meat as usual, then cut into strips or cubes. Serve in its sauce or gravy, heaped on a mound of rice or noodles. Garnish with parsley, watercress, tomato slices, or cherry tomatoes. To stretch a side dish of rice, add a can of peas, diced carrots, pimiento, or sliced mushrooms.

Finally, even if you aren't serving single-portion items, you can still fill out the meal by adding an extra canned appetizer or canned soup course. Always have these meal extenders on hand.

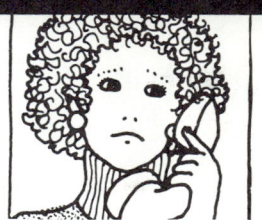

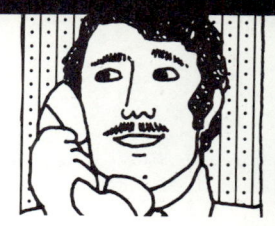

unwanted dates
he keeps calling you for dates...

SITUATION
Although you've told him "no" more than once, a man you don't want to date keeps on calling.
SOLUTION
Why not stop making excuses and tell him the truth: that you think the two of you are just too different to go out with each other. Don't get embroiled in a long discussion about why you're different—he'll only try to convince you you're not, or that a degree of contrast is good for a relationship. Instead, just tell him it's too complicated to explain, so you'd better not even try—and change the subject.

vegetarian
you're a vegetarian invited to a friend's "meat and potatoes" feast

SITUATION
You and your boyfriend are invited to dinner at a new friend's house. You're both vegetarians and your friend doesn't know it. How can you adhere to your diet without offending the hostess?
SOLUTION
The best way to handle this kind of problem is to tell the hostess that you're both vegetarians at the time the invitation is extended. This way, she can plan her menu accordingly or at least be prepared for you to pass up the meat. Assure her that you're used to coping with the situation so that she doesn't feel she has to serve everyone a vegetarian meal. If you and your boyfriend are the only guests or it's not a big party, she'll probably plan her menu around you.

If you didn't tell the hostess before you arrived, simply refuse the dishes you don't want and explain why. The less fuss made about it, the better. This will put an embarrassed hostess at ease.

wedding
what to do when wedding guests ask if they can bring someone else to the reception

SITUATION
You're having a big wedding and a smaller, expensive reception at which dinner will be served. What do you do when a couple of the guests ask to bring a date (often a man or woman you and your fiancé don't know) to the reception? You feel the wedding can expand, but because of expenses, you don't want to expand the reception guest list.
SOLUTION
If you know the person fairly well, there's no reason not to explain that because of costs, you've limited dinner to closest friends and the family. If the person is an honored guest of the family and you don't feel personally close enough to say this, tell him or her that the seating arrangement at the dinner is limited and it's impossible to expand at this time.

S summer

summer

beach
13 things to do on a beach blanket

First, pick the cleverest or prettiest blanket you can find—then *do* something on it. Any of the following practically shouts, "Join me."
- Embroider a tic-tac-toe form or checkerboard on your blanket or towel. Use a tapestry needle and colorfast yarn. Play either game with small beanbags, which won't blow away, instead of checkers or X's and O's.
- When you go with a group of friends, set up your own "casino." Some of you can play blackjack, or twenty-one, while others spin a roulette wheel. Small shells or pebbles make good chips.
- Outline a huge giraffe in the sand near your blanket. Scoop up a trough around the giraffe, piling the sand from the trough onto the giraffe's "body" and patting it to shape features. Lots of people can work on a large animal sand sculpture—so be prepared for enough company to create an entire zoo.
- Give your man a massage while you're rubbing suntan lotion on his back or neck.
- If you like to lie on your stomach and read while you tan, bring along a clear plastic book holder, the kind usually sold as a cookbook stand. Pick a book that genuinely interests you—maybe a biography of Howard Hughes, a foreign language novel, or a best-selling thriller. Chances are someone else who is really interested will happen along. Even if no one does, sand won't spill out of the pages later.
- Make a kite with a toy store kite-making kit, then fly it.
- If you're bringing toddlers along, buy a set of plastic sand molds in a dime or department store—maybe castle molds with fortifications that separate to be used individually. Surround three sides of your blanket with a turreted ridge and moat.
- If you want to be close to nature, learn to identify shells or the tracks of shore birds—such as terns and herring gulls—relying on a trusty paperback.
- Set your beach blanket with a beautiful lunch for you and him. You might include wine, cold chicken or shrimp, exotic fruits, and cheese.
- Take a portable cassette recorder and tapes, instead of a transistor radio.
- String beads for yourself or for Christmas presents.
- Create a "sand pillow" for your head(s). Decide which direction you want to face, then kick up a mound of sand along that end of the blanket. Pack firmly with your foot and lay the blanket over it. Good exercise, too.
- Bring along a deck of Tarot cards, and if you've learned to read them, you're likely to have people waiting in line to hear what you predict for the future.

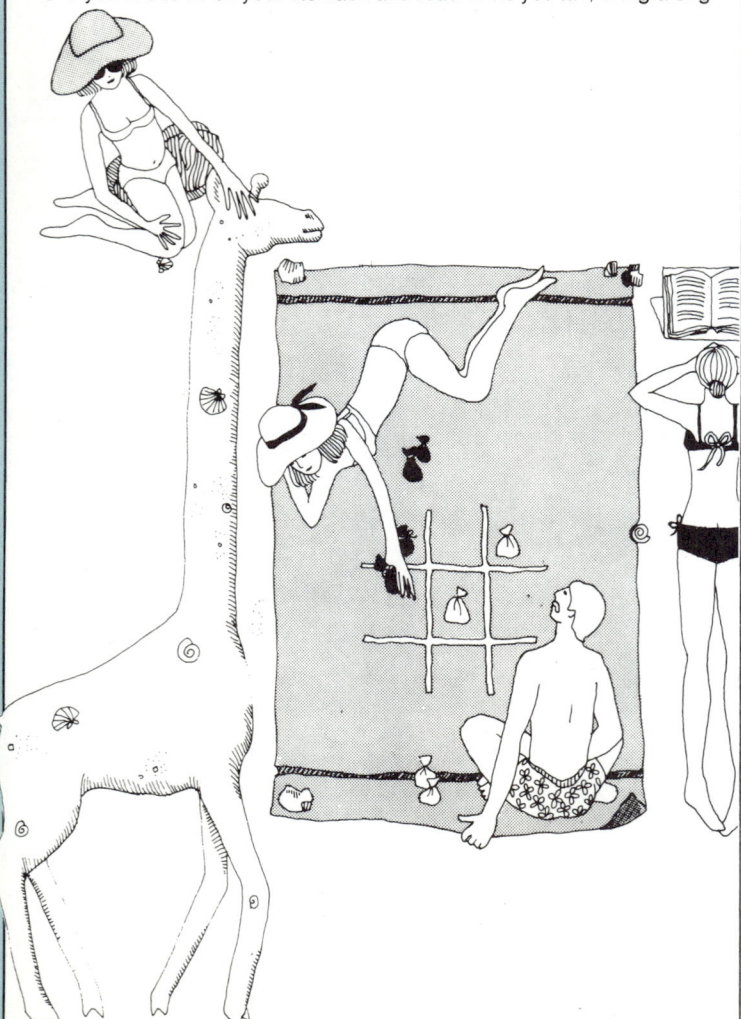

beachcombing
what you'll see of nature's glory

The best time for beachcombing is early morning—ideally, an hour or two after daybreak.

To collect shells, walk along the tide line, looking for shells freshly washed up by the most recent high tide. Prize finds are especially likely to turn up after a full or new moon, which brings unusually low tides, and right after a storm or high winds, which rip shells from their moorings.

Birds tend to cluster near the surf. Two of the most common are gulls and terns (below left), which dive head first into the water after their prey, mostly minnows. The most common gull is the herring gull, (below right); the largest is the great black-backed gull, which has a distinctive black back and wings. Both leave three-pronged, webbed tracks, much like a duck's, in the sand.

Like other birds, terns and gulls also forage for food among piles of seaweed and dead fish or birds that collect along the tide line, so keep an eye open as you pass such piles. (Masses of wet seaweed are food for small crustaceans known as sand hoppers or beach fleas; you'll spot holes they've dug in the surrounding sand.)

What about the folk saying: "Sea gull, sea gull, sitting in the sand/ Always foul weather when you're on land?" According to The Naturalist's Almanac, *the behavior of fish and birds has often been used to forecast weather changes, with questionable validity. However, this predictor may contain some truth. As air pressure drops and a storm approaches, the Almanac says, it's possible that lower-pressure or "thinner" air is harder to fly in—and the gulls may choose to sit out.*

Finally, you may also want to do some "armchair beachcombing," by reading Anne Morrow Lindbergh's classic Gift From the Sea, *or* The Naturalist's Almanac and Environmentalist's Companion *by John F. Gardner.*

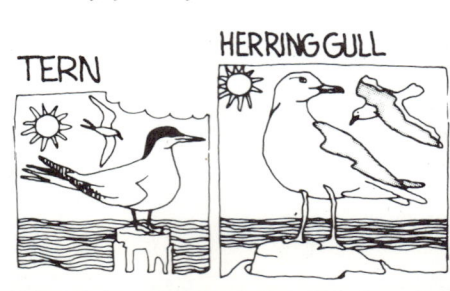

summer S

change
how to be a quick-change artist on the beach

If all you can say is "ugh" to the prospect of going home from the beach in a wet sandy bathing suit, liberate yourself and become a quick-change artist. The sketches here show you how to get dressed so you can go home or on to the next activity, but you could reverse them and get into a suit on arrival at the beach. A drawstring or elastic-waist skirt and a tube top are the best things to wear, but any full skirt and bare top would work. Pull skirt on over head, and let it rest on shoulders while you maneuver bathing suit top and bottom off and maneuver underwear on. Pull top on over your head and work it under skirt and into place, then pull skirt down to waist. That's it; you're decent and it sure feels better than sand in your suit.

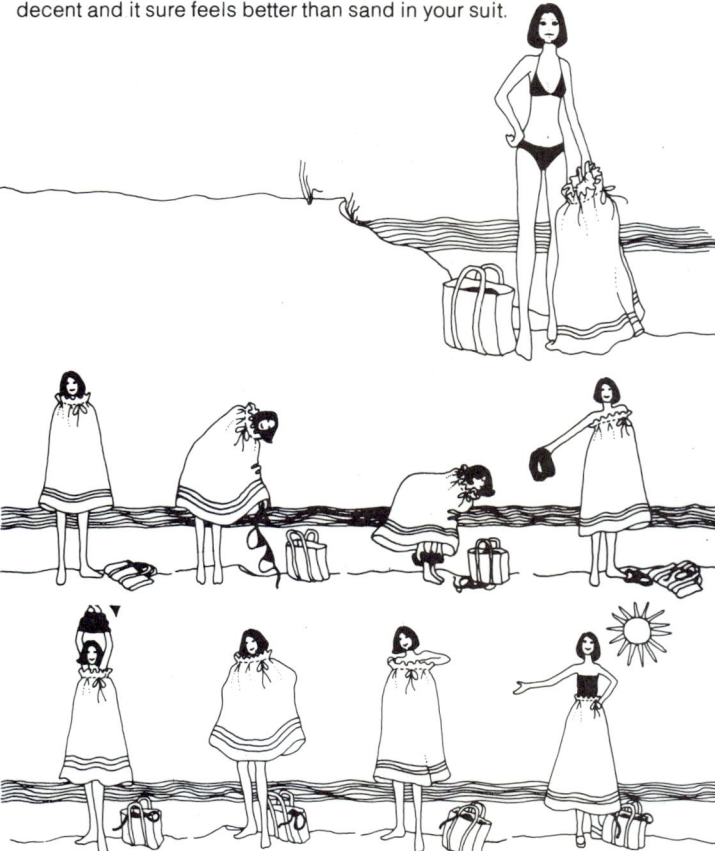

clam digging
a clam digger's quick guide

Summer tastes like strawberries, sweet purple clover, and clam bakes. So grab a bucket, roll up your jeans, and head for the beach. If you know how to follow the sea gulls and a few other practical bits of beachcombing lore, you can dig the juiciest clams on the seashore. Here's how:

- First, check with state environmental officials to see if you need a license. Some states, for example, may not require one unless you dig more than a half bushel per person, while others may require permits just for nonresidents. Some states also set minimum-size standards or hours when you may dig. City governments may also issue permits, so stop in city hall on the way to the beach. While you're there, ask a public health official for pollution information.
- Everybody knows how to dig for hard- and soft-shell clams. But few go after surf clams—most sunbathers carry their triangular shells home for ashtrays, leaving behind the meaty adductor mussels, which are tastier than scallops. They also don't know that tiny California bean clams make great chowder. Burrowing razor clams are excellent, but must be eaten the day they're caught.
- Rake the beach at low tide for hard- and soft-shell clams. Bait shops sell 6–8" pronged rakes for clamming. (A garden variety rake won't go deep enough, but you can use a spade to turn mud and sand.) You can also use your feet. Hard clam "treading" is simply poking your toes in the sand until you feel a clam. To "tread" for soft-shells you walk across tidal flats, watching for the little squirts that signal clams below. A toilet plunger works for underwater (3' to 4' deep) hard- and soft-shell clamming.
- Just use your hands to hunt surf clams, which lie just below the surface at low tide. Dig a day or so after a full moon, when gulls lead you straight to the most plentiful spots.
- For razor clams, slip a little salt in their burrows to bring them to the surface. Use your hands or tongs and a garden spade to pull them out, but move fast, because razors burrow as fast as fish swim.
- Bean clams can be shoveled up, about twelve to the shovelful of sand. Fill a wire mesh basket with sand and clams, then dip up and down in the sea to wash.
- Once you get home, de-sand clams by putting them in a pot of clean sea or fresh water and sprinkling in a handful of cornmeal. Soak soft-shells for two days, changing the bath twice a day. Razors lose their grittiness in a two-hour bath. You can de-mud and de-sand almost any other variety of clams by suspending them in a tightly covered wire basket from the end of a pier in clean sea water for two to three days—just make sure they stay in the water during low tide.

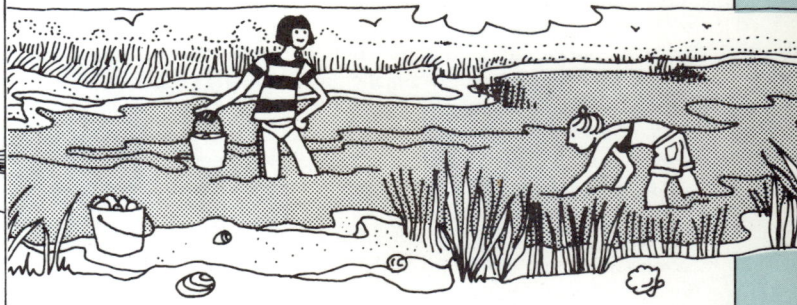

cool
14 ways to keep your cool during the hottest days of the year

- Give yourself a facial with chilled sour cream. Mix 5 tablespoons sour cream with 2 of oatmeal; massage into skin for deep cleansing and removal of dead skin cells. Leave on for 20 minutes. Rinse with hot water, then stroke skin with an ice cube.
- Turn off the heating element in your waterbed for a few hours. Even when room temperature is well over ninety degrees, the unheated water will reduce your body temperature. But don't go to sleep with it off or you'll probably wake up feeling cold no matter how hot the weather is during the night.
- So that you can manage at the hairdresser's when you vacation in Europe, write down these translations:

	● French	● Italian
shampoo	shampooing	shampoo
trim	coupe d'entretien	taglio
set	mise en plis	messa in piega
manicure	manucure	manicure
casual	souple	semplice

189

S summer

	● German	● Spanish
shampoo	Waschen	champu
trim	Haarschnitt	cortado
set	Legen	peinado
manicure	Manikure	manicura
casual	zwanglos	simple

- Consult *Barefoot in the Kitchen,* a little summertime cookbook by Marcia Wallace that has wonderful recipes for easy, make-ahead dishes, many of them served cold. Plus menus for the summer weekends, with a special for Labor Day.
- Help clean a pond or stream—your ecological contribution.
- Sew without needles or thread. Try out the sensational paper-thin web, Stitch Witchery® by Stacy—irons on to make a hem or to apply facings, appliqués, trims. At notion or fabric counters.
- Put your underwear in a plastic bag, then into the refrigerator in the morning or overnight. It's a brief but great coolant at the end of a day's worth of heat wave or beach, or as a starter after a sweltering night. Besides, Marilyn Monroe did it.
- Start on the diet you've been putting off. During a heat wave it's too hot to eat much anyway, and dieting will give you a sleek figure for fall.
- Keep your cool and your figure by getting a book on yoga exercises and *doing* them. They don't call for frantic activity, but they smooth and soothe the body and spirit.
- Go on a wild food treasure hunt and perhaps give a party with what you find growing free in the countryside. Euell Gibbons's *Stalking the Wild Asparagus,* which one critic described as "a walk in the country with a friend," is a fine guide to wild food cuisine.
- Store anything that looks wintery and smothery in a big, old-fashioned trunk. Choose one in a color or paint over your old black one. Top it with bright pillows for extra sitting space.
- For the ultimate in chiller-thrillers, read *A Catalogue of Crime,* Jacques Barzun and Wendell Hertig Taylor's learned and witty 900-page hodgepodge of information on crime and suspense, fiction, true crime tales, Holmesian literature, ghosts stories, etc.
- Use beautiful see-through oval cakes of soap that are made from flowers, fruits, vegetables—cucumber (a deep green), rosewater and glycerine (ruby), or honey and lemon (amber). Just looking at them makes you feel cool.
- Use as shirts or night dresses the airy, transparent, embroidered cotton kurtas that Indian men wear—you can find them for several dollars and up in most any Moroccan or Eastern shop or boutique, in the filmiest white, pastels, jewel tones, or prints.

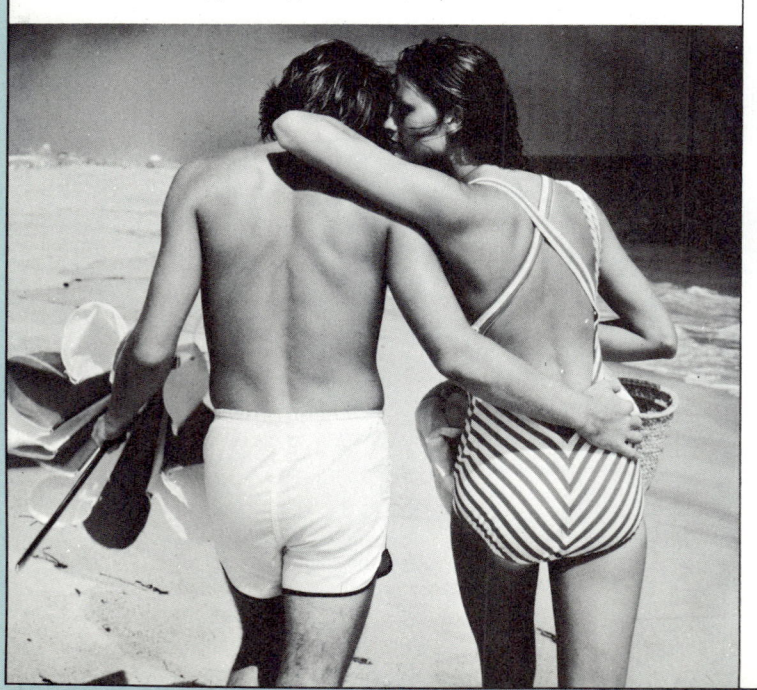

happy ending
if the summer hasn't been all you hoped for, give it a happy ending

If August comes, hot and sultry, it might seem that the summer's slipped by without your getting much fun out of it. Give it one last chance to live up to its original promise—and it could turn out to be the best of all your summers.
- It's not too late to make something exciting happen. Plan a weekend of an activity that you usually tell yourself you're too unadventurous for—like camping out, gliding, canoeing, mountain climbing, spending a night on the water in a sailboat; or too grown-up for—like trying out every ride at the carnival, even the gravity-defying "round-up." You could set out with a friend for a place you've never visited before.
- There's nothing in the world like starry-night skies in summer, and in case you've been too busy to notice them, August still has many to offer. With a blanket, some wine and cheese, and the kind of man summer nights were made for (or your neighborhood pal), have an evening picnic. The Perseids Meteor Shower occurs at night about August twelfth—the earth passes through the debris of a now-dead comet, and you can observe as many as fifty meteors an hour. According to Mihran Miranian of the Naval Observatory, the best time to look for falling stars is after midnight, and instead of letting your eyes roam the sky, concentrate on the area straight overhead.
- If your summer wardrobe starts to wilt, give it a lift with something brand new. Behind all those "back-to-school" and new fall collection clothes are sales racks with nifty things you can wear right into fall—crisp cotton shirts, a dapper lightweight blazer, a sexy maillot swimsuit that's great for the beach and for laps in indoor pools year round.
- Take up a new sport. If you didn't learn it at twelve, you'll never be able to learn it? Well, according to Dr. Joan Nessler, associate professor of health and physical education at Pennsylvania State University, if you have a solid all-around background in sports, you have a chance of becoming reasonably successful at a new sport you take up as an adult—but you've got to find the energy and time to work at it.
- Put down *War and Peace* or whatever classic you promised yourself you'd finish this summer (and are still struggling through) and pick up some light and breezy "hammock reading" that you can polish off in no time—detective thrillers by Raymond Chandler and Dashiell Hammett, some wit like *Crazy Salad* by Nora Ephron or Alan Coren's hilarious *Golfing for Cats.*
- Discover the mai tai, an exotic drink that tastes especially good if you drink it on a patio or beach at twilight. All you need is dark rum and packaged mai tai cocktail mix. Then garnish, as they do at famous Trader Vic's Polynesian restaurant, with a sprig of mint, a twist of lime peel, a cherry, and a chunk of pineapple.

heat don't talk about the heat, do something about it

First, take this true/false quiz so you'll know what to do about the heat, what are old wives' tales, and what are the cool facts. Then follow the latter.
1. You'll feel the heat more at the start of a long hot summer than later on.
2. You can beat the heat by watching your weight.
3. If you're pregnant, you'll feel warmer.
4. A cold shower is more refreshing than a lukewarm bath.
5. You should eat light foods to stay cool.
6. On hot days your thirst always tells you when and how much to drink.
7. Running cool water over your wrists—or dangling your feet in a lake—can give you a quick pickup on hot days.

summer

8. It's just your imagination if you can't concentrate when it's hot.
9. You'll tolerate heat better if you're rested.
10. You probably perspire less than your boyfriend.
11. Always wear less to feel cooler.
12. You'll always feel hot if you're overheated.
13. Salt tablets are great in summer.

● **answers**

1. TRUE—Your body needs one to three weeks to adjust to hot weather.
2. TRUE—Toting extra pounds is like carrying a heavy suitcase—you'll exert yourself doing it. The body loses heat through the skin; a heavier person has less skin surface per pound and has a harder time cooling off.
3. TRUE—You have the same problem keeping cool that a heavier person does, and the fetus also produces heat.
4. FALSE—The icy water tricks your brain into thinking you're chilled, not overheated; like a thermostat, you start warming up, not cooling off.
5. TRUE—Light salads are refreshing in summer because the body produces less heat digesting fruits and vegetables than high-protein steaks or chops. You'll feel better eating several small meals instead of a few big ones.
6. FALSE—Don't risk heat exhaustion by waiting for thirst to drink up. If you perspire a lot, drink small amounts of cool (not icy) water regularly.
7. TRUE—You lose (or gain) the most heat through hands and feet, so spot bathing can help you cool off fast.
8. FALSE—Studies have shown that when temperature and humidity are uncomfortably high, most people find it more difficult to perform routine tasks because more blood than usual is going to the skin to reduce your body temperature, which is a distraction.
9. TRUE—You're better able to handle stress, including heat stress, if you're rested and in good physical condition.
10. TRUE—Once acclimatized to heat, men perspire about three times more during moderate exercise than women, who rely on other mechanisms to adapt, according to Dr. Steven Horvath, director of the Institute of Environmental Stress at University of California at Santa Barbara.
11. FALSE—Out in the sun or exposed to bright pavements or a reflecting lake, you're best off with a lightweight cover . . . preferably clothes that are white or pastel, loose-fitting, and made of fabric that "breathes," like cotton.
12. FALSE—Heat exhaustion, caused by water and salt lost through sweating, makes you feel cold and clammy.
13. FALSE—Salt tablets are usually unnecessary and irritate the stomach. An extra dash of salt at meals can make up for most salt lost through perspiration.

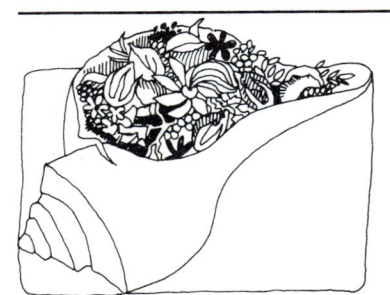

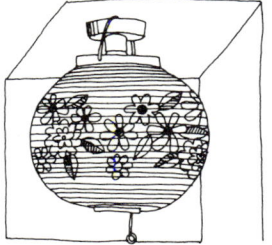

indoors
how to bring summer inside

1. Scent your surroundings by putting potpourri in large seashells, pretty glass apothecary jars, or Mason jars.
2. Buy or make cotton pillow shams that bring nature inside—flower prints, shell or sea or greenery patterns. Change a heavy winter bedspread for a light throw with a summery feeling; dark lampshades for white parchment, straw, monk's cloth. Fill containers with cut green leaves. They last for weeks.
3. Buy a few goldfish and house them in a pretty bowl. For the sounds of summer, get a pair of canaries (they sing more when they have company).
4. Substitute matchstick or split-bamboo shades for draperies. Let them hang alone now, frame with curtains in cooler months.
5. Bare your floors, or cover them with grass area rugs.
6. Really splurge and have beige or white duck slipcovers made for heavy upholstered chairs and sofas.

For brightening rented beach houses:

1. Substitute paper lanterns, white or printed, for ugly ceiling fixtures.
2. Cuts of boldly printed fabric, hung on poles, make great banners—an effective, inexpensive way to cover a wall.
3. With your landlord's permission, deck-paint a floor—solid or patterned—or stencil a pattern on the floor, around a door or molding.
5. Invest a few dollars in dime-store mirrors. Hang them everywhere to multiply the bright summer light.
6. Hang wind chimes wherever a breeze plays.

makeup
look born free in summer—with special tips for traveling

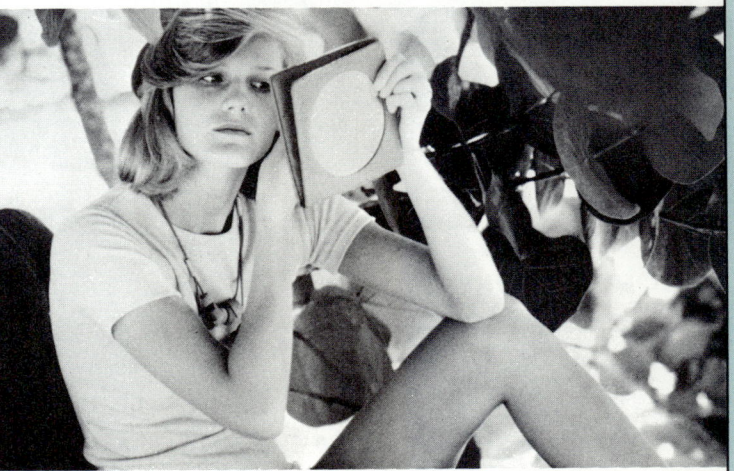

A major reason why so many women find summer hard on their looks is that they don't take advantage of the special freedom the season has to offer—that welcome relief from winter's formality and routine. That "vacation feeling" is part of summer days and your looks will be wonderfully natural if you follow some of these tips:

● Give yourself a summer-long vacation from your hair. Either get a new wash-and-wear cut or visit a good salon for advice on making your present one work in a casual, no-fuss style. If you've been setting your hair all along, try finding a no-set look now, either blown dry if it's short or medium, or pulled back simply with combs or in a ponytail if it's longer. You'll enjoy the freedom, and your hair can always use the rest from electric rollers and curling irons.

● Go easy with setting lotions and hairsprays in summer. Humidity combined with these kinds of products can make hair feel sticky and appear dirty faster.

● Compensate for your hair's extra exposure to sun, salt, and chlorinated water by deep conditioning it a little more often. Every three weeks is about average for this time of year unless you have very oily hair, which should be deep-conditioned once a month.

● Give your face a carefree summer makeup. Find new, clear, bright lip and cheek colors that make the most of whatever you have, and concentrate on these.

● Have your fresh-faced look by counteracting your skin's tendency to act up in hot weather. Most skin gets oilier in hot weather, so try out a cleanser made especially for oily skin and change from a mild skin toner to a slightly stronger astringent. If you don't usually use either

191

S summer

toner or astringent, use one now. Start with a toner; if your skin still seems very oily, try an astringent. Then apply light moisturizer around eyes and neck. This new routine should help you cope with an increased tendency to break out. A mask every week helps, too.
Special travel tips
- Don't experiment with new makeups or treatment products while traveling. Pack only those you know agree with your skin. Sun exposure combined with large doses of sea- or chlorinated water can make sensitive skin more so and increase your chances of an adverse reaction.
- A change of routine combined with lots of sun can make skin break out. Pack something to help conceal the blemishes.
- Don't rely on new or way-out clothes or makeup colors when you travel. If you don't feel comfortable wearing them, you won't be able to reach into your closet for an old standby.
- To play up that special feeling a vacation gives, treat yourself to a professional manicure and/or pedicure before you go. It will probably outlast the do-it-yourself one.

swimming

eating
fact and fallacy about swimming after you eat

No matter what your mother told you, it's not always true that you should never go into the water within an hour after eating "because you might get stomach cramps." Safety experts now say that how long you should wait depends on several factors. In general, if you have eaten a full meal and plan to do some strenuous swimming, waiting an hour is still advisable. If you have eaten only an ice cream cone or plan only to get wet in the water, you don't need to wait. Here are other factors:
- First, your physical tone. If you are in top condition, you need less time than if you're flabby. Some Olympic swimmers drink a milkshake before each race with no adverse effects.
- Second, the water temperature: Swimming in water under 70 degrees is more strenuous than swimming in warmer water, because your body has to adapt to the coldness as well as the strain of swimming. You need to wait longer for the icy waters of northern Maine than you do for a warm backyard pool.
- Third, the reason to wait after eating is not that you might get stomach cramps; it is that you are much more likely to encounter nausea, fatigue, and indigestion when you swim too soon after a meal. According to the American Red Cross's Life Saving and Water Safety, there is "not one iota of scientific evidence" that proves that a person may suffer a stomach cramp and drown as a result of going in too soon after eating. "No one knows exactly what happens in cases of stomach cramp and plenty of doubt still exists concerning its causes." It is reasonable to suspect, the American Red Cross adds, that many drownings attributed to "stomach cramps" have been heart failures due partly to overexertion.
- In any case, whether or not you need to wait a full hour, you can rarely go wrong if you do. Since swimming too soon after a meal forces your body to cope with strenuous physical activity along with the digestive process, you will almost always have more energy if you wait a while.

swimsuit
12 things anyone can do now to look better in a swimsuit

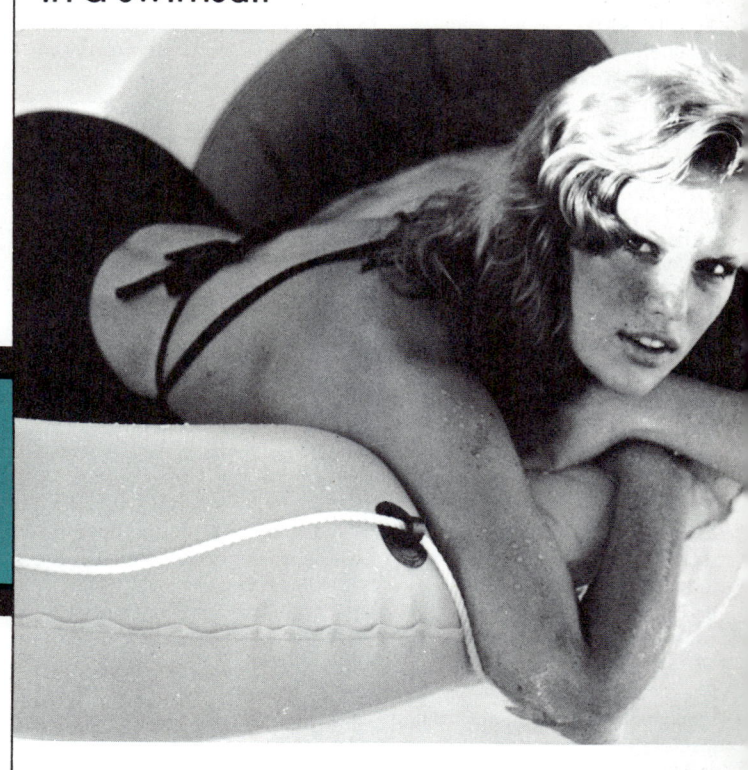

Crash shape-ups take tremendous willpower—strict diet, exercise, hours of beauty planning, and so forth. If you have that kind of willpower, you're probably in good shape already and don't need any help. But if you're an ordinary person like most of us, here are some concrete things you can do. They don't take forever and they will help you look and feel better when you first take that bare-body, summer-exposure plunge.
- Try one of the good body sloughing products to get rid of the winter-dry dead layer of skin on arms and legs. Or buy a loofa sponge and go to town in the bath or shower to scrub away the scales. Then use a rich body moisturizer faithfully each day. You'll be amazed at how much more effective the moisturizer is when the top layer has been removed.
- Don't just polish over a winter's worth of callouses on feet. Go to the dime store and invest in smoothing equipment—such as a special file made to remove callouses, and a pumice stone. Then get to work. After feet are smooth, use a good cuticle lotion or cream around toenails to soften them; trim any rough hangnails; shape toenails, and polish.
- If you don't already have a wash-and-wear haircut, consider getting one. An easy workable hairstyle is a must for a carefree summer. You might also consider investing in a curling iron for quick "sets" after a day outdoors.
- Almost everyone's hair needs some extra conditioning after exposure to central heating all winter. Take time to give yourself two deep-penetrating conditioning treatments two weeks apart. With this head start, you'll have a shiny head of hair going for you.
- If you know you won't follow an allover exercise-program, why not do one exercise for thighs or hips? Pick a favorite from your collection of exercises and do it once a day.
- Last, but not least, if you want the ultimate in motivation, try this dieter's trick. Hang a bikini from a shelf in your refrigerator as a reminder of "a moment on the lips, forever on the hips" when you're tempted to snack.

teeth

teeth
tennis
Thanksgiving
tipping
travel
TV

teeth

capped
if you've ever thought of having your teeth capped, what you should know

Having one or more teeth crowned, or "capped," is a major investment, in both money and looks. However, it needn't be scary—or even as major—as you might imagine it to be.

A crown is simply a tooth "jacket" made of porcelain, plastic, gold or a gold-and-steel alloy, or a combination of porcelain or plastic plus gold. A dentist attaches a crown to an existing tooth by filing the tooth down and then cementing the crown to it. When properly in place, the crown reaches 1/16" to 1/8" under the gum.

Most teeth—even badly broken ones—can be capped. If, however, a tooth is missing, the dentist must fit you instead with a "bridge," which is a false tooth that is cemented to those adjoining it and usually is joined to one or more crowns for stability. Why might you have your teeth capped? Perhaps the most common reason for getting a crown is that teeth have been chipped or broken. However, capping can be done on teeth that are crooked, discolored, asymmetrical, prone to decay, or for other reasons your dentist can point out.

Tooth crowning is actually a fairly simple process, done in the dentist's office, that takes about forty-five minutes to an hour per tooth for preparation, plus return visits for fitting and cementing the crown in after it's made. In most cases, it's no more painful than having a tooth filled (which means that in some cases it's completely painless), and the usual anesthesia is a "local" such as Novocain. The cost ranges from about $150 to $400 per tooth, depending on such things as where you live, what kind of material is used for the crown, and variations in dentists' fees.

If you are thinking of having your teeth crowned, your first step should be to talk with your dentist, who may refer you to a specialist who can fabricate the shapes and colors best suited to you. For example, porcelain caps are usually used on front teeth, while gold ones (which are harder) are usually good on back molars that get a lot of grinding. In any case, your crowns should match your other teeth perfectly or nearly perfectly. Once in place, a good crown usually lasts ten to fifteen years.

Finally, you may want to ask your dentist about a new method involving "composite resin" materials, which can be attached to teeth with less filing than with the traditional method. This procedure is also less expensive than crowning. Some dentists have started using them; others consider that while attaching them may be easier, they are stopgaps that won't last as long as traditional crowns.

dentist
how to find a good dentist or know you have one

Dr. Jack Maltz, a dentist on the staff of Mount Sinai Hospital in Toronto, Canada, sent us these tips for finding a reliable dentist:
● Word of mouth, says Dr. Maltz, is not the best way to find a good dentist. The person recommending the dentist may know no more than you do. A better idea is to call the closest dental school and ask for

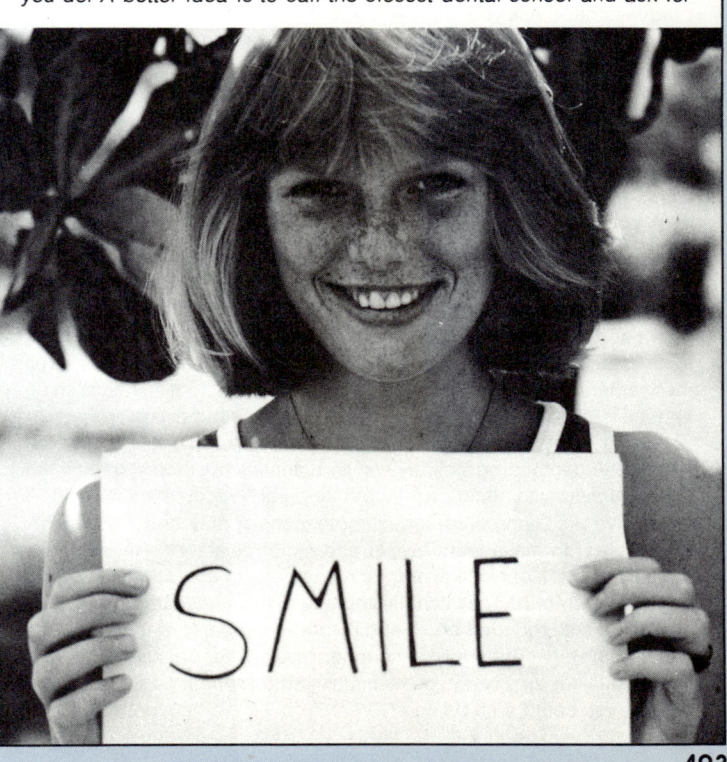

teeth

recommendations. If there's no school close by, look in the phone book for a dentist who is a specialist—an orthodontist, for example. Call, preferably early in the morning when your chances of speaking to the dentist personally are good, and tell him that you need a good dentist, not a specialist. He will know several and can give you a few good ones to choose from.

- If you're going to a new dentist or you already have one, he should be interested in preventing future problems as well as taking care of those that exist now. A good dentist will give you details of how to care for your particular mouth between visits. He'll recommend equipment such as a Water Pik or special flossing techniques if you need them. His concern should be for your entire mouth, not just your teeth. He should examine your gums, check the inside of cheeks, lips, and tongue for indications of disease.
- If you're going to a new dentist for the first time, notice whether he asks questions about your general health. If he doesn't, be suspicious. Teeth are definitely related to overall health.
- If your dentist X-rays your mouth periodically (some dentists are getting away from this practice because of the danger of yearly X-rays), notice how new the equipment looks. If you have doubts or questions, ask him how new it is and how often he plans to X-ray.
- If you're having long-range work—root canal, capping—done, discuss how much the entire job will cost and ask how much the final price may vary from the estimate. If you think the price is high, ask him to explain how he arrived at the fee.

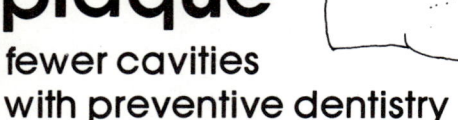

plaque
fewer cavities with preventive dentistry

The key stop to cavities—not less but none—and gum disease is plaque control. Ask your dentist to show you how. If he isn't concerned about plaque control, you might decide you want a dentist who is. Call the dental school of a local university, or write to the American Society for Preventive Dentistry, 435 North Michigan Ave., Suite 1717, Chicago, IL 60611, enclosing $1 (for postage and handling) for their list of preventive dentists in your area and for the brochure "How To Select A Preventive Dentist."

If you follow a plaque-control routine faithfully, your teeth can be virtually guaranteed for a lifetime. That is, of course, if the present damage hasn't gone too far already or if it isn't caused by other diseases that affect the mouth, such as diabetes. Plaque is an invisible matte that forms on your teeth, produced by certain substances in saliva and the bacteria in your mouth. It is the single greatest cause of tooth loss, cavities, and gum and bone diseases in the mouth. It traps the bacteria that cause deterioration and tenaciously holds them against teeth. Brushing after every meal reduces but doesn't eliminate plaque. It forms every twenty-four hours and you have to interrupt the process. A dental program devised by a dentist can help you learn the skills necessary to clean your mouth thoroughly, around each tooth. A preventive program could, for example, consist of fluoride treatments twice a year to make teeth harder and more resistant to decay and a dental visit once or twice a year for a checkup, in addition to your own do-it-yourself help. That usually includes brushing correctly once a day with a soft, rounded brush and fluoride toothpaste, and skillful use of dental floss where the brush cannot reach. After following this routine for as little as a week, gums usually stop bleeding. After a period of time, you could also be cavity-free because a clean tooth does not decay. The program also clears up bad breath problems that originate with food particles that get lodged between teeth.

A bit of diet-watching is essential for plaque control. One way to reduce dental plaque is to deprive the mouth's bacteria of its food, which is primarily refined sugar. Plaque absorbs sugar like blotting paper does water and deposits it next to teeth where it causes decay. A lot of sugar in the diet also weakens the internal resistance of teeth and gums to disease. Preventive dentists also advise high-protein, low-carbohydrate eating, including one piece of hard fruit a day—good for chewing—a fresh salad and two green vegetables each day, poultry and fish as often as possible.

wisdom
a coward's guide to wisdom teeth— what to expect

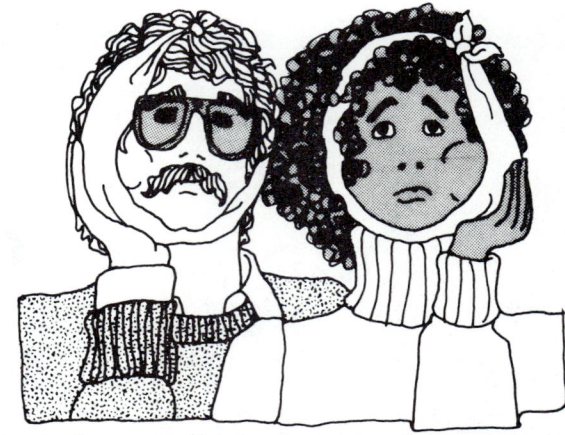

Wisdom teeth are excess baggage you usually pick up in your late teens or early twenties. Jaws are often too small to allow them room, so they may be cramped and poorly developed, or small, badly positioned, and less resistant to decay than other teeth. They're also cavity-prone because they're far back and hard to clean—or may erupt (come out) just part way and be covered with a flap of gum that traps food and germs.

"If your wisdom teeth are a persistent source of trouble—and you have all other twenty-eight teeth—you'd better take them out," says Dr. Myron M. Lieb, director of the Institute for Graduate Dentists in New York. Even before a wisdom tooth appears, an X-ray can tell if it's "impacted" (jammed against bone or another tooth) or just "un-erupted" (not out yet, but in a good position). Impacted teeth usually cause trouble and are sometimes extracted before they appear in the mouth, to avoid damage to the jawbone or other teeth. Unerupted ones may never bother you, but recent studies have shown that it is advisable to have all your wisdom teeth removed if they have not erupted by age twenty-five to avoid problems later on.

- **the tooth emergency—what to do**

What if you are in pain from an infected wisdom tooth? Chances are your dentist won't suggest pulling it until the infection subsides and will prescribe antibiotics, plenty of fluids, and frequent hot rinses to swish around your aching jaw. He probably will advise a rinse made from 2 to 3 parts water plus one part 3-percent hydrogen peroxide solution—available over the counter. Or he might tell you to use strong salt water—use a half glass of either rinse three or four times a day, and make it as hot as you can stand without burning your mouth.

- **a tooth extraction**

What can you expect if you have a wisdom tooth extracted? About an hour of silence while you bite on gauze or a moist tea bag to stop bleeding. Some pain—but that's relieved by aspirin, an ice pack, and maybe antibiotics. You'll start rinsing with warm salt water about two days after the tooth is out and the wound should heal within six weeks.

tennis

One sign to watch for a few days after extraction is pain—from a "dry socket," which means clotting was poor and bone or nerves are exposed. Your dentist can handle this, but see him immediately.

One tooth can be extracted right in your dentist's office under local anesthesia. If you're stoic, you may save money having two or more teeth extracted in a hospital, usually under general anesthesia. (Expect some swelling, discoloration, and discomfort.) This way, a medical insurance plan that doesn't normally cover dental work might help with the expense.

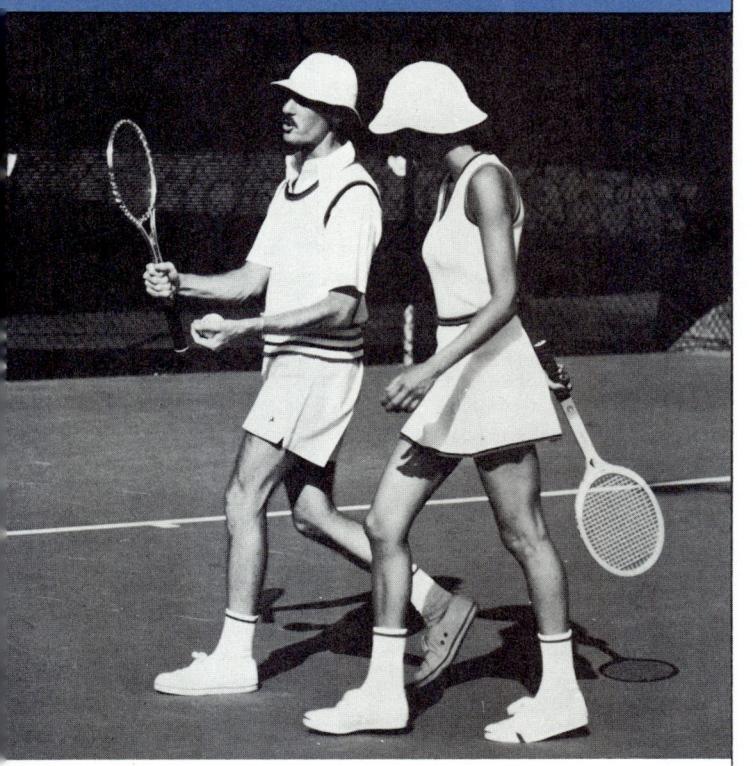

tennis

balls
how to buy the right ones for you

Different tennis balls do different things for your game. If you're a beginner, here's a rundown with some tips that might come in handy:
Unpressurized balls: These are heavier, easier-to-control balls that don't give as much speed. As a beginner, this is the kind of ball you'll probably like best. Also, they last longer. Tretorn and Slazenger are good ones to try.
Pressurized balls: Because of the highly compressed air inside these balls, they give a lot more speed to the game. When you're ready for a fast-paced game, you'll probably turn to them. Dunlop, Wilson Extra Duty, and Spalding Championship are all quality pressurized balls. You can extend their life, which can be as little as two weeks, with two devices. Nu-Ball 2 is a plastic can with an attached pump that keeps balls in a pressurized atmosphere. The Edgeroy Ball Press locks air into balls when they are stored. Both can be bought in most tennis shops.
Color: Yellow balls have been proven to be the most visible, especially under lights. If you play on a lighted court often, you might want to try them.

racquet what to look for
when you buy a tennis racquet

If you're just taking up tennis and checking around for a good racquet, consider the following points before you buy. Most reputable sporting goods stores carry demonstration models for you to try out.

● **type**
Racquets come in wood; metal—aluminum or steel; and composite—aluminum and fiberglass. Metal and composite racquets generally feel lighter and give more strength to your stroke, while wood racquets give you a little more control but a little less power. This means that with the same swing, a ball will go farther with a metal racquet than with wood.

● **grip**
The correct grip ensures the best hold on your racquet and helps make your strokes strong and sure. Take a ruler and measure from your second palm line to the end of your ring finger. This length is your grip size. (See sketch below.) Another way to determine your grip size is to make sure your thumb and forefinger touch comfortably without stretching or overlapping.

● **flexibility**
The more flexible the racquet is, the more power it adds to your shots because it has a greater spring action. More flexibility can result in less control over the ball, but more power in your shots, so consider your playing level when you buy. Wood racquets, which aren't terribly flexible, are a good choice for beginners.

● **balance**
Racquets can be "head- or handle-heavy" or about evenly balanced. A knowledgeable salesperson can help you tell the difference. Avoid a head-heavy racquet if you're a beginner—it requires more control.

● **cost**
A good racquet costs from about $25 to $50, unstrung. Ask for a good-quality nylon string (the service and string costs from $8 to $15), strung at about 55 lbs. Tighter strings give more power to your shots, but you have to hit the ball in the center of the racquet to get it.

● **is bigger better?**
Most racquets come in one conventional size, but one of the exceptions is the Prince Racket (about $75, unstrung). It has a hitting area 50 percent larger, but the entire racquet is no heavier, longer, or differently balanced than normal racquets.

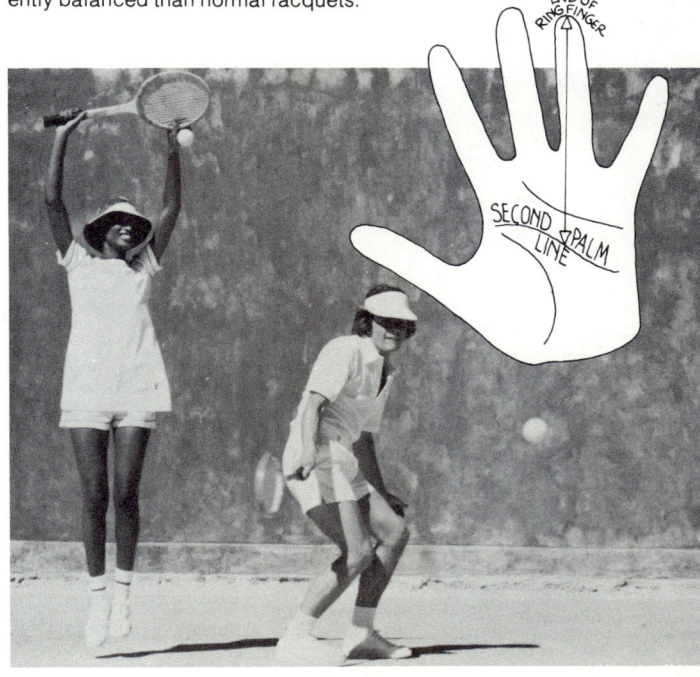

Thanksgiving

Thanks-giving

diversions
how not to eat yourself under the table

If the family Thanksgiving vacation means a week or four days of watching television, napping, and eating yourself one size bigger in boredom and body, try some of these rewarding distractions:
- Instead of slouching in front of the tube, start a ritual of your own that everyone will enjoy—get outdoors and plant tulip or crocus bulbs to bloom in the spring, especially nice if you're just visiting home and live somewhere else. They'll be a reminder of you.
- Study up on the heavens and go with whoever's interested on a long starry walk the night before the holiday.
- If you're going home from the city where you work or have moved to, make the holidays a time for old friends. If you find that get-togethers too often get bogged down with questions like "What have you been doing all year?" plan your reunion around a specific activity (such as ice skating) and let that spark the old sense of camaraderie.
- Let yourself guiltlessly enjoy the spirit of eating by eating light the day or days before and after the big day.
- If you get tired of the constant jumping from friend to friend's house, write ahead and ask your family to phone and invite your friends to a casual party.
- Get involved with the family dinner ritual by creating one dish that's different from the usual season specialties and that's yours alone.
- Find out what plays and events will be in town and mail ahead for reservations.
- Escape those terrible day-after-the-holiday blues by planning something to look forward to for that day—the theater or a museum.

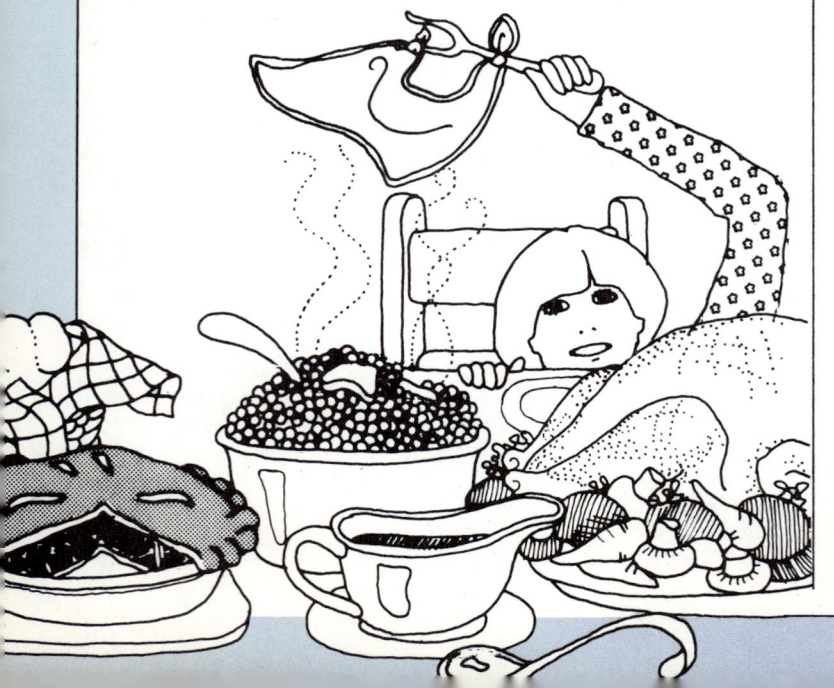

family or in-laws
how to survive Thanksgiving dinner with your family or in-laws

If a family Thanksgiving dinner has ever left you vowing to eat next year's turkey under a palm tree in the Caribbean, take heart. You aren't alone, and maybe you shouldn't go home for the holiday. (As a good rule of thumb: When the trip home is always so rushed—or expensive—that no one seems to enjoy it very much, it's time to consider alternatives.) On the other hand, if you know you want to go home, here are some ways to brighten the day.
- Having trouble making conversation with new in-laws or dimly remembered great-aunts? Don't forget the obvious topic: the holiday. There's almost no one who won't open up to, "How did you celebrate Thanksgiving when you were growing up," or, "Of all the Thanksgivings you can remember, which stands out most in your mind?"
- You're seeing less of your family now—and suddenly wish you knew the people in it better? "Oral history" techniques can help. With a cassette tape recorder, put together a narration to go with slides or home movies; family members take turns describing scenes as they remember them.
- Want to avoid the end-of-the-day arguments that result from everyone's "good behavior" wearing off? Take materials for a project to work on after dinner—maybe a needlepoint kit your mother can help with, or materials for a terrarium or collage you can make together. Oddly enough, many arguments start not because there's any real disagreement between people—but simply because they've run out of topics to discuss and start belaboring ones that should have been dropped early.

table ideas
that will start new holiday traditions in your house

Around Thanksgiving, holiday eating begins in earnest—and for the most part, it will be done around traditional bunches of bronze mums, red carnations with green candles, or maybe a floating poinsettia or two.

"Traditions are lovely, but not if they get stodgy," says Jack Bangs of New York's The Gazebo. Here, he gives you some really original centerpiece ideas; they're bound to start table conversation and some new holiday traditions in your home!
- Vegetables and fruits look beautifully down-to-earth and bountiful. Arrange a head of purple cabbage and leafy, deep green romaine, a bunch of broccoli, an artichoke, and a red onion. (Be sure everything is dripping clean.) One short-stemmed lily (hide its water supply among the vegetables) growing out from this rich green and purple earthiness will be a lovely surprise.
- Combine shades of brown eggs, cauliflower, and white onions in a pale straw basket, scatter with a few bronze-colored daisies.
- Put a clay-potted English ivy or two in the center of your table, trailing them over and around each other. Splurge at your best fruit market and scatter huge red strawberries as if they were growing on the vine.
- Look around your house for things that are dear to you, things that would intrigue your guests, make them laugh, or remember good times together. Shells collected at the beach last summer with a single orchid set into them. Heirloom family pictures arranged on a hand-laced doily with old-fashioned flowers like a bunch of lilacs or lily of the valley.
- Antique or old childhood books—one with a pop-up scene would

tipping

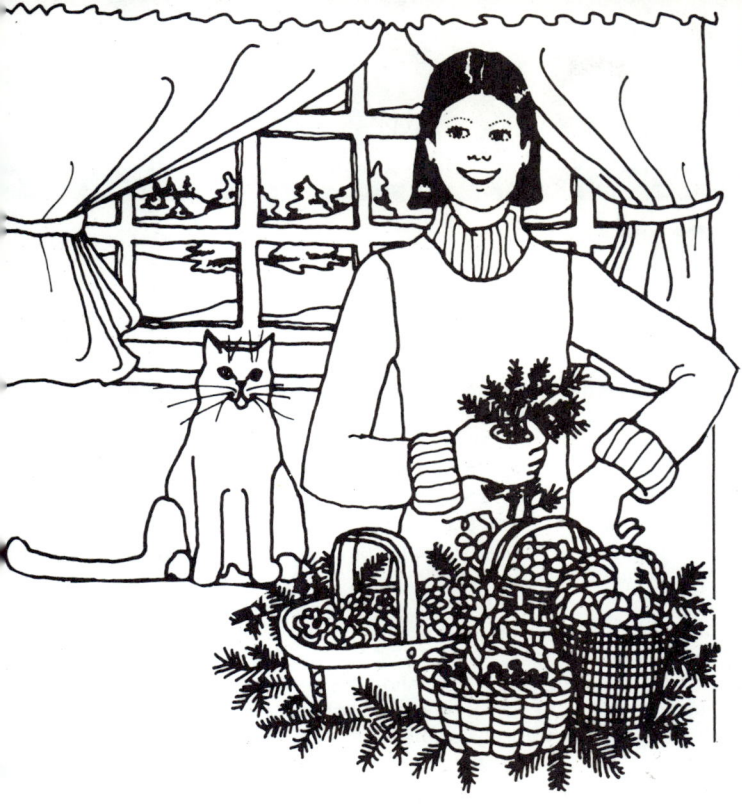

be delightful—arranged with cheese and fruit, along with a lit candle in a wine bottle. You can eat the cheese and fruit for a cozy, reminiscent dessert.
- Another centerpiece you can eat is the stuffings of a collection of small baskets—nuts and berries, such as walnuts, pecans, cashews, hazelnuts, acorns, pine cones, cranberries, and green and red grapes —most of which are edible. Any collection—rocks, antique toys, music boxes, perfume bottles—can be a lovely conversation piece.
- Around Christmas you might do an arrangement of small packages wrapped with foil papers, bits of calico, embroidered ribbons, lace, and tiny flowers. At the meal's end, everyone opens one to find a chocolate, praline, or other goody.
- Another warm, homespun table look is an old patchwork quilt used as a table cover. With a few hand-dipped bayberry candles, it carries the table on its own.
- The variegated tablecloth is another strikingly festive way to decorate your table but still saves the room a centerpiece might have taken up. Lay pieces of fabric, lengths of ribbon, crocheted dresser scarves, old curtain lace, and handkerchiefs over your table in a new design for every party.
- Think of your table as a still life. For instance, a blue deco water pitcher with a single long-stemmed lily in it and a green pear beside it would be smashing. Be a bit of an artist. Enjoy yourself and give others a chance to enjoy your treasures.
- Also remember that a single flower can be more impressive than dozens. Put a rose by everyone's place. Or a flower chosen for each individual. Adults are still charmed by the excited birthday party feeling when everyone gets a favor.

big city
small-time spender's guide to big-city tipping in the U.S.

Tipping customs vary in different parts of the U.S., but general guidelines do exist. They're simply the usual minimums, so feel free to give more or less when the service warrants it.
- *Airport porter*—50 cents a bag; taxi dispatchers do not have to be tipped.
- *Bartender*—15 percent if he serves you at the bar, nothing if the waiter or waitress brings your drink to the table.
- *Bell hop*—50 cents.
- *Chambermaid*—Nothing if you stay only one or two nights in a hotel and never see her; $1 to $2 and up if you stay longer and/or she performs extra services.
- *Hotel or apt. doorman*—25 cents if he hails a cab; otherwise, nothing.
- *Hat check attendant*—25 cents per person.
- *Ladies' room attendant*—25 cents, optional unless she performs a service.
- *Taxi driver*—20 cents minimum, usually 20 percent of the bill.
- *Red cap* (in bus terminals)—There is usually a fixed cost (about 35 cents) per bag, and the Red Cap is tipped on top of this, usually 25 cents or so.
- *Restaurant personnel*—Sometimes a service charge is tacked on to a restaurant bill. If the service was exceptionally good, you may want to leave an additional 5 percent; if the service was not special, then you are not obliged to leave anything. If the service charge is not included on the bill, the waiter should get 15 percent of the total bill; the headwaiter, $1 to $5 if he reserved you a special table; the wine steward, 10 percent of the beverage bill, with a dollar minimum.

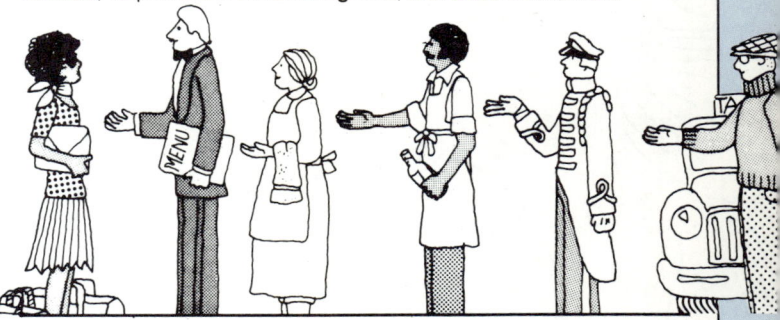

Christmas how much and to whom?

There aren't any rules, so don't feel uneasy about breaking them. Except one—if you didn't like a gift you got last year, passing it on to your manicurist this year isn't likely to please her either. There are, however, some guidelines we picked up by spot-checking tipping customs in cities, towns, and suburbs throughout the U.S. If you've just moved into a suburb, check with your neighbors; some suburbs specialize in tips of money, others in actual gifts. In the suburbs, tips might go to garbage collectors, the mailman, milkman, newsboy, and regular laundry deliveryman. City and suburb apartment dwellers may face a sizable building staff: super, elevatorman, doorman, mailman. Women who go often to beauty salons can add the hairdresser (plus assistant if he or she has one) and manicurist. Below is a checklist of what affluent middle-class tippers often choose to give.

Newsboy	$2
Milkman	$5
Mailman	$5
Garbage collectors	$3 to $5 each
Laundry truckman	$5

tipping

Garage attendant	$5 to $10
(if he parks your car, etc.)	
Doorman	$10
Superintendent	$10
Elevatormen	$5 each
Hairdresser	$5 to $10
Manicurist	$3
Cleaning help	a week's pay
Regular sitter	$5

Don't let the list intimidate you. Chances are you might tip only the garbage collector or the mailman and super. Four women sharing an apartment wouldn't try to match tipping standards with the penthouse family of many years' residence, much less be expected to. It's the right time to be fair and realistic about who helps you the most and whom you need to count on through the rest of the year.

hairdresser
who gets how much?

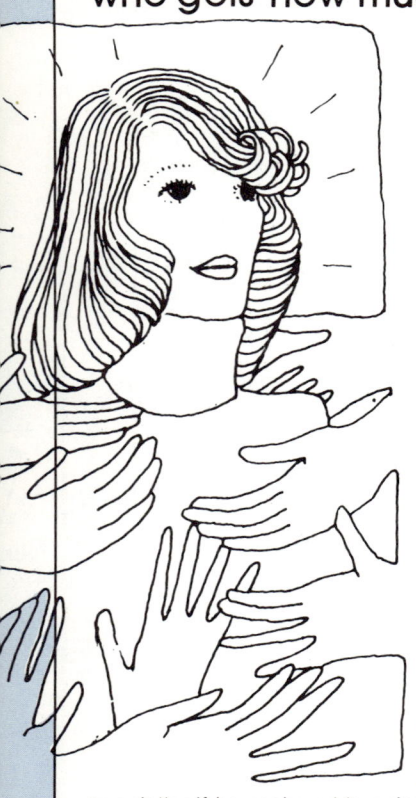

Trying to decide how you want your hair cut or set can be hard enough without worrying about how much you should tip the hairdresser. If you live in a small town or suburb, you probably have at least a rough idea of how much to tip at a salon in your area. But when you're visiting a salon in a large city, your usual guidelines may not apply, which is why we've worked out the following tipping suggestions with the help of top hairdressers and the people who use them. Feel free to give more if you've received great service or nothing if the person who shampooed you poured a chestnut rinse over your ash blonde hair. These suggestions are simply the usual minimums for a working woman who's watching pennies but doesn't want to be chintzy.

- 25 cents to the checkroom attendant.
- 25 cents to the person who brings you lunch or a snack.
- 50 cents to the person who just shampoos your hair; add 50 cents to a dollar if he or she adds a rinse or conditioner or gives a superb shampoo.
- $1 and up to the person who sets or blow dries your hair. If you can figure his or her part of the bill separately from the cut, color, and the rest, it's usual to give about 20 percent.
- 20 percent of the cost of the cut to the person who cuts your hair.
- 20 percent of the cost of a permanent, straightening, coloring, to the person who performs the service.
- 20 percent of the bill for facials, massages, etc.

The old rule about not tipping the owner of a salon doesn't always hold true—but some salon owners still feel offended if you even *try* to offer them one; they feel it implies that their business isn't doing too well, and therefore they *need* to accept tips! To be safe, ask the person at the desk whether the owner does or doesn't accept tips. Most people simply slip tips into attendants' pockets, but another solution is to use the small envelopes some salons have at the cashier's desk. Calculate each tip, put the money in separate envelopes, and write each attendant's name and your name on it.

travel

ads
know what a travel ad really means

You've seen them—the travel ads that promise "$49.95 a week in the resort hotel of your dreams"—and thought, "Wow! What a good deal!" Well, it may not be as good a deal as it appears at first glance, and the way to find out is to read the small print to the left of, to the right of, and below the come-on price.

Daily per-person double-occupancy means you'll pay this price only if you share a double room with another person. If you go by yourself, it can cost up to twice as much.

15 of 355 rooms means you should have made your reservations a month ago because this price applies to only 15 rooms in the hotel and they're probably gone.

Nearby tennis (or beach, golf, shopping) means it is not right on the hotel premises and may or may not be within walking distance.

Tennis available means you'll have to pay to play. If tennis is free and unlimited, the ad will probably say so.

Standard room means this price applies only to the cheapest accommodations in the hotel. If you want a deluxe room with a view, you'll pay more.

Mountain view or garden view is usually a euphemism for "back side of the hotel." If all rooms in a beach resort are ocean-front, the ad will say so.

8 days really means 7 nights and you'll probably have to check out of your room by noon on the 8th day.

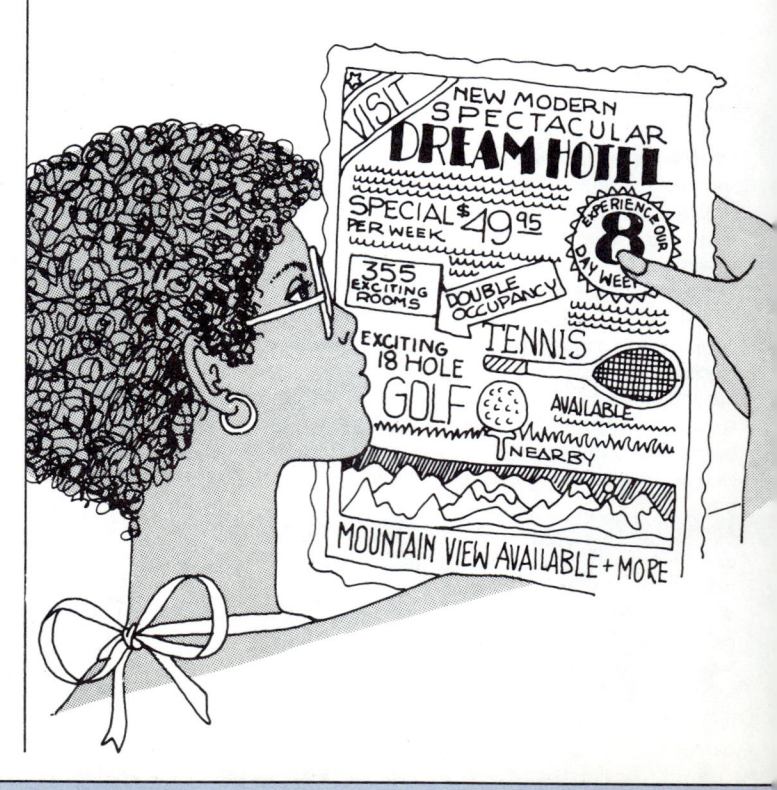

travel

agents
what a travel agent can do for you and how to pick one

If you've never used a travel agent because you didn't know what he or she could do or what it would cost—much less how to find a good one —here are answers.
- **an agent can**
 . . . help choose the right vacation spot, so you don't spend your time sightseeing when your real love is sailing, or lying on a beach when you really want to be seeing museums.
 . . . give you detailed information on fares, discounts, stopovers.
 . . . book and issue tickets for planes and ships to get you there, car rentals and bus excursions when you arrive, or all-inclusive packages.
 . . . reserve hotel rooms, tell you whether the price includes bath, meals, and so forth.
 . . . give information on sightseeing, local transportation, entertainment, sports, tipping, currency, clothing.
 . . . direct you to the proper authorities for passports, visas, shots.
- **what an agent charges**
- There should be no fee for booking transportation, tours, or most hotels, according to the American Society of Travel Agents, since these companies pay the travel agent a commission. If you want a complicated trip arranged for you, there may be a service charge.
- **how to choose one**
- Check with friends.
- Ask the agent about his or her own travel experience; he or she should have first-hand knowledge of major tourist areas.
- Be sure the agency is a member of major transportation conferences like the International Air Transport Association (IATA) and the Air Traffic Conference (ATC).
- Find out if the agency is a member of the American Society of Travel Agents (ASTA), since, among other standards, ASTA membership requires at least three years of business experience and appointment to at least two major transportation conferences.

airport security
how to pass airport security checks with a minimum of red tape

All airlines have tightened up their security in the past few years, so you may find some surprises at your nearest terminal. These tips will help you get through them.
- Arrive at the airport about fifteen minutes earlier than usual to allow enough time for required screening procedures. These are: (1) the inspection or X-raying of all your hand luggage; and (2) that you must walk through a device known as a magnetometer, which detects metal on your person or in your pockets (a hand-held metal detector is sometimes used). To speed up these checks, keep hand luggage to a minimum, don't lock it, and don't wrap any packages you're carrying.
- If you're carrying metal objects, such as a lot of keys, heavy metal belts, necklaces, or other devices that might set off the metal detectors, you'll probably be asked to remove them. Metal objects can be packed in your hand luggage or in the suitcases you check through. According to the Federal Aviation Administration, checked luggage is usually not examined, but screening procedures are used to detect explosives.
- If you are carrying rolls of film in your purse or hand luggage, you can request a physical inspection instead of the X-ray. The FAA claims that X-rays used at U.S. airports will not harm ordinary film, but damage is occasionally reported. You can also pack camera and film in a lead-laminated pouch called FilmShield, available for $5 at all good camera shops.

appliances
make sure your hairdryer, electric curlers, or iron will work abroad

Electrical systems (voltage, cycles, and plugs) differ from country to country, so when you travel abroad you may not be able to use normal American heating appliances like hair dryers, electric curlers, and irons. There are two solutions: you can buy "travel appliances," which have dual voltage (110 for the U.S., 220 for many countries abroad) and two plugs (one to fit American sockets, one to fit European and other sockets); or you can use your own heating appliances with an adapter. An adapter—a $10 to $15 device weighing about 10 ounces that plugs into the wall—is designed to reduce foreign voltage so your appliances won't burn up. There are several things to keep in mind when you buy an adapter. First, if you buy it here, the plug will probably consist of two round prongs, the standard in Europe; however, there are exceptions like England where the plug has three prongs— so make sure you check out the chart below for the type of plug used in the country you're visiting. Next, always choose an adapter according to the number or watts (not volts) specified on the bottom of the appliance (an average hair dryer uses approximately 750 watts, for instance; an iron, 1000). In the case of hair dryers only, see how many cycles are specified; if marked "50–60 cycles," the dryer will work with an adapter; if just "60 cycles," it won't. Below is a chart of volts, plugs, and cycles for various foreign countries. Use it to help you choose an adapter or dual-voltage appliance appropriate to your needs.

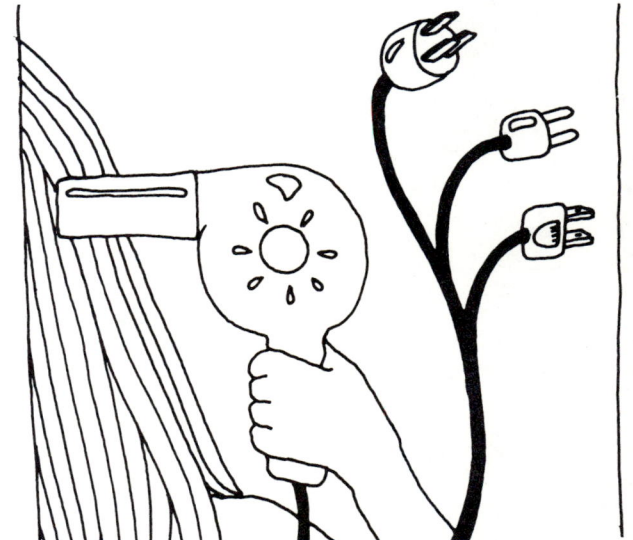

● country	● volts	● cycles	● type of plugs
U.S., Canada, Puerto Rico, Bermuda	110	60	2 flat prongs
Jamaica	110	50	2 flat prongs
Bahamas	120	60	2 flat prongs
Barbados	110	55	2 flat prongs
Antigua	220, 110	60	2 flat prongs
Mexico	125, 220	50, 60	2 flat prongs
France, Belgium, the Netherlands, Germany, Switzerland, Austria, Denmark, Sweden, Norway, Portugal, Greece, Martinique, Guadeloupe	220	50	2 round prongs
England	220	50	not standardized— 3 flat prongs or 3 round prongs
Italy	120 to 280	50	2 round prongs
Spain	110, 115, 220	50	2 round prongs

travel

baggage
if an airline loses your baggage...

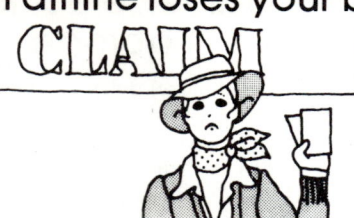

Statistics show that the amount of baggage lost each year by airlines is infinitesimal compared to the amount shipped. But if you are the one left standing at the baggage claim without a bag, such statistics are meaningless. To minimize such a possibility, always take these precautions:

- *Check in at least a half hour before departure for domestic flights, a full hour for international flights.*
- *Remove old baggage tags so your bag won't be sent to last year's vacation destination.*
- *Watch to make sure the check-in clerk attaches a new baggage tag and puts your bag on the conveyor belt.*
- *Put your name on the outside (this is required). In addition, put your name, address, and telephone number on the inside of each bag.*

If these precautions fail and your baggage is lost, take the following steps:

- *Report your lost bag to airline personnel immediately so that they can double-check the plane you arrived on. You are required to report the loss within four hours, but it's smartest to do it immediately.*
- *Take time to fill out a "loss or damage" report form. Give full details on how the bag was lost; describe the bag and its contents.*
- *If you are continuing your trip and want the baggage to catch up, give full details of your itinerary: airlines, flight numbers, destinations, addresses where you will be staying. If you change flights or airlines, fill out a new form and give this information to each airline at each airport so your baggage will follow the same route you do.*
- *If the carrier cannot find your baggage within three days, they will send you a claim form. Complete and return it as soon as possible. This claim must be filed with the airline within forty-five days of the loss. You can expect settlement of your claim within four to six weeks, but don't expect to receive full value: domestic airlines are liable for a maximum of $750. You can also be reimbursed for incidental expenses (like toiletries and other personal items) caused by baggage loss or delay.*
- *Hold on to your baggage claim check until you have received your bag; it is your only proof the bag was lost.*

brochure
reading between the lines of a travel brochure

A travel brochure may tell you only half the story about the tour you'll be taking or the hotel you'll be checking into. These pointers will help you put together the rest:

- Think twice about phrases that sound vague or contrived. For instance: "Transportation into town can be arranged." It usually means you're not within walking distance of most stores. (And if that's what you want, fine.) The "transportation" itself may be a hotel owner's pickup truck or its 5 A.M. milk run, or it may mean you pay for a parade of taxis to and from. To be sure, write to the hotel to ask if transportation is by regular bus, train, or taxi.
- Dig deeper when you read a description like "only steps from the beach." How many steps are between you and the water—a few paces across eight lanes of thruway? A fifteen-minute scramble down the face of a cliff?
- "Easter egg hunt" or "Sabbath eve services in our lounge" should tell you something about clients' religious backgrounds. Others may provide a clue to the racial or ethnic mix that you'll find.
- If you're not sure about any phrase in the brochure, ask a travel agent, the hotel's representative, or someone who has stayed there. If that's not possible and you're downright suspicious, you can write, call, or cable the hotel for details.
- Scrutinize the pictures. A hotel brochure should show fairly recent shots, both inside and out. An artist's sketch may mean the hotel is under construction. If so, expect a few minor flaws in your surroundings—perhaps you'll be awakened each morning to the hum of a buzz saw. If there's only a photo of the entrance or lobby, the rooms may leave something to be desired. Or it may mean that there's no restaurant or it isn't very promising. A hotel that claims a private beach or tennis courts usually shows them in the photo *with* the building—otherwise they may be miles apart.
- *Read the fine print*—especially legal-sounding phrases under a heading such as "General Conditions." In a tour folder, these conditions should explain what is included in the bargain price quoted on the cover. All transportation? Three meals a day? Tips and taxes? What recourse you have if all or part of the tour is canceled should be stated, as well as luggage quotas and any requirement made of you to drive a car.

The fine print should make clear also exactly what kind of accommodations you'll have in the hotels you'll be staying in. For example, will you have a private bath or will you have to share with everyone else on the floor?

Check this section to see how many, if any, meals are included, if the rates vary from high to low season and, for solo travelers, if there's a surcharge for a single room.

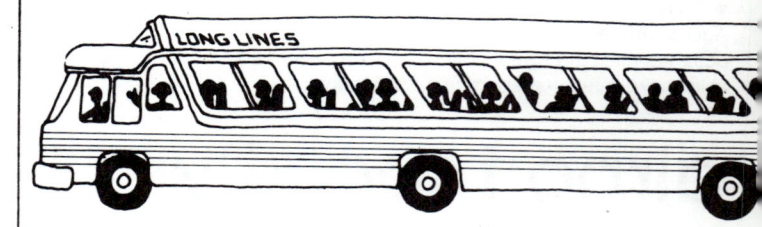

bus trip
how to plan a long bus trip

1. If you are planning a summer trip across the U.S. and Canada, look into special deals like Greyhound's Ameripass, which gives you fifteen days, one month, or two months of unlimited bus travel for a flat rate.
2. Find out about and take advantage of discounts available to Ameripass holders: discounts in motels, on sightseeing tours, and most important, at Post House Restaurants, often found in bus stations.
3. Pack as few clothes as possible. If you take one carry-on bag, you'll be able to change plans and directions more easily than if you have to retrieve two suitcases from the luggage compartment.
4. In any case, at least keep a small bag containing a lightweight blanket, extra sweater, washcloth, towel, soap, toothbrush, toilet paper, tissues, and moistened towelettes under your seat.
5. Instead of carrying around a standard pillow, buy a small inflatable plastic one—they're available in vending machines in most large bus stations.
6. To kill time during long rides on dull highways, take along a supply of paperback books, a deck of cards, a miniature chess or backgammon set, or even some stationery to catch up on letters.
7. Sit in the front of the bus for the best panoramic views of the scenery.
8. Sit in the back of the bus if you will be riding overnight—you can make a fairly comfortable bed out of the three rear seats if the bus isn't crowded.

travel

9. Better still, at least every other night, plan to stay over in a motel. You'll spend more money but be better rested.
10. Keep your eye on the bus driver during rest stops so he doesn't take off without you.
11. Have your ticket validated as far ahead as you are sure you are going, to avoid spending time in ticket lines at each town along the way.
12. Bus stations are often lurking grounds for undesirables, so if you're alone and your bus pulls in at 3:30 A.M. and you're not leaving again until 7 A.M., stay at an all-night diner or motel.

clothes what to pack for 2 weeks away from it all

If you're like most summer vacation travelers, you make one of two mistakes when you pack. Either you throw everything into a suitcase, burdening yourself with unnecessary clothes, or you pack so sparingly you don't have enough variety. You don't have to make either mistake if you think through the kind of vacation you're taking and what things you're likely to be doing most. We've pulled together a list of basic clothes plus some tips, and if you plan well, you should wear everything and not feel bored.

The following list shows you the basics. A C in front of an item means you should take it if you're planning a city-oriented trip. An R means you should take it if it's a resort-oriented trip. If you're going to spend time in both, try to gauge what proportion of your trip is city-oriented and what's resort and split your clothes accordingly. You'll also find many clothes work for both—as our list indicates.

● **clothes list**

R	caftan
C, R	cardigan
C, R	casual skirt
R	cover-up
C, R	dressy sandals
C, R	dressy top
C, R	espadrilles
R	halter
C, R	heavy wrap for cool climates
C, R	jeans
C, R	long dress
C, R	long skirt
C	raincoat
C	shirtdress
R	shorts
R	swimsuit
C, R	tailored shirt
C, R	T-shirt
C	walking shoes

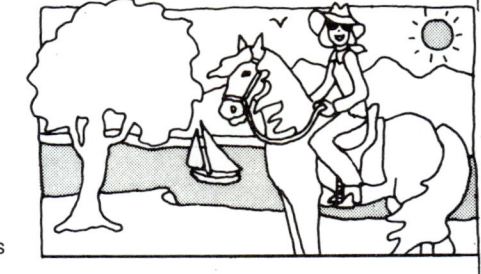

● **city tips**

In almost any city you visit for as long as two weeks, except maybe in very hot tropical climates, a lightweight raincoat is a necessity. A classic trenchcoat can go over most anything. If you find a raincoat cumbersome, an alternate might be a light, safari-type jacket. If you're going to a cool climate, say, Scandinavia or parts of the northwest U.S., you'll need a heavy wrap sweater. T-shirts, tailored shirts, plus sporty pants or skirts should take care of daytime activities. Try to limit yourself to neutrals and two colors so that everything works together. Count on a minimum of two pairs of pants and one skirt or three pairs of pants—add another pair of pants or a skirt if most are pale colors. A half dozen or so assorted T-shirts and regular shirts will vary the bottoms. For evenings, a long skirt or dressy pants and a dressy shirt or bare dressy top should take care of the splurge restaurant or dancing times. If you plan on doing a lot of this, you'll want two looks, either long skirts or pants or a long slinky jersey dress. A silky shirtdress would be good, too. Shoes: Take one pair of dressy sandals, plus two pairs of comfortable walking shoes for city sightseeing.

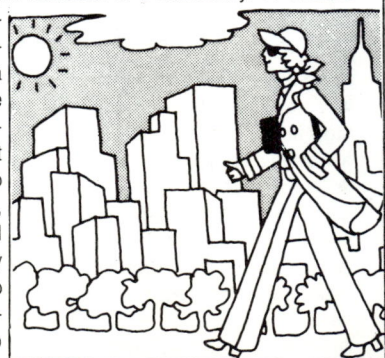

● **resort tips**

By resort, we mean primarily a beach or lake area where casual dress is expected. For most places, when you're not in a bikini, shorts or pants and a bare top or T-shirt are standard for day. Some sort of cover-up for your bathing suit is useful, too—for grabbing lunch or getting to and from your hotel. A shirt or one of the pretty Indian gauze tops would do. For evenings, resort dress-up is usually more casual than city. A long caftan is great, as is a caftan-type top with wide-legged pants. A pretty, sheer shirt worn over a stretch strapless top or a scarf tied like a bra top plus wide-legged pants looks fabulous—and you can wear the same shirt closed with pants for day. Another evening dressy shirt option: Tie your shirt at the midriff over wide-legged or straight pants. For a two-week trip, count on a minimum of two bathing suits, three pairs of casual pants or a couple of pairs of pants and a pair or two of shorts or a casual skirt. A half dozen T-shirts or regular shirts and T's mixed, plus a couple of fun bare tops, halters, or tubes should see you through. A long skirt is fun, too. Two pairs of espadrilles (plus a pair of sturdy sandals if you can squeeze them in) and a pair of bare sandals for evening should take care of the shoes.

● **general tips**
● Don't pack fragile, easily wrinkled clothes. Cotton or synthetic knits are good; synthetic mix fabrics are, too.
● When you're checking the temperatures of a spot, don't be fooled by an "average" of 70 degrees. That could mean torrid at noon and cool at night. Check into the specifics if you can, and be prepared for variations.
● Try to pack one spare outfit in your carry-on luggage so that if your suitcase doesn't make it when you do, you have at least one change until it's located.

customs what you can and can't bring back with you from a foreign trip

You can bring back $100 worth of articles for your personal use duty-free *if* (1) you carry them with you; (2) you have been abroad more than forty-eight hours; (3) you have not used any of your $100 exemption within the past thirty days. (For articles bought in the U.S. Virgin Islands, American Samoa, and Guam, there is a $200 exemption.)

Within your $100 exemption you are allowed: 1 quart of alcohol (1 gallon from the U.S. Virgins, American Samoa, and Guam) if you are twenty-one or over; 100 cigars; unlimited cigarettes for personal use.

Some articles are duty-free no matter how much they cost: antiques more than 100 years old, original paintings, books. On any item that exceeds your $100 exemption, you must pay duty, which

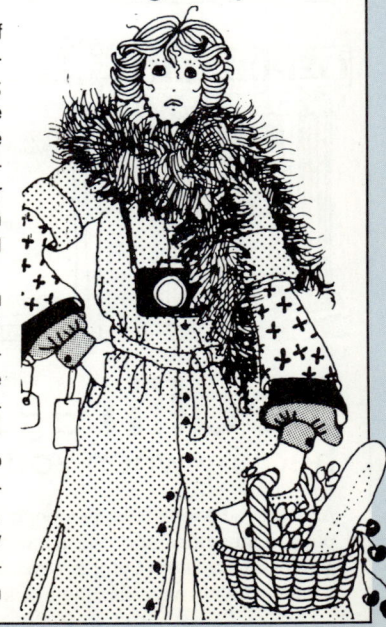

travel

varies with the item: 5 percent on records, 21 percent on cotton knit dresses, for instance. The only things you can mail duty-free are under-$10 gifts to family and friends (each person can receive only one gift a day). Mark them "Unsolicited gift enclosed—value under $10."

If you think that U.S. Customs officials don't know how to catch a thief, think again. Not only can they tell that you paid $150 for your fun fur in Oslo, but they also know the difference between amphetamines and aspirin. To be safe, carry copies of prescriptions for any drugs you're taking. Since the Agriculture Department tries to keep out any carriers of foot-and-mouth, Dutch Elm, or other diseases, Customs will detain or confiscate plants, animals, seeds, and most foods. Before going abroad, read *U.S. Customs Trademark Information* and *Know Before You Go*—free from the U.S. Customs Service, P.O. Box 7188, Washington, DC 20044.

foreign sizes
how to know which dress and shoe sizes are right for you

Whether you're going to Europe yourself or a friend offers to do some shopping for you there, you'll want to know how clothing sizes compare with what you normally buy in the U.S. Check the chart below.

● shoe sizes *

United States	Great Britain	France	Spain	Italy	Germany
5½	4	37		35½	36½
6	4½	37½	36	36	37
6½	5	38		36½	37
7	5½	38½	37	37	38
7½	6	39		37½	38½
8	6½	39½	38	38	39½
8½	7	40		38½	39½
9	7½	40½	39	39	40

● dress sizes

10	12	40	40	40	38
12	14	42	42	42	40
14	16	44	44	44	42
16	18	46	46	46	44
18	20	48	48	48	46

* Shoe widths vary greatly from country to country in Europe, but they are generally wider than in the U.S.

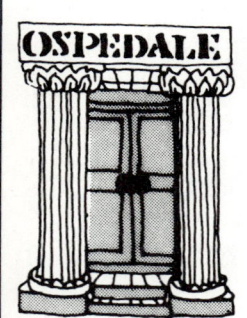

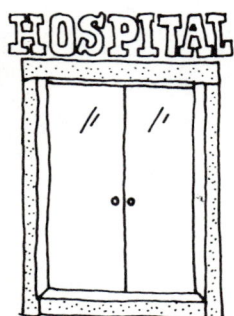

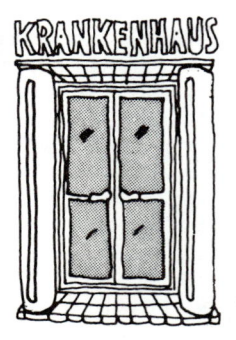

health a guide to staying healthy when you travel anywhere

Although a traveler to outer Mongolia or the Amazon jungle should look beyond these dos and don'ts for medical advice, anyone vacationing in the U.S., Western Europe, Mexico, or the Caribbean can avoid most common health hazards. Some tips:

● **in the U.S. and abroad**
● If you are flying, DO drink plenty of fluids to combat the dryness of most airplane cabins, but DON'T go overboard on food or alcohol. DO keep a nasal decongestant, chewing gum, and if you're prone to airsickness, some pills for motion sickness, in your purse; flight attendants are not always able to provide them. If you are pregnant, check with your doctor before any plane trip. And DON'T fly if you have a bad cold. (If cabin air is not properly pressurized, it can result in severe pain and other problems in ears, noses, and throats already blocked up by a cold.)
● DON'T forget a medical kit with items like your doctor's telephone number (and any special instructions he or she may have for another doctor who treats you); a Red Cross first-aid booklet; assorted bandages; cotton; thermometer; sunburn lotion; antihistamines; insect repellent; water purification tablets; extra glasses and pills for motion sickness, colds, diarrhea.
● DO take a copy of all drug prescriptions, too—and not only because you might need a refill. They also help prove to suspicious Customs officials you aren't trying to smuggle illegal drugs into or out of the country.
● DO avoid buffet tables at your destination that have been sitting out for hours. Flies, which are frequently disease carriers, may have contaminated the food, and salads and seafood may have spoiled.
● **in any foreign country**
● DON'T panic about getting last-minute smallpox, tetanus-diphtheria, polio, or typhoid inoculations—they're no longer required. On the other hand, they're always a good idea. DO keep on the lookout for cholera or other epidemics and get the appropriate inoculation.
● DON'T eat rare beef (never steak tartare) or undercooked pork in foreign countries. DO eat well-cooked fish, but avoid smoked or raw seafood. DON'T eat raw vegetables. DO wash and peel fruit yourself before eating it. DON'T touch items like mayonnaise salads, cream-filled pastries, or custards that have been unrefrigerated for any length of time.
● DO eliminate all milk products (ice cream, custards, etc.) in any area where the milk is not pasteurized. DON'T drink local-brand soft drinks in underdeveloped countries. Bacteria multiply in the sugar-water mixture they're made from. DO stick to beer when you're in doubt about water or soft drinks.
● Although the tap water in major Western European cities is usually safe, the chemicals in it may still upset your stomach, so DO drink bottled water (make sure it's sealed) if you're sensitive. In underdeveloped countries, play it safe and don't drink the tap water. DON'T count on alcohol killing germs in ice cubes from local water; if the water is unsafe, so is ice. DO brush your teeth with bottled water.
● DON'T go swimming in fresh-water rivers in tropical countries. Some are snail-infested and can cause schistosomiasis, a disease that can affect intestines, bladder, and liver. DO watch out for sharks, barracuda, and especially prickly sea urchins when swimming.

hotels
make sure you get a hotel room — and a good one at that

Keep the following tips in mind when you make reservations:
● To get one of the best rooms—one with an ocean view or one on a high floor away from street sounds—make your reservations as far in advance as possible.
● Specify whether you want a double or single room—with or without bath. This is especially important if you will be staying in an old European establishment or a small country hotel.
● Give the approximate time you will be arriving so that the hotel can make sure your room is ready—or not give it away if you're arriving late.
● Phone ahead if you are delayed en route, or pay one night's deposit

travel

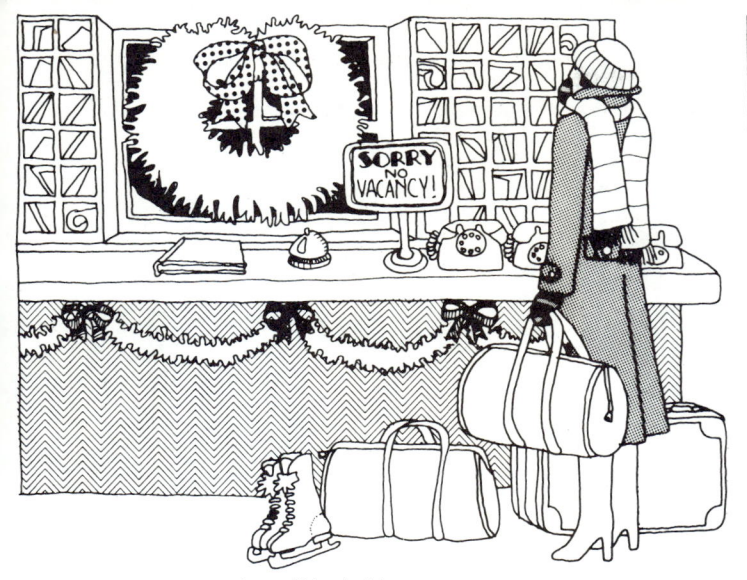

so that your reservation will be held.

● Ask the hotel to send you a written confirmation. Hotels sometimes overbook during the holidays, so it is a good idea to have proof of your reservation.

● If for some reason you cannot honor your reservation, be sure to let the hotel know so that they can rent your room to someone else. DON'T BE A NO-SHOW!

● Vacate your room at the official check-out time so you are not charged extra. The reception desk will store your luggage until you leave if necessary.

making friends
how to help a beautiful stranger find you in transit

When you walk into a packed airport or board a bus or train, how you look—and how your luck is running—play only partial roles in determining whom you'll meet there. Meeting people, and especially meeting men, depends mainly on how approachable you appear—and, of course, on how willing you are to approach and be approached. Here are tips to help with both.

Schedule your trips at peak traveling times, when the number of people traveling is on your side. If you want to meet businessmen, take into account that many executives prefer to depart on Sunday evening or early Monday morning so they can schedule a full day's work wherever they're headed. If you're a student, you'll find many more of your kind traveling on the Sunday after Thanksgiving than you will on the Tuesday after it.

Don't arrive just as your plane, train, or bus is revving up its engines. Try to get maximum exposure buying a ticket, picking out a magazine, and perhaps talking to other passengers before boarding.

Wear or carry something that says a little about you and invites questions: Try luggage tags or decals from interesting places, a campaign button on your sweater or canvas carryall, a book cover bearing your college crest, a T-shirt or pendant with a funny design or motto, even a newspaper from your hometown. If you're going from, say, Old Sandwich to Albuquerque, keep the Old Sandwich Citizen-Defender in plain view. Lots of camera equipment hanging around your neck fascinates many men, and wearing or carrying camera gear is safer than packing it in a suitcase, where it's likely to get bounced from one ramp to another.

Avoid traveling in packs. Who wants to walk up to a group that looks like a tri-state cheerleaders' convention? To give yourself a chance to be singled out, travel with one other person at most.

Talk to a variety of people—that friendly, bespectacled man who sells you a pack of gum, your bus driver, the kindly woman at the Traveler's Aid booth. Hearing your voice may give a man the opening he needs to say that "An accent like yours could only come from Louisiana" or "Where in Boston did you grow up?"

If trying to start conversations with strangers makes you clutch, just ask questions. Find out where you can store your luggage while waiting for your train or bus. If a loudspeaker announces that your turbojet plane's arrival will be delayed "due to hydraulic failure," ask anyone what that means. And does he really think the plane will only be delayed fifteen minutes, or is the airline using a stalling tactic? Don't hesitate to volunteer information you know either. If you know Puddle-Jump Airlines never gets off on time but serves delicious breadfruit on board, tell people.

Keep in touch with your sense of humor. One woman met half the male population of New England when her bus got a flat tire in the middle of the Massachusetts Turnpike, and after twenty minutes she remarked cheerfully that it was the most free time she'd had all semester.

No matter how shy or unhumorous you may be, you can always offer a stick of gum, candy, a Dramamine pill, or the sports pages of your Citizen-Defender to a person nearby—or ask him for the same.

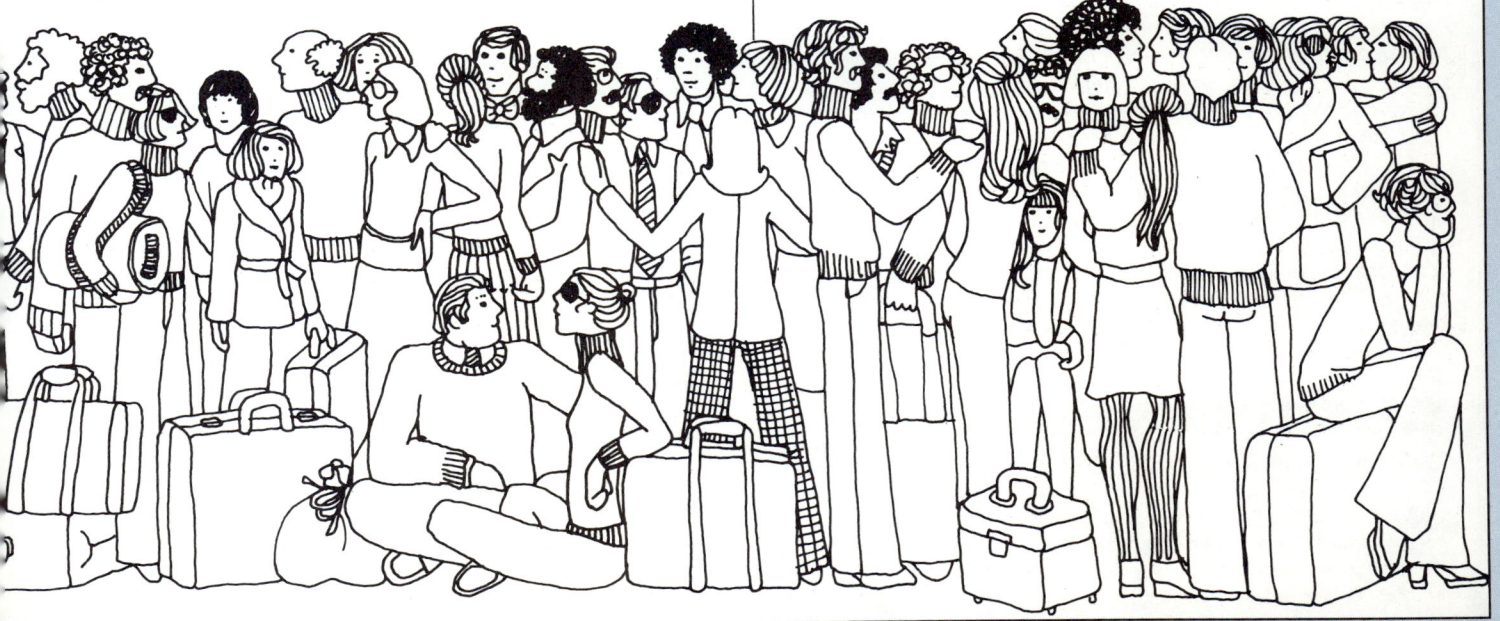

travel

meal plans
what do these initials get you?

All those confusing abbreviations in travel articles, guidebooks, and hotel rate schedules can tell you a lot about what you're getting for your money—if you know what they mean. Here's a rundown of the most popular hotel/meal plans:

EP—European Plan—room only, no meals
AP—American Plan—room plus three meals; in Europe, called *full pension*
MAP—Modified American Plan—room with breakfast and dinner
CP—Continental Plan—room and continental breakfast of rolls and coffee
BP—Bermuda Plan—room with a full-course breakfast; in England this plan is B & B (bed and breakfast)

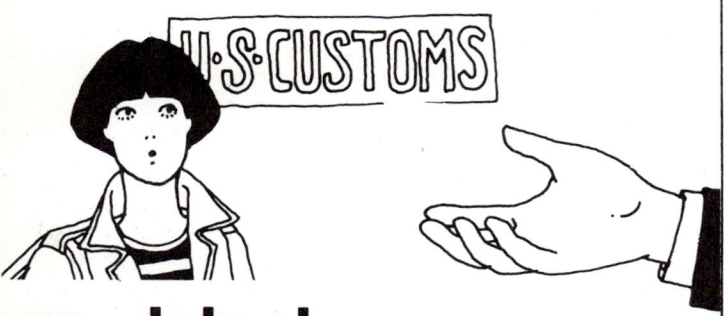

registering
avoid a hassle at customs— register valuables before you leave the country

Any new-looking foreign-made items such as jewelry, watches, and cameras may be subject to duty unless you can prove you didn't buy the item while abroad. To play it safe, register such pieces before you leave. The nearest Customs house is listed in the phone book, or use the Customs office at the airport. Registration practices vary at the particular ports. Some may register only those items with serial numbers or items that can be marked; others take pictures to provide a photographic record of certain items. It's best to check with the Customs Department beforehand to find out about its procedures. Some "new-looking" items you might want to register are: furs; leathers and suedes; fairly expensive imported clothes; real jewelry; firearms (must always be registered, especially those taken by travelers on hunting trips); any items the country you're visiting is famous for (e.g., Spanish suede and leathers; English or Irish tweeds and woolens; French clothes and leather goods; Oriental digital watches, cameras, and expensive calculators).

Registering is free and usually doesn't take much time, but it's a good idea to do it a couple of weeks before you leave, to avoid delays. If you have many things to register, call the Customs Department beforehand to learn if you should make an appointment. Once something is registered, you'll get a receipt and can show it when you go through Customs.

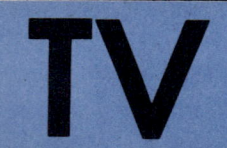

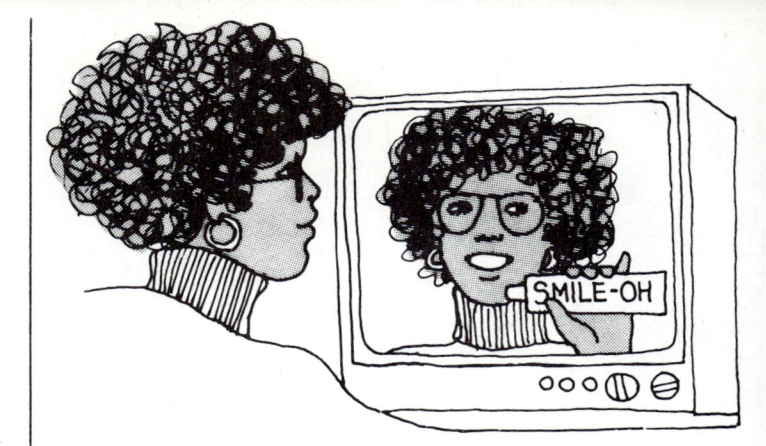

TV

commercials how you can get into TV commercials

The woman endorsing toothpaste in the TV commercial looks down-to-earth enough to be your next-door neighbor. So does the man eating the hot dog. More and more commercials are featuring "real" looking actors, nonmodel-type models, and, in some cases, even people right off the street.

So if you think your face could sell anything from deodorant to dog food (and you live in a large metropolitan area where there are ad agencies and film production companies), here's the way to try to break into the business:

● First you'll need an 8" X 10" glossy head shot, a good picture of your face that shows what you *really* look like. Stay away from glamorous or pretentious poses. For starters, one shot—with a number of copies of it —is all that's necessary.
● On the back of each copy of your photograph, attach a résumé. Include your vital statistics (height, weight, hair and eye color, measurements, sizes) and any theatrical experience (most recent first).
● Using the Yellow Pages as a guide, draw up a list of ad agencies. When you visit, ask to see their casting directors and talent agents—and then leave your picture and résumé with each. Keep notes on where you've been and when.
● In a few days, follow up each visit with a phone call, requesting an interview. Be persistent but not pushy (a little ingenuity might help, too). If you get an interview with an agent and he likes you, he'll send you to casting directors for commercial auditions. Many TV-commercial actors try to work through several agents in order to get called to as many auditions as possible.

For more pointers, pick up a copy of *How YOU Can Appear in TV Commercials* by actors Ron Milkie and Ray Carlson.

game shows
hit the jackpot on TV game shows

TV game shows have been offering cash prizes large enough to pay next semester's tuition, tide you through a period of unemployment, or send you packing on a glorious vacation. Some are fairly begging for you to win them. "Most people seem to think that the studios are overrun with swarms of eminently qualified people, who line up for months waiting to appear," says Ed Fishman, a TV contestant scout and author of *How to Strike It Rich on TV Game Shows*. "This is not the case."

Game shows fall roughly into two groups; those involving mainly luck, such as "Let's Make a Deal," and those involving a skill, such as "Jeopardy." Choose the kind of show you think you'd do best on. Bear in mind that in order to limit the number of times you may appear on one of their shows, all major TV networks eliminate the "professional contestant." (For example, a network might allow contestants to appear on only one show per year and not more than two in five years.)

Then, several weeks before you'd like to appear on a show, write to its "contestant coordinator." Addresses are usually given at the end of a show, or you can write directly to the network on which it appears. *Be brief,* including the basic facts about yourself; why you'd like to be a contestant; when you are available; and, if possible, a recent photo that needn't be returned. Some shows will offer you an interview on the basis of a letter; others will request that you attend a taping and sign up there.

During an interview, remember that all shows look for contestants with lively personalities. Dress attractively, but not flashily. Ed Fishman points out that most shows are looking for the species he calls *"Americana Domesticus"*—not, say, the female Alice Cooper.

"The best contestant is one whom you'd really enjoy having in your home," says Jim McCrell, host of "Celebrity Sweepstakes." "We look for a naturalness and ability to play the game without getting uptight about it."

The more complex skill games have other requirements, too. "For our shows, you need to be outgoing—to have what we call pizzazz," says Edythe Chan, who works for Bob Stewart Productions as associate producer of "Jackpot!" and contestant coordinator of "The $25,000 Pyramid." "You also need a good general knowledge of the facts everyone learns in school. You should know, for example, that Marie Antoinette said, 'Let them eat cake.' You should also know that Pierre Trudeau is the prime minister of Canada and that Ohio is 'the Buckeye State.' In other words, since our shows involve questions and answers, you should be up on what's going on in the world." ("Jackpot!" includes a written general-knowledge test as part of its screening procedure.) A 25-year-old copywriter who won $5,047.50 on "Jackpot!," Teri Kestenbaum adds, "Above all, you need to be able to think on your feet."

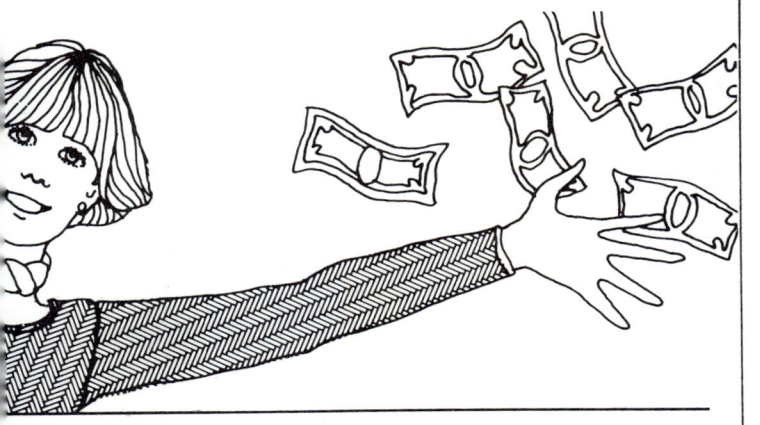

TV table
you can make

The average TV table from an appliance or department store is not only plain but expensive. Making your own is easy and much less expensive, about $15 for the one here. You'll need two 16" x 12" x ¾" pieces and two 20" x 12" x ¾" pieces of unfinished pine, strong wood glue, twelve 1¼" finishing nails, a nail punch, plastic wood, stain or paint, polyurethane finish, four L-shaped support brackets, and four small casters. (Check the size of your TV to be sure it fits these measurements. If not, alter to fit your set.) Starting with one 16" side, glue, then nail both 20" pieces to it. When secure, glue, then nail other 16" side in place (see sketch). Countersink the nails with a nail punch. Then fill holes with plastic wood. Sand rough areas. Screw the brackets under the top shelf for extra support. Stain or paint. Coat with polyurethane for protection. Add casters.

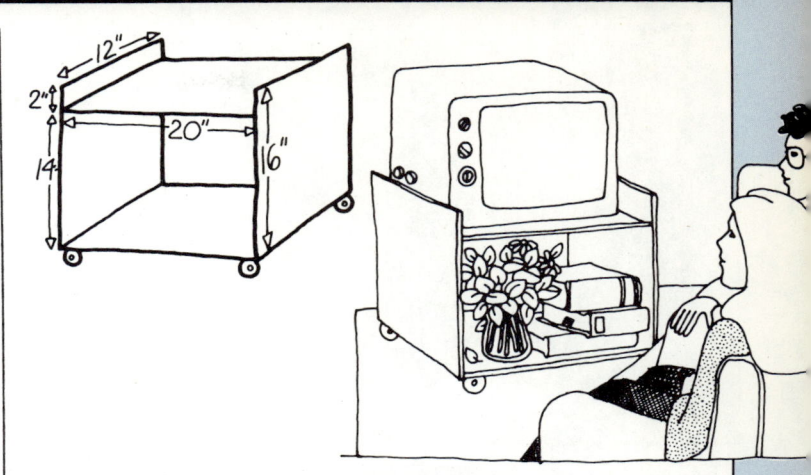

watching TV
nobody has to tell you how to watch TV—or do they?

If there's one thing most of us should be experts on, it's watching TV, especially with a bumper crop of new shows appearing every season.

But few of us actually are experts, so rate your television-watching habits by taking the true/false test below.

● **true or false**
1. *It's best to watch in darkness or semi-darkness.*
2. *TV sets should be at eye level.*
3. *It's a myth that you shouldn't sit very close to the screen; sit anywhere.*
4. *The best chair to watch from is soft, squishy, and lets you curl up cozily.*
5. *You shouldn't exercise, do needlepoint, or iron while you're watching TV.*
6. *A color TV set with an "instant-on" feature (which means electricity is running through the set constantly) should be switched permanently to its "vacation" or "defeat" switch, which cuts off the current.*

● **answers**
1. FALSE—Vision specialists recommend normal room lighting. You aren't a bat, and the sharp contrast of a bright set in a dark room is uncomfortable for viewing.
2. TRUE—It's easiest on your eyes and avoids wear-and-tear on your neck, lower back, etc. (One habit to break is watching TV on your stomach, chin in hand, with neck craned up at a set several feet higher.)
3. FALSE—Your mother was right . . . sit back. The American Optometric Association recommends that you view from a distance of at least five times the screen's width.
4. FALSE—Anything that encourages a pretzel or wet-noodle position is a minus. According to Dr. Joseph Simeone of New York University Medical Center's Institute of Rehabilitation Medicine, it's best to sit on a chair with two arms and good back support. Put your knees out straight and prop legs up parallel to the floor, or higher. Have your upper back rest on the chair, your lower back away—this helps straighten lower back.
5. FALSE—You'll give your eyes a break from zombie-eyed viewing if you look away occasionally to do something else. Experts recommend a break for at least five minutes every hour or so to water your philodendrons or do a few exercises.
6. TRUE—The U.S. Consumer Product Safety Commission is developing mandatory safety standards for all TV sets, including ones with "instant-on," but recommends this step in the interim especially if you're away for a while. They urge you not to unplug the set after each use; you might break wire strands in the cord, posing fire or shock hazards.

u umbrellas

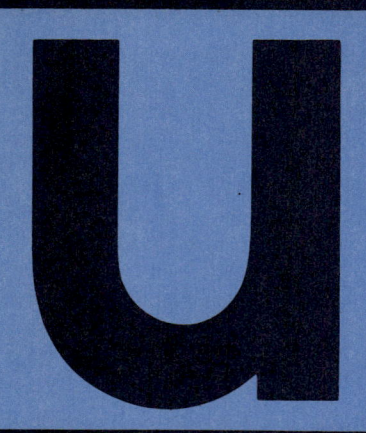

umbrellas

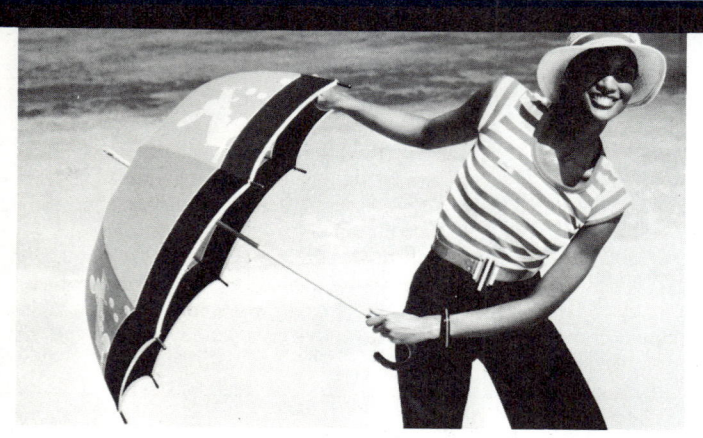

buying — buy an umbrella that will last

Any time during the year is a good time to buy an umbrella, and it makes a great, useful gift. Here are some pointers from the Association of Umbrella Manufacturers & Suppliers to help you, whether you're buying a gift or just rainy-day protection for yourself.
- Tensile strength of the umbrella frame is very important. To test one, open umbrella and gently bend one of the ribs by grasping the tip and bending it slightly. When you let go, you should notice a good "spring back" quality in the rib.
- Examine the ribs to see if they're channeled. A channeled rib, one with a groove running the length of it, gives more strength without excessive weight.
- Open the umbrella and hold it up to the light. If you see lots of tiny openings, the rain may spatter through them in a downpour.
- If the umbrella has a patterned cover, notice whether the pattern is matched at the seams. Matching is usually an indication of quality.
- If you're picking a see-through vinyl umbrella, check to see that the vinyl is heavy enough not to puncture easily.
- Make sure the umbrella opens and closes easily. This is especially important if you're buying a folding umbrella. Many of the inexpensive ones don't open up completely unless you use three hands to grasp the ribs!
- Probably the most important thing to remember to make a good umbrella last is to keep it open while it is drying. If you don't, the fabric may shrink a bit and put a strain on the ribs, weakening them and ultimately weakening the fabric. Also, the wood may swell and then the umbrella won't open.

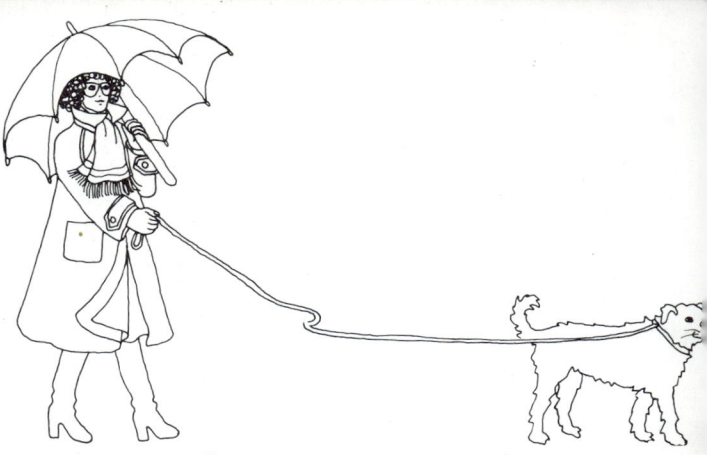

carrying — turn your umbrella into a shoulder-strap model

Instead of trying to keep your umbrella from poking and nipping everyone in crowded buses and subways, turn it into an easy-to-carry shoulder-strap model like the one sketched here.

Buy a yard of narrow upholstery webbing or sturdy trim in the notions department of a five-and-ten or department store. Place one end of the trim on one side of your umbrella head; then place the other end on top of it, forming a loop. Adjust the length of the loop until you get a size that's comfortable for you—about 14" is good. Cut off excess webbing and machine-stitch two ends together. Using a good-quality contact cement, attach the trim or webbing loop to the umbrella handle. Now cut another piece of webbing just long enough to wrap around the circumference of the handle plus ½". Glue or tack this over the ends of the loop you've formed, turning under the raw edges to give the strap a finished look. If your umbrella handle is wood, a couple of brass-headed upholstery tacks will give the strap a professional-looking finish. If you're glueing, do as neat a job as you can and be sure you've allowed enough time for glue to dry before you use the strap.

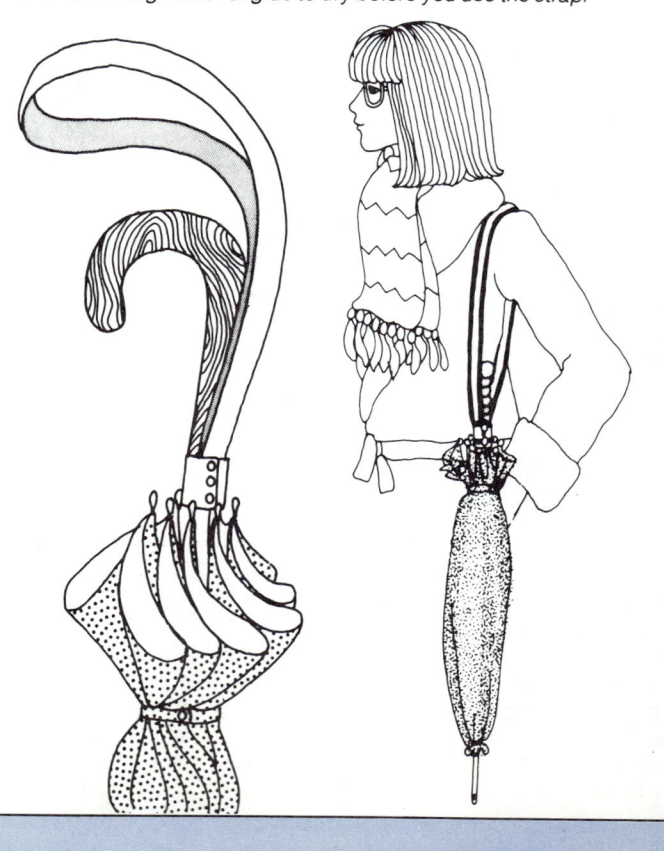

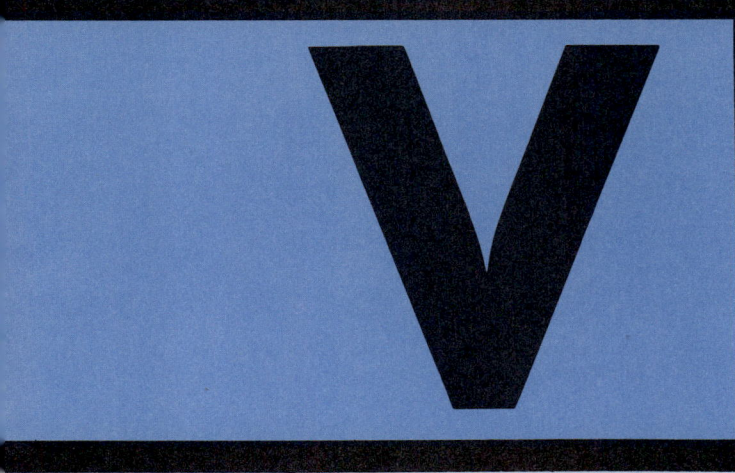

vacations

vacations
voice

vacations

backpacking
under 10 pounds all over this country and others — what to take

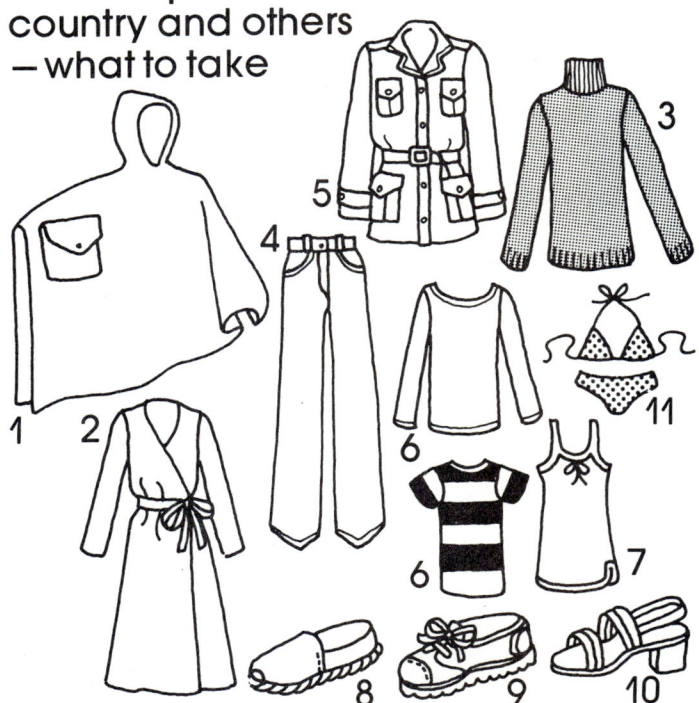

If you're walking or biking or thumbing or just traveling with the least fuss, backpacking is the answer. With a well-stocked rucksack, you can get along on the road or in the woods or even show up in the middle of a city without looking like you're lost.

The secret is a basic hiking wardrobe plus one city outfit—a bright, no-iron synthetic dress is best—that you can forget about most of the time and still expect to look great when you need it.

Depending on where you're going and how, you may have to make adjustments in the pack plan, but this basic wardrobe can take you hiking down the Appalachian Trail for a week with Saturday night in town or across Europe for the whole summer. By rolling each piece of clothing separately before you stow it, you'll end up with a neater pack; rolling also makes it easier to pull out one thing at a time as you need it.

HOW TO PACK
Put the clothes you'll use least often—in this case, a city dress (2) and city sandals (10)—on the bottom. If you've picked an almost weightless synthetic knit, it can stay rolled for days. In the middle go jeans (4), T-shirt tops (6), and a pullover (3). Tuck in a safari-type jacket (5) that you can wear on the road or over your city clothes.

Try to get by with a minimum of underwear and undershirts (7), which can double as nightgowns. Roll all your underwear and at least two pairs of socks (wool is more absorbent, better for hiking) into tiny balls to fit into any available corners, along with your bikini (11).

For comfort, the most important pieces of gear are a pair of well-broken-in hiking shoes (9) and espadrilles (8). When you're not wearing them, they wedge snugly down the side of your pack or tie to the outside of the bag.

A fold-up nylon poncho (1) takes up little room in a pack and makes a great raincoat—even covers your bag and protects your bike if you're pedaling. Keep it on top to pull out in a hurry.

Sort out your cosmetics and beauty supplies, and decide what you really can't live without. Leave everything else at home. (Keep in mind that the faster and simpler your beauty routine at campsites, the better.) Pack beauty supplies, toothbrush, toothpaste, soap, and cold-water laundry soap in side compartments.

Pack maps, a paperback guidebook, and extras such as suntan lotion and sunglasses go in easy-to-get-at top zipper compartments.

Then practice packing and unpacking the whole business a few times before you start out so that you're sure your system will be fast and practical on the road.

countdown
a summer vacation countdown to help you avoid last-minute headaches

12 WEEKS BEFORE
● Read about destination; plan your itinerary.
● See a travel agent and make all reservations.
10 WEEKS BEFORE
● Apply for a passport and an International Student Identity Card.
8 WEEKS BEFORE
● Get necessary inoculations.
4 WEEKS BEFORE
● Get necessary visas.
3 WEEKS BEFORE
● Buy luggage, clothes, anything else you plan to take.
2 WEEKS BEFORE
● Get tickets and confirmations in hand.
1 WEEK BEFORE
● Make a list of everything you want to pack.
● Check to be sure all clothes are clean and in good repair.
3 DAYS BEFORE
● Make arrangements to have the post office hold your mail—or confirm arrangements to have a friend pick it up.
2 DAYS BEFORE
● Arrange transportation to airport.
1 DAY BEFORE
● Pack suitcase, checking each item off list as you pack it.

V vacations

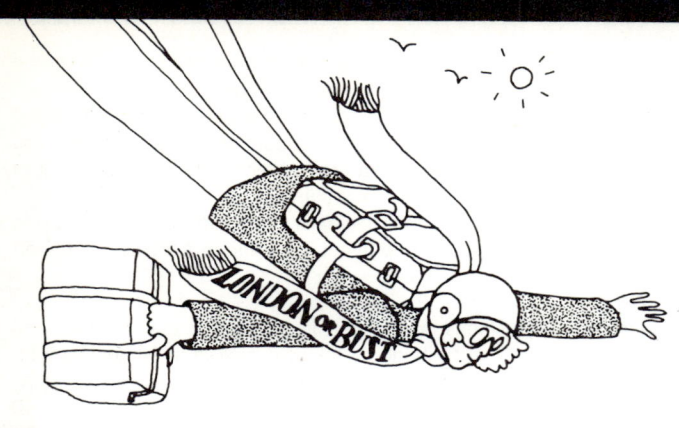

family abroad
how to stay with a family abroad

For an insider's view of what it's like to live in a foreign country, why not spend part of your vacation living with a native family? If you're over 21, you can set it up through the Adult Homestay Program run by The Experiment in International Living. Homestays of one to four weeks can be arranged in about thirty countries—including India, Thailand, Japan, and most of Western Europe and South America. Homestays are usually set up in smaller towns or rural areas, rather than cosmopolitan centers such as Paris or Rome. Costs vary by country and length of stay; for example, you'd pay about $40 in India or $180 in France for a two-week stay. You should apply six to eight weeks before your trip. Keep in mind that some countries won't accept homestays during their busiest tourist months; for France or Italy, this means July and August; for Argentina, it's January and February. For more information, write to Inquiries Secretary, The Experiment in International Living, Brattleboro, VT 05301.

home
how to get back to normal after a vacation

The end of a great vacation means back to work and settling into a routine; it can be hard to get back to normal. These tips can help you keep that special vacation feeling while you get functioning again.
● Allow yourself a day at home before returning to work. It will help you shift from an unstructured vacation situation to a routine. ● Don't try to do all the dirty laundry or unpacking the minute you're back. All the frantic activity will destroy the leisurely, relaxed mood a vacation is supposed to create. Speed up your pace gradually; try to do only the unpacking the first day, then relax. ● If you have vacationed with someone else, even your husband, try to give yourself some private time and space the first week you're home. Constant togetherness with a vacation partner can be a strain; getting back in touch with yourself privately can be good for your mental health. ● Many people find they can get around the letdown feeling that comes at the end of a vacation by saving one last treat for home. Even if your budget is flattened, it can be a smart psychological move to scrape together enough to take yourself out to dinner the first night back, see a movie, or do something that makes you feel that the fun isn't all over. ● Don't plan any big projects at home or work the first week after a vacation; your energies won't be at a peak. The second week is a better choice.
● Surprisingly, many people feel a kind of "first-day-on-the-job" shyness when they return from a vacation, especially if it's been two weeks or longer. To help you avoid the awkwardness you feel when everyone flocks around asking how the vacation was, try to get to the office early so you can compose yourself over coffee and cope with people one by one as they come in.

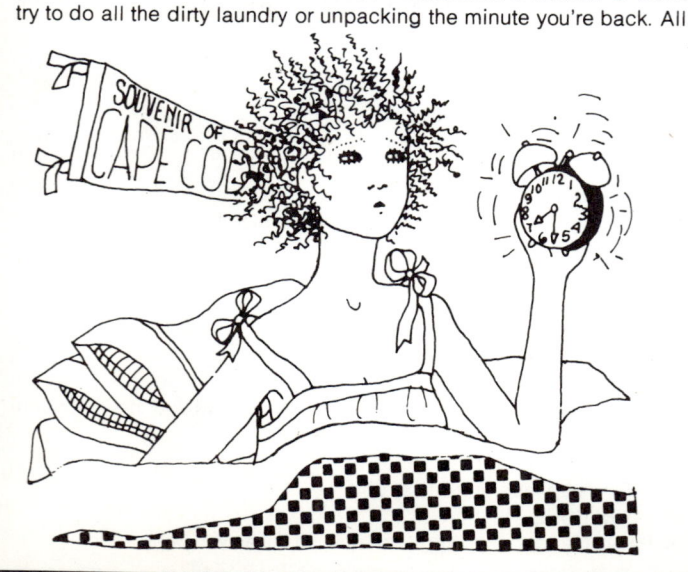

voice

what is your voice saying about you?

It's a scene that's familiar to most of us. You're at a party and have just been introduced to someone you've had your eye on since you walked in. Then you begin to speak—and a voice you barely recognize comes out . . . all wrong, it seems, for the impression you're hoping to convey.

Actually, it may not have so dire an effect as you might think, says voice and drama coach Liz Dixon. "There are some people who are terrific in spite of their voice, and in any long-range acquaintance, the woman behind the voice will come through," says Ms. Dixon. But how can you make sure your voice will be a short-range hit, too? Here are some tips from Ms. Dixon, of the Alfred Dixon Speech Systems in New York City.

● *First, try the acid test. Tape your own voice on a cassette recorder placed near the phone or another spot that will catch you in easy, spontaneous speech. Then "diagnose" your own voice. Do you sound too breathy? Too squeaky? Too fast? If so, you may be able to do some minor voice-editing yourself; for example, by speaking more slowly, if you normally speak at a breakneck clip. Remember, though, that a tape recorder usually magnifies the flaws in your voice—so don't be too hard on yourself!*
● *If you don't like the way you sound, work a little on your voice each day. Practice reading into a tape recorder, especially from lyrical poetry such as that of Keats or Shelley. Good speakers, Ms. Dixon says, are like good singers: "They tend to emphasize the vowel sounds, while they touch on the consonants and run."*

These tips can help at parties:
● *Sounding good begins with a relaxed mind-set—so try above all to hang loose, both mentally and physically.*
● *Don't try to scream over the high-decibel level of the music. Without talking more softly, lower the pitch of your voice.*
● *Timing is also important. "There's always a brief pause between the time one person finishes speaking and the time her words register in the minds of others," Ms. Dixon says. "You have to allow for that brief conversational 'beat' before you start to speak. Otherwise, you'll be talking into people's thought processes, and what you have to say won't sink in, because people are still digesting what someone else has said."*

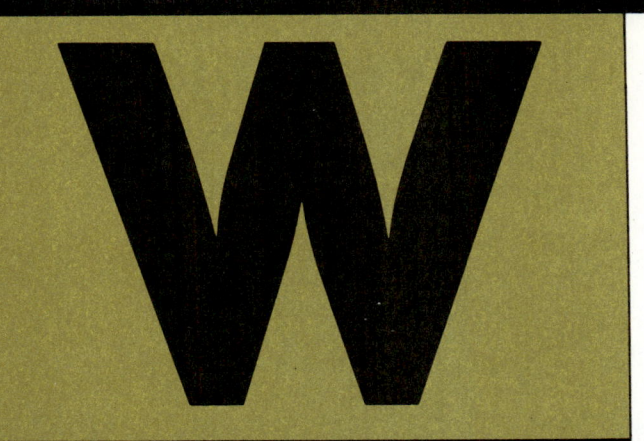

weather

weather
weddings
wine
winter
women's rights

weather

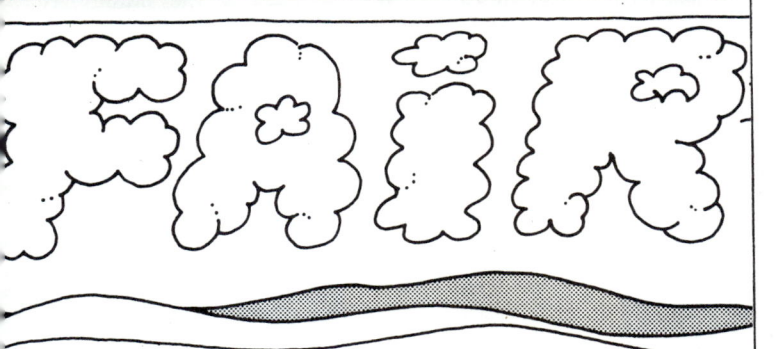

forecast
be your own weather forecaster

Clouds write weather messages in the sky. Learn to read them and you'll be on your way to predicting weather like the pros (keeping in mind *their* unpredictability). The following guide, worked out by amateur weatherwoman Marie Cicchinelli, will start you off.

- **cloud type and appearance**

CIRRUS: Thin, curved, feathery wisps. Sky is blue or rose; crimson or light mauve at sunset.
Weather to be expected: Fair, with little change for the next twenty-four hours.
CIRROSTRATUS: Thin, weblike sheets. Sky has a milky look. Halos form around sun and moon.
Weather to be expected: Fair. Rain or snow in six to twelve hours if clouds thicken.
CIRROCUMULUS: White, rippled, fibrous bands like sand on a beach. Blue sky.
Weather to be expected: Sun becomes hazy. Steady rain in a few hours.
ALTOSTRATUS: Gray sheets. Sky looks like layers of frosted glass.
Weather to be expected: Fair. Rain or snow within twenty-four hours if clouds lower and thicken.
ALTOCUMULUS: Light gray patches of small fluffy cotton balls arranged in rows, separated by blue skies.
Weather to be expected: Fair. If clouds change to layers, rain or snow in six to twelve hours. Then warmer with partly cloudy skies.
STRATUS: Smooth, gray layers like fog. Sky has heavy, leaden, wet look.
Weather to be expected: Sky should clear. Clouds break up. If clouds lower and thicken, expect drizzle.
NIMBOSTRATUS: True rain cloud in dark gray layers.
Weather to be expected: Steady rain or snow if these clouds formed beneath altostratus.
STRATOCUMULUS: Long gray rolls in layers or patches. Soft outline. Blue sky shows between patches.
Weather to be expected: No change for one to two days. Short hard rain may fall if clouds come together, but if they break, it will be cooler and clear.
CUMULUS: Large, thick white puffs with cauliflower tops and flat bottoms. Sky is blue.
Weather to be expected: Fair. When these clouds build into solid banks, hard rain or thunderstorms can occur.
CUMULONIMBUS: Thunderhead. Flat bases and tops that pile high and spread out into anvil shapes.
Weather to be expected: Severe thunderstorms, high winds, and possibly hail. Watch for tornadoes.

summer
do you know enough about the weather to keep cool... and/or out of the rain?

Is it really true that it's cooler in the shade, a ring around the moon means rain, and counting the seconds after a lightning flash tells you where the bolt has struck? Test your knowledge of some of the most common summer weather ideas against the facts.

- **true or false**

1. It's not summer heat but humidity that makes you uncomfortable.
2. On hot days, the air temperature may be 15 or 20 degrees cooler in the shade.
3. To tell where a lightning bolt has struck, count the seconds between the lightning flash and the subsequent roll of thunder; every five seconds equals one mile.
4. Whether the barometer says "stormy" or "very dry" is more significant than whether it is rising or falling.
5. During a summer storm, one of the safest places to be is in a car.
6. A ring around the moon heralds rain.
7. Crickets chirp faster in hot weather.
8. Birds tend to cluster on the ground when a storm is approaching.
9. "Singing" telephone wires signal a change in the weather.

- **answers**

1. TRUE. Warm air holds more moisture than cool air; so you'll feel stickier on hot days than on cool ones. How much stickier? Keep an ear tuned for the "THI" (or Temperature-Humidity Index) on weather forecasts. The National Weather Service reports that few people feel uncomfortable when the THI is 70 or below. About half of us feel

W weather

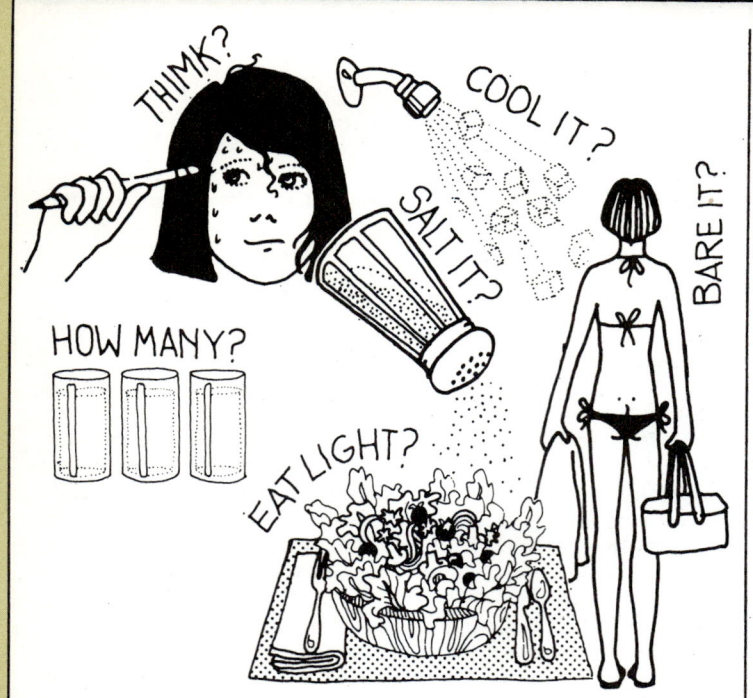

uncomfortable by the time the THI reaches 75, and almost everyone swelters by the time it hits 79.

2. FALSE. Contrary to popular belief, the temperature of the *air* is the same whether taken in the shade or sun. Although a thermometer placed in the sun will record a higher temperature than one in the shade, it is because the thermometer indicates not the temperature of the air but of the glass and mercury, which become hotter in sun than in air. *You* feel warmer in the sun because your clothing and skin, like the glass and mercury of the thermometer, are warmed to a temperature above that of the air.

3. TRUE. Since light travels faster than sound, the flash always precedes the thunder. You can gauge the distance in miles to the lightning stroke by counting off seconds after the flash, with every five seconds equaling one mile.

4. FALSE. More significant than any specific reading is the tendency of the barometric pressure within a given period. A rapidly rising barometer usually means clearing skies; a suddenly plummeting one, a spell of foul weather.

5. TRUE. If caught in a sudden storm, seek the lowest ground possible. Cars are among the safest places to be, because the rubber tires help insulate against electricity. Most likely to be damaged are such nonconductors as brick and wood, materials that crack and break easily from the heat generated by the lightning.

6. TRUE. The sun and moon sometimes appear to be ringed when there are high ice clouds in the atmosphere. This condition can signal rain or snow.

7. TRUE. Crickets chirp at a rate that increases with the temperature. You can count the number of chirps in 15 seconds, add 37, and come out with the correct air temperature!

8. TRUE. The low-pressure area that accompanies a storm makes flying more difficult for birds.

9. TRUE. A rising wind, often signaling the coming of a storm, causes a high whining sound when it blows across telephone wires.

weddings

anniversaries
11 great ways to celebrate your parents' 25th wedding anniversary

Your parents have been together twenty-five years, and after all the "forgotten" loans and listening and party dresses and, in the end, valued advice, you'd like to do something special for them.

● Toast them from your present of a 25-year-old bottle of Scotch or wine. It's their year and better than ever for the aging.

● Needlepoint a big, bold numeral 25 in pop art graphics.

● If you've got a family of patchworkers, assign each a patch or two in a communal quilt with a 25 motif. It's common in early American needlework to find bits and pieces of the maker's life, often in picture form. To give this familiar, almost historic feeling to your quilt, include the hem of a wedding dress, a patch from a child's outgrown pajamas.

● Send for the front page of The New York Times of their wedding date. It's $3.00 unframed and $10.50 for a wood-framed 7" by 9" mini-Times. Address your request (check included) to Microfilming Corp. of America, 21 Harristown Rd., Glen Rock, NJ 07452. (Allow four weeks for delivery.)

● Plant for your parents a silver maple tree, for twenty-five more years of watching it grow. If smaller is better, substitute an aluminum plant. Its luminous silver leaves respond quickly to light, and if the plant is turned every few days, your parents will have a sparkling reminder of their twenty-fifth.

● Get a humorous, warmly remembered family photo blown up into a poster. Mount it and letter in "Twenty-five Great Years" at the bottom. The poster can be matted and framed (in chrome) for a range of prices. Or, for more traditional types, get a favorite old family portrait or snapshot restored. Take it to a commercial or portrait photographer, then have it framed.

● If the family lives at far distances and you can't be together, send a tape around among all the members—maybe you can even get a recording of a grandchild's first words. Then give your parents their own recording machine (everyone could chip in) to play back the tape now and for years to come.

● Put together a two- or three-projector slide show of old family pictures. You can borrow or rent the extra projectors from a camera shop or rental store. Provide background for the slides with records popular at the time they were married or a tape of music interspersed with narration by family and friends.

● Throw a "This Is Your Life" party by telephone. Contact old friends your parents haven't seen for years and assign each a specific time during the evening to phone your parents at your home. Invite others over for a small gathering of close-to-home family and friends.

● If their hearts are set on a second honeymoon, but neither you nor they can foot the whole bill, buy them one-way airfare or take care of their hotel bill in advance. If the trip is their gift to themselves, make it extra special with flowers in the hotel room when they arrive; add the names of some good restaurants or of a club where one of the big bands happens to be appearing.

● Give a romantic day or evening for two. Send flowers and champagne for breakfast, tickets to their favorite entertainment—baseball, theater, whatever—and arrange for dinner out.

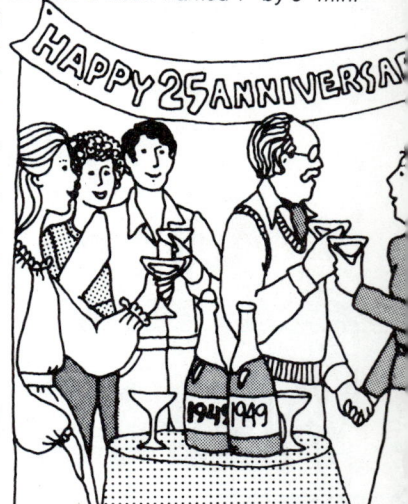

weddings W

bridesmaid
dresses that will really be worn again

If you're planning a wedding that includes bridal attendants, remember that you might be putting a financial cramp on friends by expecting them to pay for expensive dresses and headpieces in addition to transportation and wedding gifts. Here are tips for cutting the cost.

1. When shopping for dresses with your bridesmaids, don't stick to the bridal salon. Check out regular evening dresses, sportswear, even sales racks.
2. Since many bridesmaid dresses have a two-piece effect, why not put the pieces together yourself? Choose full-, ankle-length, or mid-calf-length skirts in awning stripes, gingham, Indian print, or a bright solid. Pair them with dressed-up blouses, camisoles, or halters, depending on the style of your wedding. For a casual one, consider a wrap-around apron look with bold-colored T-shirts.
3. You might let bridesmaids make their own dresses or have someone who can sew make them. Besides costing less than dresses off the rack, these let you give your wedding exactly the look you want. For example, one bride who wanted an old-fashioned wedding wore a quilted patchwork dress, and each of her attendants wore a long skirt in the fabric from one of the patches.
4. Cut down on trimmings. Don't insist that your attendants have matching shoes; just suggest a particular style, heel size, and basic color like beige that they can wear with anything. And instead of fancy hats, give your friends a ribbon, a wreath of flowers, or a single gardenia for their hair.
5. If you do decide on an expensive bridesmaid ensemble in hopes that your friends "really can wear it again," let them help choose it. And decide if it looks too "bridesmaidy" by trying it on yourself. Would *you* wear it again?

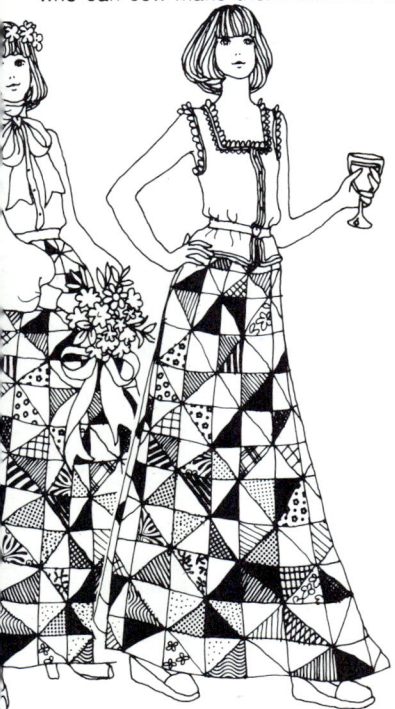

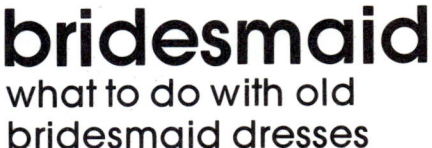

bridesmaid
what to do with old bridesmaid dresses

With so many shorter, bare evening dresses around for parties, you might be able to get one "free" from the fabric of a long bridesmaid dress that you don't plan to wear again. (If the dress is velvet, satin, or brocade, think ahead to the Christmas season.) First make an approximate measure of how much fabric is in the skirt before you buy a pattern—a strapless one or one with spaghetti straps would be good—then you'll know if you have enough for your pattern. Slit the stitching at the waist seam to free the skirt fabric, a small job compared to the great dress you'll make.

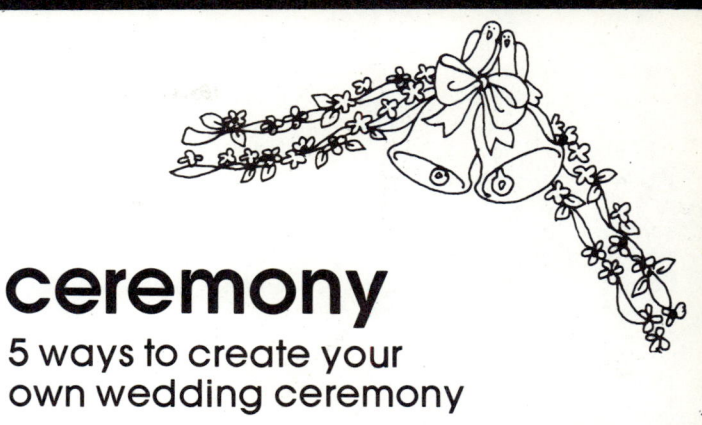

ceremony
5 ways to create your own wedding ceremony

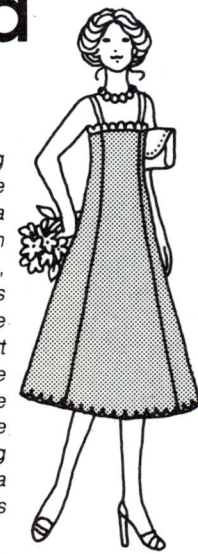

Perhaps the most important thing to remember about writing your own wedding ceremony is that legally, there is nothing you are required to say in it. However, there may be quite a bit that you are required by your religion to say; so your first step should be a talk with your minister, priest, or rabbi about which words and rituals you must include, which ones you may eliminate, and what you may add of your own. (Obviously, if you are having a civil ceremony, you may say anything you like.) Then begin planning the ceremony, using these tips:

● As soon as you know you're getting married—or even before—start keeping a file of ideas, quotes, passages, and so on for possible use. If you wait until a few weeks before the ceremony, you may not have time to track down an obscure sonnet you once loved.

● Try to hunt up a quotation, verse, prayer, or piece of music used in the wedding of your parents or married brothers and sisters, and incorporate that into yours. Many couples have found that this gives a feeling of continuity from one generation to another—especially when fewer and fewer women are wearing Mother's dress or Grandmother's veil—and starts a tradition of their own.

● For twelve complete wedding ceremonies you can use or adapt, see *The New Wedding*, by Khoren Arisian. The book also contains a list of musical selections—such as Arlo Guthrie's rock version of the hymn "Amazing Grace," and Bach's Brandenburg Concerto No. 2 in F —plus prose and poetry selections that you can read in the ceremony. They range from the Old Testament Song of Songs ("This is my beloved and this is my friend") to Mark Twain and Simone de Beauvoir.

● See *The Underground Wedding Book*, by Diane Reed, for ideas for very above-ground ceremonies. Example: Ms. Reed suggests placing a large, colored candle at each of the two family pews. After you have recited your vows and kissed, you and your partner then light a taper from each of your family's candles and return to the altar. There you light a single, pure white candle to symbolize the formation of one new family, as the person officiating explains your gesture to the guests.

● Consider carefully who will say whatever is in the ceremony when you're writing it. For example, why not include lines or parts for your parents, grandparents, or close friends, as many couples are doing? And why not divide any reading that you and your partner do—of a poem, say—so that you read the first few lines, he reads the next, and you read the conclusion together.

collage
a charming under-$5 gift for anyone who's getting married

If you're not much of a camera buff, but you'd still like to give a friend some visual momento of her wedding, here's how to put together a really special wedding collage with just a smidgen of collecting and paste-up skills.

You can start by gathering interesting bits and pieces for the collage long before the ceremony. The wedding invitation, directions on getting to the church or hall—maybe with a snip from a hand-drawn map

211

W weddings

—and material from the hem of a bridesmaid's dress all make great starters. After the reception, you can complete your collection with parts of the bride's or maid-of-honor's bouquet, clips from paper doilies or guest towels, the flowers that you usually find tied around the handle of the cake knife, champagne wrappers, even cocktail picks, and labels from the tin cans tied to the honeymoon car.

Your next step is to buy a clear plastic box frame. Remove the cardboard box from its plastic frame, then wrap the box in decorative material, such as dotted Swiss, secured with a few dabs of rubber cement. With this as background, experiment with different collage arrangements by pinning on the odds and ends you've collected; aim for eye-catching contrasts of shape, color, and texture. Once you've settled on a final design, secure the pieces with a dab of rubber cement, and slip the box into the frame. For the back surface, you'll need a sheet of plain stationery plus some India ink, or colored paper and contrasting tinted ink. Title the collage, write in who it's to and from, and then identify all the things you've included. If your penmanship is less than legible, have a friend with a more decorative handwriting—maybe even a flair for calligraphy—help you out. Center the sheet and then cover with a frame of colored matboard from an art supply store.

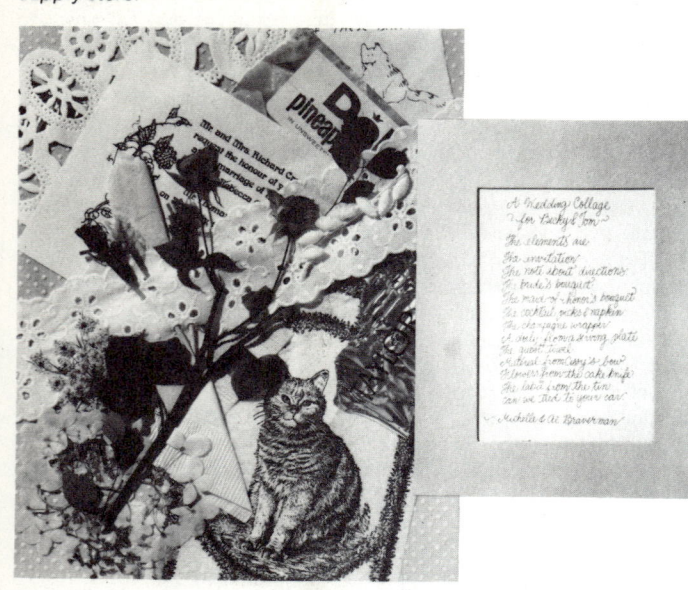

low-cost
have the wedding of your dreams, with up to 75 guests

Do-it-yourself weddings surprise almost no one these days, but their costs sometimes do—unless you plan to spend carefully from the start. These tips can help:

- **invitations**

Through a process called photo-offsetting, you can create your own beautiful but inexpensive invitations. Just take several boxes of attractive stationery and whatever you'd like to have printed on it—maybe a hand-lettered message plus a drawing or quotation—to any photo-offset shop, listed under Offset Reproductions in the Yellow Pages. The shop will reproduce the message and design on your stationery in any color ink for about $10 to $20 per hundred sheets.

- **location**

The least expensive place to have the wedding, or at least the reception, is at home—and preferably in a garden where people will expect and accept informality. Borrow a friend's backyard if you need to, or call your city parks department to find out if it has a special area for outdoor weddings. A church or synagogue wedding adds anywhere from $50 on up to your cost.

- **wedding dress and veil**

If you have a family dress tucked away in an attic, a dressmaker will usually be able to make it fit you. If not, a friend or relative may be willing to make you one. Even if no one can, you'll find many beautiful and inexpensive wedding dresses in import shops, especially Mexican. Instead of a veil, try a lace mantilla or a wreath of fresh flowers.

- **attendants**

Every bride claims that she wants her attendants to have dresses "they'll wear more than once," so choose two-piece outfits—such as long print or gingham skirts and white lace blouses that attendants choose for themselves—then they'll be able to mix and match parts later on. A friend or attendant may be able to whip up all the skirts from one easy pattern.

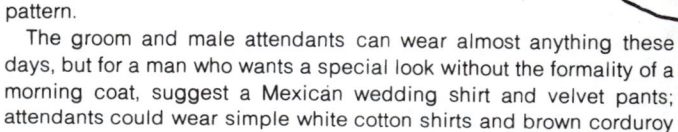

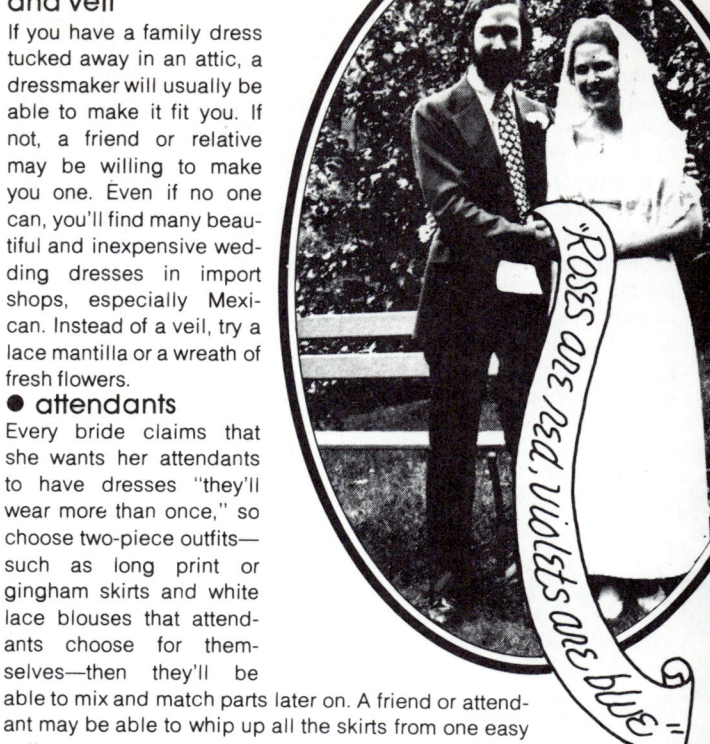

The groom and male attendants can wear almost anything these days, but for a man who wants a special look without the formality of a morning coat, suggest a Mexican wedding shirt and velvet pants; attendants could wear simple white cotton shirts and brown corduroy slacks.

- **flowers**

For your bouquet, a simple spray of garden flowers—maybe white lilacs and daisies or ferns—will avoid a big florist's bill. If these aren't available, you can save by buying unarranged flowers from the florist. Attendants can carry these, too—and one bride even had each bridesmaid carry a single brilliant paper flower that she made herself.

- **rings**

Plain 14-karat gold rings generally give you the most for your money when you have only a small amount to spend, since you don't have to pay for the hand labor that goes into more intricate designs. However, you might also want to consider a less traditional ring, such as the 14-karat gold flexible mesh ring, which is less expensive.

- **photography**

Professional photography may cost $500 or more for a small wedding; instead, why not enlist the aid of friends with photographic experience? Their services can be a wedding gift.

- **wedding cake**

For about $5, you should be able to buy a three- or four-tiered cake pan set in the dime store or from mail-order specialty houses. If you'd prefer a bakery to do the work, don't even whisper the word "wedding" when you order; wedding cakes usually cost more than similar cakes without the bride and groom on top.

- **music**

The easiest way to provide music at the ceremony or reception is to have friends play. You may also find a few talented and willing music majors at a local college.

- **food**

To feed a swarm of guests with really filling food, consider a simple meal such as baked ham, gourmet baked beans, a salad, rolls, and cake.

- **punch**

A traditional open bar could rack up $250 on liquor alone. But the

weddings

punch recipe that follows is for a traditional German wedding punch called *Bohle*, which is inexpensive and delicious.

3 qts. fresh or 3 16-oz. bags frozen whole strawberries
⅘ pt. bottle dark rum
⅘ pt. bottle brandy
1 case domestic champagne
4 gal. domestic white wine (e. g., Sauterne)
12 28-oz. bottles soda water
2 very large punch bowls with ladles

Chill all ingredients overnight. Three hours before the wedding, put berries, rum, and brandy in a bowl. Refrigerate. When ready to serve, make punch by mixing three bottles of champagne to one bottle of wine to three bottles of soda, plus ice. Combine with part of the fruit mixture (save some for refills) and serve.

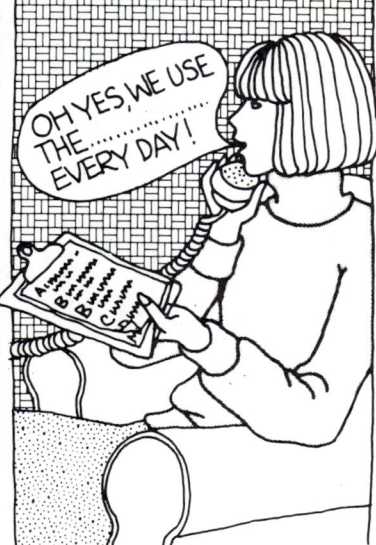

presents
how to keep track of wedding presents

The scene: Six weeks after your wedding. Great-aunt Sally calls to find out how you liked her wedding present. You and your husband stand there looking helplessly at each other—neither of you can remember whether she gave you the sterling silver picture frame or the hand-crocheted place mats.

Particularly for newlyweds who've received an avalanche of wedding presents all at once, this kind of scene might seem unavoidable—and yet, in most cases, it isn't. The trick, as one bride discovered, is to keep a list (preferably alphabetical) of who gave you what next to the phone during the first year or so of marriage; then you can instantly locate someone's gift and thank him or her for it.

Two other ideas for dealing with lots of presents: Instead of writing formal notes, you might try another bride's solution. She had her favorite black-and-white photo duplicated in wallet-size, then wrote a line or two of thanks on the back of each and tucked it into a small envelope. (Sample: "Tom and I are smiling in this picture because we like the camping pack you sent so much. . . . Please come see us soon.")

Or, if your creativity seems to run dry after the forty-ninth note, remember that what everyone really wants to know is simply that her gift will be put to good use. So try to include at least that in each. For example, "The cookbook has a great *coq au vin* recipe we can't wait to try," or, "We've put the check toward a watercolor we were hoping to buy to hang over the sofa," or even, "We're still debating whether to fill your bowl with potpourri or shells from our honeymoon." Note that you don't have to have done anything with the presents yet; just telling someone how you hope to use it will help them see the present in the same context you do.

showers
give a shower that's in tune with a couple's life-style

Today's free-form weddings have inspired a whole new attitude toward showers. "Dos" and "don'ts" for both have almost disappeared as rules have taken a back seat to imagination.

You've probably spotted some of the same trends we have. First, showers have gone strongly coed. Second, they're moving outdoors. We've heard of picnic and barbecue showers—even showers at the beach. Third, they're becoming off-beat; at one "Age of Aquarius" shower, the engaged couple received an astrological forecast for the next twenty years. Most of them, even baby showers, include drinks (mixed at night, milk punch in the afternoon, champagne for brunch).

If you assume that a shower means twenty-five females armed with dish drainers and potato peelers, consider any of the following variations:

● Ecology shower: Send invitations to this outdoor shower on recycled paper. For refreshments, you might serve an "organic" cake from a reliable health food store; for munching, try gold and dark raisins mixed with nuts. As presents, give plants in clay pots, a candle-making kit, or a cookbook such as *The New York Times Natural Foods Cookbook*—its recipes include "Consciousness III Cookies."

● Entertainment-for-two shower: A young couple today may not need the "basics" a shower usually provides. So find out how well supplied the two of them are, and if they already have everything, then splurge. For refreshments, have each guest bring a crock of pâté, a jar of caviar, or brandied apricots. Chip in to give the couple tickets to a play, concert, or sports event; records or cassette tapes; a gift certificate for dinner out.

● Liberated shower: Invite both sexes. Decorate a cake with something like "Congratulations Mr. and Ms. Smith-Jones," or whatever names they plan to use. Wrap a mixture of traditionally female gifts (potholders) with traditionally male gifts (pliers). See that each of them opens both kinds of gifts.

● Do-it-yourself shower: Motivated either by poverty or creativity, many couples prefer to make, build, or grow what they'll need early in marriage. You might carry out the theme by serving food the guests can put together themselves: maybe an assortment of breads with unusual sandwich fillings, or an array of butters. You can buy apple, prune, and cashew butter at many markets, or you can make olive butter by mashing chopped black olives into soft butter to spread on black bread. Give paint rollers and pans, tools, hardware, a subscription to a home improvement magazine, or a tool chest.

● A traditional shower with a twist: If you give an all-female shower at night, you might show home movies of friends' weddings; in the afternoon, give a shower at a swimming pool; in the morning, serve a champagne brunch on a patio or even in a kitchen. Let each guest make food and bring the recipe as a gift.

● When you're giving lots of small presents, it's thoughtful not to include givers' names on packages. When all are given anonymously from people in attendance, you spare the bride having to write thank-you notes for twenty-five tiny items.

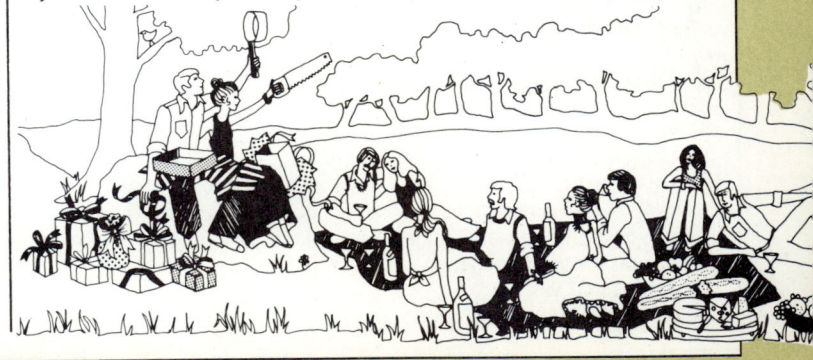

213

wine

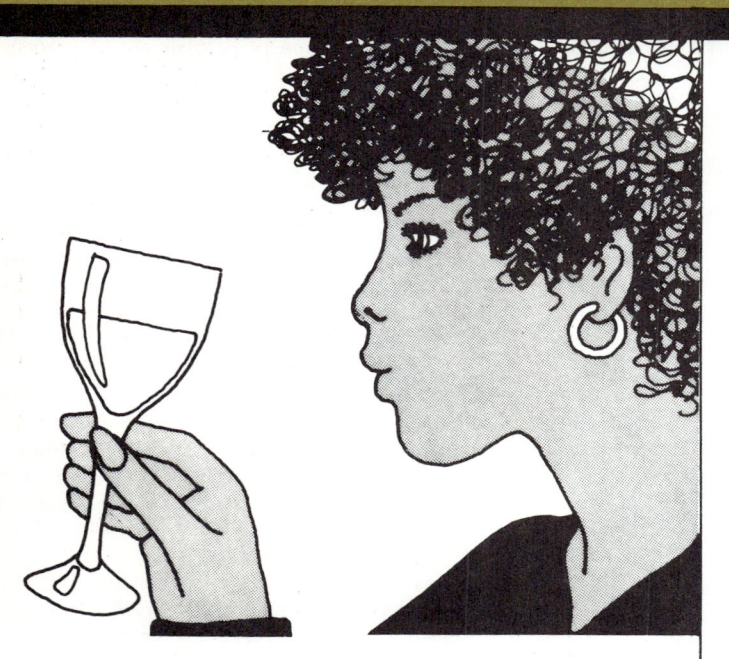

decanting
how to make a $2 bottle of wine taste like more

Decanting is one good trick with wine worth learning. According to wine connoisseur William Houlton, it can make a good, inexpensive (about $2) bottle of red wine taste even better. Decanting is basically just transfering wine from its original bottle to another container that has no top or cover—a crystal decanter or a plain glass carafe.

By decanting a young red wine (less than five years old) an hour or two before serving, you expose it to the air and give it a chance to "breathe" and develop a bit. The reaction that occurs because of the contact with air will improve the taste and fragrance, or bouquet. Decant a white wine about fifteen minutes before serving to bring out the freshness.

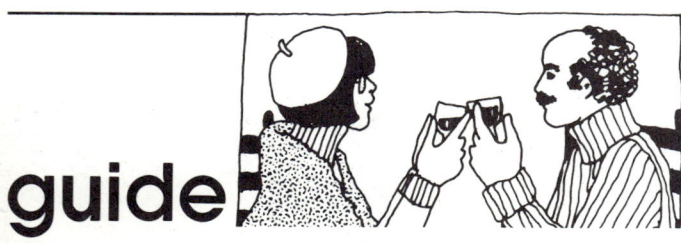

guide
to buying, storing, and serving wine

Whether it's because poets and kings have sung its praises or because we know wine snobs who drink nothing but the best, many of us feel it's hard to understand and serve wine correctly. It isn't. Once you've learned a few basic facts about how to buy, store, and serve wine, you can try dozens of inexpensive kinds without fear of making mistakes in wine etiquette.

● **types of wine**
Although there is an enormous variety in types of wine, whether white or red, most fall into three main categories: *dry, mellow,* and *sweet.* Within these three categories, there are still wines and sparkling wines, such as champagne and sparkling Burgundy. For example, Burgundy (red) and Chablis (white) are dry wines; Rosés are generally mellow; and Sauternes are usually sweet—not as much as the sweetest dessert wines such as Cream Sherry or Port, but slightly sweet, not too much so to be served with meals.

After a while, your taste buds will be able to pick up these distinctions, but in the beginning you may have to ask an experienced friend or liquor store owner to help you tell the difference.

Besides being either dry, mellow, or sweet, wines are also classified as either *appetizer* (or *aperitif*), *table,* or *dessert* wines. Appetizers include dry Sherry and dry Vermouth and are generally served before (or between) meals. Dessert wines, including Port and Tokay, make good after-dinner or party drinks. Table wines are served with meals; some of the most common reds are Burgundy and Claret; the common whites are Chablis, Sauterne, and Rhine wine.

Which table wine you should serve with any meal depends, of course, on what you're eating, but many people prefer to play it safe by adhering to the old rule of serving red wine with red meat and white wine with fish, chicken, turkey, and white meat (such as veal). There is a reason behind that rule—namely, the fuller-bodied red wines usually complement the hearty flavor of roasts and stews, while the white wines won't overwhelm a delicately seasoned filet of sole. But your taste buds should ultimately be the judge of which wine you serve with which dish. (While you're still learning, you're unlikely to go wrong if you tell your liquor store proprietor what you're cooking and let him guide you.) Remember that a good rosé is a wine that can go with almost anything.

● **storage**
Most experts agree that light and heat affect wine; so it's best to store wine in an area that isn't brightly lighted and has a temperature less than 65 degrees. A closet or cabinet shelf is usually safe. If the bottle has a cork, store it on its side or the cork may dry out and allow air to enter, possibly affecting the wine.

● **serving**
Whether or not you chill wine should be as personal a choice as which wines you serve with which foods. Most Americans prefer red wines at room temperature, white and sparkling chilled. But since we tend to overheat our homes, and since red wine shouldn't be warmer than 70 degrees, some people place red wine on a cool windowsill to get it to "room" temperature before serving. If you prefer wine chilled, an hour or so in the refrigerator is usually sufficient.

To give table wine maximum exposure to air—that is, to bring out its full flavor—always serve it in untinted, tulip- or bowl-shaped glasses that hold at least 8 ounces and are about 3" in diameter, as in the sketch. (A clear glass lets you appreciate different wine colors by holding the glass up to the light or by looking through it onto a white tablecloth.) It's also important to use a glass with a stem and to hold the glass by the stem (see sketch), since wrapping your fingers around the bowl of the glass will take the chill off the wine in minutes. A stem also lets you test for the "body"—that is, the lightness or heaviness of a wine—by twirling the stem gently between your fingers, so that the wine swishes around in the glass. A robust or full-bodied wine will fall down the side of the glass in sheets, while light wines will break into runny legs. And obviously, you can't do this if your glass is filled to the brim, which is one reason that you shouldn't fill it more than half to two-thirds full. Another is that with a glass that's two-thirds full or less, you can absorb the wine's bouquet. Just put your nose over the edge of the glass, tip the glass upward, and take a good, long sniff.

wine

tasting

One way to sample the flavor of a wine is by the process known as "whistling in." To do this, take some wine in your mouth and draw a breath of air in as you hold the wine on your tongue. This usually produces a gargling noise; the flavor of the wine will swell in your mouth, remaining there after you have swallowed it. You may have to practice this a few times before you get the knack.

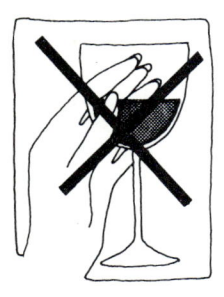

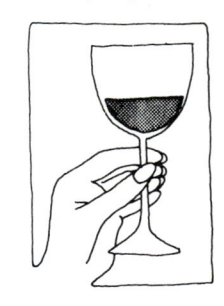

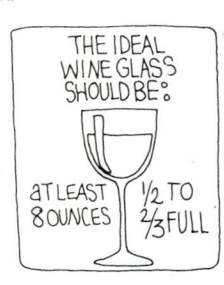

THE IDEAL WINE GLASS SHOULD BE: at least 8 ounces, 1/2 to 2/3 full

health
is wine a health drink?

"To your health" is a toast that goes along with many a glass of wine, but does wine actually have any health value? Well, a glass of wine isn't mother's milk, but it does have substantial nutritional value.

The alcohol in wine is metabolized very rapidly; therefore, it's a quick energy source. While it has little vitamin B1, a glass of wine can supply up to 18 percent of the daily requirement for B2, 52 to 94 percent of B6, 5 to 14 percent of niacin, and 2 to 5 percent of pantothenic acid. (Amounts of vitamins differ with different kinds of wine.) Wine also contains all of the thirteen major mineral elements considered necessary for maintenance of life. Surprisingly, wine contains a very large part of the minimum daily requirement of iron.

So the next time someone drinks to your health, believe it.

labels
how to read a wine label

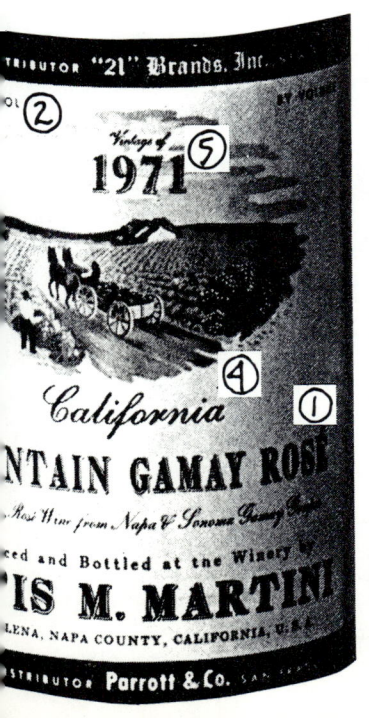

If you'd like to start building up some wine expertise of your own, you might begin with the labels on the wine bottles. Following are some of the facts you'll find on the label on the front of any wine bottle—and don't forget to check for a back label, too. Many California wine bottles, for example, have back labels containing information on when and how to serve the wine—and they alone might be enough to help you pick the wine for any meal you're having.

- *The name of the wine* (1), which is usually in the largest type, and its *alcohol content* (2). Among table wines, or those you'd drink with a meal, this usually ranges from 7 to 14 percent, with the average being 12 or 12.5 percent. A higher alcohol content—say, between 15 and 21 percent—means the wine is an apéritif or dessert wine, one you'd drink before or after a meal instead of along with it.
- *The liquid ounces, or an equivalent, in the bottle.* Most wines (except for jug wines) are sold in bottles containing 25.6 fluid ounces. This size is known as a "fifth" (meaning four-fifths of a quart) and provides six average dinner servings. A half-gallon jug has 64 fluid ounces, for about sixteen dinner servings.
- *Whether the wine is carbonated.* If it is, this will be indicated by either the word "champagne" or a term such as "sparkling," "crackling," *spumante* (on Italian wine labels), or *mousseux* (on French wines).
- *The name of the producer or bottler, shipper or importer* (3). Ardent oenophiles, or wine lovers, can make a near-religion out of studying bottlers and shippers. However, if you're a beginner, and especially if you drink mostly American wines—which are usually produced and bottled by the same company—simply make a note of the producers (that is, brands) of wine that you've enjoyed. The name is usually enough to ensure you'll get a wine of comparable quality the next time you buy.
- *The country of origin of the wine—and often the region or state* (4). Sometimes the region in which the wine originated is the name of the wine itself, as with Burgundy, Bordeaux, and Beaujolais in France; Chianti in Italy; Tokay in Hungary; and the Rhine and Moselle wines from the Rhine and Mosel valleys in Germany. In this case, the wine is known as a *generic* wine, as opposed to a *varietal*, whose name is derived from the primary grape from which it is made. (Common grapes are the Gamay, Pinot Noir, Zinfandel, Chenin Blanc, Chardonnay, Johannisberg Riesling, and Cabernet Sauvignon, the last of which is generally acknowledged to be the best grape grown in the United States.) In addition, there is a third kind of wine, that with a special trademarked name—often for a blend of several grapes or years—which has been coined by the producer. In the United States this includes Almaden's Grenache Rosé and Mountain Red Burgundy, Paul Masson's Baroque, and Taylor's Lake Country Red. A good way to keep all these regions, grapes, and blends straight when you're trying several different wines, is to keep a record of those you like best, perhaps steaming the labels off the bottles and saving them as an additional reminder.
- *The vintage year—not included on all wines* (5). Vintage simply means "harvest," or all the grapes gathered in a particular year. Commonly, the term is used to refer to an exceptionally good year, but in the strictest sense, every wine that's not a blend of grapes from several years is a vintage wine. While the vintage can make a great deal of difference among, say, French wines, where an early frost or other natural conditions can have a major effect on the grape crop, it is less important among California wines, which make up 75 percent of those sold in the U.S. This is because California's relatively stable temperature makes the crops less vulnerable to the whims of nature and more uniform from one year to the next. Remember, though, that the best red wines improve with a few years of aging in the bottle; so their prices usually go up as their ages do.
- The shape of a wine bottle often tells you what kind of wine is in it, as it does for each of the wines shown below.

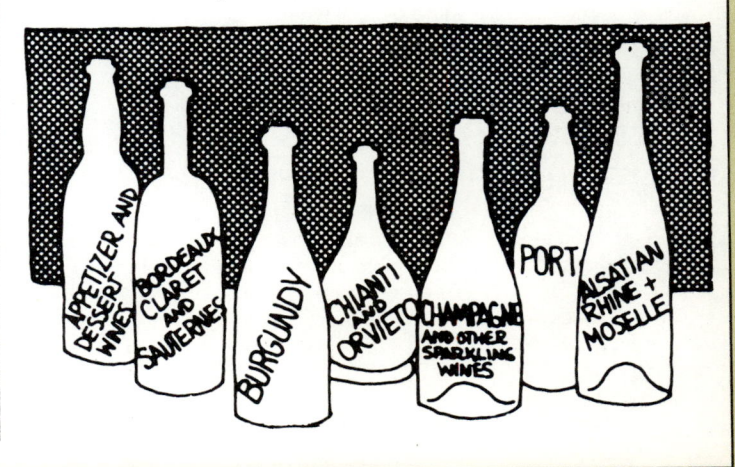

APPETIZER AND DESSERT WINES | BORDEAUX CLARET AND SAUTERNES | BURGUNDY | CHIANTI AND ORVIETO | CHAMPAGNE AND OTHER SPARKLING WINES | PORT | ALSATIAN RHINE + MOSELLE

W wine

lingo
bouquet, body, richness and all that jazz— but what does the wine taste like?

To help you translate the confusing language of wine, we've provided some clues about what is inside the bottle. First, a few basics.

● **wine terms**

Bouquet: Means fragrance. To savor any wine's bouquet, bring your glass slowly to your nose and sniff gently. You will notice a characteristic scent. Although you can't taste the "bouquet," it's definitely a part of the pleasure of drinking wine.

Body: A wine's substance is called "body." Think of it as the opposite of thin and watery.

Richness: Basically it's how mature the flavor is. You might think of richness as being on one end of the scale and "lightness" as being on the other.

Crispness: This usually describes white wine, and means the degree of dryness, the bounce. Think of it as the opposite of sweetness, but with no trace of "pucker-your-mouth" sourness.

● **wine types**

If you're aware of a few of the basic wine types and their general flavors, buying will be easier. Here are some French wines and the corresponding California grapes with similar flavors.

Bordeaux: Probably the most famous French wine region, producing both red and white wines. The reds are full-bodied dry wines with a rich, mature flavor; some well-known examples are Médoc, Saint-Emilion, and Pomerol. Because of their robust flavor, they are excellent with roasts and steaks. California equivalents are Cabernet Sauvignon, which fetches top prices, and Ruby Cabernet, not as expensive. White Bordeaux—Graves is an example—are dry but not super-dry, mellow, and pleasant to drink. They are excellent with delicate fish dishes. The other white wine from the Bordeaux region is Sauterne, a dessert wine.

Burgundy: Red wines from this region are dry, full flavored, and rich, but generally lighter than Bordeaux. Some typical examples are Côte de Nuit and Côte de Beaune. They can be served successfully with most meat dishes. A comparable California wine is the Pinot Noir. Some of the famous French white wines from Burgundy are Chablis (bone dry, crisp, with a tingle of acidity) and Pouilly-Fuissé. Pinot Chardonnay is a California counterpart.

Beaujolais: Actually part of the Burgundy region, Beaujolais wines have a character all their own, light, fruity, lovely. They are best drunk within three years of vintage. Gamay or Gamay Beaujolais are comparable California wines.

Loire Valley: The wines here are mostly white; they're light and pleasantly dry. Muscadet is a popular one.

Note: This is very basic information. There are many other excellent American, French, and European wines that are worth trying once you've become familiar with the basic types.

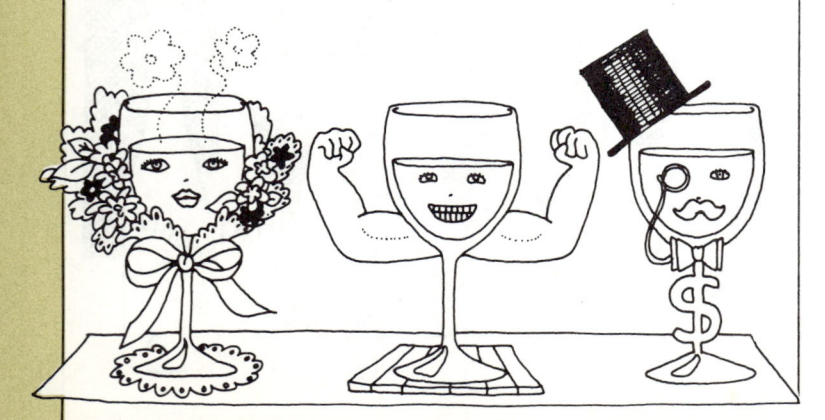

winter

blues
outsmart the midwinter blues

If your mood matches the weather on those gray midwinter days, you've got plenty of company. Psychologists say most people have a few more blue days at that time of year. The postholiday letdown and the confining weather with no prospect of relief for several months, are two of the reasons. Facing the blues, admitting that they're not just in your imagination, then taking some positive action can help you outsmart them. Here are some suggestions:

● February is the start of a new semester in many adult and continuing education courses. Sign up and get interested in something new. It will take your mind off the weather and give you the prospect of making some new friends. Try something for the pure fun of it. Pottery, jewelry design, even exercise at the local "Y" will provide stimulation.

● Combat that sluggish, low-energy feeling that comes from being cooped up. Overheated rooms and little exercise can actually lower the oxygen level in your blood, causing you to feel blah and lazy. Use your lunch hour for an invigorating walk, or open the window near you a crack. The fresh, chilly air will help replenish your oxygen and your energy. Psychologists say we're most productive in a room of about 68 degrees. That's a lot colder than most homes and offices.

● Make the psychology of color work for you. Dr. K. W. Schaie, professor of psychology at the University of Southern California, rates gray as a negative color—a neutralizer. So it's no wonder that continually gray skies can dampen and repress your sunnier needs and responses. Compensate for the winter gray by adding color to your life. Buy a lush green plant, splurge on an occasional bunch of fresh flowers, or consider painting your bedroom a nice cheery yellow to brighten your mood all year long.

● Try not to get sick. Dr. D. L. Walker, a professor at the University of Wisconsin Medical School, reports that many human viruses grow best at one or two degrees below body temperature. Cold weather exposure, especially when you're tempted to underdress on the first non-frigid days, could lower body temperature just enough to permit the growth of inactive viruses you've been harboring.

midwinter pickup
5 fun things you probably wouldn't have thought of doing

January and February tend to be months of marking time for many people. Often you find yourself doing little more than riding out the winter on a suddenly slack schedule. Almost everyone needs a lift at those times—but almost no one has much money or energy left over from the holidays. And that's where the following ideas come in. Any one might be just the postholiday pickup you need to take the edge off a harsh midwinter day:

● Have a snow picnic with some friends your own age or a few of your favorite toddlers. You'll need a plastic tablecloth, food that mittened hands can grasp (no silverware), and an insulated bottle—full of hot cinnamon-spiced cider for children or mulled wine for adults. Afterward, unpack your ice skates and light out for a nearby pond, or make snow sculptures. If light, feathery snow won't "pack," pile snow in a bucket and wet with a garden hose. To make colored snow for eyes,

women's rights

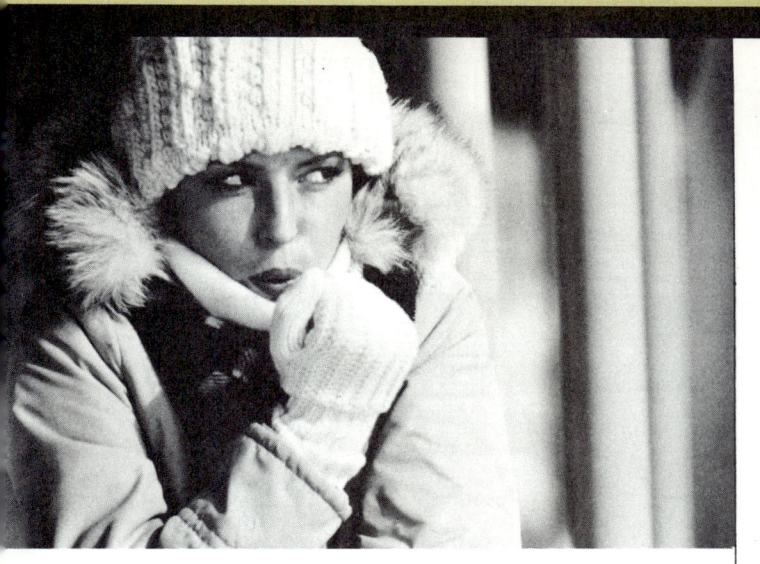

hair, or other accents on the sculptures, add food coloring to the bucket.
● Recycle your closet contents while you support a favorite fund with a tag-sale party. Go through your closet—and get a group of friends to do the same—setting aside any casual clothes you haven't worn in a year, and dressy or evening clothes you haven't worn in two. Sift through old books, jewelry, and buttons, too. Then invite friends in for a party sale with refreshments. Tag each item with a low price, and publicize the recycling center or "hot-line" that will benefit.
● Give any room a face-lift with fine sheets, pillowcases, towels used in imaginative ways. January white sales offer terrific designer sheets at reduced prices; you might make a lampshade or wastebasket to match. Buy extra pillowcases and use them to cover the wastebasket or lampshade, with all-purpose glue. To make curtains out of sheets, hem and slip them over a spring rod; or for a great shower curtain, sew vertical buttonholes at the top, and back the curtain with an inexpensive shower curtain liner from the dime store. If you've found a batch of pretty towels, why not frame them?
● Visit a winter carnival, or make travel plans and reservations for one that's coming up. Winter carnivals are a combination of the Winter Olympics and Mardi Gras, often with a torchlight parade or a ski competition.
● Plan a Chinese New Year party to celebrate the lunar new year. You might have a light supper at which everyone helps cook one easy dish, such as walnut or gold coin chicken, using a recipe from any Chinese cookbook. And try to buy or borrow a wok, the traditional pan used in Chinese cooking. Decorations: paper lanterns, paper dragons and lions, and red scrolls wishing friends happiness and prosperity.

women's rights

black women
help for the black woman who wants woman-power in her community

If you're a black woman looking for advice on starting or continuing a worthy project in your community, the National Council of Negro Women, Inc., may help. It can assist you in overcoming racism through its national office and more than 170 local sections. One example of its work: NCNW Women's Center for Education & Career Advancement is designed to further the career potential and earning power of minority working women in clerical and administrative positions. Another program tries to place more women in the health-care field, while Operation Sisters United (SU) provides an alternative to detention for girls between the ages of eleven and seventeen who are caught up in the criminal justice system. The Council also has programs in three countries in southern Africa. For more information, write to the National Council of Negro Women, Inc., 1346 Connecticut Ave. N.W., Washington, DC 20036.

changing role
guide to the changing role of women in sports, education, business

Changes in the role of women have been occurring in so many areas and at such a rapid clip, that nothing short of a computer could keep track of all of them. The next best thing to a computer, however, might be an informative booklet called "Woman's Changing Place: A Look at Sexism" by Nancy Doyle. The twenty-eight-page guide sums up the progress of the past few years in sports, business, law, and education, among other fields. So if you're a student doing a term paper on women or simply someone who'd like an aerial view of the changes, send 50¢ to Public Affairs Pamphlets, 381 Park Ave. So., New York, NY 10016, requesting booklet # 509. Sections of the pamphlet deal with the effects of these changes on black women, children, older women, and female executives, to name a few.

credit
good news for women: single, married, or divorced, you get a real credit boost

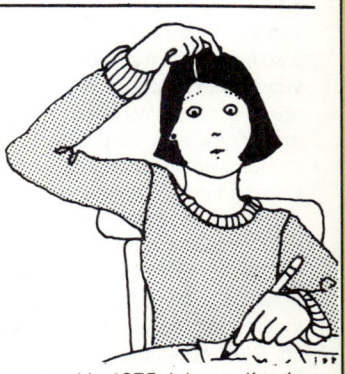

The Equal Credit Opportunity Act was passed in 1975. It bans discrimination on the basis of sex or marital status in all areas of credit and entitles you to up to $10,000 in damages if you can prove discrimination in court. Specific regulations and key proposals include: Credit rating should not be affected simply because you're female—single, married, or divorced; if married, you should be able to apply for credit on your own. To obtain more information or to register complaints, write to: E.C.O.A. Task Force, Federal Reserve Board, Washington, DC 20551. Or write to the Consumer Credit Project, a private consumer advocacy group, 261 Kimberly, Barrington, IL 60010, for information.

women's rights

President
YOU have a chance to become President

Hold on to your hat—and get ready to throw it into the political ring! A qualified woman running for President has a much better chance of winning now than ever before, says a Gallup Poll taken in August, 1975: 73 percent of Americans would vote for her compared to only 31 percent in 1937, 48 percent in 1949, and 66 percent in 1971—the last previous poll taken.

The word is even better for other top offices: 88 percent of Americans would vote for a qualified woman for Congress; 81 percent for governor; and 83 percent for mayor. (The survey involved 1,515 people from more than three hundred areas across the country.)

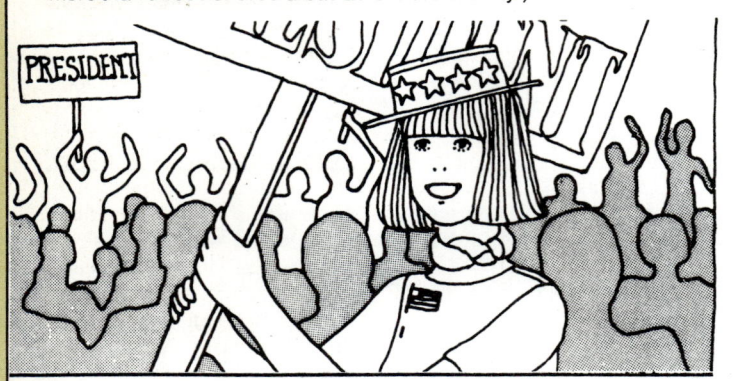

rape
facts that every woman should know about rape

As more becomes known about rape, misconceptions become clearer. Sgt. Gladys Polikoff, commanding officer of the Sex Crimes Analysis Unit of the New York City Police Department, feels that the following are some of the most common misconceptions and that awareness will provide women with some protection.

FICTION: Most women who are raped "ask for it."
FACT: Rape victims have been anywhere from ten months to ninety years old, says Sgt. Polikoff, which tends to disprove this myth. Rapists also tend to pick a spot and wait for someone to approach; they select victims not because they're sexy but because they're vulnerable. A rapist almost always attacks a woman alone—rarely two women, no matter how sexy they look. So your best protection is to have another person with you in any potentially dangerous situation; for example, if your campus has periodic "rape scares," suggest that an all-night escort service be set up.
FICTION: Most rapists rape to fulfill sexual desire.
FACT: Most rapists are motivated not by sexual desire but by hostility toward society as a whole or toward women. In fact, many rapists are married and have active sex lives at the time of the crime.
FICTION: Your best defense is usually to fight.
FACT: There is no best response. "Every woman has to make up her own mind about the best avenue of escape," Sgt. Polikoff says. If a weapon is involved, you might not want to fight. Try to stay calm and think. One woman prevented a rape by telling the rapist she would get money for him. She went to the kitchen and ran out the back door.
FICTION: Rapists are older men who strike out at unknown victims.
FACT: By one estimate, 53 percent of rapists are under 25, and over 30 percent of all victims are known, if only peripherally, to the rapist. So be cautious. "Women are very trusting of anyone who claims to be a repair or delivery man, common poses that rapists use," says Sgt.

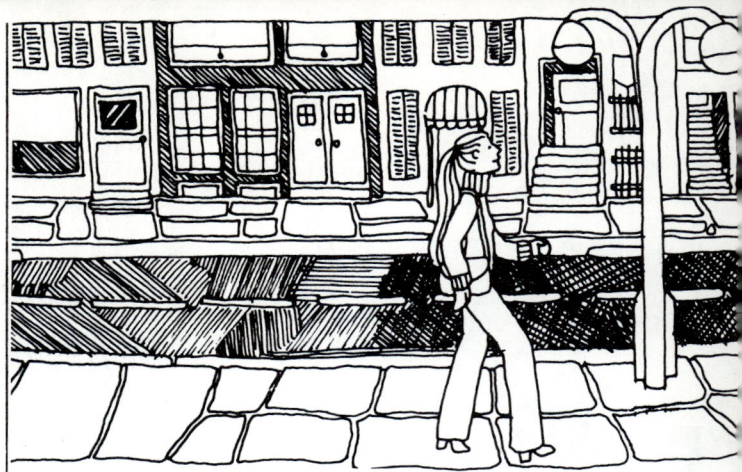

Polikoff. Even if you're expecting a delivery, ask any strange man to slip his identification under the door or ask for the name and phone number of his company and call to see if they have a man by his name. Note: *The Sex Crimes Analysis Unit, a subdivision of the New York City Police Department, is headed by a female commanding officer and staffed by a supervisor and eleven investigators. For a copy of their suggested preventive measures and checklist for rape victims, write to: Sex Crimes Analysis Unit, Room 1312, One Police Plaza, New York, NY 10038. Sgt. Polikoff also reminds any rape victim to call the police immediately, then get medical attention, including tests for VD and pregnancy. Do not wash or douche prior to a doctor's examination, and keep the clothing worn at the time of the rape.*

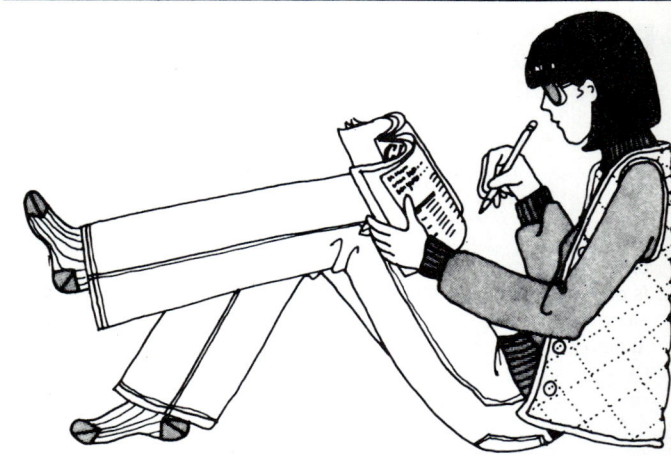

special-interest
3 extra-special-interest books for women — all for $5 or less

In *The New Woman's Survival Sourcebook*, editors Susan Rennie and Kirsten Grimstad cover the gamut from money, child care, religion, and life-styles to education and sex, and more. It's packed with useful information, addresses, and everything else a woman needs to survive in a liberated way.

How to love and live happily ever after with small children is what *The Mother's Almanac* is all about. Besides a lot of sound advice on parenting, it's full of noncooking recipes, games, and crafts for children. By Marguerite Kelley and Elia Parsons.

Job hunting, or thinking about it? Look into a paperback that tells you how to make it less painful. *Woman's Workbook*, by Karin Abarbanel and Connie McClung Siegal, tells how to get your first job, re-enter the job market, and lots more.

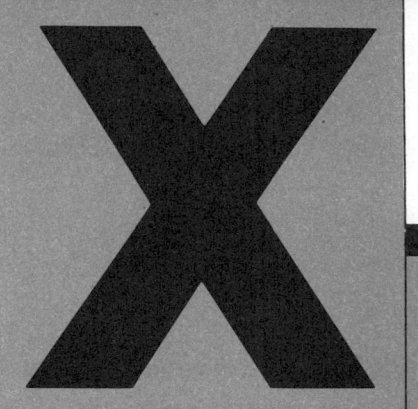

X-rays

X-rays

Xerox art X-rays

Xerox art

push-button art from a Xerox machine

If you can't think of a Xerox copier without thinking of dull business letters you've run off, you might track down one of the Xerox color copiers. A local Xerox office can steer you to a dime store, stationery shop, or other copy center that has one. And you can use it to run off all kinds of bright, unpredictable graphics—from party invitations to wall art—for about 35 cents to 80 cents each.

A color copier works much like a regular black and white machine, with a start button and a dial to set the number of copies you want. There are also four color buttons—"full color," magenta, yellow, and cyan (blue)—that you can use for different effects. The "full color" button gives a glossy, multicolor copy; magenta, yellow, and cyan produce prints in just those colors; or you can press two together for green, red, or dark blue.

You place whatever you're copying on the glass plate, press the start button, and let light scan the glass one to three times, depending on which color buttons you use. Each scan means a new colored powder is being set down on the paper. Heat then fuses the powders to the paper to make the print.

Props for Xerox art can be anything from crumpled string or fabric to photographs and jellybeans. For example, you can run off a magenta income tax form for a post-April 15th party invitation, or an arrangement of leaves and wildflowers from a memorable camping trip. Here are other tips:

● Make rainbow-striped print by flapping the copier lid over the plate as light scans it. For a spiral design, run soft tissue from side to side along the moving light beam.
● Copy a photograph in different colors to suggest different moods. Or make a still photo really "move" by copying it in one position, then shifting it slightly before light scans a second or third time.
● Copy juice, soup, or other labels for pop-art prints.
● Make a collage of favorite travel photos, and if relatives have helped finance your trip, why not send them copies as a thank you?
● Ask the Xerox machine operator to load the copier with different kinds of paper; for example, textured stationery, rice or construction paper—any twenty-pound stock cut 8" x 10" or 8½" x 11". Or try color transparencies (clear plastic sheets) for "instant stained glass." Design on them as you would on paper, then hang copy in a sunny window.

some types of X-rays to think twice about before having

X-rays are an important tool in the diagnosis and treatment of injury and disease, but according to Priscilla Laws, Ph.D., author of *X-rays: More Harm Than Good?* X-rays are neither necessary nor beneficial in many of the circumstances in which they're used. Therefore, medical and dental patients are sometimes needlessly exposed to low levels of radiation—and cumulative doses of this kind of radiation are considered to be potentially hazardous. Here are some points of information from Dr. Laws's book, which is based on a consumer guide on X-rays that she did for Ralph Nader's Health Research Group.

DENTAL: According to Dr. Laws, the major hazard of dental X-rays is probably economic. Many dentists automatically order X-rays of a patient's mouth at every routine checkup, in some cases even before a thorough examination. The Environmental Protection Agency has stated, however, that dental X-rays should not be a standard part of every dental exam and should be taken only after the dentist has examined the patient and established by clinical indication the need for X-rays. You should question your dentist about the reason for any X-ray examination.

CHEST: There is mounting evidence that some types of diagnostic X-rays, such as the yearly chest X-ray offered by tuberculosis associations to the general public or by companies to their employees, do not result in improved medical care for people with no symptoms or signs of trouble. In certain instances, you don't have a choice when it comes to chest X-rays (as in a pre-employment physical or a hospital outpatient examination). However, when it is your right to say yes or no, always check with your doctor first about what to do. (There is now a simple skin test for detecting TB.)

DURING PREGNANCY: Exposing pregnant women to X-rays is known to be potentially hazardous to the unborn child. A developing fetus or embryo is even more sensitive to radiation than an adult. If you know you are pregnant or think there is a possibility of your being so, avoid all X-ray examinations of the lower back or abdominal region unless there are strong indications of a serious condition. You should also be wary of an X-ray exam to determine the size of the pelvis during pregnancy (pelvimetry).

MAMMOGRAPHY: Mammography is a special X-ray examination usually involving two or three X-ray films of each breast. It became popular with the public's growing awareness of the high incidence of breast cancer in this country. However, the fact that the female breast is very susceptible to cancer also makes it more sensitive to radiation-induced cancer, and the National Cancer Institute recently discontinued the routine use of mammograms as a screening tool for symptom-free women under fifty years of age with no family history of breast cancer. Breast self-examination on a monthly basis is recommended for women under fifty, with an examination by a gynecologist at least once a year. If signs of trouble are present, your doctor may recommend a mammogram.

y yogurt

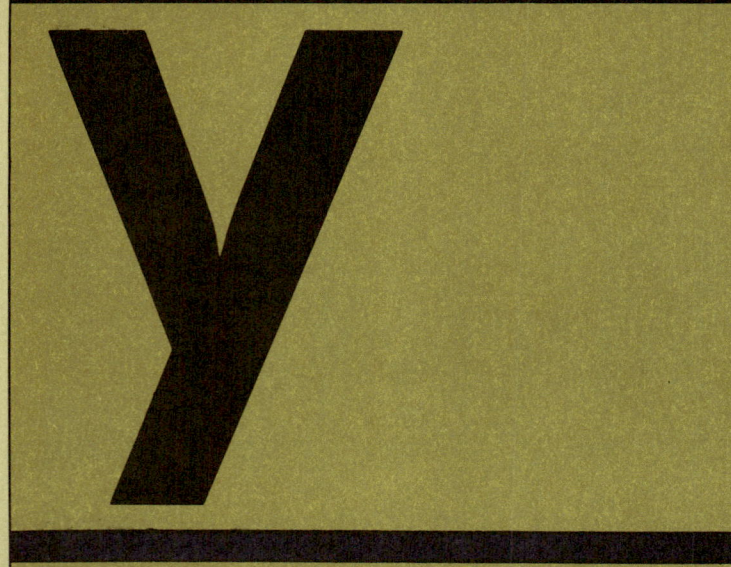

yogurt

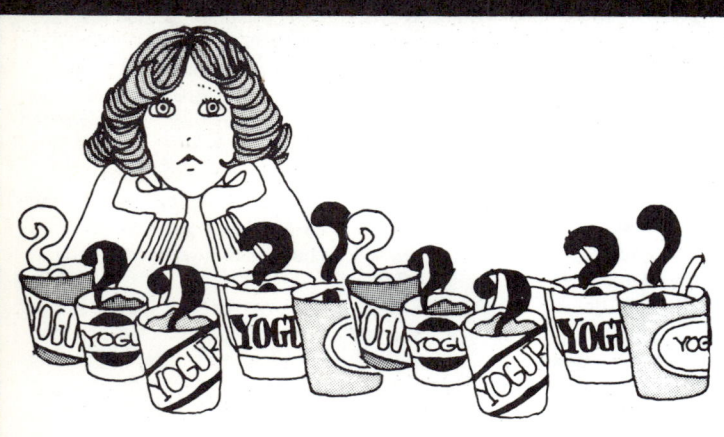

calories
a countdown on yogurt calories — from apricot to peach melba

If you're a dieter who thinks of yogurt as a staple food, take a look at the chart below to see how fattening your favorite flavors really are—or aren't.

● **calorie counts**
per 8-oz. portion; counts are approximate

● **Breakstone**
Swiss Parfait
apricot	250	strawberry	260
black cherry	256	*Sundae style*	
blueberry	286	apricot	220
honey	276	blueberry	252
lemon	254	cinnamon apple	228
lime	242	pineapple	220
Mandarin orange	264	plain	140
peach	254	prune whip	232
peach melba	268	raspberry	250
red raspberry	264	strawberry	224
		vanilla	196

● **Colombo**
black cherry	250	pineapple-orange	210
blueberry	240	plain	150
cold duck	210	raspberry	230
honey/wheat germ	200	strawberry	230
lemon	210	vanilla-honey	210
peach melba	230		

● **Dannon**
apricot	258	pineapple-orange	260
blueberry	258	plain	136
boysenberry	258	prune whip	258
cherry	258	red raspberry	258
coffee	200	strawberry	258
Dutch apple	260	vanilla	190
peach	260	2½ oz. frozen pop	120

● **Johnston (western states)**
Fruit Sundae / *Fondae*
banana	284	apricot	226
blueberry	279	boysenberry	226
boysenberry	289	cherry	224
cherry	280	Mandarin orange	211
chocolate	326	peach	226
cranberry	223	raspberry	227
French apple	304	strawberry	226
Mandarin orange	282	*Frozen Fruit Bokae—*	
peach	286	aerated, less yogurt	
pineapple	286	per volume	
plain	159	boysenberry	182
prune	293	cherry	185
pumpkin	208	Mandarin orange	180
raspberry	287	peach	180
strawberry	286	pineapple	180
vanilla	236	raspberry	184
		strawberry	180

● **Sealtest Light n' Lively**
apricot	256	peach	252
black cherry	256	peach melba	244
blueberry	257	pineapple	241
grape	245	red raspberry	225
lemon	229	strawberry	234
Mandarin orange	234		

flavors dream up your own new yogurt flavors

Have you ever heard of butter maple or Cheri-Suisse yogurt? Probably not, because they and the other mouth-watering concoctions here are the results of a *GLAMOUR* yogurt-tasting party. A group of yogurt fans came up with these treats, which you can duplicate at home. Or ask friends to invent their own for a tasting at your place. They're all based on 8 ounces of plain yogurt (approximately 135 calories) plus unique flavorings. (If you use the yogurt concoctions as refreshing desserts, try garnishing them with something appropriate, such as orange peel or slivered almonds, for an extra-festive look and taste.) To 8 oz. of plain yogurt add:

● **chocolate yogurt**
½ tsp. chocolate extract
Sweeten to taste with sugar, honey, or artificial sweetener.

● **chocolate-orange yogurt**
¼ tsp. chocolate extract
1 or 2 drops orange extract
Sweeten to taste with sugar, honey, or artificial sweetener.

● **chocolate-almond yogurt**
½ tsp. almond extract
¼ tsp. chocolate extract
Sweeten to taste with sugar, honey, or artificial sweetener.

- ### chocolate-mint yogurt
½ tsp. chocolate extract
¼ tsp. mint extract
Sweeten to taste with sugar, honey, or artificial sweetener.
- ### orange-vanilla yogurt
¼ tsp. orange extract
⅛ tsp. vanilla extract
Sweeten to taste with sugar, honey, or artificial sweetener.
- ### butter-maple yogurt
½ tsp. artificial maple flavor
½ tsp. artificial butter flavor
Sweeten to taste with sugar, honey, or artificial sweetener.
- ### Cheri-Suisse yogurt
1 tsp. Cheri-Suisse liqueur
Sweeten to taste with sugar, honey, or artificial sweetener.

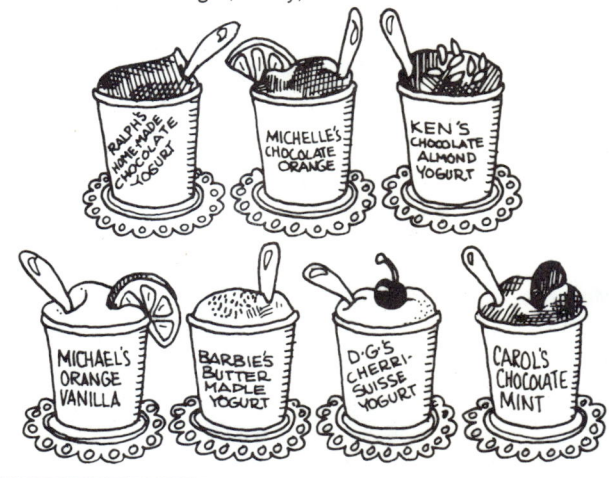

health — what's so great about yogurt?

Yogurt is nutritious but, you may be surprised to know, not much more so than the milk from which it is made. A cup of it has slightly more protein than milk—but not enough to be significant. Aside from considerably more calcium in yogurt, you get the same nutritional benefits from a cup of whole or skimmed milk.

What's misleading is yogurt's popular image as a dietary food. But, claims New York weight specialist Dr. Morton B. Glenn, "It is just not a substitute for the protein needed at breakfast, lunch, and dinner." Nor is it a diet substitute for skimmed milk or between-meal snacks, because it's high in calories. Yogurt labels claiming "low-fat" or "98–99 percent fat-free" don't mean much in terms of calories—low-fat, plain yogurt averages 135 calories per eight-ounce container. That's about 53 more than a cup of skimmed milk. The flavored yogurts (vanilla, coffee, fruit) have high calorie-counts because of their high sugar content: about 210 calories for a container of vanilla or coffee, and around 270 for the fruit flavors. A snack of strawberry yogurt can have more calories than a small piece of chocolate layer cake (235).

Why isn't there a dietetic yogurt? First, because if yogurt were made only from skimmed milk to cut the calorie count, it would be watery. Most commercial yogurt is made partly from whole milk and partly from skimmed to create the puddinglike texture. Second, a sweetener is necessary to take out some of yogurt's sourness.

Contrary to popular claims, the Food and Drug Administration does not recognize any medical properties for yogurt, although some proponents believe it aids digestion, prevents vitamin B deficiency, and prolongs life. However, some physicians recommend yogurt to control diarrhea and other unpleasant side effects sometimes caused by antibiotics.

You may love yogurt's unique flavor and consistency, but if you're dieting, it's not necessarily the best choice.

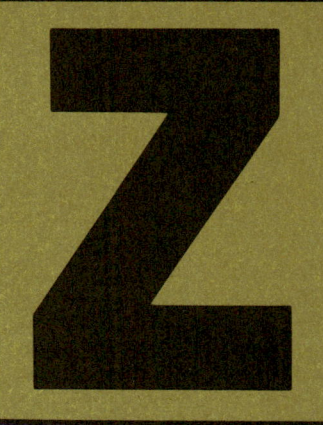

zuppa inglese

a great Italian dessert

A long time ago, an Italian chef concocted this luxurious dessert, whose name means English soup, for homesick English diplomats who missed their tea-time "trifles." Here's an easy way to try this delight:

9" x 5" x 3" sponge cake
½ c. dark rum or sherry
1 10-oz. pkg. frozen mixed fruit or raspberries, thawed and drained
1 pkg. egg custard or vanilla pudding (2 c.), prepared and at room temperature
¼ c. bittersweet chocolate, grated
3 egg whites
Salt
⅓ c. sugar
Slivered almonds
Canned or brandied cherries or candies

1. Cut cake into ½" slices; sprinkle with liquor just to moisten.
2. Line the bottom of a 9" pie pan with one layer of cake. Arrange half the fruit over it. Then, pour just enough custard over the fruit to spread it to the edges of the sponge cake.
3. Make another, smaller layer of cake on top of the first, and sprinkle with chocolate, then with enough custard to cover the layer. Alternate the layers of cake with fruit or chocolate and custard, making a pyramid.
4. Cover with plastic wrap and refrigerate several hours, or overnight, until the cake is firm and set.
5. Two hours before serving, preheat oven to 450° F. Beat egg whites (at room temperature) with a pinch of salt till they hold soft peaks. Add sugar, beat till stiff but not dry.
6. Swirl the meringue into soft peaks over the dessert. Sprinkle with slivered almonds and bake 5 minutes—do not let the meringue overbrown. Cool to room temperature one hour and refrigerate until serving. *Don't* cover.
7. Garnish *zuppa inglese* with a ring of canned or brandied cherries or candies; cut with a knife dipped in water.

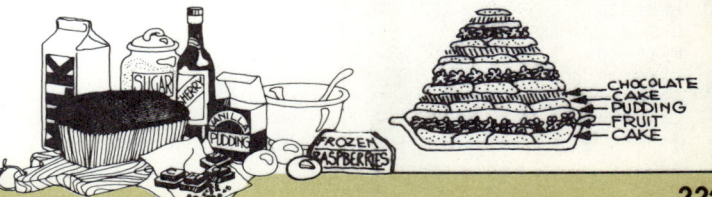

index

a

Acne, 170
  makeup, 114
Advertisements
  apartment, 6
  travel, 198
Agencies, travel, 199
Airline complaints, 35
Airport security, 199
Alcoholic drinks, 58–60
  for parties, 133
Anniversaries, wedding, 210
Antihistamines, 93
Antique auctions, 10
Apartments, 6–9
  ads for, 6
  checklist for, 6–7
  first days in, 8–9
  landlord-tenant problems, 104–5
  moving out of, 7
  renting, 7
  safety in, 7, 110
  searching for, 8
Appliances
  complaints, 35
  sales, 163
  travel with, 199
April, 122
Aquariums, 134–35
Arrests, 106
Art, 9
  Xerox, 219
Art deco, 9
Aspirin, 89–90
Astringents, 11–12
Auctions, 10
August, 124
Automobile complaints, 35
Automobiles, See Cars
Autumn flowers, 10–11
Avocados, 74–75

b

Backpacking, 207
Back scrubber, 42
Back soothers during pregnancy, 141
Baggage during travel, 200
Balls, tennis, 195
Bangs, 81
Bank credit cards, 47
Bathing suits, 72, 192
Bathtub exercises, 60
Bath wrap, 42
Beach, 188
  beachcombing, 11, 188
  changing clothing at, 189
Beach volleyball, 175–76
Beads, 100–1
Beauty care for outdoors, 132
Beauty products, 11–12
  cleansers, 11
  cosmetics, 11–12
  perfumes, 12
  shopping for, 159
  storage of, 12
Beverages, 76
Bicycles, 13–14
  buying, 13
  safety on, 13
  tuning, 13–14
  winter care of, 14
Birds, 130
Birthday cakes, 75
Black women
  hair care for, 81
  makeup for, 114
  rights of, 217
Blonding, 82

Blow dryers, 82–83
Blusher, 114
Body
  massage, 15
  rhythms, 14
Books, 16
  women's, 218
Boots and boot care, 155–56
Bows, Christmas, 27
Bras, 65
Breast exam and health, 90
Bridesmaids, 211, 212
Brochures, travel, 200
Brushes, hair, 83
Bugs, plant diseases and, 138
Burglars, 109
Bus trip ideas, 200–1
Buying, See Shopping smart

c

Cakes
  birthday, 75
  Poundcake, 41
Calculators, 158
Calendar of annual sales, 163
Calendar for men, 116
Camping gear, 17
Candles, decorating with, 49
Canoeing, 176
Careers, 18–19
Carryall, 42–43
Cars, 20–23
  accidents and, 20
  driving, 20
  extras for, 20–21
  gas for, 21
  owner's manual for, 21–22
  renting, 22
  signals with, 22–23
  small, 23
Casts, injury, 167–68
  exercises with, 61
Cats, 135
Ceilings, decorating, 49
Chair sling, 43
Cheese, 77–78
  for dieting, 53
Children, 23–27
  books for, 16
  clothes sizes for, 23
  dressing, 23–24
  early development of, 24
  men with, 116–17
  nightmares of, 25
  photographs of, 25
  puppets for, 25–26
  sneakers for, 26
  time away from, 26
  toys for, 26–27
Chinese food, 56
Chopsticks, 56
Christmas, 27–30
  bows, 27
  dinner, 28
  gifts for men, 28–29
  high-calorie foods of, 27
  package wrappings for, 30
  tipping at, 197–98
  traps, 29
  trees, 29
Cigarette smoking, 174–75
Clam digging, 189
Closets, decorating, 49–50
Clothing
  at the beach, 189
  for college, 32
  for cross-country skiing, 168–69
  for pregnancy, 142
  sales, 163
  shopping for, 158
  size charts for, 164
  sizes for children, 23
  for traveling, 201, 202

  See also Fashion; Sewing
Clothing care, 30–31
  of down, 31
  and dry cleaning, 30
  fabrics and, 31
Clubs
  book, 16
  record, 143
Coats, 65
  fur, 68
Coffee, 38
Colds, 91–92
Collage, wedding, 211–12
College, 31–35
  abroad, 31–32
  clothing, 32
  cramming, 32–33
  diet in, 33
  essentials, 33
  going back to, 33
  health on campus, 33–34
  insurance for, 97–98
  notetaking, 34
  questions in, 34
  tests, 34–35
Color, hair, 84
Colors, fashion, 66
Commercials, 204
Complaints and hotlines, 35–36
Convenience foods, 75
Conversation, 36–37
Cooking, 37–42
  coffee, 38
  crises in, 38–39
  desserts, 39, 76, 220, 221
  dinners after skiing, 167
  gourmet forgeries, 39
  leftovers, 40
  with meat steamer, 40
Cosmetics, 11–12
Costumes, Halloween, 88–89
Coughs and colds, 91–92
Counseling, pre-marriage, 118–19
Country auctions, 10
Crafts, 42–47
  back scrubber, 42
  bath wrap, 42
  buying, 163
  carryall, 42–43
  chair sling, 43
  desk folder, 43–44
  frames, 44
  hammock, 44
  hassock, 44–45
  makeup case, 45
  needlepoint, 46
  painting, 46
  pillows, 46
  ribbon bags and pillows, 47
  selling, 45
Cramming in college, 32–33
Cramps, exercises for, 61
Credit cards, 47–48
Credit, women and, 217
Crime prevention, 109–10
Croquet, 176
Cross-country skiing, 168–69
Crossword puzzles, 79
Customs, travel and U.S., 201–2

d

Dates, weekend, 120
Decanting wine, 214
December, 126
Decorating, 49–52
  with candles, 49
  ceilings, 49
  closets, 49–50
  desks, 50
  fireplaces, 50
  with plants, 138–39
  wall arrangements, 51

  wall hangings, 51
  windows, 51–52
Dental emergencies, 194
Dentists, 193–94
Depilatories, 12
Desk folders, 43–44
Desks, decorating, 50
Desserts, 39, 76, 220, 221
Diamonds, 101
Diet and health in college, 33–34
Dieting, 52–55
  cheese, fruit and, 53
  low-calorie substitutes, 54
  lunches for, 54
  sandwiches for, 54–55
  snacks for, 55
  vitamins and, 55
Dining out, 56–58
Divorce, 105
Documents, legal, 105
Dogs, 135–36
Doors and locks, 110
Down, care of, 31
Dreams, 172–73
Dresses
  bridesmaid, 211, 212
  long, 69
  sewing, 149–50
Dried flowers, 10–11, 74
Drinking, 58–60
Drinks for parties, 133
Driving, 20
Drugs, shopping for, 159
Drugstores, types of, 159
Drug use, health and, 92–93
Dry cleaning, 30
  complaints about, 35

e

Early childhood development, 24
Eating out, 56–58
Eating and swimming, 192
Elderly people, 110
Embarrassing situations, 184–187
Employment agencies, 18–19
Espadrilles, 156–57
Exercises, 60–64
  bathtub, 60
  casts and, 61
  for cramps, 61
  five-minute, 62
  for headaches, 62–63
  for new mothers, 63
  during pregnancy, 63–64
  for trouble spots, 64
Eyeglasses, 80

f

Fabric care, 31
Facials, 170
Factory outlets, 160
Fall fashions, 66–67
Family jewels, 101
Family trees, 145–46
Fashion, 65–73
  See also Clothing
Fast foods, 53
February, 121
Feelings during pregnancy, 141
Fencing, 176
Fertilizing plants, 139
Fireplaces, decorating, 50
Flatware, 95
Flowers, 73–74
  arrangements, 73–74
  cut, 74
  drying, 10–11, 74
  romance and, 144
Flu, 93
Foods, 74–78
  avocado, 74–75

222

index

birthday cakes, 75
Christmas, 27-28
convenience, 75
fruits and vegetables, 76
for parties, 133
peanut butter, 76-77
for picnics, 77
salads, 77
wine, cheese, and fruits, 77-78
Foreign languages, 78
Frames, 44
French food, 57
Frisbee, 177
Fruits, 75, 76, 77-78
dieting and, 53
Fur coats, 68
Furniture complaints, 35
Furs, buying, 160

g

Games, 79-80
Game shows, television, 204-5
Garbage disposal, 110-11
Gasoline, 21
Gifts
Christmas, 28-29
for men, 117
wedding, 213
wrapping, 27, 30
Glasses, 80
Grass rugs, 95-96
Guitars, buying, 161
Gymnastics, 177

h

Hair and hair care, 81-88
bangs, 81
for black women, 81
blonding, 82
blow dryers, 82-83
brushes for, 83
color for, 84
cutting, 84-85
henna rinses, 85-86
products for, 83-84
removal, 86
split ends, 86-87
streaking, 86, 87
styles of, 87-88
wet sets, 88
Haircuts
children's, 24
men's, 117
Hairdresser
choosing, 84
tipping, 198
Halloween costumes, 88-89
Halters, 99, 150
Hammock, 44
Hangovers, 59
Hardware necklaces, 102
Hassock, 44-45
Hay fever, 93-94
Headaches, exercise for, 62-63
Health, 89-95
aspirin, 89-90
and beauty care products, 159
breast exam, 90
cigarette smoking and, 174-75
clubs, 91
colds, 91-92
drugs, 92-93
flu, 93
hay fever, 93-94
pills, 94
during pregnancy, 141
travel and, 202
venereal disease, 94-95
yogurt and, 221
Health and diet in college, 33-34

Health of pets, 136-37
Health of plants, 138
Heart disease and smoking, 174
Heat, summer, 190-91
Hems, sewing, 150-51
Henna rinses, 85-86
Herb butters, 39-40
Hiking, 177
Home furnishings, 95-96
flatware, 95
grass rugs, 95-96
mattresses, 96
sales for, 163
sofas, 96
wicker, 96
Home movies, 127
Horseback riding, 178
Hotels, 202-3
complaints, 36

i

Ice skating, 178
Illness, see Health
Infants
clothing, 23
insurance, 97
See also Children
Injuries, skiing, 167-68
In-laws, 118, 196
Insomnia, 97
Insurance, 97-98
college, 97-98
newborn, 97
tenant's policy, 98
Interviews, employment, 18
Italian foods, 57
Italic writing, 98

j

January, 121
Jeans, 99-100
Jewelry, 100-2
beads, 100-1
diamonds, 101
family, 101
hardware necklaces, 102
original, 102
spice necklaces, 102
Jobs, 18-19
Jogging, 178-179
July, 124
June, 123
Junk mail, 113

k

Kitchen crises, 38-39
Kites, 103
Knickers, 99, 169
Knives, 103

l

Labels, wine, 215
Lampshades, 107
Landlords and tenants, 104-5
leases, 104
rip-offs, 104-5
Lawyers, 105
Leases, apartment, 104
Leather, sewing, 152
Legal matters, 105-6
arrests, 106
divorce, 105
documents, 105
lawyers, 105

small-claims courts, 106
wills, 106
Legal rights
for moving, 128
for shopping, 162
of women, 217-18
Light casts, 168
Lighting fixtures, 107-8
globe, 107
lampshades, 107
string lamps, 108
study, 165
Lighting for plants, 140
Liquor for parties, 133
Living problems, 108-12
alone, 108
burglars, 109
crime prevention, 109-10
doors and locks, 110
for elderly, 110
garbage, 110-11
parents, 111-12
pickpockets, 112
roommates, 112
weekend kit for, 112
Living together, 118
Locks and doors, 110
Low-calorie substitutes, 54
Lunches for dieters, 54

m

Maiden names, 129
Mail, 113
shopping by, 161
Mail-order complaints, 35
Makeup, 114-16
acne, 114
for black women, 114
blusher, 114
eyeglasses and, 80
for Oriental women, 114-15
party, 115-16
summer, 191-92
white uniforms and, 116
Makeup case, 45
March, 122
Massage, 15
Maternity clothes, 142
Mattresses, 96
May, 123
Meal plans, travel, 204
Meat steamer, 40
Memory, 146
Men, 116-20
calendar for, 116
with children, 116-17
gifts for, 28-29, 117
haircuts for, 117
in-laws, 118
living together with, 118
mitten to share with, 118
pre-marriage counseling and, 118-19
reading aloud with, 119
secrets of, 119-20
weekend dates, 120
Metric system, 120
Midwinter pickups, 216-17
Modeling, 18-19
Moisturizers, 11-12
Monopoly, 79
Motorcycles, buying, 161-62
Movies, 127
Moving, 7, 128
Mystery books, 16

n

Names, 129
remembering, 146
Nature, 130
Necklaces, 102
Needlepoint, 46

Nerves, party, 133-34
Newborn, insurance for, 97
Nicknames, 129
Nightmares, children's, 25
Nonsmokers, 174
Notetaking in college, 34
November, 126

o

October, 125
Oktoberfest, 131
Oriental women, makeup for, 114-15
Original art, 9
Original jewelry, 102
Ornaments, Christmas, 29
Outdoors, 131-32
Owner's manual, car, 21-22

p

Paddleball, 179
Paintings, originals, 9
Pants, 69-70
sewing, 152-53
Parents, 111-112
Parties, 133-34
fashions for, 70
food and drink for, 133
makeup for, 115-16
nerves, 133-34
rentals for, 134
Peanut butter, 76-77
Perfumes, 12
Pets, 134-37
aquarium, 134-35
cats, 135
dogs, 135-36
illnesses, 136
veterinarians, 137
Pharmacies, 159
Photographing children, 25
Pickpockets, 112
Picnics, 77
Pillows, 46
Pill use, 94
Plants, 137-41
accessories for, 137
buying, 138
cures for, 138
decorating with, 138-39
feeding, 139
free, 139-40
lighting for, 140
repotting, 140
terrariums, 140-41
Platform tennis, 179
Poncho, rain, 153
Pool, 180
Pregnancy, 141-42
back soothers for, 141
exercises for, 63-64
feelings during, 141
wardrobe for, 142
Pre-marriage counseling, 118-19
Presents, see Gifts
Problem skin, 170-71
Pumpkins, 89
Puppets, children's, 25-26
Puzzles, 79

q

Questions in college, 34
Quilts, 142
Quirks, body, 15

r

Racquets, tennis, 195
Railroad complaints, 36

index

Rape, 218
Reading aloud, 119
Receivers, stereo, 165
Recipes
   Almond-Crusted Cheese Pie, 39
   Artichoke Heart Salad, 37
   Bleu Cheese Burgers, 37
   Brown Sauce, 37–38
   Café Diable, 42
   Chicken in Beer, 37
   Christmas Turkey, 28
   Cornish Hens Alexis, 41
   German Potato Salad, 131
   Hamburger Stroganoff, 167
   herb butters, 39–40
   Hollandaise Sauce, 39
   Hot Chocolate-Nut Sundae, 37
   Hot Wine, 167
   Mousse, 41
   Party Pudding, 39
   Pâté, 39
   Poundcake, 41
   Sabayon Sauce, 42
   Steamed Meatballs, 40
   Zuppa Inglese, 221
Record albums, 143
Registering, travel and, 204
Rentals, party, 134
Renting
   apartments, 7
   cars, 22
   movies, 127
Restaurants, 57–58
   complaints, 36
Résumés, 19
Ribbon pillows and bags, 47
Rights, shoppers', 162
Romance, 144
Roommates, 112
Rugs, grass, 95–96
Running, 180

S

Safety
   in apartments, 7, 110
   on bicycles, 13
Salary, 187
Sales, shopping, 162–63
Sandwiches, 76
   for dieters, 54–55
Scarves, 70–71
Scrabble®, 79–80
Secrets, 119–20
Seeding plants, 139–40
Self-improvement, 145–49
   courses, 145
   family tree, 145–46
   memory, 146
   shyness, 146–47
   singles groups, 147
   sulking, 147
   time, 148
   volunteering, 148
   world records, 148–49
Selling craft items, 45
September, 125
Serving wines, 214–15
Sewing, 149–55
   apron jumpers, 151
   dresses, 149–50
   halters, 150
   hems, 150–51
   leather and suede, 152
   nightgowns, 152
   pants, 152–53
   rain poncho, 153
   shirts, 153–54
   skirts, 154
   tops, 154
   vests, 155
Shirts, sewing, 153–54
Shoes, 155–57
   boots, 155
   buying, 156
   comfort in, 156
   espadrilles, 156–57
   repair, 157
   sneakers, 157
Shoppers' rights, 162
Shopping, Christmas, 29
Shopping smart, 158–67
   for calculators, 158
   for clothes, 158
   for drugs, 159
   in drugstores, 159
   fashion, 71–72
   for furs, 160
   for guitars, 161
   by mail, 161
   for motorcycles, 161–62
   sales, 162–63
   sales calendar, 163
   for sewing machines, 163–64
   size charts, 164
   for sports gear, 165
   for stereos, 165
   for study lights, 165
   for typewriters, 166
   warranties, 166
   for watches, 166–67
Showers, wedding, 213
Shyness, 146–47
Signals, car, 22–23
Silk tree, spring, 183
Singles groups, 147
Size charts, 164
Skiing, 167–69
   casts for injuries, 167–68
   cross-country, 168–69
   gear for, 169
   knickers for, 169
   parties after, 167
Skin and skin care, 170–72
   acne, 170
   facials, 170
   outdoors, 132
   problems, 170–71
   soaps, 171
   in summer, 171
   sunlamps, 172
Skirts, 154
Sledding, 180
Sleep, 172–74
   dos and don'ts, 172
   dreams, 173–74
   morning, 173
   night, 174
Sleeping bags, 17
Small-claims courts, 106
Smoking, 174–75
   heart disease and, 174
   nonsmokers and, 174
   quitting, 175
Snacks for dieters, 55
Sneakers, 157
   for children, 26
Snorkeling, 181
Snowshoeing, 181
Soaps, skin care and, 171
Sofas, 96
Softball, 182
Speakers, stereo, 165
Spice necklaces, 102
Split ends, 86
Sports, 175–83
   beach volleyball, 175–76
   canoeing, 176
   croquet, 176
   fencing, 176
   Frisbee, 177
   gymnastics, 177
   hiking, 177
   horseback riding, 178
   ice skating, 178
   jogging, 179
   paddleball, 179
   platform tennis, 179
   pool, 180
   running, 180
   sledding, 180
   snorkeling, 181
   snowshoeing, 181
   softball, 182
   squash, 182
   walking, 182–83
Sports equipment, 163, 169
Sports gear co-ops, 165
Spring fever, 183
Spring silk tree, 183
Squash, 182
Stereos, buying, 165
Storage of cosmetics, 12
Storing wines, 214
Streaking hair, 86, 87
String lamps, 108
Study lights, buying, 165
Suede, sewing, 152
Sulking, 147
Summer, 188–92
   beach, 188
   beachcombing, 188
   clam digging in, 189
   cooling off in, 189–90
   heat, 190–91
   ideas for, 190
   indoors, 191
   makeup for, 191–92
   skin care, 171–72
   swimming and eating in, 192
   swimsuits, 72, 192
   weather, 209–10
Summer flowers, 144
Sunlamps, 172
Survival kits, moving, 128
Swimming and eating, 192
Swimsuits, 72, 192

t

Table ideas, Thanksgiving, 196–97
Tables, television, 205
Teeth and teeth care, 193–95
   capped, 193
   dentists, 193–94
   plaque control, 194
   wisdom teeth, 194–95
Telegrams, romantic, 144
Television, 204–5
Tennis, 195
Tents, 17
Terrariums, 140–41
Tests in college, 34–35
Thanksgiving, 196–97
Thrift-store fashion, 72
Time, use of, 148
Tipping, 197–98
Tops, 73
   jean, 100
   sewing, 154–55
Toys for children, 26–27
Travel, 198–204
   ads, 198
   agents, 199
   airport security, 199
   appliances abroad, 199
   baggage, 200
   brochures, 200
   bus trips, 200–1
   clothing for, 201
   foreign clothing sizes, 202
   foreign languages and, 78
   health and, 202
   hotels, 202–3
   mail forwarding, 113
   meal plans, 204
   registering and, 204
   sales, 163
   U.S. Customs, 201–2
   weekend kit for, 112
   See also Vacations
Treasure hunting, 11
Tune-ups, bicycle, 13–14
Typewriters, buying, 166

u

Umbrellas, 206
Underwear, 73
Unmarried couples, 118

v

Vacations, 207–8
   backpacking, 207
   with a family abroad, 208
   getting home from, 208
   preparing for, 207
   See also Travel
Valentines, romantic, 144
Vegetables, 75, 76
Venereal disease, 94–95
Vests, 155
Veterinarians, 137
Vitamins, 55
Voice, 208
Volunteer work, 148

w

Walking, 182–83
Wall arrangements, 51
Wall hangings, 51
Wardrobe, pregnancy, 142
Warranties, 166
Watches, buying, 166–67
Weather, 209–10
Weddings, 210–13
   anniversaries, 210
   bridesmaids, 211, 212
   collage for, 211–12
   low-cost, 212–13
   presents, 213
   showers, 213
Weekend kits, 112
White uniforms, makeup and, 116
Wicker furniture, 96
Wills, 106
Windows, decorating, 51–52
Wines, 77–78, 214–16
   buying, storing, and serving, 214–15
   Hot Wine, 167
   labels, 215
   terms, 216
Winter, 216–17
Winter care of bicycles, 14
Wisdom teeth, 194
Women's rights, 217–18
Woods, 130
Work, outdoor, 132
World records, 148–49

x

Xerox art, 219
X-rays, 219

y

Yogurt flavors and calories, 220–21

z

Zuppa Inglese, 221